GROWTH OF THE HEART
IN HEALTH AND DISEASE

Growth of the Heart in Health and Disease

Editor

Radovan Zak, Ph.D.

Professor of Medicine and
Pharmacological and Physiological Sciences
University of Chicago
Chicago, Illinois

Raven Press ■ New York

Raven Press, 1140 Avenue of the Americas, New York, New York 10036

Made in the United States of America

Library of Congress Cataloging in Publication Data
Main entry under title:

Growth of the heart in health and disease.

Includes index.
1. Heart—Hypertrophy. 2. Heart—Growth. I. Zak, Radovan. [DNLM: 1. Heart—Growth and development. 2. Heart enlargement. WG 200 G884]
RC685.H9G76 1984   616.1′29   83-24804
ISBN 0-89004-734-0

The material contained in this volume was submitted as previously unpublished material, except in the instances in which credit has been given to the source from which some of the illustrative material was derived.

Great care has been taken to maintain the accuracy of the information contained in the volume. However, Raven Press cannot be held responsible for errors or for any consequences arising from the use of the information contained herein.

Materials appearing in this book prepared by individuals as part of their official duties as U.S. Government employees are not covered by the above-mentioned copyright.

Preface

Growth of the heart has been studied by physicians and biologists for more than one hundred years. The principal motives of this search have been to understand when and why an enlarged heart fails as a pump and then how to assist it when it does fail. A remarkable compendium of data has accumulated, yet we are still far from understanding all aspects of heart disease. The relatively biggest advance has been made in the treatment of heart failure, its diagnosis and timing. However, we know practically nothing about the reasons why the failure occurs.

Cardiac hypertrophy is clearly an adaptive response, but for a limited time only. The process that first allows an organism to survive eventually leads to its death. Is the sign of death present from the onset of adaptive growth, or is it an "adaptive energy" (a term used by H. Selye in his germinal treatise on the adaptive syndrome) that eventually becomes exhausted? To differentiate these two possibilities, it is necessary to examine and compare the growth of the heart in both health and disease. This is the strategy that we have adopted in developing this volume.

In the first section a review of the growth of the heart from the viewpoint of molecular and cellular biology, anatomy, embryology, morphology, and experimental morphology is presented. The second section gives specific examples of cardiac growth associated with disease. In the final section an analysis of the relationship between the size of the heart, the characteristics of the functional demands placed on it, and its function as a pump are discussed.

The reader will soon discover that it is not only the failure of the enlarged heart that eludes our understanding, but the processes which regulate growth as well. Yet the understanding of growth has been the central concern of biological studies since the cell theory was advanced. Is the size of an organ in a healthy individual predetermined? Is there a limited number of cell divisions for each cell? What factor(s) determines when a cell is to divide? Is an enlarged organ that is composed of more cells functionally better off than when its constituting cells are larger than normal? These questions, descriptive in nature, are fundamental to cell theory.

As far as the causal relationship is concerned, we would like to know what factors regulate the size of an organ. Is it the performed function that provides the growth-regulating signal? Or is it the level of the humoral factor(s) (altered depending on the organ's use or disuse) that predetermines the organ's size?

At the mechanistic level, a knowledge of how the putative signals regulate the activity of genes is valuable. The rapid advances made in cellular and molecular biology in recent years hold promise for elucidation of these fundamental questions. Genes for specific cellular constituents have been isolated, and their structure is currently being determined. The complexity of gene regulation in higher organisms is bewildering at present, although in a few instances the switching of specific genes is already being accomplished. Insight into these basic steps of growth will enable us to study causal and descriptive aspects of growth in a more meaningful way. There is great promise that the physician in this era of cellular and molecular cardiology will be able not only to use better probes to delineate physiological and pathological growth, but to provide lasting assistance to the heart in failure.

R. Zak

Contents

Growth of the Normal Heart

Growth of the Heart During Functional Overload

Consequences of Functional Overload

Contributors

Norman R. Alpert
Department of Physiology and
  Biophysics
University of Vermont
College of Medicine
Burlington, Vermont 05405

Sanford P. Bishop
Department of Pathology
University of Alabama, Birmingham
University Station
Birmingham, Alabama 35294

Edward B. Clark
Department of Pediatric Cardiology
University of Iowa
Hospital and Clinic
Iowa City, Iowa 52242

Victor J. Ferrans
Department of Pathology
National Heart Institute
National Institutes of Health
Bethesda, Maryland 20205

Jose M. Icardo
Department of Anatomy
Faculty of Medicine
Polignono de Cazona, s/n
Santander, Spain

Robert R. Kulikowski
Departments of Anatomy and
  Physiology
Milton S. Hershey Medical Center
Hershey, Pennsylvania 17033

Joan W. Lacktis
Department of Anatomy
University of Chicago
947 East 58 Street
Chicago, Illinois 60637

Francis J. Manasek
Department of Anatomy and
  Pediatrics
University of Chicago
947 East 58 Street
Chicago, Illinois 60637

Louis A. Mulieri
Department of Physiology and
  Biophysics
University of Vermont
College of Medicine
Burlington, Vermont 05405

Atsuyo Nakamura
Department of Anatomy
University of Chicago
947 East 58 Street
Chicago, Illinois 60637

Quynhchi Nguyenphuc
Department of Pediatrics
University of Chicago
947 East 58 Street
Chicago, Illinois 60637

Suzanne Oparil
Department of Medicine
University of Alabama, Birmingham
1012 Zeigler Building
Birmingham, Alabama 35294

David George Penney
Department of Physiology
Wayne State University
School of Medicine
Detroit, Michigan 48201

Karel Rakusan
Department of Physiology
University of Ottawa
School of Medicine
Ottawa, Ontario, Canada

Thomas F. Schaible
Department of Medicine and
*   Physiology*
Albert Einstein College of Medicine
Montefiore Hospital and Medical
*   Center*
Bronx, New York 10467

James Scheuer
Department of Medicine and
*   Physiology*
Albert Einstein College of Medicine
Montefiore Hospital and Medical
*   Center*
Bronx, New York 10467

James F. Spann
Department of Medicine
Temple University
Health Center
Philadelphia, Pennsylvania 19140

Radovan Zak
Department of Medicine and
*   Pharmacological and*
*   Physiological Sciences*
University of Chicago
950 East 59 Street
Chicago, Illinois 60637

Growth of the Heart in Health and Disease,
edited by Radovan Zak. Raven Press,
New York © 1984.

Overview of the Growth Process

Radovan Zak

*Department of Medicine and Pharmacological and Physiological Sciences,
University of Chicago, Chicago, Illinois 60637*

One of the most important properties of the heart is its ability to adapt to an altered hemodynamic load. On a short-term basis the heart is able to cope with an enhanced load by increasing its ability to develop pressure via the Frank-Starling mechanism. However, when the overload is repeated or long-lasting, a second mechanism becomes activated, leading to an altered expression of cardiac genes. This adaptive response can take three forms: (a) an increased rate of synthesis of cardiac components resulting in enlargement of the organ; (b) altered rate of synthesis of some cellular components with a resulting change in the composition of the heart, e.g., an increase in the amount of mitochondria observed within the first few days of aortic constriction; and (c) a change in the characteristics of cardiac proteins, e.g., replacement of the low-ATPase myosin by a molecular variant of high-ATPase myosin which takes place during thyroid-induced cardiac enlargement. In essence, the growth of the overloaded heart can be viewed as a change in the orderly temporal regulation of cardiac genes which takes place during myogenesis and growth in the normal animal. For this reason, in this chapter we review our current understanding of the strategies of gene regulation in eukaryotic cells.

CELLULAR BASIS OF ORGAN GROWTH

The growth of an organ can result from two processes: an increase in the number of cells by their division (cellular hyperplasia) and the enlargement of existing cells (cellular hypertrophy) (Fig. 1). On the basis of these two modes of growth, the cells of mammalian tissues can be divided into two categories: (a) cells which are unable to undergo hypertrophy, e.g., fibroblasts; and (b) cells that do undergo hypertrophy, e.g., myocytes. In the nonhypertrophy category the cells remain mitotically competent throughout the life of an individual, although the rate of division gradually declines with age. When a growth stimulus is applied to these cells, the synthesis of nuclear DNA becomes readily activated irrespective of age.

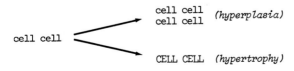

FIG. 1. Two possible modes of organ growth. The size of an organ can increase either by increasing the number of its cells or by increasing cell size.

The cells that do undergo hypertrophy also multiply by mitosis, but only during early ontogeny. Later, the DNA synthesis is gradually repressed, and eventually the cells become mitotically quiescent. The time when this occurs depends on the type of cells involved (Fig. 2). The response of these cells to the growth stimulus depends largely on their ability to synthesize DNA at the time at which the stimulus is applied. For example, in young rats when the rate of DNA synthesis is high, the heart enlargement produced by both volume (47) and pressure (22) overload is accompanied by activation of DNA synthesis. This activation is demonstrated by the incorporation of (^{3}H)thymidine into muscle nuclei as well as by the increase in the activity of the DNA polymerase α (11). As no change was found in the frequency of multinucleated cells, nuclear division appears to be followed by cellular division. Measurements of cell volume corroborate these conclusions (40). Thus the compensatory enlargement of hearts in young animals has the same basis as that observed in normal postnatal development, i.e., a combination of hypertrophy and hyperplasia.

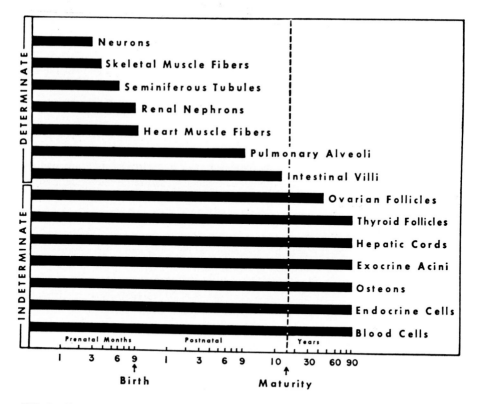

FIG. 2. Duration of hyperplasia in various types of cells. Those cells which cease dividing before birth have a determined number of structural units. Those cells which retain their ability to divide throughout the life span of the individual potentially can grow without limits and therefore have an indeterminate number of structural units. (From Goss, ref. 30.)

In contrast, when similar stimuli are applied to the adult animal, in whom DNA synthesis is already low, the only results are the labeling of previously quiescent nuclei of connective tissue cells and an increase in their number. No activation of mitotic activity of the myocytes is evident, and the compensatory growth of the heart is carried out by the hypertrophy of existing muscle cells (68). A similar loss of mitotic response with age was also described for other cells in this category, e.g., pulmonary alveoli in lungs which have become enlarged as a consequence of unilateral pneumonectomy (31). Despite this lack of hyperplastic growth, the ability to synthesize DNA is not necessarily lost in adult cells. This is indicated by the fact that the number of nuclei containing more than one set of chromosomes (polyploidy) increases in myocytes of the adult heart when it is undergoing hypertrophy (2,50). The significance and consequence of such endoreplication of DNA, however, remain undetermined. The shift toward a higher frequency of polyploid nuclei is quite prominent in primates, although in other animal species this repression of DNA synthesis in the adult is more stringent and endoreplication of DNA occurs to only a very small degree.

Additional support for the belief that DNA synthesis in nonmitotic cells is repressed rather than lost came from studies of multinucleated fibers of skeletal muscle. In these, replication of DNA was induced in mitotically inactive nuclei by infection with polyoma and SV40 viruses (68). The factors possibly responsible for the loss of mitotic activity during compensatory growth are discussed in *this volume* (R. Zak).

GROWTH AT THE MOLECULAR LEVEL

The growth of an organ, either by hyperplasia or hypertrophy, is accompanied by the coordinated accumulation of cellular components that maintain the functional capacity suitable for a given developmental stage. Among the individual organelles, myofibrils, mitochondria, and sarcoplasmic reticulum have been studied in the greatest detail.

In the case of myofibrillogenesis, two approaches have been used: the morphological description of sarcomeres and physicochemical studies on the structural properties and assembly of individual myofibrillar proteins. Under an electron microscope, the assembly of myofibrils was studied extensively in embryonic cardiac and skeletal muscles and their cultured cells. During the early stage of development, both the thick (15 to 20 nm diameter) and thin (6 nm diameter) filaments coexist individually and in clusters (26). Both thin (49) and thick (58) filaments are claimed to be detected first in electron micrographs of developing muscle cells. However, in biochemical studies, the synthesis of myosin and actin, which are the main constituents of thick and thin filaments respectively, was found to be initiated simultaneously (21). Hence controversy still exists over which class of filaments appears first.

Immediately after their appearance, the filaments assume a parallel orientation toward the cell membrane. Their aggregates grow, both in width and length, and eventually exhibits the double hexagonal latticework typical of the adult myofibril. The first completed myofibrils have been noted primarily in the periphery of the cell (6,42). This is particularly the case where the thin filaments have been clearly observed to be inserted into the filament attachment area in the vicinity of the intercalated discs (fascia adherens). With continued development, new sarcomeres are added to the ends of the incomplete myofibrils. Eventually, long rows of sarcomeres are seen spanning the entire length of the muscle cell. As the cell size continues to increase, previously formed myofibrils move to the central portion of the cell and are displaced by newly assembled myofibrils at the cell periphery (6).

The nature of the forces which stabilize the nascent sarcomeres is unclear. Some investigators believe that the prior deposit of Z-band material is a prerequisite for the formation of sarcomeres (42), but others do not (25). Although it is clear that the electron-dense material analogous to the Z-band material of adult myofibrils is abundant in areas where sarcomeres are seen forming, the double hexagonal arrangement of thick and thin filaments, which has proceeded naturally in the absence of Z-bands, has also been observed and described by other investigators (26).

Support for the view that self-assembly of myofilaments can take place in the absence of Z-bands was found in studies in which reconstruction of the double hexagonal lattice occurred in cultured cells after the Z-bands (and α-actin) were removed by proteolytic digestion (27). As longitudinal growth of newly formed myofibrils did not take place in the absence of Z-bands during these experiments, it is conceivable that Z-band material is necessary for the end-to-end attachment of adjacent sarcomeres, even though the interaction between thick and thin filaments can take place in its absence.

The assembly of sarcomeres has also been investigated using purified myofibrillar proteins. From these studies it appears that both myosin and actin have information encoded into their amino acid sequence which allows for the orderly interaction of individual molecules. For example, when the ionic strength of the myosin solution is gradually decreased, bipolar tapered aggregates occur which are remarkably similar to the native thick filaments (37,39). Individual molecules are then assembled in pairs along the long axis of the aggregate. Successive pairs are displaced exactly by 14.3 nm and are rotated 120° relative to each other. The molecules reverse their polarity in the middle of the filaments, resulting in a bipolar filament and an antiparallel arrangement of the myosin molecules at both of its ends.

When the amino acid sequence for the rod portion of its molecules was studied, the remarkable stringency of the myosin aggregation became evident (45a). The sequence data suggest that the ionic interactions are the most important force involved in the assembly of thick filaments as the outer surface of the myosin rod contains a high density of charged groups and lacks hydrophobic amino acids. Acidic and basic residues are clustered at regular intervals; and if the neighboring molecules are displaced by 14.3 nm, interactions between the positive and negative regions of adjacent molecules become possible. Currently, though, we still do not know what forces determine the bipolar nature of the myosin aggregate.

Recent advances in the techniques of molecular biology have allowed study not only of thick filaments but also of the myosin molecule itself. Myosin contains two classes of subunits held together by noncovalent forces: heavy and light chains. Each molecule is a dimer of heavy chains with dissimilar light chains attached to it. The heavy chain contains two structural parts. The tail portion of the molecule (rod), which contains the C-terminus of heavy chains, is an α-helical coiled coil and is responsible for the aggregation properties of myosin discussed above. Light chains are localized in the head region of the molecule, which is mostly globular and constitutes a cross bridge with the ATP and actin binding sites. At the present time, neither the nature of the noncovalent interactions or the exact localization of light chains in the head portion of the myosin molecule is known. It was established, however, that the chains are synthesized on different sets of polysomes (59). Moreover, the kinetics of labeling with trace amino acids indicates that the synthesis of heavy and light chains is not coordinated, and consequently the unassembled pool of one of the light chains exists in the cytoplasm (73).

As far as the interaction of the two heavy chains that constitute the myosin molecule is concerned, sequence analysis has revealed that there exists a pattern of amino acids repeated along the polypeptide in which the hydrophobic amino acids occupy every third and seventh position (45a). Similarly, periodicity in the linear deposits of hydrophobic residues were found in other supercoiled proteins, e.g., tropomyosin (45). Apparently, all coiled-coil α-helices are stabilized by hydrophobic interactions between the inner surfaces of the two strands of the supercoil. (In the case of myosin, the strands are the two heavy chains.) Such clustering of hydrophobic residues at the inner surface of a coiled coil is predicted by the model of seven amino acid repeats in which the hydrophobic residues alternate at the third and seventh positions. This model is an attractive one as it also explains the absence of hydrophobic residue at the outer surface of the molecule mentioned during the description of thick filament aggregation.

Less is known about the assembly of the remaining myofibrillar proteins. Actin is the second most abundant protein (next to myosin), and it is known to exist in two forms: monomeric, or globular (G-actin), and polymerized, or filamentous (F-actin). The structural features of F-actin and thin filaments are similar. Each is composed of two strands of G-actin wound around each other to form a double helical filament. The pitch of the helix is exactly 38.5 nm with seven G-actins per turn.

The conversion of G- to F-actin can be induced in the test tube by adding salts in physiological concentrations. The process proceeds in two steps. First, the condensation of several actin monomers must occur in order to form a polymerization nucleus. Secondly, successive additions of monomers must take place in order to result in the formation of the long filaments of F-actin (64). The elongation appears to be unidirectional, with the new monomers being added to the end, which ultimately becomes attached to the Z-band. This is important because it is known that the thin filaments are anchored into the Z-band in such a way that the polarity of the G-actins in the helix is opposite on the right and left sites of the Z-band. A similar kind of polarity was also noted in developing muscle cells when the filaments were decorated with heavy meromyosin in order to highlight their polarity (60). Additional support for the polarity in the actin-myosin interaction was obtained when purified G-actin was polymerized in the presence of myosin filaments (34). The resulting copolymer consisted of one myosin filament complexed with six actin filaments arranged in a hexagonal array. Most interestingly, the polarity of actin at each end of the aggregate was reversed. These data suggest that the actin filament begins forming at the middle of the sarcomere, with crossbridges acting as organization centers for the assembly and with polymers growing unidirectionally toward each end of the myosin spindle and ultimately toward the Z-band of the sarcomere.

The mechanisms leading to the assembly of regulatory proteins into the thin filaments are poorly understood. Tropomyosin is a unique protein in that it is completely helical. The molecule is a dimer of helical chains wound around each other, forming a two-stranded coiled coil in which the two chains are cross-linked by a single intramolecular disulfide bond (51). Within the supercoil the chains are oriented in the same direction, with little or no staggering, and are bonded noncovalently head to tail. The resulting cable-like structure spans the entire length of the thin filament as well as the groove created by the two strands of the actin helix in which it lies.

At the present time, we can only infer that the newly synthesized tropomyosin is assembled within the myofibrils at its characteristic position from the very beginning of sarcomere formation. Evidence for this inference is derived from immunofluorescence studies with antibodies raised against subunits of troponin (49). Through this approach it has been shown that the nascent myofibrils are stained with antitroponin consisting of 40 nm periodicity typical of adult myofibrils. As tropomyosin is known to anchor troponin to the thin filament, it follows that tropomyosin must also be present in nascent myofibrils. Thus it is evident that the regulatory proteins have an inherent tendency to self-assemble. Yet the nature of the forces involved in the actin-tropomyosin-troponin interaction remain largely obscure.

The second most prominent organelle in the heart cell is the mitochondrion. Its biosynthesis is very complex and involves the interaction between two genetic systems: the nucleocytoplasmic system and the mitochondrial system. Mitochondria are the only animal cell organelles that contain their own unique species of DNA from which all the mitochondrial RNAs are transcribed. This includes the mitochondrial messenger RNA (mRNA), which codes for about a dozen hydrophobic mitochondrial proteins, e.g., the several subunits of cytochrome oxidase and the apoprotein of cytochrome b. Mitochondrial mRNA is transcribed within the mitochondria by its own ribosomal system. The remaining 90% of mitochondrial proteins, however, are coded by nuclear genes translated on cytoplasmic ribosomes and subsequently incorporated into the mitochondria. In addition, all mitochondrial lipids and carbohydrates are also synthesized outside the organelle. The intimate interaction between the nuclear and mitochondrial genetic systems is evident from the fact that the synthesis of some multisubunit proteins is directed by both systems. For example, cytochrome oxidase is composed of seven subunits, four of which are synthesized in the cytoplasm and three in the mitochondria (57).

The introduction of proteins into the mitochondria is a formidable task as it involves not only translocation across the membrane but also deposition of the translocation protein in a precise location within the organelle. Mitochondria consist of two distinct membranes: an outer membrane and a highly infolded inner membrane. The folds of the inner membrane constitute the cristae, which house the machinery of oxidative phosphorylation. Within the boundaries of these membranes are two mitochondrial compartments. The space referred to as the intermembrane is located between the outer and inner membranes. The central compartment bounded by the inner membrane is referred to as the mitochondrial matrix.

In a typical case the protein destined for the mitochondria is synthesized on the free cytoplasmic ribosomes as a precursor, which is a few thousand daltons larger than the mature polypeptide. The precursor is then imported across both mitochondrial membranes in a reaction that requires an electrochemical potential across the inner membrane. This step results in the precursor spanning the inner membrane with its NH_2 terminus sequences protruding into the matrix compartment. In a second step, the protruding segment is removed by the action of chelate-specific matrix protease. Finally, a short sequence of amino acids at the newly formed amino terminus is cleaved by the action of a second protease. In the case of cytochrome b_2, the cleavage products are released in soluble form into the inter-mitochondrial space. In the case of cytochrome c_1, the mature protein remains anchored in the inner membrane via a hydrophobic sequence localized close to the carboxyl end (19).

Most of the steps of mitochondrial assembly described above were elucidated in studies of yeast. However, there is no reason why similar steps might not also apply to the heart, where most of the knowledge of mitochondrial genesis has been accomplished through electron microscopy. Early development of muscle cells is characterized by the sparse presence of mitochondria. Upon maturation, the mitochondria become more abundant as well as more densely packed with cristae. These changes appear to be accelerated at birth and reflect the increased dependency of cardiac myocytes on oxidative metabolism (42).

The third cellular component whose assembly has been examined in some detail is the sarcoplasmic reticulum (SR). This is an intracellular membrane system which regulates the concentration of ionized calcium. In primary cultures of chick skeletal muscle the first sign of SR formation was noted in myotubes. Here it appeared to form as a tubular extension of the rough endoplasmic reticulum (24). These electron microscopic observations are in agreement with biochemical studies, which also indicate that the endoplasmic reticulum is involved in the formation of SR proteins. The two most abundant and best characterized proteins examined are Ca^{2+}/Mg^{2+}-ATPase and calsequestrin. The ATPase is an intrinsic protein which comprises about 75% of the total SR proteins. Its globular molecule is anchored in the hydrophobic interior of the membrane and is asymmetrically oriented so that a portion of it projects to the outside of the SR. Calsequestrin is an extrinsic protein localized in the inner lumen of the SR membrane. In cultured rat cell muscles, both proteins were found to be formed on membrane-bound polysomes (32). The expression of the respective genes for the two proteins during differentiation of cultured muscle cells is not coordinated in time, the synthesis of calsequestrin being initiated about 20 hr before the ATPase. These data indicate that there are separate mechanisms of gene regulation for the proteins of SR (35,71). The insertion of nascent SR proteins into the lipid bilayer must be as complex a process as that of mitochondria, but no studies examining this process are available to date.

CONTROL OF GENE EXPRESSION IN EUKARYOTES

In addition to cell proliferation and assembly of cellular components, the phenomenon of biological growth requires knowledge of the mechanism by which the expression of genes is regulated. Fortunately, during the last decade most of the reaction steps involved in the translation of genetic information encoded in the nucleotide sequence of the DNA molecule into the amino acid sequence of a polypeptide chain have been elucidated. It thus has become possible to examine the regulatory mechanisms involved in turning the individual genes off and on during cell differentiation and growth.

The basic schema of gene expression, shown in Fig. 3, allows us to postulate the following levels of regulation:

1. Transcriptional regulation, i.e., control of the synthesis of mRNA on the DNA template by the action of RNA polymerase

2. Posttranscriptional regulation, i.e., control of the number of functionally competent mRNA molecules available for translation in the cytoplasm

3. Translational regulation, i.e., modulation of the output of proteins directed by the existing amount of mRNA

4. Degradation of the gene product

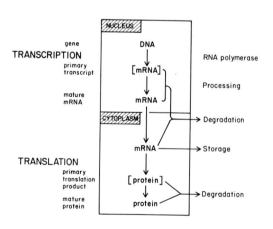

FIG. 3. Gene regulation. The processes which include processing of primary transcript (involving its degradation) plus the transport of mature mRNA into the cytoplasm are referred to as posttranscriptional. The processes prior to translation (i.e., transcription, posttranscriptional, cytoplasmic degradation, and "storage" of mRNA) are sometimes referred to as pretranslational. See text for details.

DNA Organization and Gene Structure

Although the information available about the regulation of gene expression in eukaryotes is still fragmentary, indications are that the regulatory mechanisms are much more complex than in prokaryotes. The major difference is that in eukaryotes the information encoded in the DNA molecule is about three orders of magnitude larger than in the prokaryotes. This is understandable because cell differentiation does not result in loss (or addition) of genetic information. The vast diversity of cells in the animal body contains identical genomes, but an individual cell expresses only a small part of its full genetic potential. Consequently, at any given time only a small portion of total DNA serves as a template for the synthesis of mRNA.

The complexity of gene regulation is suggested by structural features of the DNA molecule in higher organisms. In contrast to prokaryotes, the DNA in eukaryotic chromosomes combines with two classes of protein: the highly basic histones and the mildly acidic nonhistones. The resulting nucleoprotein material is referred to as chromatin. The single molecule of DNA is arranged along the chromatin fiber in repeated units called nucleosomes. Each nucleosome consists of several hundred base pairs wound around an octamere of histones. The nucleosomes are held together by another segment of the same DNA molecule called a linker DNA. Thus the resulting chromatin fiber is a flexible chain of an uninterrupted and unbranched DNA molecule with beads of nucleosomes formed along its length. The association of nonhistones with chromatin is less clear, but it is believed that the nonhistones do not function as building blocks as the histones do.

The third difference between eukaryotes and prokaryotes is that the amount of DNA in the haploid eukaryotic nucleus vastly exceeds the number of genes needed. One of the reasons for such an excess is that the genomes of higher cells contain segments of repeated nucleotide sequences distributed throughout the length of the DNA fiber. As a consequence, the genes which exist as single copies per genome are interdispersed with nontranscribed, repetitive sequences, which are about 300 base pairs long.

The fourth peculiarity of the eukaryotic genome which contributes to the observed excess of DNA is that some genes are clustered and tandemly repeated many times. The best examples of this organization are the genes coding for ribosomal RNA and histones. The reiterated genes are separated by spacer segments of DNA which, similar to repetitive sequences mentioned above, are not transcribed. (Moreover, there are other known segments of DNA which are not transcribed. These are the pseudogenes, segments of DNA located in close proximity to transcribed genes but having a nucleotide sequence slightly different from the gene itself.)

The fifth difference between the proeukaryotes and eukaryotes lies in their genomic organization. In eukaryotes nearly all the genes are split; that is, the expressed nucleotide sequences (exons) are interdispersed by silent intervening sequences (introns). This is not the case with prokaryotes. In general, the intervening sequences are longer than the expressed sequences, further contributing to the excess of DNA in the eukaryotic genome. In contrast to the spacers and repetitive sequences, the introns are transcribed but do not appear in mature mRNA. This is further described in the section on posttranscriptional regulation.

At present, the significance of the complex organization of eukaryotic genomes is not understood completely. Undoubtedly, however, this organization is related to the need to process a large amount of DNA-encoded information.

Transcriptional Control

The actual process that leads to the opening of repressed genes for their transcription by RNA polymerase remains largely obscure. From our current knowledge of gene organization (see above), one can postulate the interplay of three factors: (a) the conformation of chromatin; (b) the regulatory nucleotide sequences of the DNA molecule; and (c) the activity and/or amount of RNA polymerase.

In regard to the conformation of chromatin, it is generally believed that some uncoiling or loosening of the DNA fiber within the chromatin is necessary for the transcription to occur. It is known that the chromosomes display two regions after staining with basic dyes. These regions are the nonstaining euchromatin and the staining heterochromatin. The former corresponds to active genes, the latter to inactive ones. This classic observation has been more recently refined by the discovery that DNase I cut some regions of DNA more easily than others. The DNase I hypersensitive regions are associated with transcriptionally active regions of chromatin and apparently correspond to a more open structure of DNA, which makes it accessible to the action of the splitting enzyme (67).

Concerning the actual mechanisms of chromatin loosening, it is believed that histones act as the blocking agents and inhibitors of RNA synthesis on the DNA template (62). The high degree of homology between different types of cells and among different physiological states, however, makes it unlikely that histones are specific regulators of gene expression. The nonhistones of chromatin are more likely to play such a role. They are highly heterogeneous in molecular weight, bind preferentially to homologous DNA, are cell type specific, and stimulate transcription of isolated DNA and chromatin. Moreover, several examples of their reversible covalent modification are known. These include phosphorylation by cAMP-dependent nuclear protein kinase. The extent of phosphorylation appears to be correlated with the transcriptional activity of various tissues (72). The second example of nonhistone modification is ADP ribosylation (described in more detail in Chapter 7).

Considerable progress has been made recently in determining the role of nucleotide sequences of DNA in the regulation of its transcription. The current view of gene structure is shown in Fig. 4. The gene consists of a series of exons and introns which are bound on either side by untranslated (i.e., noncoding) regions that demarcate the points where transcription of RNA polymerase is initiated and terminated, respectively. Genes are flanked on either side by nontranscribed regions. Of special interest is that the DNase-hypersensitive region mentioned above is localized in front (i.e., upstream) of the active genes (i.e., it precedes the

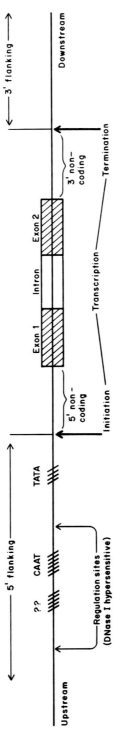

FIG. 4. Gene structure. This is a 1983 version of a split gene which is typical of higher organisms. The structure and function of regulation sites are still tentative.

initiation site). Moreover, two DNA sequences of unusual nucleotide composition were found to precede the gene. These are the TATA and the CAAT which is localized further upstream in the DNase I hypersensitive region. (These sequences are referred to by some as "boxes.") Currently it is believed that the TATA box helps to determine the exact starting point for transcription, whereas the CAAT and perhaps even more remote segments of the DNA determine the efficiency of transcription.

Although sequences of DNA have been identified which are clearly associated with gene transcription, it remains to be explained how these remote regions actually influence the association of RNA polymerase with the initiation site. It is possible that, analogous to the prokaryotic operon model, the eukaryotic regulatory sequences are the target for transcription-stimulating molecules. Attachment of a stimulating molecule somehow results in a conformational change which allows transcription to take place.

The above concepts are fully compatible with the older theory of gene regulation in higher organisms proposed by Britten and Davidson in 1969 (Fig. 5) (8). Their model postulates the existence of several regulatory genes in addition to producer genes which code for cellular proteins. A producer gene can be transcribed only when an activator molecule recognizes the adjacent receptor sites. The activator molecule is postulated to be RNA. This species of RNA is synthesized only when a special DNA segment (referred to as an "integrator gene") is turned on by an adjacent sensor site. This site corresponds with a segment of DNA which recognizes the particular agent that influences gene expression.

The essential feature of the above theory is the postulate that the receptor site and the integrator genes are repeated many times throughout the genome. Thus the function of a substantial portion of the DNA molecule is to regulate the activity of its remaining segment. This postulate is consistent with the observation of repeated DNA sequences mentioned above. The most important consequence of this model is that it explains why a small number of molecules are capable of activating a large number of genes. Unlike the original Jacob and Monod operon models, the entire control mechanism can be operative within the nucleus because RNA rather than

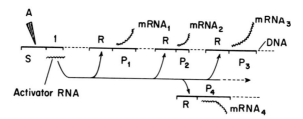

FIG. 5. Britten-Davidson model of gene control in nucleated cells. Interaction of an activator molecule *(A)* with the sensor gene *(S)* opens the adjacent integrator gene *(1)* for transcription of activator RNA. The activator RNA, in turn, interacts with a receptor gene *(R)*, which results in transcription of mRNAs from the adjacent producer genes (P_1, P_2, P_3, and P_4). This model explains how a single activator molecule can influence the expression of several genes.

protein serves as the regulatory mechanism. Undoubtedly, this simple scheme will be refined with time. Nevertheless, it serves as a very useful framework for future inquiry into the mechanisms of gene regulation.

One additional possible mechanism for gene regulation deserves to be mentioned. In several studies an inverse correlation has been found between the level of methylation of cytidine residues in the vicinity of genes and the activity of those genes. Specifically, the demethylation of 5-methylcytosine was found to be associated with the increase in gene transcription (9).

In addition to changes in template activity, control of transcription could also involve modulation of the activity of RNA polymerase. Of the three types of this enzyme, only one (type II) is involved in the synthesis of mRNA. The remaining types (I and III) transcribe the genes coding for ribosomal, transfer, and 5S RNAs. The transcription of DNA template by RNA polymerase is a complex reaction which requires, in addition to the four ribonucleotides, divalent ions (Mg^{2+} and Mn^{2+}) and several protein factors which participate in the initiation, elongation, and termination of the polynucleotide chain (7).

Polymerase II is associated with chromatin and in reconstitution experiments was found to form a complex specifically with the nucleosome core which consists of DNA and the histone octamere (see above). Of particular interest is the observation that the nucleosome core undergoes reversible conformational change upon binding to polymerase II (5). Such a change is consistent with the loosening in the chromatin structure needed for DNA transcription.

In the myocardium the DNA-dependent RNA polymerase has been studied in nuclei of muscle cells obtained from hearts following constriction of the ascending aorta (17). The polymerase activity increases rapidly and reaches a peak value on the second postoperative day. Additionally, the elevation of polymerase activity lags behind the increase in RNA synthesis, which can be noted 4 hr after aortic constriction. Changes in chromatin may account for the early rise in RNA synthesis, whereas an increase in the activity or amount of polymerase takes place later, during the development of compensatory hypertrophy.

Posttranscriptional Control

The second level of gene control includes the processes which determine the amount of mature mRNA in the cytoplasm. These processes include: (a) modification of mRNA nucleotides; (b) excision of introns and splicing of split genes; and (c) transport of mRNA from the nucleus to the cytoplasm.

The primary transcripts range in size between 2 and 20 kilobases and accordingly are referred to as heterogenous nuclear RNA (hnRNA). The processing of hnRNA begins prior to its completion. Two enzymes catalyze the modification steps which involve both ends of the nucleotide chain. The 5' end becomes methylated by the addition of 7-methylguanosine, a process referred to as capping: a polyadenyl tail about 200 nucleotides long is added to the 3' end by the action of poly A polymerase. The exact role of these two modifications is not known. Some data, however, suggest their stabilizing effects on the processed mature mRNA.

The primary transcript is usually several times the size required to code for its corresponding polypeptide as extensive cleavage and splicing is necessary for the production of mRNA. These processes are carried out after capping and polyadenylation by the concerted action of endonuclease and ligase. This kind of processing leads to the production of mature mRNA, which codes for a single polypeptide (i.e., is monocistronic) and has the following structure:

(5′ End) cap–untranslated region–translated region
–untranslated region–poly A (3′ end)

The exact role of the untranslated regions is not known. It is believed that the one localized in the 5′ portion of the molecule is involved in the initiation of translation, which is known to proceed in the 5′-to-3′ direction.

The complexity of mRNA processing, briefly outlined above, suggests several possible control steps. These include a change in mRNA stability via differential capping and polyadenylation, or differential splicing and the discard of particular hnRNA sequences (18). None of these possibilities has been unequivocably proved to regulate gene expression in muscle, however.

The final step of possible posttranscriptional control includes the transportation of mRNA from the nucleus into the cytoplasm. Very little is known about the nucleocytoplasmic transport of RNA, except that numerous pores of appropriate size for RNA passage exist in nuclear membranes, including those of normal and hypertrophic hearts (28). Moreover, the participation of a special class of proteins has been suggested by a study of poly A-containing ribonucleoprotein particles detected in both the nucleus and the cytoplasm (56).

Translational Control

The rate at which the mRNA is translated represents yet another level of gene regulation. One can postulate three mechanisms of such control: (a) rate of mRNA degradation; (b) storage or masking of mRNA; and (c) modulation of protein output by the mRNA-ribosomes complex.

Concerning the rate of mRNA degradation, there are several well-documented cases of changes in mRNA half-life after induction of protein synthesis (18). For example, in primary cultures of skeletal muscles, the half-life of myosin heavy-chain (HC) mRNA increases from 10 hr to 50 hr after fusion of myoblasts to form myotubes (10). It is at the time of fusion that the synthesis of myosin increases dramatically.

In regard to the second regulatory mechanism, comparison of the rate of myosin heavy chain (HC) synthesis with the level of its mRNA indicates that not all of the newly synthesized mRNA is being translated (55). Because myosin HC mRNA isolated from prefusion myoblasts is translationally inactive when tested in a cell-free system (10), it appears that storage (or masking) of mRNA occurs. The inactive mRNA seems to be associated with a protein when forming a ribonucleoprotein particle. Additional experimentation suggests that there is also a special class of

RNA which regulates translation of mRNA. For example, ribonucleoprotein particles containing low-molecular-weight RNA species [referred to as inhibitory (i) RNA] have been isolated from homogenates of chicken embryonic muscles. The particles were found to be a potent inhibitor of *in vitro* protein synthesis (59).

The pathway of protein synthesis is highly complex, consisting of three steps: polypeptide initiation, elongation, and termination. In addition to the availability of active mRNA discussed above, the following factors might determine protein output: the activity and amount of several protein-soluble factors involved in each step of translation; the activity of several enzymes, e.g, peptidyl transferase and aminoacyl-tRNA synthetase; the availability of high-energy phosphate (addition of each amino acid requires hydrolysis of four high-energy phosphates: one molecule of ATP for amino acid activation and three molecules of GTP for translation itself); and the functional state of ribosomal subunits including changes in their conformation and phosphorylation.

Many examples of modulated protein output can be found in the literature. In regard to the heart, the initiation appears to be affected by insulin (46), whereas elongation is the primary target of energy depletion during anaerobiosis (38).

It is of particular interest that phosphorylation of several classes of protein is able to regulate translation of mRNA. This includes the initiation factor responsible for placing the first methionyl-transfer RNA (tRNA) on the ribosome, one of the proteins of smaller (40S) subunits of ribosomes, and aminoacyl-tRNA synthetase (15).

Control of Protein Degradation

Since the demonstration that all proteins undergo continuous degradation and resynthesis (a process referred to as turnover), it has become evident that the level of a protein within a cell can be determined not only by synthesis but by degradation as well. Indeed, under some situations (e.g., with the liver during a nutritional shift), decreased degradation of total proteins was found to accompany tissue growth (16). The contribution of protein degradation to the control of gene expression can be evaluated only when a well-characterized single protein is measured. Only a very few examples of such studies can be cited. In one of these studies involving the heart, degradation of cytochrome was found to decrease during the early phase of developing hypertrophy (3).

Very little is currently known about the pathways of protein degradation, but it appears that in muscle cells there are three classes of enzyme characterized by acidic, neutral, and alkaline pH optima.

Lysosomes are not very prominent structures in muscles; nevertheless, biochemical studies have provided convincing evidence for the presence of membrane-sequestered acidic proteases (61). Current available data indicate that their activity increases when the muscle mass decreases, e.g., during starvation (4). In normal muscles, however, the contribution of acidic proteases to protein turnover is less clear.

Two neutral proteases have been characterized to some extent. One is the calcium-activated neutral protease (CANP), present in sarcoplasm, which preferentially removes Z-lines and α-actinin when incubated with isolated myofibrils (53). The physiological role of CANP remains uncertain as its activity requires 2 mM Ca^{2+}, a concentration which exceeds values normally found in the sarcoplasm. Recently, though, an enzyme similar to CANP was found which is active in the presence of a physiological concentration of calcium (20). Possibly this enzyme is derived from CANP via posttranslational modification. The second neutral protease detected in muscle appears similar to the ATP-dependent degradation system found in reticulocytes (23). The role of both neutral proteases in protein degradation remains to be clarified.

There is also considerable uncertainty about the role of alkaline protease in the degradation of muscle proteins. Although the enzyme can be clearly detected in muscle homogenate, it is likely to be derived from nonmuscle cells (e.g., mast cells) which have a very high proteolytic activity at alkaline pH (66).

MYOCYTE DIFFERENTIATION

Biological growth at the molecular level can be defined in terms of DNA replication and altered transcription of specific genes. To apply this approach in a meaningful way to the study of the heart (and other multicellular organs as well), one must be able to identify individual types of cells and specific gene products. This is not an easy task as pure cell lines of cardiac myocytes are not yet available, and the fractionation procedures yielding an enriched population of muscle cells are still to be perfected. Regarding the products of specific genes, a complication arises from the fact that many muscle proteins are members of multigene families. As a consequence, even "typical" muscle proteins, e.g., myosin, cannot be considered unequivocal markers of the myocytic genome, as myosin variants are also expressed in nonmuscle cells, e.g., fibroblasts.

Molecular Diversity of Muscle Proteins

The overall muscle characteristics—e.g., in the sarcomere structure, the pathways of ATP hydrolysis, or the response of regulatory proteins to calcium—are similar between cross-striated muscles. Nevertheless, the speed of shortening and metabolic activity vary widely not only among animal species but between different muscles of the same animal. Such diversity results, in large part, from the existence of multiple molecular forms of muscle proteins. Although the structure and function of individual proteins are similar, these proteins are products of multiple genes. As a consequence of slight differences in amino acid sequence, called microheterogeneity, the biological activity between members of each gene family differs. So far, polymorphisms were detected for myosin, actin, tropomyosin, troponin, and some sarcoplasmic proteins (70). Various terms are used to indicate molecular variants, e.g., isozymes, isoproteins, and isoforms, or more specifically, isoactins, isomyosins, etc.

The studies of myosin polymorphism have so far attracted the most attention, and at present about 10 variants have been described. There are two broad classes of myosin in cross-striated muscles. One is present in fast muscles and the other in slow and cardiac muscles. The polymorphism of myosin resides in both light and heavy chains, and is reflected in the rate of ATP hydrolysis and in its pH optima. Electrophoretic analysis carried out under denaturing conditions revealed that the light chains of myosin obtained from fast, slow, and cardiac muscles are all polypeptides of different molecular weight. The heavy chains, on the other hand, have rather similar molecular weights, but numerous studies have shown that their amino acid sequences differ. Moreover, myosin of fast muscles contains methylated histidines and lysine residues as a consequence of posttranslational modification (see ref. 70).

A new insight into myosin polymorphism was gained when conditions for electrophoresis in the native state was developed. In this case, the variants of myosin are separated on the basis of their charge. Using this procedure, the previously identified classes of myosin have been resolved into additional variants. Thus three isomyosins were detected in fast muscles and two in slow muscles. Additionally, cardiac myosin has been resolved into two atrial isomyosins and one to three (depending on animal species and age) ventricular isomyosins. Not all the details of myosin diversity have been clarified, but it is known that the three fast muscle isomyosins have identical heavy chains. They differ only in their light chains (LC). Thus we have two homodimers of LC-1 and LC-3, respectively, and one heterodimer. In the ventricle there are two homodimers of heavy chains (alpha and beta, respectively) and one heterodimer, whereas the set of light chains is identical in all three isomyosins. In addition to the isomyosins present in adult muscles, distinct forms have also been found in embryonic and neonatal skeletal muscles.

Less is known about the remaining muscle proteins. Amino acid analyses have demonstrated that the actins of various origin are similar but not identical molecules. The amino acid substitutions are reflected in the overall charge of the molecule which allows resolution of three broad groups of actins which, in order of decreasing isoelectric points, are denoted as α, β, and γ isoforms. The α-isoactins are typical of the contractile apparatus, whereas the β and γ variants are localized in the cytoplasm. Within the α-isoactins at least two variants are known: skeletal and cardiac. In contrast to myosin, there is no significant divergence in the biological activity of isoactins. Yet the microheterogeneity in their primary structure clearly indicates that the isoactins are products of a multigene family.

Within the regulatory proteins two forms of tropomyosin are known. They are homodimers of subunits α and β, respectively. The α_2 form is present in fast and cardiac muscles, whereas the β_2 form is present in slow fibers. The troponin subunits T and I differ in their amino acid sequence between fast, slow, and cardiac muscles, although the sequence homology is very high. Cardiac troponin I differs in one additional feature, the presence of a short amino acid sequence in which the serine residues are reversibly phosphorylated. The cardiac and slow muscle variants of troponin C are identical and differ from the one present in fast muscles.

Several aspects of polymorphism observed within the contractile proteins are noteworthy. First, both skeletal and cardiac muscles contain discrete populations of cells which express one isoprotein in preference to another one. For example, in the ventricle some myocytes contain the heavy-chain α, others contain the heavy chain β, and still others contain both. Secondly, the cell complement of the isoprotein is not static but changes depending on the developmental stage and the hormonal and functional status of the muscle. For example, administration of a high dose of thyroid hormone results in simultaneous activation and repression of genes for heavy chains α and β, respectively. Finally, the expression of each protein appears to follow its own theme. For example, myosin and troponin C are very similar in cardiac and slow muscles. In contrast, the tropomyosin of the heart is identical to that in fast muscles, whereas troponin T and I differ in all three types of muscle. Each set of genes thus appears to have its own regulatory signals.

Cell Differentiation Programs

The generation of specific types of cells requires the selection of a specific program that differentiates the information stored within the DNA molecule. The mechanisms controlling the expression of a particular set of genes, however, must account not only for the generation of diversity between cells but also for mainte-nance of the phenotype between proliferating stem cells. There are currently two schools of thought about the mechanism by which a given phenotype is selected over another (36).

One group of investigators view cell differentiation as embryonic induction mediated by cell-cell interaction or by exogenous molecules. The stem cells are visualized as being undifferentiated and able to initiate transcription of any set of genes. For example, the zygote is said to be a multipotent cell which can be induced to differentiate into cell types A, B, C, etc. The selection of a given phenotype does not require DNA synthesis and is dependent on the cell microenvironment, which in turn changes with developmental time and cellular density. The accumu-lating putative signals then activate a particular set of genes via their effect on DNA regulatory sequences by a mechanism similar to those outlined under "Tran-scriptional Control," above.

The second group of investigators stresses intracellular time-dependent changes that alter chromosomal structure and, thereby, expression of cell-specific genes. The differentiation programs of a cell are thus viewed as inherited and consequently limited. The cells can undergo two types of division: (a) one in which the daughter cells are identical to mother cells (proliferative mitosis); and (b) one that generates cells with phenotypes different from those of their ancestors (quantal mitosis). Thus there are no multipotent, undifferentiated cells; rather, all cells belong to a predetermined lineage. For example, after a certain number of proliferative mitoses the zygote undergoes quantal mitosis, which results in two transient phenotypes (A and B), each of which eventually gives rise to cell lines C,D, and E,F, respectively.

The first theory receives its support from the experiments in which differentiation and cell proliferation were influenced independently of each other by manipulating the growth environment. In one such study, the differentiation of mesenchymal cells derived from the limb bud was examined (12). The mesenchymal cells are progenitors of three cell lines: myoblasts, chondroblasts, and fibroblasts. Depending on the energy status of the cultured cells, the mesenchymal progenitors could be shunted directly into any of these three lineages. This indicates that the phenotypic options of mesenchymal cells are open.

The advocates of the second theory have cultured single cells derived from the same source (1). The obtained subclones were found to be bipotent only, yielding either myoblasts/fibroblasts or chondroblasts/fibroblasts. No subclone was found which would produce both myoblasts and chondroblasts, indicating that the phenotypic options are predetermined.

There are several possibilities for reconciliation of these opposing sets of data. For example, the cellular microenvironment might influence the proliferation and/or survival of one cell type but not another. Alternatively, the cells which are induced to proliferate more rapidly can reach their quantal mitoses earlier than the other cells. However, more definitive answers to these all-important questions about the control of gene expression can be obtained only when well-characterized probes for the cell-specific genes become available. In this direction, studies of myosin and actin have already been initiated, but the data are not complete and are often contradictory. It is clear, nevertheless, that there is a definitive transition in the expression of the myosin phenotype during myogenesis. For example, the presumptive myoblasts were found to synthesize myosin light and heavy chains, which are distinct from those found in overtly differentiated myotubes (13,14).

The results of trying to determine the earliest form of cross-striated myosin are somewhat contradictory. In one study chicken myotomal-stage skeletal and cardiac myosins were found cross-reacting with antibodies for cardiac, fast, and slow myosin heavy chains, indicating simultaneous expression of all types of myosin during the early stage of overt myogenesis (44). In other studies, however, the earliest detectable myotomal-stage myosins as well as cardiac myosins were found to react only with antibodies to ventricular myosin. The same data were obtained for embryonic postmyotomal muscles. These data are consistent with the expression of cardiac-like myosin, which is typical of striated muscles in their epithelial stages of development. After the myotomal tissue loses its epithelial character and divides into individual muscle masses, and cells begin to form multinucleated myotubes, another form of myosin heavy chain appears (referred to as embryonic myosin). This variant is clearly distinct from that found in adult skeletal muscles. Embryonic myosin in turn is replaced by neonatal and, later, adult fast or slow variants of myosin heavy chains, leading to a myosin complement typical of a given muscle cell (69). The adult phenotype is not static, however, often varying depending on numerous factors, e.g., the type and extent of contractile activity and the hormonal and developmental state. For example, of the three isomyosins identified in the rabbit ventricle, the V3 variant predominates during the late embryonic period. After birth, however, the synthesis of V1 isomyosin is increased and that of V3 repressed with consequent predominance of V1 which has high ATPase activity.

During the period which follows, the trend reverses again so that in ventricles of old animals V3 is the main species of myosin.

From the described experiments the complexity of gene regulation during muscle differentiation and growth appears bewildering. The fragmentary data indicate that there are several independent differentiation cues. Sorting out which one is permissive and which is obligatory will require the additional characterization of gene products as well as the development of more definitive probes.

PHYSIOLOGICAL VERSUS PATHOLOGICAL GROWTH

The change in the pattern of gene expression produced by the functional load is characteristic of many, if not all, cross-striated muscles. As far as we know, it is only in the heart that sustained hemodynamic overload leads to diminished contractile function and eventual heart failure; this occurs when the overload is prolonged or exceeds some as yet unspecified limit. This loss of ability to cope with functional requirements has led to several attempts to classify various phases of the compensatory growth of the heart. For example, Meerson (45b) divided hypertrophy into three stages corresponding to Selye's phases of the general stress syndrome: stage of damage (alarm reaction), stage of stable hyperfunction (resistance), and stage of progressive cardiosclerosis and gradual exhaustion (exhaustion). The major drawback of these generalized stages is the lack of unequivocal and measurable indices of growth response of the heart, e.g., the extent of damage, hyperfunction, resistance, or exhaustion. Therefore more appropriate terminology is that which is compatible with an experimental description of compensatory growth: phase I—developing hypertrophy; phase II—compensatory hypertrophy; and phase III—heart failure. As indicated in Fig. 6, the workload exceeds the mass of the heart in phase I, which is typical for the life style of that species. During phase II, the induced growth has compensated for the increased workload established in phase I. In phase III, the workload per unit of cardiac mass increases again due to progressively decreasing force generation and consequent dilatation of the heart. From the above description it is apparent that what is at first an adaptive physiological response that allows the individual survival eventually becomes a pathological process. So far we have only a few clues about the transition, or distinction, between physiological and pathological growth and the nature of pathological lesions. Several generalizations, however, can be made. First, the intermittent overload of the heart through exercise results in hypertrophy without phase III. Phase III is typically reached only when the overload is sustained because of systemic hypertension or valvular lesions. The second consistent observation is that during phases II and III the ratio of mitochondrial to myofibrillar volumes in cardiac myocytes is decreased. Whether the relative loss of energy-generating units, together with other mechanisms, contributes to the aberrant expression of genetic information in the failing heart remains to be elucidated.

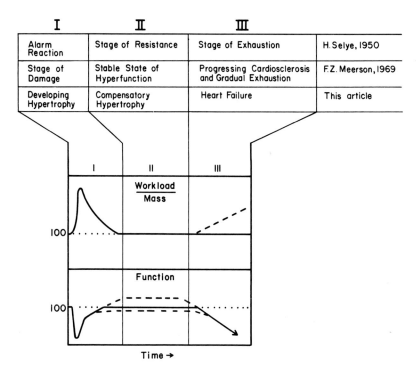

I	II	III	
Alarm Reaction	Stage of Resistance	Stage of Exhaustion	H. Selye, 1950
Stage of Damage	Stable State of Hyperfunction	Progressing Cardiosclerosis and Gradual Exhaustion	F.Z. Meerson, 1969
Developing Hypertrophy	Compensatory Hypertrophy	Heart Failure	This article

FIG. 6. Phases of cardiac overload and terminology used by various investigators. In the lower part of the diagram, *100* and the *dotted line* indicate normal values (i.e., prior to the imposition of a work overload). The *full line* indicates the generalized response of the heart. The *interrupted line* indicates that conflicting data have been obtained in various experimental models. (For example, in phase II the "function" of the heart was reported to be normal, increased, and decreased.)

CONCLUSION

During the last decade cellular and molecular biology experienced remarkable progress. However, our understanding of organ growth remains rudimentary. Estimates of cell populations become more accurate after application of quantitative stereological techniques and measurements performed on isolated cells. As far as the biogenesis of cellular components is concerned, the accumulation of information about protein amino acid sequences provides a good start for the analysis of forces involved in the assembly of multiprotein complexes. The mechanism controlling expression of the gene in nucleated cells was discovered to be immensely more complex than in the prokaryotes. Our concept of cellular differentiation will undoubtedly undergo further refinement because of the fact that the muscle phenotype is not fixed but continually adapts to functional and metabolic demands placed on the organism. Despite unraveled complexities, however, our ability to assay not only specific gene products but also the structure of genes themselves holds considerable promise for the rapid advancement of our understanding of such a complex biological phenomenon as organ growth.

REFERENCES

1. Abbott, J., Schiltz, J., Dienstman, S., and Holtzer, H. (1974): The phenotypic complexity of myogenic clones. *Proc. Natl. Acad. Sci. USA*, 71:1506–1510.
2. Adler, C. P. (1976): DNA in growing hearts of children: biochemical and cytophotometric investigations. *Beitr. Pathol.*, 158:173–202.
3. Albin, R., Dowell, R. T., Zak, R., and Rabinowitz, M. (1973): Synthesis and degradation of mitochondrial components in hypertrophied rat heart. *Biochem. J.*, 136:629–637.
4. Amenta, J. S., and Brocher, S. C. (1980): Mechanisms of protein turnover in cultured fibroblasts: differential inhibition of two lysosomal mechanisms with insulin and NH_4Cl. *Exp. Cell Res.*, 126:167–174.
5. Baer, B. W., and Rhodes, D. (1983): Eukaryotic RNA polymerase II binds to nucleosome cores from transcribed genes. *Nature*, 301:48.
6. Bishop, S. P. (1983): Ultrastructure of the myocardium in physiologic and pathologic hypertrophy in experimental animals. *Perspect. Cardiovasc. Res.*, 7:127–147.
7. Biswas, B. B., Ganguly, A., and Das, A. (1975): Eukaryotic RNA polymerases and the factors that control them. *Prog. Nucleic Acid Res. Mol. Biol.*, 15:145–184.
8. Britten, R. J., and Davidson, E. H. (1969): Gene regulation for higher cells: a theory. *Science*, 165:349–357.
9. Brown, D. (1981): Gene expression in eukaryotes. *Science*, 211:667–674.
10. Buckingham, M. E., Caput, N., Cohen, A., Whalen, R. G., and Gros, F. (1974): The synthesis and stability of cytoplasmic messenger RNA during myoblast differentiation in culture. *Proc. Natl. Acad. Sci. USA*, 71:1466–1470.
11. Bugaisky, L., and Zak, R. (1979): Cellular growth of cardiac muscle after growth. *Tex. Rep. Biol. Med.*, 39:123–138.
12. Caplan, A. I., and Rosenberg, M. J. (1975): Interrelationship between poly(ADP-rib) synthesis, intracellular NAD levels and muscle or cartilage differentiation from mesodermal cells of embryonic chick limb. *Proc. Natl. Acad. Sci. USA*, 72:1852–1857.
13. Chi, J. C., Fellini, S. A., and Holtzer, H. (1975): Differences among myosins synthesized in non-myogenic cells, presumptive myoblasts, and myoblasts. *Proc. Natl. Acad. Sci. USA*, 72:4999–5003.
14. Chi, J. C., Rubenstein, N., Strahs, K., and Holtzer, H. (1975): Synthesis of myosin heavy and light chains in muscle cultures. *J. Cell Biol.*, 67:523–537.
15. Clemens, M. (1983): Protein phosphorylation and translation of messenger RNAs. *Nature*, 302:110.
16. Conde, R. D., and Scornik, O. A. (1976): Role of protein degradation in the growth of livers after a nutritional shift. *Biochem. J.*, 158:385–390.
17. Cutilletta, A. F., Rudnik, M., and Zak, R. (1978): Muscle and non-muscle cell RNA polymerase activity during the development of myocardial hypertrophy. *J. Mol. Cell. Cardiol.*, 10:677–687.
18. Darnell, J. E. (1982): Variety in the level of gene control in eukaryotic cells. *Nature*, 297:365–371.
19. Daum, G., Gasser, S. M., and Schatz, G. (1982): Import of proteins into mitochondria: energy-dependent, two-step processing of the intermembrane space enzyme cytochrome b_2 by isolated yeast mitochondria. *J. Biol. Chem.*, 257:13075–13080.
20. Dayton, W. R., Schollmeyer, J. V., Lepley, R. A., and Cortes, L. R. (1981): A calcium-activated protease possibly involved in myofibrillar protein turnover: isolation of a low-calcium-requiring form of the protease. *Biochem. Biophys. Acta*, 659:48–61.
21. Devlin, R. B., and Emerson, C. P. (1978): Coordinate regulation of protein synthesis during myoblast differentiation. *Cell*, 13:599–611.
22. Dowell, R. T., and McManus, R. E. (1978): Pressure-induced cardiac enlargement in neonatal and adults rats: left ventricular functional characteristics and evidence of cardiac muscle cell proliferation in the neonate. *Circ. Res.*, 42:303–310.
23. Etlinger, J. D., Speiser, S., Wajnberg, E., and Glucksman, M. J. (1981): ATP-dependent proteolysis in erythroid and muscle cells. *Acta Biol. Med. Ger.*, 40:1285–1291.
24. Ezerman, E. B., and Ishikawa, H. (1967): Differentiation of the sarcoplasmic reticulum and T system in developing chick skeletal muscle in vitro. *J. Cell. Biol.*, 35:405–420.

25. Fischman, D. A. (1967): An electron microscope study of myofibril formation in embryonic chick skeletal muscle. *J. Cell. Biol.*, 32:557–577.

26. Fischman, D. A. (1970): The synthesis and assembly of myofibrils in embryonic muscle. *Curr. Top. Dev. Biol.*, 5:235–280.

27. Fischman, D. A., and Zak, R. (1971): Assembly of myofibrils in the absence of protein synthesis. *J. Gen. Physiol.*, 57:245.

28. Goldstein, M. A. (1974): Nuclear pores in ventricular muscle cells from adult hypertrophied hearts. *J. Mol. Cell. Cardiol.*, 6:227–235.

29. Gorza, L., Sartore, S., Triban, C., and Schiaffino, S. (1983): Embryonic-like myosin heavy chains in regenerating chicken muscle. *Exp. Cell Res.*, 143:395–403.

30. Goss, R. J. (1966): Hypertrophy versus hyperplasia: how much organs can grow depends on whether their functional units increase in size or in number. *Science*, 153:1615–1620.

31. Goss, R. J. (1967): The strategy of growth. In: *Control of Cellular Growth in Adult Organisms*, edited by H. Their and T. Rytomaa, pp. 4–27. Academic Press, London.

32. Greenway, D. C., and MacLennan, D. H. (1978): Assembly of the sarcoplasmic reticulum: synthesis of calsequestrin and the $Ca^{2+}Mg^{2+}$-adenosine triphosphatase on membrane-bound polyribosomes. *Can. J. Biochem.*, 56:452–456.

33. Grove, D., Zak, R., Nair, K. G., and Aschenbrenner, V. (1969): Biochemical correlates of cardiac hypertrophy. IV. Observations on the cellular organization of growth during myocardial hypertrophy in the rat. *Circ. Res.*, 25:473–485.

34. Hayashi, T., Robert, B., Ip, W., Cayer, M. L., and Smith, D. S. (1977): Actin-myosin interaction: self-assembly into a bipolar "contractile unit." *J. Mol. Biol.*, 111:159–171.

35. Holland, P. C., and MacLennan, D. H. (1976): Assembly of the sarcoplasmic reticulum: biosynthesis of the adenosine triphosphatase in rat skeletal muscle cell culture. *J. Biol. Chem.*, 251:2030–2036.

36. Holtzer, H., Biehl, J., Payette, R., Sasse, J., Pacifici, M., and Holtzer, S. (1983): Cell diversification: differing roles of cell lineages and cell-cell interactions. In: *Limb Development and Regeneration*, pp. 271–280. Alan R. Liss, New York.

37. Huxley, H. E. (1963): Electron microscope studies on the structure of natural and synthetic protein filaments from striated muscle. *J. Mol. Biol.*, 7:281–308.

38. Jefferson, L. S., Wolpert, E. B., Giber, K. E., and Morgan, H. E. (1971): Regulation of protein synthesis in heart muscle. III. Effect of anoxia on protein synthesis. *J. Biol. Chem.*, 246:2171–2178.

39. Kaminer, B., and Bell, A. L. (1966): Myosin filamentogenesis: effects of pH and ionic concentration. *J. Mol. Biol.*, 20:391–401.

40. Korecky, B., and Rakusan, K. (1978): Normal and hypertrophic growth of the rat heart: changes in cell dimensions and number. *Am. J. Physiol.*, 234:H123–128.

41. Legato, M. J. (1972): Ultrastructural characteristics of the rat ventricular cell grown in tissue culture, with special reference to sarcomerogenesis. *J. Mol. Cell. Cardiol.*, 4:299–317.

42. Legato, M. J. (1979): Cellular mechanism of normal growth in mammalian heart. II. A quantitative and qualitative comparison between the right and left ventricular myocytes in the dog from birth to five months of age. *Circ. Res.*, 44:263–279.

43. Masaki, T., and Yoshizaki, C. (1972): The onset of myofibrillar protein synthesis in chick embryo in vivo. *J. Biochem. (Tokyo)*, 71:755–757.

44. Masaki, T., and Yoshizaki, C. (1974): Differentiation of myosin in chick embryos. *J. Biochem.*, 76:123–131.

45. McLachlan, A. D., and Stewart, M. (1976): The 14-fold periodicity in α-tropomyosin and the interaction with actin. *J. Mol. Biol.*, 103:271–298.

45a. McLachlan, A. D. and Karn, J. (1982): Periodic charge distributions in the myosin rod amino acid sequence match cross-bridge spacings in muscle. *Nature* 299:226–232.

45b. Meerson, F. Z. (1969): The myocardium in hyperfunction hypertrophy and heart failure. *Circ. Res.* 25:(Suppl. II), 1–163.

46. Morgan, H. E., Jefferson, L. S., Wolpert, E. B., and Rannels, D. E. (1971): Regulation of protein synthesis in the heart muscle. II. Effect of amino acid and insulin on ribosomal aggregation. *J. Biol. Chem.*, 246:2163–2170.

47. Neffgen, J. F., and Korecky, B. (1972): Cellular hyperplasia and hypertrophy in cardiomegalies induced by anemia in young and adult rats. *Circ. Res.*, 30:104–113.

48. Obinata, T., Shimada, Y., and Matsuda, R. (1979): Troponin in embryonic chick skeletal muscle cells in vitro: an immunoelectronmicroscope study. *J. Cell Biol.*, 81:59–66.
49. Obtinata, T., Yamamoto, M., and Maruyama, K. (1966): The identification of randomly formed thin filaments in differentiating muscle cells of the chick embryo. *Dev. Biol.*, 14:192–213.
50. Pfitzer, P. (1971): Polyploide Zellkerne im Herzmuskel des Schweins. *Virchows Arch. [Cell Pathol.]*, 9:180–186.
51. Phillips, G. N., Jr., Lattman, E. E., Cummins, P., Lee, K. Y., and Cohen, C. (1979): Crystal structure and molecular interactions of tropomyosin. *Nature*, 278:413–417.
52. Pollard, T. D., and Craig, S. W. (1982): Mechanism of actin polymerization. *Trends Biochem. Sci.*, 7:55–58.
53. Reddy, M. K., Rabinowitz, M., and Zak, R. (1983): Stringent requirement for Ca^{2+} in the removal of Z-lines and α-actinin from isolated myofibrils by Ca^{2+}-activated neutral proteinase. *Biochem. J.*, 209:635–641.
54. Reid, G. A., and Schatz, G. (1982): Import of proteins into mitochondria: extramitochondrial pools and posttranslational import of mitochondrial protein precursors in vivo. *J. Biol. Chem.*, 257:13062–13067.
55. Robbins, J., and Heywood, S. M. (1978): Quantification of myosin heavy chain mRNA during myogenesis. *Eur. J. Biochem.*, 82:601–608.
56. Roy, R. K., Lau, A. S., Munro, H. N., Baliga, B. S., and Sarkar, S. (1979): Release of in vitro-synthesized poly(A)-containing RNA from isolated rat liver nuclei: characterization of the ribonucleoprotein particles involved. *Proc. Natl. Acad. Sci. USA*, 76:1751–1755.
57. Rubin, M. S., and Tzagoloff, A. (1973): Assembly of the mitochondrial membrane system. X. Mitochondrial synthesis of three of the subunit proteins of yeast cytochrome oxidase. *J. Biol. Chem.*, 248:4275–4279.
58. Saetersdal, T. S., Myklabust, R., Skagseth, E., and Engedal, H. (1976): Ultrastructural studies on the growth of filaments and sarcomeres in mechanically overloaded human hearts. *Virchows Arch. [Cell Pathol.]*, 21:91–112.
59. Sarkar, S., Mukherjee, A. K., and Guha, Ch. (1981): A ribonuclease-resistant cytoplasmic 10 S ribonucleoprotein of chick embryonic muscle. *J. Biol. Chem.*, 256:5077–5086.
60. Shimada, Y., and Obinata, T. (1977): Polarity of actin filaments at the initial stage of myofibril assembly in myogenic cells in vitro. *J. Cell Biol.*, 72:777–785.
61. Smith, A. L., and Bird, J. W. C. (1975): Distribution and particle properties of the vacuolar apparatus of cardiac muscle tissue. *J. Mol. Cell. Cardiol.*, 7:39–61.
62. Stein, G., Spelsberg, T. C., and Kleinsmith, L. J. (1974): Nonhistone chromosomal proteins and gene regulation. *Science*, 183:817–824.
63. Sweeney, L. J., Clark, W. A., Zak, R., and Manasek, F. J. (1983): Evidence for a primordial striated muscle myosin. *J. Cell Biol.*, 95:369a.
64. Wegner, A. (1976): Head to tail polymerization of actin. *J. Mol. Biol.*, 108:139–150.
65. Whalen, R. G., Butler-Browne, G. S., and Gros, F. (1976): Protein synthesis and actin heterogeneity in calf muscle cells in culture. *Proc. Natl. Acad. Sci. USA*, 73:2018–2022.
66. Woodbury, R. G., Everitt, M., Sanada, Y., Katunuma, N., Lagunoff, D., and Neurath, H. (1978): A major serine protease in rat skeletal muscle: evidence for its mast cell origin. *Proc. Natl. Acad. Sci. USA*, 75:5311–5313.
67. Wu, C. (1980): The 5' ends of Drosophila heat shock genes in chromatin are hypersensitive to DNase I. *Nature*, 286:854–860.
68. Zak, R. (1974): Development and proliferative capacity of cardiac muscle cells. *Circ. Res. (Suppl. V)*, 35:17–26.
69. Zak, R. (1981): Contractile function as a determinant of muscle growth. *Cell Muscle Motil.*, 1:1–32.
70. Zak, R., and Galhotra, S. S. (1983): Contractile and regulatory proteins. In: *Cardiac Metabolism*, edited by A. J. Drake-Holland and M. I. M. Noble. Wiley, New York.
71. Zubrycka, E., and MacLennan, D. H. (1976): Assembly of the sarcoplasmic reticulum: biosynthesis of calsequestrin in rat skeletal muscle cell cultures. *J. Biol. Chem.*, 251:7733–7738.
72. Zak, R., and Rabinowitz, M. (1979): Molecular aspects of cardiac hypertrophy. *Annu. Rev. Physiol.*, 41:539–552.
73. Zak, R., Martin, A. F., Prior, G., and Rabinowitz, M. (1977): Comparison of turnover of several myofibrillar proteins and critical evaluation of double isotope method. *J. Biol. Chem.*, 252:3430–3435.

Growth of the Heart in Health and Disease,
edited by Radovan Zak. Raven Press,
New York © 1984.

Assessment of Cardiac Growth

Karel Rakusan

*Department of Physiology, University of Ottawa, School of Medicine,
Ottawa, Ontario, Canada*

Growth, in contrast to development and maturation, is a quantitative phenomenon. Therefore a careful application of proper quantitative methods is of utmost importance. The aim of this chapter is to review the basic quantitative methods available for the assessment of cardiac growth. Needless to say, these methods are applicable for the evaluation of cardiac growth both inside and outside its normal limits. Cardiac growth is usually assessed at three hierarchical levels: the level of the whole organ (macrostructure), the tissue level (microstructure as examined by light microscopy), and the level of a single cell (microstructure as examined by electron microscopy).

Before we proceed to a description of the available methods at the three levels described above, some issues common to several of these methods are discussed. The main question concerns site and size of sampling. The goal of each quantitative study is to obtain a representative sample, which means a sample that "faithfully" reflects the real situation. Most stereological methods are based on the concept of random sampling. Cardiac tissue, however, is composed of heterogeneous regions with a definite orientation. Sometimes, in order to circumvent the sampling problem at the organ level, sampling is limited to a restricted, well-defined region of the heart. The overall results and their validity always depend on the chosen design of sampling (e.g., random, stratified, or systematic sampling). This topic was discussed recently in depth by Weibel (44) and Cruz-Orive and Weibel (11).

In addition to where and how we sample, the "representativeness" of the sample is determined by its size. Often we see reports based on a very small number of measurements which do not reflect the real situation. At the same time, however, it is relatively easy to estimate the number of measurements necessary for any preset accuracy by using either graphic methods or simple calculation. In the former case, "running averages" are plotted as a function of the number of measurements. These plots are examined to see if the running average is stable over the last third of the sample. If this is not the case, the sample size is increased until this stability requirement is met (12). In the latter case, the number of measurements *(N)* necessary (e.g., to reduce a sampling error to 1% of the mean values) is calculated from the mean value ($\overline{X}$) and standard deviation (SD). The mean and standard deviation are derived from the measurement of a relatively small sample in a pilot study. If 1% of the relative standard error of the mean (SEM) equals 100 SEM/$\overline{X}$, which in turn is $(SD/\sqrt{N}/\overline{X})100$, then the number of measurements necessary to achieve such an accuracy is $N = (100 \ SD/\overline{X})^2$.

Finally, whenever possible, only directly measured data should be compared, not the derived parameters. For instance, even a relatively small error in direct measurement of the cell diameter is amplified when used for computation of the three-dimensional volume of the muscle cell.

ORGAN LEVEL MACROSTRUCTURE

Cardiac Dimensions

The values of the *external dimensions* of the heart were reported extensively in the older morphological literature. The most important measurements of external dimensions were the cardiac length, breadth, and width and the ventricular circumference. Cardiac length was defined as the distance from base to apex, the width as a maximal distance perpendicular to the length, and the breadth as a maximal distance between the anterior and posterior surfaces of the heart.

At present, it is mainly the *internal dimensions* of the heart that are being used. They are obviously dependent on the method used to dissect the heart and its fixation. An investigation of factors likely to result in differences between clinical estimates of cardiac size and its postmortem appearances was reported by Eckner et al. (13). An excellent review and detailed description of the methods for measuring the internal dimensions of the heart from autopsy was published by Lev et al. (21). These authors proposed standard measurement of 16 well-defined internal dimensions.

The first reported measurement of the ventricular volume was published as early as 1733 by Hales, who ran wax into the isolated heart and calculated the volume. The capacity of the cardiac ventricles was estimated using similar principles by many authors, including Kyrieleis (20), who investigated changes of the ventricular volumes in human hearts by filling previously fixed hearts with a known amount of water. Volume can also be estimated indirectly on the basis of the internal dimensions of the heart (21,39).

In clinical medicine cardiac dimensions can be measured using noninvasive techniques. These involve mainly the application of roentgenographic and echocardiographic methods. Detailed descriptions of such techniques are out of the scope of this chapter. The interested reader is referred to an abundant cardiology literature on this topic.

The ventricular dimensions in experimental animals *in vivo* can be assessed by pulse-transit ultrasonic methods as described and validated by Rankin and co-workers (36). Computer-assisted reconstruction of the cardiac size and shape was recently described by Janicki and co-workers (15).

Cardiac Mass

Cardiac mass is traditionally described as cardiac weight. The term cardiac weight is in turn often used to describe the mass of both ventricles, excluding the cardiac atria. The cardiac atria have only an auxiliary function in cardiac pumping; their composition differs in many respects from that of ventricular tissue, and it is quite difficult to separate accurately the big vessels from the atria. In addition, the atrial contribution to the total cardiac weight is relatively small. The cardiac ventricles are usually divided into the septum and the free walls of the right and left ventricles. In the adult heart, the septum is, in many morphological and functional aspects, a part of the left ventricle. Therefore the weight of the septum is often combined with the weight of the free left ventricular wall in order to obtain the left ventricular weight. An alternate approach is to divide the weight of the septum and assign it proportionally to both ventricles according to the weights of their free walls. This consideration is important when evaluating the right or left ventricular preponderance, which changes during the early stages of postnatal development as well as in various pathological situations.

In human section material, proper care should be taken to remove epicardial fat, which may influence cardiac weight to a varying degree. Measurements of cardiac weight in experimental animals in most cases allow one to determine the dry weight; this is done by weighing a piece of tissue before and after drying to a constant weight. This is especially important when variation in the tissue water content is expected (e.g., tissue edema associated with cardiac failure).

The absolute cardiac weight, expressed in milligrams or grams, is closely related to the weight of the body mass which must be supplied by the pumped blood. The fact that the growth rates of the organs do not always correspond to the growth rate of the total organism was recognized as early as 1762 by Haller, who described "incrementum inaequale" of the organs in contrast to "incrementum universale" of the whole organism. The relationship between organ weight and body weight may be analyzed by the allometric formula which describes the organ weight y as a power function of body weight (x):

$$y = bx^\alpha \qquad (1)$$

The constant b is the value of y when $x = 1$ and α is the slope of the line on the double logarithmic scale, which indicates the rate of organ growth with respect to body growth. The easiest way to determine the constants b and α is to transform the allometric formula to its logarithmic form:

$$\log y = \alpha \log x + \log b \qquad (2)$$

which is subsequently treated as a standard linear equation.

The relative cardiac weight denotes simply the absolute cardiac weight expressed as a fraction of body weight. It is a useful index for comparing pathological cardiac growth in subjects or experimental animals of similar body weights. It may be misleading, however, when the body weights of the experimental and control groups differ significantly, as is often the case. For instance, in situations where body weight is significantly reduced because of the experimental procedure, as in hyperthyroidism or during exercise, an increased relative cardiac weight is partly a reflection of a decrease in body weight per se because the relative cardiac weight even in normal animals is higher in low-body-weight groups and decreases with growth. The proper comparison should be made using body weight controls obtained either directly or by using expected cardiac weights calculated from data collected on a large sample of the normal population. For similar reasons, several authors have tried to avoid the variability in body weight by searching for a reference parameter which is not influenced by physiological, nutritional, or environmental factors. They have, for instance, compared cardiac weight to body length in autopsy material (47) or to the tibial length in adult and old rats (46).

TISSUE LEVEL: MICROSTRUCTURE AS EXAMINED BY LIGHT MICROSCOPY

The most prominent features at the tissue level are coronary capillaries and cardiac myocytes (i.e., muscle cells—called muscle fibers in the older literature). These are the structures which are usually evaluated quantitatively by different methodical approaches. The rest of the tissue has seldom been analyzed to any great extent. It is customary to measure the extracellular tissue space by applying the point-counting method to histological cross sections. In addition, the contribution of the "nonmuscle" nuclei to the total population of the myocardial nuclei may be counted on histological sections. The "nonmuscle" cell population data are sometimes subdivided into the contribution of nuclei from connective tissue cells and that from endothelial cells.

Myocardial Capillary Supply

Some of the methods used for determining myocardial capillary density and its functional evaluation, as well as some of the older results on changes in the capillary density under normal and pathological conditions, are summarized in our 1971 review (32).

The number of capillaries is often related to the number of cardiac myocytes, called the cell/capillary ratio. This index, however, ignores the size of the individual cells. For instance, in the heart of neonatal rats, four cells are supplied by a single capillary, although the cell/capillary ratio is 1:1 in hearts from adult animals. On the other hand, the capillary density (i.e., the number of capillaries per square unit) is higher in young rats, with an unfavorable ratio of four cells per capillary, than the capillary density found in adult animals.

A more suitable index of capillarization, introduced by Krogh (19), is the radius of the tissue cylinder supplied by a single capillary. This radius, sometimes called the diffusion distance, is defined as the mean half-distance between two capillaries in a cross section. It is derived from the number of capillaries counted per square millimeter of cross section N, assuming a square array. The square root of the capillary number in this case corresponds to the number of intercapillary distances per millimeter (e.g., 1,000 μm) and the mean diffusion distance R_1:

$$R_1 = 10^3/2\sqrt{N} \tag{3}$$

where R_1 is the diffusion distance (in μm) and N is the number of capillaries per square millimeter. Using this parameter, however, we do not include all portions of the tissue. The area on the cross section which is not covered by the circles of radius includes the parts of the tissue which are first prone to hypoxia. In order to avoid this omission, Thews (41) proposed a new model of the capillary supply based on the assumption that the area supplied by one capillary has a hexagonal shape. In this case all the tissue area is covered, and the diffusion distance (R_2) equals the side of a hexagon. The new diffusion distance (R_2) can be calculated from the number of capillaries (N) and the size of the area (A) as:

$$R_2 = (2A/3\sqrt{3N})^{1/2} \tag{4}$$

R_1 represents the minimal diffusion distance, calculated on the basis of a square array which leaves approximately 21% of the tissue outside the cylinder. On the other hand, R_2 represents the maximal diffusion distance calculated on the basis of a hexagonal arrangement, and in this case a similar fraction of the issue is included in two neighboring cylinders. As a compromise between these two extremes, it is possible to calculate an "average" diffusion distance $(R_3$, in μm) from the number of capillaries per square millimeter as:

$$R_3 = 10^3/\sqrt{N\pi} \tag{5}$$

A different approach was proposed by Roberts and Wearn (38), who estimated the capillary surface area per unit volume of tissue, which they related to the volume of muscle cells in the same tissue unit. The capillary surface area was calculated from the number of capillaries per cross section with a unit diameter of 8 μm, which is equal to the size of a red blood cell. A similar approach was used recently by Anversa et al. (3) and Wiener et al. (45). In their method the capillary cross sections were measured directly by the point-counting method. The capillary lumen, however, is influenced by perfusion of the tissue at the time of sacrifice and by its subsequent fixation and embedding. In addition, both of these methods assume that capillaries have the form of cylinders which run parallel to the long axis of the myocytes. This is probably not always the case, and the degree of capillary tortuosity can be measured on longitudinal sections (9).

All the methods described so far lead only to an average index of the capillary supply. However, the degree of heterogeneity of the capillary spacing is probably even more important (42). The variability of the intercapillary distances can be obtained from direct measurements on the surface of the beating heart (26). Alternatively, it can be derived indirectly from the measurements obtained by the method of concentric circles (Fig. 1). This approach was proposed by Loats et al. (23) for skeletal muscle and applied by Rakusan et al. (34) to measurements in heart muscle. It provides a means of estimating the tissue distribution at different

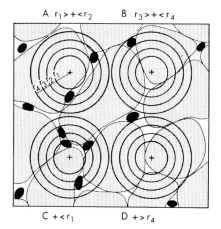

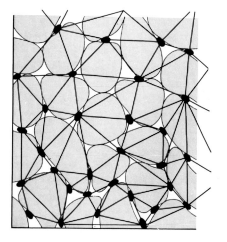

FIG. 1. Method of concentric circles. A system of concentric circles of known radii is randomly applied to the tissue, and the distance from the center point to the nearest capillary is recorded.

FIG. 2. Intercapillary distances as measured from the capillary connections forming the network of closed triangles.

distances from the nearest capillary. In this method, a system of concentric circles of known radii is randomly applied to the tissue. For each center point in the above array, the largest circle around it which contains no capillary is recorded. In this fashion, the percentage of the points corresponding to the percentage of the tissue which is beyond or within a certain distance from the nearest capillary can be determined.

Finally, intercapillary distances can be measured directly on histological sections by drawing the lines from each capillary to surrounding capillaries on a tracing of the field to form a network of closed triangles, with no lines crossing between the points (Fig. 2). This approach was used by Renkin and co-workers (37) for evaluating the heterogeneity of the capillary distribution in skeletal muscle. To our knowledge, it has not yet been used in the assessment of capillarity in heart muscle.

An alternative approach is to measure the capacity of the terminal vessels using the radioisotope technique as described by Myers and Honig in 1964 (27). They injected experimental animals with a suspension of red blood cells marked by ^{51}Cr and plasma marked by ^{131}I. On the basis of comparison between the activity of the blood and the activity of the tissue samples with no visible vessels, they calculated the capacity of the terminal vascular bed. In order to avoid any distortion of the results arising from different degrees of heart contraction, Rakusan and Rajhathy (33) stopped the hearts in diastole by injecting KCl. It was assumed that the vascular capacity in any part of the heart truly reflects the number of terminal vessels open at the time of death. Their results proved to be very close to those derived from independently measured capillary density on histological sections in a parallel series of experimental animals.

Cardiac Myocytes

Quantitative evaluation of cardiac myocytes includes the measurement of cell size (dimensions) and cell number. The knowledge of cell number and its changes is essential for evaluating the type of growth, which can be either hypertrophic or hyperplastic. This question was reviewed recently by Rakusan et al. (33). The size of the myocyte may be estimated by biochemical analysis of the myocardium or by quantitative morphologic methods. The latter may be applied either to isolated myocytes or to tissue sections. Similarly, estimates of the number of cardiac myocytes can be based on both of these approaches.

Methods for Estimating Cell Size

Biochemical analysis of the myocardium

For biochemical analysis of the myocardium, the size of the cardiac myocyte is estimated indirectly by measuring the DNA content of the tissue and relating the cardiac weight or amount of protein to the DNA. Indices such as protein/DNA or weight/DNA may serve as a measure of cell size. The tissue is easy to sample, no subjective judgment is involved, and standard biochemical analysis is applied. This method, however, does not take into account variations in DNA content per nucleus (varying degrees of polyploidy) or the variations in the number of nuclei per cell (the percentage of bi- and polynucleated myocytes); it also does not distinguish between the DNA of cardiac myocytes and the DNA of remaining "nonmuscle" cells.

Further improvements to the biochemical approach have been offered by Cheek (8), who suggested correcting the cardiac weight for its extracellular component, i.e., to use muscle weight minus the chloride space as a measure of cellular mass. Furthermore, he proposed measuring the DNA unit as a functional replacement of the size of the muscle cell. It was suggested that each nucleus within the myocyte has jurisdiction over a certain volume or mass of cytoplasm to form a DNA unit. On the basis of the DNA concentration in the tissue, one can measure the number of diploid nuclei per gram. If 1 g of muscle minus the extracellular fluid in that gram is divided by the number of nuclei, the size of the DNA unit is obtained. It should be stressed, however, that even in its improved form the biochemical approach yields only an estimate of the average size of the myocyte without any indication of its variability.

Measurements based on isolated myocytes

The isolation technique consists of perfusion of the coronary vascular tree with hyaluronidase and collagenase, and subsequent mechanical separation of adhering cells. In this case, cell width and length are measured either on spontaneously contracting cells observed under phase contrast microscopy or on fixed cells using normal microscopy. Cell width can be measured quite easily, whereas the subjective element of averaging the irregularities of the intercalated discs is involved when estimating cell length. The volume of the myocyte is then calculated using the above parameters and an assumed cylindrical configuration. This method is relatively fast and yields estimates of the variability of cell dimensions. It contains, however, a subjective error and a potential sampling error due to the varying yield of cells. The cell volume is calculated using the cylindrical model, which is certainly only a crude approximation of cell shape. This method has been used by several authors for evaluating cell size in the heart (6,16,17).

Histometric methods

The definitive histometric approach is to reconstruct the muscle cells from serial sections, which is feasible using a computer-assisted three-dimensional reconstruction system (25). This approach, however, is time-consuming and requires the knowledge of computer imaging techniques. For more common usage several alternative methods are available which can be subdivided as follows.

Measurements on cross sections. It is possible to measure the cell diameter either directly on the cross sections of the individual myocytes or to estimate its average value indirectly. Direct measurements can be done either using an eyepiece micrometer or by measuring the distances on micrographs. These methods presuppose cross sections perpendicular to the long axis of the cells. Even in this case, however, the cross sections of the myocytes are not circular but, rather, resemble ellipses. If one presumes the cylindrical configuration of the muscle cells, the ellipsoid shape of the cross section is the result of the distortion due to an angle of the section which is not precisely perpendicular to the long axis. The more this angle differs from 90°, the greater is the difference between the long and short axes of the ellipsoid on the cross section. The short axis, however, does not increase, and it corresponds to the diameter of the cylinder.

In the second approach, the departure from the ideal cylindrical configuration is assumed to be real and the average diameter is determined as the mean of the shortest diameter and one perpendicular to it, or as the mean of the shortest and longest diameters. The best solution of this approach is presented in Aherne's method (2) based on two theorems in geometrical probability. The computing formula is $A = L \times I$, where A is the mean cross-sectional area of the cell, L is the mean value of measurements made across the cell from the most lateral point on one side to the most lateral point on the other side, and I is the mean value of the measurements made at random across the cell profile (i.e., the mean chord). For details see Fig. 3.

This methodological approach calls for strictly perpendicular sections; it is relatively time-consuming and requires a large number of measurements in order to obtain representative sampling. Calculation of the cell volume assumes the cylindrical model and a constant width/length ratio or, alternatively, additional measurements of the cell length. On the other hand, it provides in addition to the average values an estimate of their variability.

The indirect estimation of the cell diameter on a cross section is based on the following approach: First, the total cross-sectional area of the muscle cells per unit area is measured and then divided by the number of cell profiles in this area. The result is equal to the mean cross-sectional area of a single myocyte. The area of the muscle profile may be measured planimetrically, or, more conveniently, by a stereological method of point counting.

An alternative approach is to measure stereologically both volume density and surface density and to derive an average cell diameter, as suggested by Arai and co-workers (4). In this case, one assumes that individual muscle fibers are so transformed as to make geometrical cylinders without changing the surface/volume ratio *(S/V)*; the diameter of a cylinder *(D)* is then determined as:

$$S/V = \pi D/\pi \ (D^2/4) = 4/D \text{ and } D = 4V/S \tag{6}$$

This method shares some of the pitfalls of the previous one (the need of exactly perpendicular sections, length measurements, and assumption of the cylindrical model). It is, however, much faster and less subjective than measuring individual diameters. On the other hand, only average values of the cell diameters are obtained.

Measurements on longitudinal sections. The diameter of a muscle cell can be measured accurately on a longitudinal section only in a situation in which the

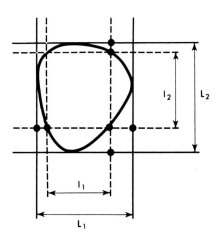

FIG. 3. Estimation of the cross-sectional area from two measurements: connection of the most lateral profiles *(L)* and connection of the intersections of a random point *(I)*. The same measurement is repeated at least once in different orientations (L_1, L_2, $I_{,1}$, I_2).

equatorial plane is located within the slice because measurements on the remaining sections would yield falsely low values. It is possible to detect the presence of the equatorial plane by focusing. If the image of a muscle cell becomes larger and smaller again when focusing up and down, its equatorial plane is located in the slice and may be measured. If by focusing in any one direction (up or down) the image keeps growing until the muscle cell disappears from the focus, its equatorial plane lies outside the slice and it is not measured. Alternatively, the cell width can be measured only at the level of the visible nucleus.

Another possible approach, although more complicated, is less subjective and less tiresome because it eliminates the need of focusing or searching for nuclei. In this case, the width of all cells is measured and the result is subsequently corrected for underestimation caused by the presence of cells which were cut outside their longitudinal axis. It is possible to calculate the degree of underestimation, which depends mainly on the ratio between the cell diameter and the thickness of the section (35).

Measurement of the diameter on longitudinal sections with subsequent corrections is faster than direct measurements on a cross section. The disadvantage is, once again, its dependence on the cylindrical model and the need of access to a computer.

Measurements based on tissue nuclear profiles. Counts of the number of myocyte nuclear profiles in several histological sections of increasing thickness can be used to derive the number of muscle cell nuclei per unit of tissue volume. Knowing the myocyte fraction of the tissue volume, independently measured by the point-counting technique, it is possible to calculate the average myocyte volume per nucleus, which corresponds to the DNA unit as described above. The average volume of the myocyte is then estimated taking into account the percentage of bi- and polynucleated cells (24).

This is a relatively fast method which therefore enables representative sampling. The subjective component is its need for distinction between muscle and "nonmuscle" cell nuclei and the ability to estimate the fraction of binucleated cells. Only average values of the volume are obtained.

Methods for Estimating Cell Number

It is relatively easy to make some indirect conclusions concerning the increase in the cell number or its absence, i.e., cell hyperplasia or hypertrophy. In most cases, judgments about the nature of cardiac growth have an indirect basis. For instance, a decrease in the density of muscle nuclei in the tissue which is proportional to an increase in cardiac weight is taken as a sign of cardiac hypertrophy (7a), whereas a higher than expected nuclear density is interpreted as a sign of cardiac hyperplasia (22). Another example of indirect conclusions could be quoted from our own old observation (31). Chronic sideropenic anemia, induced subsequent to the weaning period in rats, caused a sizable increase in cardiac weight (more than double the control values). On the other hand, the density of myocytes and capillaries remained unchanged. Therefore we concluded that the mode of growth in this particular experimental situation was hyperplasia.

The final decision about the type of growth (hypertrophic versus hyperplastic) should be made on the basis of changes in the number of cardiac myocytes per organ. It is rather difficult to find a satisfactory method for this estimation. All the pitfalls and errors involved in measuring the cell size are magnified when the cell number is estimated. Basically we can divide these methods into morphological and biochemical approaches. Both are time-consuming and have several inherent deficiencies as described below. Therefore it is not surprising that the estimates of the total population of cardiac myocytes vary by a large margin. For instance, in the case of the rat left ventricle the reported spread is 8 million to 90 million cells (7,10). Nevertheless, careful application of these methods by the same investigator may lead to comparable estimates. An example of cardiac hyperplasia, confirmed by both morphological and biochemical approaches with similar cell counts, was reported by Rakusan et al. (33).

Biochemical estimates

The biochemical approach is based on the assumption that because the amount of DNA is constant within a single diploid nucleus, it is possible to estimate the number of cells in a given organ by measuring its total DNA content and dividing the result by the amount of DNA per cell (14). This approach was subsequently refined by application of corrections for various degrees of ploidy, for various numbers of nuclei per cell, and for various proportions of muscle and nonmuscle nuclei. In this case the problem of sampling encountered with morphological methods is minimized and reliable estimates of the total DNA content may be obtained. The amount of DNA per diploid nucleus (genome) is probably constant even though its estimates vary from 6 to 7×10^{-12} g (14,29). Potential sources of error are the remaining parameters used for calculating the number of myocytes, i.e., the amount of DNA per nucleus (the degree of polyploidy), the number of nuclei per cell (the percentage of bi- and polynucleated cells), and the proportion of muscle and nonmuscle nuclei in the total population and therefore their relative contribution to the total DNA content. The last correction is probably the least reliable of these parameters. It contains all the problems of sampling inherent in the morphological methods. In addition, the distinction between the two kinds of nuclei is sometimes difficult and is unfortunately always based on subjective judgment.

Morphological estimates

Morphological estimates of the total number of cardiac myocytes are based either on counting the number of muscle nuclei in a known volume of tissue with subsequent corrections for the thickness of sections (24) or on determining the size of cardiac myocytes. The latter approach can use the cell dimensions derived from the measurements of either isolated myocytes or of myocytes in histological sections. In this case the cellular fraction of the tissue volume is first measured by a point-counting method and then divided by the average cell volume. The approach based on nuclear counting is limited by subjectivity when evaluating muscle cell nuclei and by potential changes in the number of nuclei per muscle cell. The second approach includes all the errors and fallacies involved in the estimation of cell size. All morphological estimates share a problem of representative sampling. Morphometric methods are usually time-consuming, and often insufficient numbers of measurements are collected.

Investigation of the mitotic rate and the rate of DNA synthesis by autoradiography brings additional important information concerning the type of growth and development. On the other hand, it does not quantify the growth product in a strict sense, and therefore these techniques are not discussed here in detail.

CELL LEVEL MICROSTRUCTURE AS EVALUATED BY ELECTRON MICROSCOPY

The general strategy, sampling procedure, and examples of calculations of stereological parameters in mammalian cardiac myocytes were described recently by Page (28). Cardiac myocytes are delimited by a plasma membrane, the sarcolemma. An external sarcolemma and an internal sarcolemma (T-system, intercalated discs) enclose the major subcellular components: myofibrils, mitochondria, nuclei, sarcoplasmic reticulum, and sarcoplasm. These cellular subcompartments are quantitatively described by their volume densities, as determined by the point-counting method. Surface densities of sarcolemmal, mitochondrial, and sarcoplasmic reticulum membranes can be then obtained using the method based on intersection counts. Volume density and surface density may be related either to the tissue or cell volume.

The volume fraction of a cellular compartment can be easily obtained by counting the number of "hits," i.e., the number of points (P) of the grid lying inside the compartment (c) in relation to the total number of points.

$$P \text{ hits}/P \text{ total} = \text{area } c/\text{area total} = \text{volume } c/\text{volume total} \qquad (7)$$

The surface density of randomly distributed objects (S_v) may be derived from the number of intersections within a test line (N_i) and the total length of the test line (L_T) as:

$$S_v = 2 N_i/L_T \qquad (8)$$

Most of the subcellular components, however, have a definite orientation; that is, they are anisotropic, and therefore a special stereological approach should be applied.

Sarcoplasmic Reticulum

The theoretical grounds for stereological analysis of the volume and surface of the sarcoplasmic reticulum in muscle cells were described by Weibel (43). The tubules of sarcoplasmic reticulum are highly oriented in the longitudinal direction of the muscle cells; they are lined up in parallel and are periodically arranged in relation to sarcomeres. This particular arrangement makes sampling and stereological measurements difficult. Sampling is relatively easy in longitudinal sections, but measurement is difficult as the section thickness usually exceeds the diameter of the sarcoplasmic reticulum tubules. On the other hand, measurements are relatively easy on cross sections, but the sampling of these periodically arranged structures is difficult. Weibel proposed the use of oblique sections with an orientation which is close to perpendicular to the long axis of cells. The angle of sectioning should be between 70° and 90°. In such situations the underestimation of measured surface density is probably within the error of the method (i.e., <1.5%). The volume density is independent of the angle of sectioning.

Mitochondria

A detailed description and derivation of the methods for measuring mitochondrial subcompartments and areas of mitochondrial membranes in cardiac myocytes can be found in an article by Smith and Page (40). These authors measured the size distribution of mitochondrial cross sections using the particle size analyzer. For measurements of mitochondrial membranes and subcompartments they used very thin sections of mitochondrial profiles prepared from longitudinal sections. Part of these profiles, in which the traces of cristae were sharply delineated, were used for stereological measurements after manual enhancement with colored red pencils. In this fashion they were able to distinguish the area of the cristae inner membrane as well as to approximate the fractions of mitochondrial volume contributed by the matrix, the cristae plus inner membrane, and the intercristal space.

Nucleus

Measuring the relative nuclear volume and a relative surface of the nuclear membrane by standard stereological methods does not pose any particular problems. There is some controversy concerning the number of nuclei per cardiac myocyte. A method of choice is the cell isolation technique, as described above, from which the number of nuclei per cell can be readily obtained. An alternative approach is to measure the number of nuclei per cardiac myocyte on histological material using either exact longitudinal sections (5) or serial cross sections (18). In addition, the DNA content of cardiac muscle nuclei may be determined by cytophotometry (1, 30). In this case, Feulgen-stained smears of isolated muscle cell nuclei are examined by cytophotometer and compared with a standard (e.g., spermatozoa as a control for haploid content or nuclei from fibrocytes for diploid values).

CONCLUSION

We have attempted to present a systematic overview of the methods available for quantitative assessment of cardiac growth at three levels of organization: organ, tissue, and cell. As may be seen from this review, each has some strong and weak components, and the method of choice depends on the experimental protocol and the objectives of the study.

We stressed the importance of data collection, as any conclusion, hypothesis, or model can be only as good as the entry data. Even properly collected data could be misinterpreted if not placed in the right perspective. Misrepresented measurements can lead to false conclusions. Examples of this are relatively common in the literature. For instance, a significant increase in the relative heart weight of experimental animals may be produced by fasting because the relative heart weight decreases with increasing body weight and vice versa. This can hardly be described as cardiac hypertrophy when compared to normal growing controls. Another example is the conclusion that hyperplasia of cardiac myocytes occurred in experimental cardiomegaly when it was based only on increased DNA content of the heart. (In one such case it subsequently turned out that an increase in DNA content was due entirely to an increase in the number of "nonmuscle" nuclei and that the number of muscle cells remained unchanged).

We conclude that quantitative assessment of normal and stimulated cardiac growth with adequate precision is feasible if representative samples are obtained and properly measured and the results verified, preferably by two or more analytical approaches.

REFERENCES

1. Adler, C. P., and Sandritter, W. (1980): Alterations of substances (DNA, myoglobin, myosin, protein) in experimentally induced cardiac hypertrophy and under the influence of drugs (isoproterenol, cytostatics, strophantin). *Basic Res. Cardiol.*, 75:126–138.
2. Aherne, W. (1968): A method of determining the cross sectional area of muscle fibers. *J. Neurol. Sci.*, 7:519–528.
3. Anversa, P., Loud, A. V., Giacomelli, F., and Wiener, J. (1978): Absolute morphometric study of myocardial hypertrophy in experimental hypertension. II. Ultrastructure of myocytes and interstitium. *Lab. Invest.*, 38:597–608.
4. Arai, S., Machida, A., and Nakamura, T. (1968): Myocardial structure and vascularization of hypertrophied hearts. *Tohoku J. Exp. Med.*, 95:35–54.
5. Baroldi, G., Falzi, G., and Lampertico, P. (1967): The nuclear patterns of the cardiac muscle fiber. *Cardiologia*, 51:109–123.
6. Bishop, S. P., Oparil, S., Reynolds, R. H., and Drummond, J. L. (1979): Regional myocyte size in normotensive and spontaneously hypertensive rats. *Hypertension*, 1:378–383.
7. Black-Schaffer, B., Grinstead, C. E., and Braunstein, J. N. (1965): Endocardial fibroelastosis of large mammals. *Circ. Res.*, 16:383–390.
7a. Black-Schaffer, B., and Turner, M. E. (1958): Hyperplastic infantile cardiomegaly. *Am. J. Pathol.*, 34:745–765.
8. Cheek, D. B. (1975): *Fetal and Postnatal Cellular Growth.* Wiley, New York.
9. Cluzeaud, F., Laplace, M., Rakusan, K., and Hatt, P.-Y. (1981): Hypertrophie cardiaque secondaire a une anémie par carence en fer. *Pathol. Biol.*, 29:11–18.
10. Costabel, U., and Adler, C. P. (1980): Myocardial DNA and cell number: the influence of cytostatics. II. Experimental investigations in hearts of rats. *Virchows Arch. [Cell. Pathol.]*, 32:127–138.
11. Cruz-Orive, L. M., and Weibel, E. R. (1981): Sampling designs for stereology. *J. Microsc.*, 122:235–257.
12. Davey, D. F., and Wong, S. Y. P. (1980): Morphometric analysis of rat extensor digitorum longus and soleus muscles. *Aust. J. Exp. Biol. Med. Sci.*, 58:213–230.

13. Eckner, F. A. O., Brown, B. W., Overll, E., and Glagov, S. (1969): Alteration of the gross dimensions of the heart and its structures by formalin fixation. *Virchows Arch. [Pathol. Anat.]*, 346:318–329.
14. Enesco, M., and Leblond, C. P. (1962): Increase in cell number as a factor in the growth of the organs and tissues of the young male rat. *J. Embryol. Exp. Morphol.*, 10:530–562.
15. Janicki, J. S., Weber, K. T., Gochman, R. F., Shroff, S., and Geheb, F. J. (1981): Three dimensional myocardial and ventricular shape: a surface representation. *Am. J. Physiol.*, 241:H1–H11.
16. Katzberg, A. A., Farmer, B. B., and Harris, R. (1977): The predominance of binucleation in isolated rat heart myocytes. *Am. J. Anat.*, 149:489–500.
17. Korecky, B., and Rakusan, K. (1978): Normal and hypertrophic growth of the rat heart: changes in cell dimensions and number. *Am. J. Physiol.*, 234:H123–H128.
18. Korecky, B., Sweet, S., and Rakusan, K. (1979): Number of nuclei in mammalian cardiac myocytes. *Can. J. Physiol. Pharmacol.*, 57:1122–1129.
19. Krogh, A. (1927): *The Anatomy and Physiology of Capillaries.* Yale University Press, New Haven, Conn.
20. Kyrieleis, C. (1963): Die Formveränderungen des Menschlichen Herzens nach der Geburt. *Virchows Arch. [Pathol. Anat.]*, 337:142–163.
21. Lev, M., Rowlatt, U. F., and Rimoldi, H. J. A. (1961): Pathologic methods for the study of congenitally malformed hearts. *Arch. Pathol.*, 72:491–511.
22. Linzbach, A. J. (1947): Mikrometrische und histologische Analyse hypertropher menschlicher Herzen. *Virchows Arch. [Pathol. Anat.]*, 314:534–594.
23. Loats, J. T., Sillau, A. H., and Banchero, N. (1978): How to quantify skeletal muscle capillarity. In: *Oxygen Transport to Tissue,* edited by I. S. Silver, M. Erecinska, and H. I. Bicher, Vol. 3, pp. 41–48. Plenum Press, New York.
24. Loud, A. V., Anversa, P., Giacomelli, F., and Wiener, J. (1978): Absolute morphometric study of myocardial hypertrophy in experimental hypertension. I. Determination of myocyte size. *Lab. Invest.*, 38:586–596.
25. Marino, T. A., Cook, P. N., Cook, L. T., and Dwyer, S. J., III (1980): The use of computer imaging techniques to visualize cardiac muscle cells in three dimensions. *Anat. Rec.*, 198:537–546.
26. Martini, J., and Honig, C. R. (1969): Direct measurement of intercapillary distance in beating rat heart in situ under various conditions of O_2 supply. *Microvasc. Res.*, 1:244–256.
27. Myers, W. W., and Honig, C. R. (1964): Number and distribution of capillaries as determinants of myocardial oxygen tension. *Am. J. Physiol.*, 207:653–660.
28. Page, E. (1979): Model cases from biological morphometry: mammalian ventricular myocardial cells. In: *Stereological Methods,* edited by E. R. Weibel, Vol. 1, pp. 284–288. Academic Press, London.
29. Petersen, R. P., and Baserga, R. (1965): Nucleic acid and protein synthesis in cardiac muscle of growing and adult mice. *Exp. Cell. Res.*, 40:340–352.
30. Pfitzer, P. (1971): Nuclear DNA content of human myocardial cells. *Curr. Top. Pathol.*, 54:125–168.
31. Poupa, O., Korecky, B., Krofta, K., Rakusan, K., and Prochazka, J. (1964): The effect of anaemia during the early postnatal period on vascularization of the myocardium and its resistance to hypoxia. *Physiol. Bohemoslov.*, 13:281–287.
32. Rakusan, K. (1971): Quantitative morphology of capillaries of the heart (number of capillaries in animal and human hearts under normal and pathological conditions). *Methods Achiev. Exp. Pathol.*, 5:272–286.
33. Rakusan, K., and Rajhathy, J. (1972): Distribution of cardiac output and organ blood content in anemic and polycythemic rats. *Can. J. Physiol. Pharmacol.*, 50:703–710.
33a. Rakusan, K., Korecky, B., and Mezl, V. (1983): Cardiac hypertrophy and/or hyperplasia? In: *Myocardial Hypertrophy and Failure,* edited by N. R. Alpert, pp. 103–110. Raven Press, New York.
34. Rakusan, K., Moravec, J., and Hatt, P. Y. (1980): Regional capillary supply in the normal and hypertrophied rat heart. *Microvasc. Res.*, 20:319–326.
35. Rakusan, K., Raman, S., Layberry, R., and Korecky, B. (1978): The influence of aging and growth on the postnatal development of cardiac muscle in rats. *Circ. Res.*, 42:212–218.
36. Rankin, J. S., McHale, P. A., Arentzen, C. E., Ling, D., Greenfield, J. C., Jr., and Anderson,

R. W. (1976): The three-dimensional dynamic geometry of the left ventricle in the conscious dog. *Circ. Res.*, 39:304–313.

37. Renkin, E. M., Gray, S. D., Dodd, L. R., and Lia, B. D. (1981): Heterogeneity of capillary distribution and capillary circulation in mammalian skeletal muscles. In: *Underwater Physiology. VII. Proceedings of the Seventh Symposium on Underwater Physiology*, edited by A. J. Bachrach and M. M. Matzen. Undersea Med. Soc., Bethesda.

38. Roberts, J. T., and Wearn, J. T. (1941): Quantitative changes in the capillary-muscle relationship in human hearts during normal growth and hypertrophy. *Am. Heart J.*, 21:617–633.

39. Shreiner, T. P., Weisfeldt, M. L., and Shock, N. W. (1969): Effects of age, sex and breeding status on the rat heart. *Am. J. Physiol.*, 217:176–180.

40. Smith, H. E., and Page, E. (1976): Morphometry of rat heart mitochondrial subcompartment and membranes: application to myocardial cell atrophy after hypophysectomy. *J. Ultrastruct. Res.*, 55:31–41.

41. Thews, G. (1960): Die Sauerstoffdiffusion im Gehirn. *Pfluegers Arch.*, 271:197–214.

42. Turek, Z., and Rakusan, K. (1981): Lognormal distribution of intercapillary distance in normal and hypertrophic rat heart as estimated by the method of concentric circles: its effect on tissue oxygenation. *Pfluegers Arch.*, 391:17–21.

43. Weibel, E. R. (1972): A stereological method for estimating volume and surface of sarcoplasmic reticulum. *J. Microsc.*, 95:229–243.

44. Weibel, E. R. (1979): *Stereological Methods, Vol. 1: Practical Methods for Biological Morphometry.* Academic Press, London.

45. Wiener, J., Giacomelli, F., Loud, A. V., and Anversa, P. (1979): Morphometry of cardiac hypertrophy induced by experimental renal hypertension. *Am. J. Cardiol.*, 44:919–929.

46. Yin, F. C. P., Spurgeon, H. A., Rakusan, K., Weisfeldt, M. L., and Lakatta, E. G. (1983): Use of tibial length to quantify cardiac hypertrophy: application in the aging rat. *Am. J. Physiol.*, 243:H941–H947.

47. Zeek, P. M. (1942): Heart weight. I. The weight of the normal human heart. *Arch. Pathol.*, 34:820–832.

Growth of the Heart in Health and Disease,
edited by Radovan Zak. Raven Press,
New York © 1984.

The Growing Heart:
An Anatomical Perspective

Jose M. Icardo

Department of Anatomy, Faculty of Medicine, Poligono de Cazona, s/n, Santander, Spain

Understanding the form and function of the mature heart requires a basic knowledge of the main aspects of cardiac developmental anatomy. This knowledge also serves to provide a structural framework on which to place our increasing understanding of the biochemical and molecular aspects of heart development and growth. Embryonic heart development has been a major focus of scientific interest, and much information has accumulated on the subject. Historically, much of this work has been done using the embryonic chick because it is easily available and can be studied thoroughly without the inconvenient developmental gaps present in many of the human embryo collections. Close developmental similarities between avian and mammalian hearts constitute another important advantage to the use of the chick. Although the developmental steps of cardiogenesis are not identical in chick and man, most of the processes described for the embryonic chicken can be extended to the human embryo, and it is likely that many developmental mechanisms are similar if not identical.

This chapter is an overview of the basic aspects of embryonic heart development presented in an anatomical context. It is based mainly on the chick heart; and, where necessary, developmental differences between avian and mammalian hearts are stressed. Furthermore, some examples from human embryos have been included in this study. At the end of the chapter, Tables 1 and 2 present the chronological relationship of the main events of cardiac morphogenesis in different species.

There are many conflicting points of view regarding some aspects of heart development. These conflicts arouse a great deal of controversy. I have tried to avoid most of the discussion of these conflicts, restricting myself largely to a descriptive approach. Although they may not be accepted fully and are certain to arouse further controversy (and hopefully investigation), the points of view I provide represent some of the current ways of viewing cardiac embryology.

BILATERAL ORIGIN OF THE HEART PRIMORDIA:
FUSION OF THE HEART ANLAGE

All vertebrate hearts are derived from cells arising from both sides of the bilateral embryo. Hence vertebrate hearts have both right- and left-side-derived components.

The bilateral heart primordium makes its appearance very early in development. The presence of future heart-forming cells can be recognized by prospective mapping techniques even prior to the appearance of the first pair of somites (103, 107,117). There are several techniques that have been devised to discern the embryonic origin of cells that give rise to specific structures. Such techniques result in fate maps, or maps of embryonic fields in which the future fate of cells is discerned. One of these techniques consists of transplanting small pieces of early blastoderm into the chorioallantoic membrane of older embryos (103,135). Subsequent differentiation of the grafts permits us to establish the organ-forming capacity of the transplanted cells. Another technique consists of labeling the early blastoderm with (^{3}H)thymidine (90,107). Thymidine-labeled grafts from donor embryos are then transplanted into homologous sites of homologous recipient embryos. Subsequent autoradiographic study of the host embryos allows determination of the movements undergone by the labeled areas as well as their final location in a particular organ. The use of these techniques permits identification of prospective organ-forming regions well before any morphological indication of such an organ is present.

The first visible indication of the heart anlage in most vertebrates is seen at about the three- to four-somite stage as bilateral thickenings of the splanchnic mesoderm (Fig. 1). The cells of this distinct region of the mesoderm eventually form the muscular wall of the heart. Somewhat later, the primitive endocardial cells appear between the endoderm and the thickened splanchnic mesoderm (105). The precardiac areas, situated on each side of the embryonic midline, therefore, contain mesodermal cells, pre-endocardial cells, and associated extracellular material. The subsequent development of the heart primordia is closely related to the formation of the foregut.

Cardiogenesis is linked inextricably to foregut formation. During the formation of the endodermal foregut the cardiac primordia are carried progressively toward the embryonic midline (Fig. 1). The shift in position of the heart anlage is not only the result of endodermal deformation but also appears to involve active movement of the precardiac cells relative to the endoderm (19). This relationship is suggested experimentally by the failure of normal cardiogenesis if the foregut is cut or damaged (18). Finally, the paired heart primordia contact each other ventral to the developing foregut and fuse following a rostrocaudal sequence. As a result, an unpaired tubular structure is formed at the embryonic midline.

Fusion of the heart anlage is first completed on the ventral side of the primitive tube. The right and left mesodermal layers become contiguous dorsal to the developing endocardium, but they do not fuse until later in development. They persist as a double-layered structure, termed the dorsal mesocardium. The dorsal mesocardium attaches the developing heart to the embryonic trunk during subsequent stages. A similar structure connecting the ventral aspect of the developing heart with the splanchnopleura was also formed as a result of fusion along the ventral surface. However, the ventral mesocardium is a much more transient structure than the dorsal mesocardium and is present for only a short period of time.

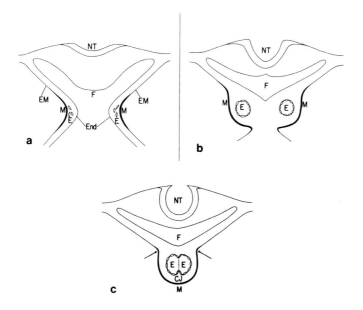

FIG. 1. Fusion process of the cardiac primordia. The prospective myocardium *(M)* arises as bilateral thickenings of the splanchnic mesoderm *(EM)*. The first endocardial cells *(E)* appear between the endoderm *(End)* and the prospective myocardium. In **b** and **c**, *E* represents the endocardial tubes. Note in **b** that the myocardium is bending toward the embryonic midline, enwrapping the endocardium. Note in **c** that dorsal to the developing endocardium the right and left mesodermal layers are not fused yet; *arrows* indicate the dorsal mesocardium. *(CJ)* cardiac jelly. *(F)* foregut. *(NT)* neural tube.

The paired origin of the heart needs to be emphasized. The fusion process of the heart primordia can be prevented by different methods, e.g., application of pressure in the embryonic midline (32), surgical intervention cutting through mid-tissues of the anterior intestinal portal (18), or interposition of a piece of tissue between the two heart anlages (106). When one of these maneuvers is made, two independent beating hearts, located on each side of the embryonic midline, are formed. These hearts differentiate synchronously (58), indicating that a midline position is not a requisite for normal differentiation.

FORMATION OF THE CARDIAC LOOP

After the initial fusion of the paired anlage, the early heart is located in the inside of the primitive pericardial cavity and presents an approximately straight tubular form. Its anterior limit is formed by the ventral aorta. Its posterior limit is formed by the two omphalomesenteric (vitelline) veins. The dorsal aspect of the heart tube is linked to the embryonic trunk by the dorsal mesocardium. This relatively straight heart next undergoes a process of bending and rotation to form a structure known as the cardiac loop (Fig. 2).

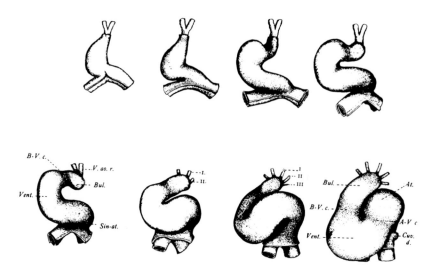

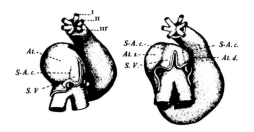

FIG. 2. Ventral views of the chick heart showing formation of the cardiac loop and the progress of regional differentiation. *(At.)* atrium. *(A-V.c.)* atrioventricular constriction. *(Bul.)* bulbus cordis. *(B-V.c.)* bulboventricular constriction. *(Cuv.d.)* ductus of Cuvier. *(Sin-at.)* sinoatrial region. *(V.ao.r.)* ventral aortic roots. *(Vent.)* ventricle. *(I,II,III)* aortic arches. (From Patten, ref. 94.)

FIG. 3. Dorsal views of the chick heart showing the formation of the sinus venosus. *(At.)* atrium. *(At.d.)* right atrium. *(At.s.)* left atrium. *(S-A.c.)* sinoatrial constriction. *(S.V.)* sinus venosus. *(I,II,III)* aortic arches. (From Patten, ref. 94.)

The ventral aspect of the heart bulges outward and rotates to the right side of the embryo (8). As a result, the straight heart acquires a C-shaped form, the ventral aspect of the primitive tube becoming the convex right side of the cardiac loop. The bending of the heart continues progressively, and the C-shape form becomes more apparent. As the bend progresses, the dorsal mesocardium breaks in the mid-region of the heart and is rapidly obliterated, freeing most of the heart from the embryonic body. The heart then twists on itself and adopts a sigmoid, S-shaped form (Fig. 2).

The various parts of the heart—sinus venosus, atrium, ventricle, and bulbus cordis (55,120)—become clearly differentiated, and regional division can be discerned during the later stages of cardiac loop formation. The sinus venosus is situated at the caudal end of the heart (Fig. 3). Separated from the atrium by the sinoatrial sulcus, the sinus venosus receives blood from all the parts of the embryo.

At the final stages of development of the cardiac loop, the atrium occupies a cranial position relative to the ventricle. This primitive atrium rapidly expands into two lateral lobes, the future right and left atria. The ventricle adopts a saccular aspect and is located in a medial and inferior position between the atrium and the bulbus cordis. This primitive ventricle represents the future trabeculated portion of the right and left definitive ventricles. The ventricular portion of the cardiac loop is separated from the atrium by a narrow and distinct region, the atrioventricular canal. A sulcus, the bulboventricular sulcus, separates the ventricle from the bulbus cordis. The bulbus cordis is the most cranial portion of the cardiac loop and represents the truncoconal portion of the heart. Its distal part, the truncus, is the future site of origin of the aorta and pulmonary artery. Its proximal part, the conus, is the prospective infundibular region. Later in development the conus forms part of the definitive ventricles.

The looping process of the heart tube is the first indication of gross morphological asymmetry observed in the developing embryo. In part because of this it has received a large amount of attention by both early and contemporary embryologists. However, the exact causes and the mechanisms involved in this deformative process remain unclear. The importance of the cardiac extracellular matrix in the formation of the cardiac loop is emphasized elsewhere in this volume.

Structure of the Heart Tube

During cardiac loop formation the heart tube is a histologically simple structure. Basically, the heart consists of an outer layer, or myocardium, and an inner layer, or endocardium. Myocardium and endocardium are separated by a sleeve of ground substance termed cardiac jelly (see Fig. 5 below) (17).

The myocardium is composed of a homogenous population (67) of developing cardiac myocytes (the successors of the cells of the precardiac splanchnic mesoderm). The most characteristic feature of these cells is the accumulation of myofibrils in the cytoplasm, i.e., the acquisition of a differentiated phenotype. Only later in development does the myocardial wall acquire other cell types, e.g., epithelial cells, fibroblasts, and smooth muscle cells.

In addition to their muscle phenotype, the embryonic myocytes have seemingly unusual characteristics. They are involved in the secretion of components of cardiac jelly and show a well-developed Golgi apparatus and large amounts of granular endoplasmic reticulum (67). Despite the accumulation of myofibrils, differentiated cardiac muscle continues to replicate DNA, as demonstrated with (^{3}H)thymidine-incorporation studies (51,133). Although it is not clear if all the cells incorporating thymidine are able to enter into mitosis, it is certain that some of them do. It had been long thought that differentiated cardiac myocytes cannot divide. However, cardiac myocytes containing myofibrils undergo mitosis not only during the stages considered here (68,109) but even during fetal and early postnatal periods (31). Another characteristic of these cells is their phagocytic capacity. Cardiac myocytes are able to phagocytose cellular debris (28,47), acting as "amateur" phagocytes.

The heart lumen is lined by endocardial cells. During cardiac loop formation, these cells present an orderly arrangement and are aligned perpendicular to the heart lumen (49). The alignment of the endocardial cells appears to be the result of motile activity of these cells.

The cardiac jelly, the ground substance interposed between myocardium and endocardium, is a heterogeneous extracellular matrix composed largely of glycosaminoglycans and glycoproteins (73,74,77). The composition and the ultrastructural arrangement of the components of cardiac jelly vary widely during the stages of cardiac loop formation (43,45,48,84). These changes are closely related to the formation of the cardiac loop (see Manasek, this volume).

Acquisition of Basic Heart Functions

Most of the basic heart functions begin during loop formation. The contractile activity of the heart starts in the chick embryo at about the 10-somite stage (97,116). As soon as the first myofibrils appear in the cytoplasm of the developing myocytes (9,63,67), the first heart contractions can be observed. The first contractions are irregular and spasmodic, restricted to the most caudal part of the heart, along the right margin of the primitive ventricle. Long quiescent periods of up to 2 to 3 min (97) are interposed between these initial contractions. Soon a rapid, rhythmic beating develops, and the entire heart becomes involved in contraction. The first contractions are ventricular in origin, and the heart rate increases to 80 to 90 beats/min with the contraction progressing from the caudal to the cranial end in a peristaltic form. When the atrium and sinus venosus develop at the end of the cardiac tube, they beat at a higher rate and take over control, causing an increase in heart rate. By the end of the sixth day of incubation, well after cardiac loop formation, the heart rate has increased up to 220 beats/min (105). Later in development the heart rate decreases somewhat, probably reflecting the influence of vagal regulation.

The functional autonomy of myocardial tissue is evident. The beginning of the heartbeat prior to innervation and the fact that the embryonic myocytes beat spontaneously when maintained as isolated cells in culture (7,60) proves that the contractile capacity of the heart is a property inherent to the cells of the embryonic myocardium. It has been demonstrated clearly that there is not a single pacemaker in the embryonic heart (2,91). Rather, the center of pacemaker activity is displaced in a caudal direction as new heart regions, with a higher rate of contraction, develop at the caudal end of the primitive cardiac tube. The adult pacemaker, the sinoatrial node, is derived from the sinus venosus, the last of the embryonic heart regions that takes control of the pacemaker function (20).

The embryonic circulation begins when the heartbeat is strong enough to move blood throughout the embryo. The blood enters the sinus venosus and is pumped through the single lumen toward the bulbus cordis. This flow, from the venous end to the arterial end, is a relationship that persists unchanged throughout life.

The circulation of the blood is well established before the heart has anatomically defined valves. From the time the circulation begins until the time distinct valvular apparatuses are formed, a valve effect, largely preventing regurgitation, is achieved by the systolic apposition of cardiac jelly. In the atrioventricular canal and bulbus cordis, specialized areas of the cardiac jelly become apposed in an alternative and rhythmic manner which prevents regurgitation of blood (98). The valve effect of the cardiac jelly is imperfect, however. Some regurgitation occurs, as demonstrated by the presence of ventricular diastolic pressure (92).

Arterial blood pressure cannot be recorded until the circulation of the blood is well established. Nonpulsatile at first, the blood pressure becomes rapidly pulsatile and rises, during the stages of cardiac loop formation, from 0.4 mm Hg to 1.0 mm Hg (125). By the time of hatching, the arterial systolic pressure has increased to 30.0 mm Hg (29).

Myocardial Trabeculation

At the final stages of loop formation the myocardium is a compact epithelial tissue layer formed exclusively of myocytes. In the ventricular region wide intercellular spaces appear between the myocardial cells, and the myocardium separates into two distinct zones: a compact outer layer and an inner spongy layer (56).

Coincident with these myocardial wall changes, the endocardium evaginates at discrete points, forming outpocketings directed toward the myocardium (Fig. 4). When the endocardial outpocketings contact the myocardial basal surface, the myocardial cells separate to form little gaps. The endocardium penetrates the myocardial wall through these gaps and expands laterally into the previously formed

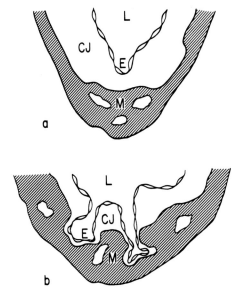

FIG. 4. Initial stages of the process of myocardial trabeculation. The endocardium *(E)* forms outpocketings that penetrate the myocardial wall *(M)* and expand into the wide intercellular spaces of the myocardium. Note the progressive decrease in thickness of the cardiac jelly *(CJ)*. *(L)* heart lumen.

intercellular spaces. A primitive trabecular pattern is thus formed. The endocardial cells that penetrate the gaps are the first nonmuscle cells observed in the myocardial wall. The continuity of the endocardial cells within the myocardium with the rest of the endocardium is patent. These endocardial outpocketings may serve as a source for myocardial nutrition when the diffusion of nutrients through the cardiac jelly does not fill the metabolic needs of the myocardial cells (75).

Later in development the myocardial trabeculae form a continually more complicated pattern. Most of these primitive trabeculae eventually disappear, but some coalesce to form the papillary muscle, or trabecula carneae, observed in the adult heart. Coalescence of the primitive trabeculae also appears to be the mechanism by which the primordium of the interventricular septum is formed. The continued formation of trabeculae has an important advantage. It prevents the ventricular wall from becoming too thick and solid and consequently unable to perform its contractile functions efficiently.

Fate of the Cardiac Jelly

The thickness of cardiac jelly in the ventricular region decreases greatly during trabeculation (Figs. 5–7). Some extracellular material remains between the endocardium and myocardium in the trabeculae located closest to the lumen, but even

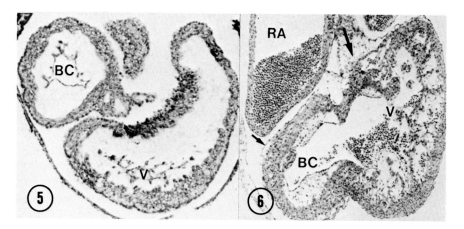

FIG. 5. Cross section of the human embryo heart at the level of the cardiac loop. Note the wide acellular space interposed between the myocardium and endocardium. *(BC)* bulbus cordis. *(V)* ventricle. (From the Kyoto Collection, 1845-H12, slide 5, section 7.)

FIG. 6. The distribution of the cardiac jelly (human embryo) has changed considerably when compared with Fig. 5. In the bulbus cordis *(BC)* the layer of cardiac jelly remains thick and has been invaded by mesenchymal cells. In the ventricular region *(V)* the thickness of cardiac jelly has decreased concomitant with the formation of myocardial trabeculae. No cardiac jelly is detectable in the right atrium *(RA)*. *Arrows* indicate the epicardium. (From the Kyoto Collection, 1127-H14, slide 6, section 3).

this disappears[1] when trabeculation is completed. The width of the cardiac jelly is also reduced in the atrial region (Figs. 6 and 7). The myocardium and endocardium are brought together progressively, and the cardiac jelly disappears from this region. This process is more apparent and rapid in the right side of the atrium; the left side retains a thin but persistent layer of cardiac jelly for a longer period of time. In other zones of the heart, however, the layer of cardiac jelly remains thick. The atrioventricular canal and bulbus cordis retain a large amount of cardiac jelly (Figs. 6 and 7).

The causes of the progressive reduction in thickness of the cardiac jelly are not known. One possible explanation is that the components of the cardiac jelly are being enzymatically digested. An increase in hyaluronidase activity has been demonstrated in the ventricular region at the stages in which trabeculation proceeds and the width of the cardiac jelly is reduced (83,89). Another possible explanation deals with the presence of hemodynamic forces. Because of the bending of the cardiac tube the blood entering the heart is separated into two streams (6) which

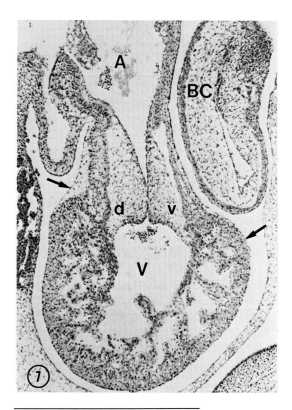

FIG. 7. Longitudinal section of the human embryo heart through the atrioventricular canal. The cardiac jelly in the bulbus cordis *(BC)* and atrioventricular canal has been populated by mesenchymal cells. *(d)* and *(v)* dorsal and ventral atrioventricular endocardial cushions. Note the progressive formation of trabeculae in the ventricular region *(V)*. No cardiac jelly is detectable in the atrium *(A)*. *Arrows* indicate the epicardium. (From the Kyoto Collection, 1290-H14, slide 6, section 3.)

[1]The term "disappears," as used here, refers to the disappearance of the cardiac jelly as the ground substance occupying the wide space interposed between myocardium and endocardium. However, at these stages the heart is growing rapidly, and the total amount of cardiac extracellular material may not be reduced. Quantitative studies have yet to be done.

follow an independent and spiraling course from the venous end to the arterial end. The spiraling course of these streams creates zones of friction or high- and low-pressure zones in the heart wall (3,10). The cardiac jelly could then be displaced from the high-pressure zones and accumulate in the low-pressure zones, if we assume that cardiac jelly can flow. In the low-pressure zones, when the friction effects of the blood flow are less intense, the heart septa develop. It is clear, however, that the net viscosity of the cardiac jelly as well as the high structural ordering of its components must present a real impediment for this displacement to occur, and it is unlikely that simplistic hemodynamic flow molding models are correct.

In the atrioventricular canal and bulbus cordis the cardiac jelly is invaded by cells migrating from the endocardium (54,98). The endocardial cells extend pseudopodia and filopodia into the cardiac jelly and are eventually seeded into the matrix (79,80). Centrifugal migration from the endocardium toward the myocardium follows the first appearance of mesenchymal cells in the cardiac jelly. With the progressive increase in cell density, the previously acellular cardiac jelly is transformed into a mesenchymatous matrix. Coincident with the process of cell migration, the cardiac jelly becomes more sharply delineated and forms rather distinct zones, the endocardial cushions (Figs. 6 and 7). As the presence of endocardial cushions is intimately related to the process of heart septation, they are described in detail later.

Most of the cells populating the cardiac jelly have their origin in the endocardium lining the atrioventricular canal and bulbus cordis. However, in the most distal part of the bulbus cordis, the source of mesenchymal cells appears to be twofold. In this distal region of the heart, cells derived from the splanchnic mesoderm enter the cardiac jelly via a craniocaudal migratory pathway (78,122,129). The extracardiac source of mesenchymal cells is limited in number, and they probably mix with the cells derived from the endocardium, contributing to the bulk of endocardial cushion cells. It is worth noting that it is not necessary that a large number of endocardial cells migrate into the cardiac jelly. The frequency of mitotic figures among the cushion cells suggests that the progressive increase in cell number is mostly due to interstitial growth rather than the continued seeding of cells from the endocardium (78).

THE HEART AFTER THE CARDIAC LOOP

External Modifications

With the completion of looping, the heart has acquired an S-shaped form. However, the sigmoid aspect of the cardiac tube can be discerned only in true ventral views (94). For convenience in description, the heart is more frequently compared to a U (Fig. 8a). The ventricle forms the bend of the U, whereas the bulbus cordis and the sinoatrial region form its right and left limbs, respectively. The saccular aspect of the ventricular region disappears progressively, and the

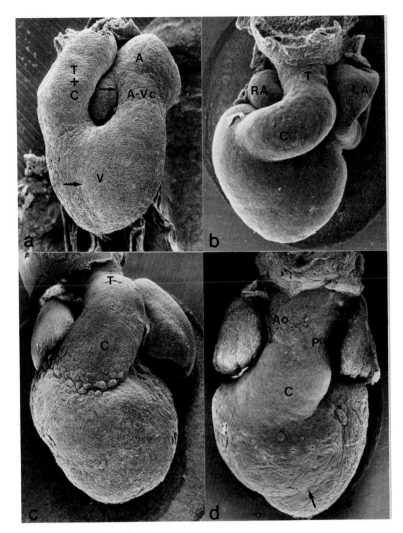

FIG. 8. Scanning electron micrographs of chick embryo hearts showing the modifications of the external form of the heart at postlooping stages (ventral views). *(A)* atrium. *(Ao)* aorta. *(A-Vc)* atrioventricular canal. *(C)* conus. *(LA)* left atrium. *(P)* pulmonary artery. *(RA)* right atrium. *(T)* truncus. *(V)* ventricle.

a: Third day of incubation. At this stage the bulbus cordis *(T+C)* cannot be separated into its two components. *Arrows* indicate the interatrial and interventricular sulci. Compare with Fig. 2. **b:** Fourth day of incubation. The bulbus is growing longitudinally and bends around a transverse axis. This is the point at which its two components, truncus and conus, can be distinguished. Compare the size of the two atria. **c:** Fifth day of incubation. Note the rapid growth of the right atrium. **d:** Sixth day of incubation. The proximal segments of the aorta and pulmonary artery are already formed. However, there is not yet external separation. Note the location of the interventricular sulcus *(arrow)*. The apex of the heart is already formed for the left ventricle.

ventricle becomes more trapezoidal (Fig. 8a–d). The atrium is expanding rapidly in a lateral direction, at first mainly toward the left side. Consequently, the left side of the atrium is initially much larger than the right side. The interatrial and interventricular grooves, or sulci, appear in the ventral aspect of the atrium and ventricle, marking the zones where the interatrial and interventricular septa will develop. The deep fissure between the right and left limbs of the U-heart is represented internally by a spur of tissue, the bulboventricular flange, located to the left of the opening of the bulbus (see Fig. 12, below).

The bulbus cordis apparently changes its position from lateral to the primitive atrium to a ventral and medial position between the right and left developing atria. This shift in position of the bulbus cordis has been classically described as bulbar rotation (5). However, it appears that neither a real nor a relative displacement of the bulbus cordis takes place (22,101,111,118). The rapid asymmetrical growth of the ventricular and atrial regions gives the impression of bulbar movement, but the spatial relationships of the bulbus cordis with the embryonic axis remain constant, at least until partitioning of the heart is completed.

The bulbus cordis increases in length, particularly because of longitudinal growth in the area of the truncus. The increase in the length of the bulbus causes this portion of the heart to bend around a transverse axis. The point of maximal bending marks the separation between conus and truncus, and it is important in regard to the origin of the semilunar valves (22,23,118,127,128). As a consequence of the lengthening of the truncus, the truncoconal junction becomes displaced progressively toward the ventricles.

As can be observed in Fig. 8, the length of the conus decreases progressively. The apparent decrease in length of the conal portion of the heart has been classically described as bulbar absorption (99), suggesting that the conus "sinks" into the definitive ventricles. It actually appears that there is no real absorption (22,34), that is, no absolute shortening of the conus occurs (101,118). The increase in length of the truncus together with the progressive formation of the trabeculae in the anterior wall of the conus gives the impression of bulbar absorption. Again, asymmetrical differential growth of the heart changes the limits and relations of the individual component parts. The relative shortening of the conus is responsible for the "displacement" of the anlage of the semilunar valves toward the ventricles and the continuity between the mitral and aortic valves.

In the dorsal surface of the heart the sinus venosus becomes increasingly differentiated. The deepening of the atrioventricular sulcus causes the sinus venosus to lose its close relationship with the left atrium. The sinus venosus now opens only into the right atrium. In the avian embryo the sinus venosus remains as a distinct structure located in the dorsal wall of the right atrium (102). Its opening is shared by the cava veins. In the human embryo the cava veins obtain independent openings, and part of the sinus venosus is transformed into the coronary sinus. The various parts of the heart have now nearly assumed the adult configuration.

During the stages just described the heart is growing rapidly. The increase in mass of any organ is accomplished by two basic mechanisms, i.e., cell division (hyperplasia) and cell mass increase (hypertrophy). Cardiac myocytes continue to divide not only during the developmental stages described above but also during the fetal and early postnatal periods (31,136). Although the number of myocytes undergoing cellular division declines progressively, centers of active cell proliferation have been described in both atria and ventricles (30,112). The outgrowth of the heart chambers seems to be determined, at least in part, by the presence of these proliferative centers. Cell division thus appears to be an important mechanism in heart growth. Muscle cell hypertrophy is a basic mechanism of heart growth during the fetal and postnatal periods (138). However, the exact role of cell hypertrophy during the developmental stages considered here has yet to be determined.

Growth regulation by increasing functional demands is a well-documented process (33). After loop formation the circulating blood volume has increased considerably (113). The myofibrillar content of the heart has also increased (40,71). The cytoplasm of the myocardial cells is loaded with tightly packed myofibrils aligned following the longitudinal cell axis. With the increasing contractile capacity, the workload of the heart and the stroke volume also increase (108). It is clear that the heart is able to grow in response to functional demands. Heart enlargement occurs when the heart is subjected to hemodynamic overload, e.g., in valvular and hypertensive diseases. Moreover, during the early postnatal period, cardiac overload increases both the cell mass and the rate of division (24,85). On the other hand, unloaded myocardium undergoes rapid atrophy (14). However, the exact role of hemodynamics in heart embryogenesis is still unclear. The fact that blood circulation does not begin until the bending of the heart tube is well advanced (94) suggests the small morphogenic importance of blood flow to loop formation. Experimental evidence (76,119) has confirmed that simple observation. At postlooping stages hemodynamic forces appear to play an active role in heart development. Changes in the size of the heart chambers have been experimentally produced by altering the blood flow through the heart (12,50,110). However, it is still unclear whether these morphologic changes are due to modifications of the hemodynamic load or to the forces generated by the altered blood flow (137). On the other hand, it has been recently reported that the distribution of the zones of proliferative activity does not change in hypoplastic developing ventricles (112).

Other mechanisms of growth must be considered during heart development. Nonmyocardial cells (e.g., epicardial cells, fibroblasts, and vascular and nerve cells) are incorporated into the developing heart (see descriptions later). These cell types have higher rates of division than the myocytes, their number increases progressively, and in the adult heart they represent 75% (136) to 87% (53) of the total cell number. Although during the stages considered here the addition of nonmuscle cells account probably for only a small part of the total increase in heart mass, their presence must be considered. There is yet another factor participating in the rapid enlargement of the atrial region. Part of the wall of the sinus venosus is incorporated progressively into the developing right atrium. In the adult heart the inner surface of the right atrial chamber presents two clearly different zones: (a) a smooth zone derived mainly from the sinus venosus; and (b) an irregular zone where pectinate muscles are present, derived from the primitive embryonic right atria. A similar process occurs in the left atrium. The wall of the primitive pulmonary vein is incorporated progressively into the atrial wall until the four definitive pulmonary veins obtain independent openings (102,105). Part of the left precava vein is also incorporated into the right atrium, especially in the region of the atrial septum. In the adult heart about 50% of the atrial septum is derived from this secondary process of incorporation (102).

Heart development is clearly a complex multifactorial process. Little is known of the mechanisms that control DNA replication and the proliferative activity of the myocardial cells. As heart form and contractile function develop simultaneously, it is difficult to distinguish between intrinsic developmental programs and the effects of extrinsic, epigenetic factors, e.g., the circulatory activity. An understanding of the factors that control the genetic expression of tissue-specific proteins is in its beginning. The presence of different types of myosin isozymes appears to be developmentally regulated. The distribution of heavy- and light-chain subunits of cardiac myosin has been shown to vary during development (64,81,134) and in response to cardiac overload (26). Moreover, different types of myosin subunits distribute differently in atrial and ventricular myocytes and in Purkinje fibers (134). Although the sequential appearance of myosin molecules during embryogenic periods is still unknown and there is much to be learned about the fetal and postnatal periods, the presence of these myosin subunits could be used in the future as an index of heart development and maturation.

Heart Partitioning

The relatively simple changes in the external form of the heart are accompanied internally by a series of successive morphogenic steps which bring about the transformation of the single heart tube into a four-chambered organ. The heart septa arise independently in the bulbus cordis, ventricle, and atrium, and become united to make two independent circulatory channels (62). In a tubular organ such as the heart, there are two basic mechanisms of septa formation (59). The first involves the growing of two opposite masses of tissue. Eventually, these masses of actively growing tissue meet each other and fuse. The septa thus formed are characteristically large and bulky, and only secondarily are transformed into thin septa (126). The second is a more passive process. A narrow portion of the heart does not increase in diameter, or does it very slowly, but the immediate segments on each side expand rapidly. This kind of septum is at first not completed. An opening, located normally in an eccentric position, is always present. This opening is eventually closed by tissue deriving from nearby structures. The septation of the bulbus cordis and the division of the atrioventricular canal are examples of the active growth mechanism. The interatrial and interventricular septa develop in a more passive form and are completed secondarily by neighboring proliferating tissue (126).

Interatrial Septum

The interatrial septum arises as a thin myocardial partitioning from the dorso-cephalic wall of the atrium (Fig. 9), between the openings of the sinus venosus and the pulmonary vein. The septum presents a comma-shaped form with a concave free edge directed toward the atrioventricular canal (Fig. 10). This initial septum is termed septum primum, and the space between its free edge and the atrioven-tricular canal is the foramen primum.

The septum primum grows rapidly toward the atrioventricular canal until its free border meets the endocardial cushions. When it fuses with the dorsal and ventral endocardial cushions, the foramen primum is occluded (Fig. 10). The partitioning of the atrium would then be completed if not for perforations that arise in the dorsal portion of the septum primum (Fig. 11). These perforations, the foramina secunda, establish a communication between the two atria that is not closed until hatching (or birth).

The foramina secunda in the chick permit the shunting of blood from the right to the left atria and act as a one-way valve that prevents backflow of blood in the reverse direction (38,95). In mammals this valvular action is achieved by the

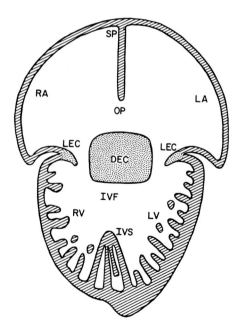

FIG. 9. Frontal section of the heart showing the formation of the interatrial septum (*SP:* septum pri-mum) and the interventricular sep-tum *(IVS)*. The foramen delimited by the free border of the septum primum and the endocardial cush-ions of the atrioventricular canal is the ostium primum *(OP)*. In the atrioventricular canal, the dorsal endocardial cushion *(DEC)* has not yet fused with the ventral cushion. The interventricular septum forms by coalescence of the primitive tra-beculae. *(IVF)* primitive interven-tricular foramen. *(LA)* left atrium. *(LEC)* lateral endocardial cushion. *(LV)* left ventricle. *(RA)* right atrium. *(RV)* right ventricle.

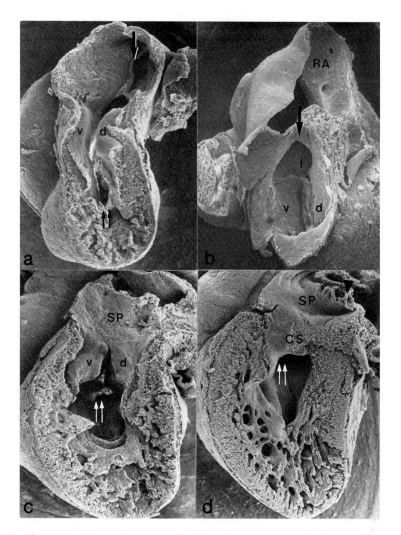

FIG. 10. Scanning electron micrographs of chick embryo hearts showing the formation of the interatrial and interventricular septa. **a, c, d:** Longitudinal sections through the left side of the atrioventricular canal (right segment of the specimen, seen from the left side). **b:** The atrial roof has been removed and the atrial cavity is exposed (seen from the top). The direction of growth of the septum primum *(SP)* is indicated by *single arrows*. The free border of the interventricular septum and the interventricular foramen are indicated by *double arrows. (CS)* cushion septum. *(d)* dorsal endocardial cushion. *(l)* right lateral endocardial cushion. *(RA)* right atrium. *(v)* ventral endocardial cushion.

   a: Third day of incubation. The interatrial and interventricular septa are beginning to form. The dorsal and ventral endocardial cushions are already present. **b:** Fourth day of incubation. The septum primum extends with a concave free border toward the dorsal and ventral endocardial cushions of the atrioventricular canal. Compare with Fig. 9. **c:** Fifth day of incubation. The septum primum has reached the endocardial cushions and fused with their dorsal aspect. The ostium primum has been occluded. The fusion of the endocardial cushions is now beginning. **d:** Sixth day of incubation. The endocardial cushions have fused, and the cushion septum has been formed. Note some of the foramina secunda, collapsed, in the dextrodorsal aspect of the septum primum *(arrowhead)*. Compare with Fig. 11.

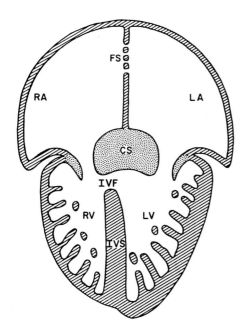

FIG. 11. Frontal section of the heart at a later stage than that shown in Fig. 9. In the atrioventricular canal, the dorsal and ventral endocardial cushions are already fused, forming the cushion septum *(CS)*. The foramen primum has been closed. The foramina secunda *(FS)* establish a communication between the right atrium *(RA)* and left atrium *(LA)*. The interventricular septum *(IVS)* now presents a compact appearance. Its free border is directed toward the right side of the atrioventricular canal. *(IVF)* secondary interventricular foramen. *(LV)* left ventricle. *(RV)* right ventricle.

formation of another septum, the septum secundum, which develops to the right of the septum primum, and appears to act as a flap valve.

Atrioventricular Canal

The cardiac jelly in the region of the atrioventricular canal expands to form two distinct zones, the dorsal and ventral endocardial cushions. The cushions thicken rapidly, projecting progressively into the lumen; they then approach each other and fuse (Figs. 7, 10–12). Fusion of the dorsal and ventral endocardial cushions brings about the division of the atrioventricular canal into two vertically oriented apertures, the right and left atrioventricular orifices. The mass of cushion tissue resulting from the fusion of the two endocardial cushions is termed cushion septum (Figs. 10 and 11).

The mechanisms of endocardial cushion fusion are still poorly understood. From a mechanical viewpoint, the continuous blood flow and the fact that the paired cushions contact and separate intermittently with each other during heart contraction has to represent an obstacle for the fusion process to occur. In the atrioventricular canal the septum primum, fused with the superior aspect of the dorsal and ventral cushions, may act as a physical template (Fig. 10c), aligning the cushions and guiding the process of fusion (35). In the bulbus cordis, where similar processes of fusion occur, no similar mechanism have been postulated. Cushion fusion does not basically involve cell fusion mechanisms (see, however, ref. 66), but the fusion of similar anatomical structures. Endocardial cells at the point of fusion extend

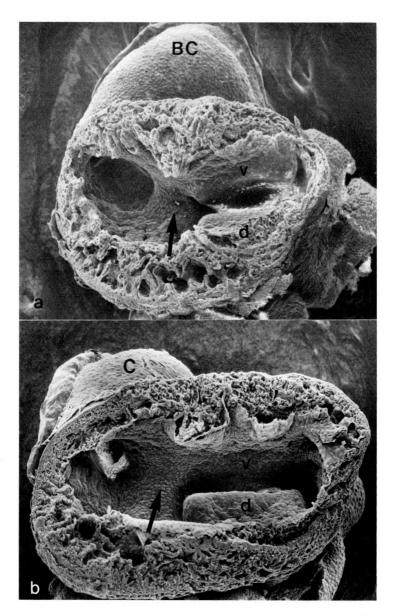

FIG. 12. Scanning electron micrographs of chick embryo hearts showing the morphological changes in the region of the atrioventricular canal and the changes in position of the bulbus cordis relative to the atrioventricular canal. The apex of the heart has been dissected away (upper segment of the specimens, seen from the apex). *(BC)* bulbus cordis. *(C)* conus. *(CS)* cushion septum. *(d)* dorsal endocardial cushion. *(IVS)* interventricular septum. *(LV)* left ventricle. *(RV)* right ventricle. *(v)* ventral endocardial cushion. *(1)* dextrodorsal conal ridge. *(2)* sinistroventral conal ridge. **a:** Third day of incubation. In the atrioventricular canal the dorsal and ventral endocardial cushions are already present. The bulboventricular flange *(arrow)* separates the opening of the bulbus cordis from the atrioventricular canal. Compare throughout this figure the changes in position of the bulbus cordis and the progressive effacement of the bulboventricular flange. **b:** Fourth day of incubation. The dextrodorsal conal ridge is barely visible in the lumen of the conus.

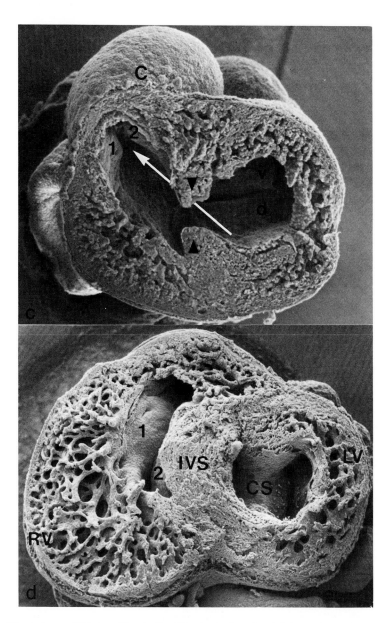

FIG. 12. cont. c: Fifth day of incubation. The dextrodorsal and sinistroventral conal ridges are growing toward each other. The endocardial cushions in the atrioventricular canal are not yet fused. The plane of the section includes the dorsal and ventral prolongations *(arrowheads)* of the interventricular septum. Note that they are directed toward the right side of the atrioventricular canal. Note also the relations between the heart chambers. The atrioventricular canal opens directly into the left ventricle. The bulbus opens directly into the right ventricle. The left ventricle communicates with the conus through the secondary interventricular foramen *(white arrow)*. **d:** Sixth day of incubation. The dextrodorsal and sinistroventral conal ridges have met each other in the lumen of the conus. The cushion septum *(CS)* is formed. The left atrioventricular aperture can be observed at the left of the cushion septum. Note the development of the interventricular septum and the trabeculated aspect of the ventricles.

finger-like projections over the opposite surfaces. Although it is difficult to demonstrate well-developed intercellular junctions between endocardial cells of opposite cushions (36,104), membranes of apposed endocardial surfaces become adherent and break down when physical stress is applied (35). As the fusion progresses, the endocardial cells that are left behind the line of fusion lose adherence and become indistinguishable from the rest of the mesenchymal cells that populate the cushion septum (35,104). The possible role of changes in cell membrane structure with subsequent changes in properties of cell recognition and adhesion has yet to be explored during cushion fusion.

Programmed cell death appears to be an important mechanism in cardiac remodeling and shaping (88,100,114). Cell death occurs in heart development accompanying other fusion processes, e.g., fusion of the primitive endocardial tubes (87). However, only scarce dying cells can be observed during cushion fusion. On the other hand, the presence of mitotic figures is a common finding that suggests the possible importance of cell proliferation and active cell behavior (36,66).

At the same time that the division of the atrioventricular canal takes place, two small masses of cushion tissue, the right and left lateral endocardial cushions, develop on the lateral margins of the primitive atrioventricular aperture. Both atrioventricular orifices are thus encroached on by cushion tissue. These masses of cushion tissue participate in the formation of the atrioventricular valves.

Interventricular Septum

The formation of the interventricular septum is related intimately to the process of myocardial trabeculation. Coalescence of the primitive trabeculae at the apex of the ventricle forms the primordium of the interventricular septum (Figs. 13 and 14). From the ventricular apex the septum grows higher and thicker and extends, with a concave free border, toward the atrioventricular canal. The orifice formed between the free border of the septum and the atrioventricular canal is the primary interventricular foramen (Fig. 9). The dorsal aspect of the free border of the interventricular septum reaches the cushion septum and fuses with its right border. However, the ventral zone of the septum remains at a distance, delineating the so-called secondary interventricular foramen (Fig. 11).

The primitive ventricular region is now divided into left and right chambers, both ventricles communicating through the secondary interventricular foramen. The aperture of the bulbus cordis lies to the right of the interventricular septum, and the bulbus communicates directly only with the right ventricle (Fig. 12c). The later development of the interventricular septum is associated closely with the process of bulbar septation. The secondary interventricular foramen never closes but is used in connecting the aorta with the left ventricle (62).

Septation of the Bulbus

The septation of the bulbus cordis is achieved in the same basic manner as the division of the atrioventricular canal. The cardiac jelly expands in the bulbus cordis

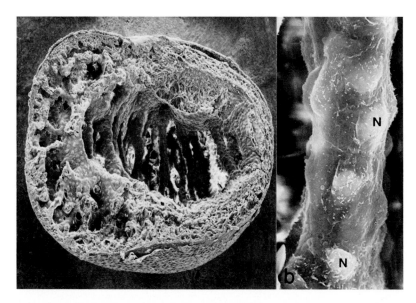

FIG. 13. Scanning electron micrographs of the ventricular apex in a 4-day chick embryo heart. **a:** Low magnification showing the aspect of the primitive trabeculae. Note their ventro-dorsal orientation. The primordium of the interventricular septum cannot yet be distinguished. **b:** Higher magnification of one of the primitive trabeculae present in **a.** The endocardial cells that cover the myocardial core are flattened, polygonal, and have prominent nuclei *(N)*. Note the interdigitations between the cells and the presence of numerous microvilli, especially in the nuclear region.

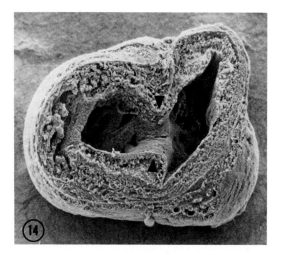

FIG. 14. Scanning electron micrograph of a 5-day chick embryo heart showing formation of the interventricular septum. The heart apex has been exposed (seen from the top). The septum forms by coalescence of the primitive trabeculae. The concave free border of the septum is apparent. The plane of the section passes through the ventral and dorsal prolongations of the septum *(arrowheads).* (Fig. 12c represents the upper segment of the same embryo.)

and forms two sets of endocardial cushions, the truncal and conal ridges (Fig. 15). Their fusion causes septation of the bulbus. The simplicity of this process is obscured by the spiraling course followed by the cushions and the "incorporation" of the conus into the ventricular region (105).

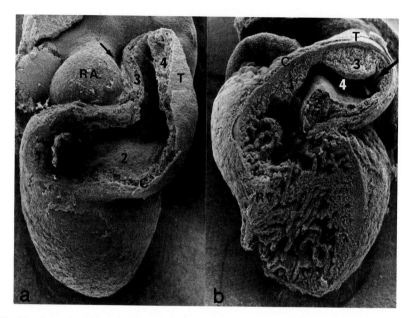

FIG. 15. Scanning electron micrographs of chick embryo hearts showing the development of the conal and truncal ridges. *(1)* dextrodorsal conal ridge. *(2)* sinistroventral conal ridge. *(3)* sinistroventral truncal ridge. *(4)* dextrodorsal truncal ridge. *(RA)* right atrium. *(RV)* right ventricle. *(C)* conus. *(T)* truncus. The right wall of the truncoconus has been dissected away (left segment of the specimen, seen from the right).
  a: Fourth day of incubation. The plane of section passes through the dextrodorsal and sinistroventral truncal ridges. The sinistroventral conal ridge is barely visible. The dextrodorsal conal ridge has been removed. *Arrow* indicates the interatrial sulcus. **b:** Fifth day of incubation. The four truncoconal ridges are present. Note the spiraling trajectory followed on one hand by the dextrodorsal conal ridge and the sinistroventral truncal ridge, and on the other hand by the sinistroventral conal ridge and the dextrodorsal truncal ridge. *Arrow* indicates one of the intercalated valve swellings.

One of the truncal ridges is located dorsally and to the right, the other ventrally and to the left. These are the dextrodorsal and sinistroventral truncal ridges. Similar structures, the dextrodorsal and sinistroventral conal ridges, arise in the wall of the conus. Truncal and conal ridges develop distally, following a spiraling course (Figs. 15 and 16) (59,128). The dextrodorsal conal ridge spirals ventrally and to the left. Its direction is followed in the truncus by the sinistroventral truncal ridge. The sinistroventral conal ridge spirals dorsally and to the right. Its direction is continued in the truncus by the dextrodorsal truncal ridge (Figs. 15–17). The spiraling trajectory of the septum, separating the aorta and the pulmonary artery, is then formed in the following manner: The sinistroventral conal ridge becomes continuous with the dextrodorsal truncal ridge, and the dextrodorsal conal ridge becomes continuous with the sinistroventral truncal ridge. Both systems cross each other at the truncoconal junction (21,23,55,127).

In the meantime, the portion of the heart connecting the truncoconus with the aortic arches has enlarged, becoming a differentiated region, the truncoaortic sac

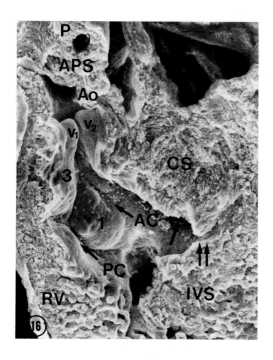

FIG. 16. Scanning electron micrograph of a 6-day chick embryo heart showing the development of the truncoconal ridges. The heart has been dissected longitudinally (right segment of the specimen, seen from the left). The dextrodorsal conal ridge *(1)* becomes continuous with the sinistroventral truncal ridge *(3)*. Before the fusion of the conal ridges, the conal portion is divided into an aortic conus *(AC)* and a pulmonic conus *(PC)*. Note the relation between the aortic conus and the interventricular foramen *(double arrow)*. The right atrioventricular canal is indicated by the *arrow*. One of the cusps of the semilunar valves (v_1) can be seen arising from the main truncal ridge; v_2 arises directly from the wall of the truncus, from the intercalated valve swelling. *(Ao)* aorta. *(APS)* aortopulmonary septum. *(CS)* cushion septum. *(IVS)* interventricular septum. *(P)* pulmonary artery. *(RV)* right ventricle.

(59). The division of the truncoaortic sac is carried out by the formation of a spur of mesenchymal tissue, the aortopulmonary septum, which originates between the fourth and sixth aortic arches (65). The aortopulmonary septum grows downward toward the truncus (Fig. 16) until it meets the truncal ridges. The aortopulmonary septum is a horseshoe-shaped structure. It is anchored in the truncal ridges by two limbs of densely arranged mesenchymal cells, the prongs of the aortopulmonary septum (57). Although the prongs of the aortopulmonary septum are present in the tissue of the truncal ridges before the process of fusion takes place, their significance relative to the fusion process is still unknown. The direction followed by the aortopulmonary septum accounts for part of the spiraling trajectory of the aorta and pulmonary artery.

Soon after the truncal and conal ridges become continuous, the truncal ridges enlarge, meet each other in the lumen of the still undivided truncus, and fuse. The fusion of the truncal ridges follows a craniocaudal direction and divides the distal portion of the bulbus cordis into an aortic and a pulmonic channel. After fusion of the truncal ridges, the conal ridges enlarge and fuse in the same manner, and the septum of the conal portion becomes continuous with the septum of the truncus (Fig. 18).

Formation of the Aortic Vestibulum

The truncal region has been divided into an aortic and a pulmonic channel. The aperture of the conus lies ventral to the atrioventricular canal and to the right of

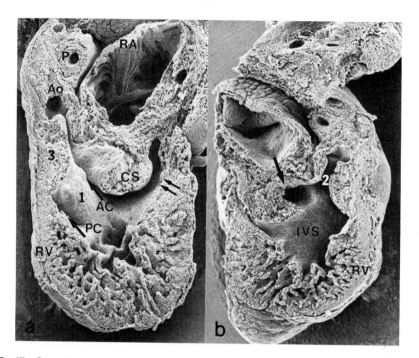

FIG. 17. Scanning electron micrograph of a 6-day chick embryo heart. The heart has been sectioned longitudinally, and both halves are presented. *(Ao)* aorta. *(CS)* cushion septum. *(IVS)* interventricular septum. *(P)* pulmonary artery. *(RA)* right atrium. *(RV)* right ventricle. *(1)* dextrodorsal conal ridge. *(2)* sinistroventral conal ridge. *(3)* sinistroventral truncal ridge.

a: Right segment of the specimen (seen from the left). The dextrodorsal conal ridge is continuous with the right side of the cushion septum. Note the presence of the aortic conus *(AC)* and the pulmonic *(PC)* conus on both sides of the conal cushions. *Double arrow* indicates the right atrioventricular canal. **b:** Left segment of the specimen (seen from the right). The secondary interventricular foramen is in the center of the figure *(arrow).* Note its aspect. Because of the thickening of the interventricular septum, the interventricular foramen has become a tunnel-like communication between the ventricles. The sinistrodorsal conal ridge is continuous with the anterior margin of the interventricular septum.

the interventricular foramen (Fig. 18). Further recession of the bulboventricular flange together with enlargement to the right of the atrioventricular canal bring about new changes in the position of these structures relative to each other. The recession of the bulboventricular flange brings the posterior (aortic) division of the conus above the interventricular foramen. The sinistroventral conal ridge then becomes continuous caudally with the anterior margin of the interventricular septum (Fig. 17). The dextrodorsal conal ridge becomes continuous with the right lateral endocardial cushion and with the right side of the cushion septum (Fig. 18). Finally, the conus septum fuses with the ventral part of the interventricular septum, and the left ventricle becomes continuous with the aortic channel.

A communication, the tertiary interventricular foramen, persists between the already formed aortic vestibulum and the right ventricle (Fig. 19). The tertiary

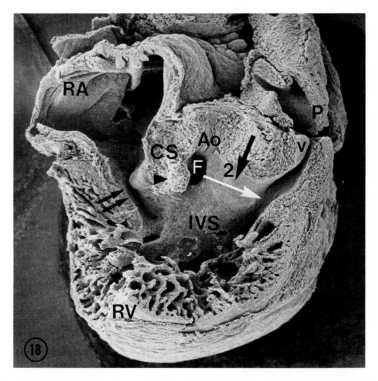

FIG. 18. Scanning electron micrograph of a chick embryo heart at the middle of the sixth day of incubation. The heart has been dissected through the right atrium *(RA)*, the right atrioventricular aperture *(double arrow)*, and the right ventricle *(RV)*. The secondary interventricular foramen is in the center of the figure *(F)*. In front of the interventricular foramen the fusion of the conal ridges has already begun, but the inferior part of the sinistroventral conal ridge *(2)* is still unfused. At this stage the dextrodorsal conal ridge blends with the right side of the cushion septum *(CS)*. The dextrodorsal conal ridge has been left out of the dissection, but the plane of the section passes through the zone of blending *(arrowhead)*. The continued fusion of the conal ridges in a downward direction *(black arrow)* together with the growing of the right side of the cushion septum along the top of the interventricular foramen (direction of growth marked by *arrowhead*) isolate the interventricular foramen from the right ventricle. Then the interventricular foramen becomes part of the aortic vestibulum, and in this sense the aorta is transferred to the left ventricle. *(Ao)* indicates the position of the aortic outflow tract (most of it has been removed). The future position of the tertiary interventricular foramen is indicated by the *white arrow*. *(P)* pulmonary artery. *(v)* valvular cusp.

interventricular foramen is enclosed caudally by the interventricular septum, ventrally by the conus septum, and dorsally by the cushion septum. Tissue deriving from these three structures will close the foramen, forming the origin of the membranous part of the adult interventricular septum.

Semilunar Valves

The primordia of the semilunar valves are formed by three pairs of small tubercles of cushion tissue. Two of these paired tubercles arise from the main truncal ridges.

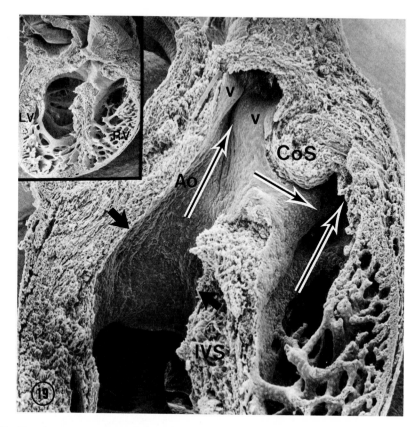

FIG. 19. Scanning electron micrograph of a 6.5-day chick embryo heart. The heart has been dissected tangentially to the interventricular septum *(IVS)*. The aortic *(Ao)* and pulmonic *(P)* outflow tracts have been exposed (the direction of the blood flow is indicated by the *white and black arrows*). The tertiary interventricular foramen *(small white and black arrow)* communicates the aortic vestibulum with the right ventricle. The foramen is delimited caudally by the interventricular septum, ventrally by the conus septum *(CoS)*, and dorsally by the cushion septum. *Arrows* indicate the approximate position of the left margin of the secondary interventricular foramen. **Inset:** Low magnification of the same specimen showing the general relations of the heart. *(LV)* left ventricle. *(RV)* right ventricle.

The third pair, the intercalated valve swellings (55), arise directly from the wall of the truncus, between the main truncal ridges (Fig. 16). When the division of the truncus is achieved, each channel receives one of the intercalated valve swellings and two of those derived from the main truncal ridges. A process of excavation by a mechanism not yet understood, at the upper surface of these tubercles, forms the cusps of the semilunar valves. The anlage of the valve cusps then adopts a pocket-like form (44,123). The space formed between the arterial face of the cusps and the wall of the arteries is the primordium of the Valsalva sinus (Fig. 20). No supporting structures, e.g., papillary muscles or chordae tendineae, develop associated with the semilunar valves. No vascular, neural, or muscular elements are

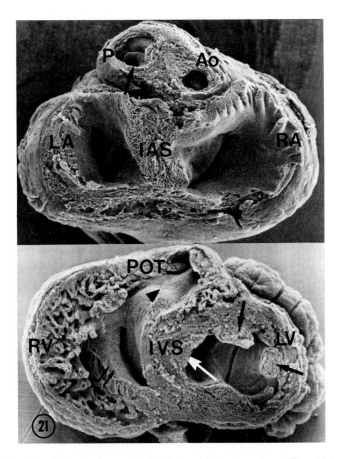

FIG. 20. Scanning electron micrograph of a 7-day chick embryo heart. The atrial walls have been removed, and the floors of the right *(RA)* and left *(LA)* atria are exposed (seen from the top). The base of the interatrial septum *(IAS)* is in the center of the figure. The semilunar valves of the aorta *(Ao)* and pulmonary artery *(P)* have been exposed. Note the three-rayed aspect of the semilunar valves when viewed from the top. *Arrow* indicates the primordium of one Valsalva sinus.

FIG. 21. Scanning electron micrograph of a 7-day chick embryo heart. The apex of the heart has been removed (upper segment of the specimen, seen from the apex). The interventricular septum *(IVS)* is in the center of the figure. In the left side of the heart, the mitral valve presents two valve leaflets with papillary muscles *(arrows)* associated. The entry into the aortic outflow tract is indicated by the *white arrow*. In the right side of the heart one single valve leaflet *(double arrow)* is present, with no papillary muscles. The pulmonary outflow tract has been exposed. A small depression *(arrowhead)* marks the closure of the tertiary interventricular foramen. *(LV)* left ventricle. *(RV)* right ventricle.

observed in the developing valve leaflets. The histological maturation of the semilunar valve tissue is not completed until advanced postnatal periods (13).

The place of origin of the semilunar valves implies a change in the structure of the muscular wall of the truncus, above the valvular level. Simple degeneration

(121) and cell death (46) have been implicated in the disappearance of the muscular cells from the truncal wall. The possibility that these muscular cells may actually undergo a process of dedifferentiation (1) is an interesting suggestion that needs to be explored more.

Atrioventricular Valves

The development and final aspect of the atrioventricular valves present great differences between chicken and human embryos. In both species the primordium of the valve leaflets is formed of cushion and muscular tissue. However, the extent of participation of both kinds of tissue is different in avian (105) and human (127,128) hearts. In mammals the muscular tissue of the embryonic valves is soon replaced by connective tissue, and only occasional muscle fibers can be found associated with the base of the leaflets in the adult heart (86). These muscle fibers, some of them probably of the conduction tissue type (41), interweave with collagen and elastic fibers, forming a loose meshwork. It has been suggested that the presence of muscle cells in the adult valves may prevent ballooning of the leaflets toward the atria during systolic contraction (15,25). Vascular and nerve elements are also found in the mature valves. The papillary muscles and chordae tendineae develop as supporting structures from the trabeculae carneae related to the ventricular aspect of the embryonic leaflets.

The mammalian tricuspid valve is represented in the chicken by a single muscular leaflet (11,16) with no chordae tendineae associated (105). The contraction of this muscular valve during systole prevents the backflow of blood toward the right atrium. The mitral orifice in the chick is guarded by two lateral leaflets with chordae tendineae associated, a situation similar to that in mammals (Fig. 21).

Formation of the Epicardium

During most of the stages of cardiac loop formation the myocytes in the outer surface of the myocardium are directly exposed to the pericardial fluid. It is later in development that the epicardial investment of the myocardium develops. The formation of the epicardium (the visceral pericardium) begins in the dorsal aspect of the heart (56,69,115,129) (Fig. 6). Mesodermal cells in the region of the sinus venosus extend over the heart and form an epithelial sheet on the dorsal surface of the ventricular myocardium. From here the epicardial sheet migrates, expanding radially, on both sides of the ventricular region. When the entire ventricular myocardium is encircled, the epicardial investment extends cranially toward the bulbus cordis and caudally toward the atrium (115). Formation of the epicardium begins at the final stages of cardiac loop formation and continues during the stages of cardiac septation. Before the septation of the heart is achieved, the entire myocardial surface is covered by the primitive epicardium.

Once formed, the epicardium is a simple one-cell-thick epithelial sheet apposed to the outer surface of the myocardium. Soon the epicardium develops a substantial subepicardial layer containing ground substance and mesenchymal cells (Figs. 6

TABLE 1. *List of landmarks of cardiac morphogenesis*

1. First "fusion" of epimyocardial layers of bilateral heart primordia
2. Completion of "fusion" of primordia of bulbus cordis and primordia of ventricles
3. First appearence of myofibrils in myocardium
4. First myocardial contractions
5. Blood flow through heart begins
6. Appearance of external atrioventricular and bulboventricular grooves or sulci
7. Earliest heart curvature apparent
8. Achievement of S-shaped curve
9. Expansion and ventromedial "rotation" of primordium of right ventricle
10. Atrial septum primum appears
11. Perforations (ostium secundum) in atrial septum first seen
12. Atrial septum secundum first definable
13. Alignment of right atrial cavity with primordium of right ventricular cavity
14. Ventral and dorsal endocardial cushions first definable
15. Ostium primum closed by fusion of septum primum with endocardial cushions
16. Ventral and dorsal endocardial cushions unite
17. Cells first seen in cardiac jelly
18. Trabeculations first seen in regions of ventricles
19. Muscular ventricular septum first definable
20. Aortic-pulmonary septum first definable
21. Internal division of aortic sac by aortic-pulmonary septum complete
22. "Rotation" of downstream (distal) segment of bulbus cordis
23. Septa or ridges of bulbus cordis first definable
24. Downstream (distal) division of bulbus cordis completed
25. Upstream (proximal) division of bulbus with closure of "interventricular foramen" complete
26. Appearance of intercalated swellings of semilunar valves
27. Semilunar valves achieve grossly mature form
28. Atrioventricular valves achieve grossly mature form
29. Aortic arches I definitive
30. Dorsal aortas fuse
31. Aortic arches I disappear
32. Aortic arches II definitive
33. Aortic arches II disappear
34. Aortic arches III definitive
35. Aortic arches IV definitive
36. Dorsal aortas between arches III and IV disappear
37. Dorsal aorta (right or left) distal to arch IV disappears
38. Aortic arches VI definitive
39. Dorsal portion of one (right or left) aortic arch VI disappears
40. Bud of main pulmonary vein projects from atrium
41. Main pulmonary vein unites with pulmonary venous plexus
42. Buds of coronary veins from coronary sinus first definable
43. Buds of coronary arteries first definable
44. Left anterior cardinal vein obliterated
45. Mesenteric portion of inferior vena cava first definable
46. Conduction system first definable histologically
47. Main conduction system organized in its major form
48. Purkinje system can be identified
49. Nervous tissue first definable histologically in heart or great arteries

From Sissman, ref. 116, with permission.

TABLE 2. *Chronology of landmarks in cardiac morphogenesis*

Landmark	Human[a]	Chicken[b]	Pig	Rabbit	Rat	Mouse	Frog[c]
1	X	9+	9 somites	10 somites	3 somites	7 days	
2	X	10		12 somites	6 somites	8 days	17
3		10					
4	XI	10		9 somites	3 somites	8 days	19
5	XI	12+			8 somites	8.5 days	
6	X	13	13 somites	11 somites	5 somites	8 days	
7	X	10	13 somites	12 somites	5 somites	7.5 days	18
8	XI	15	17 somites	21 somites	10 somites	8.5 days	19
9	XII–XVII	16–22	25 somites–6 mm	34 somites			
10	XIV	15	3.7 mm	34 somites	12.5 days	10 days	21
11	XVI	26	7 mm	12.75 days	13.25 days	11 days	⋮
12	XVI	⋮	8.5 mm	13 days	14 days		
13	XIII–XVI						
14	XIII	19		11 days	12 days	10 days	24
15	XVI	28	9 mm	14 days	14 days	11 days	22
16	XVI	28	10.5 mm	14 days	14 ± days	11 days	
17	XIII	17			12 ± days		
18	XII		3.5 mm	32 somites		9 days	22
19	XIV	23	6 mm	12 days	13 ± days	9 days	
20	XV	25	7 mm				23
21	XVII	27	10 mm		13.25 days	11.5 days	25
22	XVI–XVII	28	10–14.5 mm				⋮
23	XIII	28		39 somites	12 days		⋮
24	XV	30			15.5 ± days		⋮
25	XVIII	34	20 mm	16.5 days	16 days	13 days	⋮
26	XV	28				13.5 days	
27	40 mm	34				14.5 days	
28							

29	X	10	10 somites	9.25 days	11 ± days	8 days	19
30	XI	15	27 somites			9 days	
31	XIII	17	30 somites	10.5 days	13 ± days	10 days	20
32	XII	15	24 somites	9.5 days	12 ± days	9 days	
33	XIV	23	36 somites	11 days	13.75 ± days	10.5 days	
34	XIII	15	27 somites	10 days	12 ± days	10 days	
35	XIII	18	36 somites	11.75 days	13 ± days	10 days	
36	XVII	31		14 days	15 ± days	13 days	
37	XVIII	29	20 mm	15 days	16 ± days	14 days	21
38	XIV	23	36 somites	11.75 days	13.5 ± days	11 days	
39	XVII	...	18 mm	14.25 days	15 ± days	12.5 days	20
40	XIII	13 +	5 mm			11.5 days	25
41	XIV	17	<10 mm		12.5 days		
42			6.5 mm	12.75 days			
43	XVIII	25	10.5 mm	14.5 days			
44	60 mm	...	28 mm		...	...	
45	XX	29	6.5 mm		12.5 days	12.5 days	
46	XVI			13 days			
47	XXIII						
48	60–100 mm						
49	XIV	22	6 mm	12 days	12 days		

From Sissman, ref. 116, with permission.

a Roman numerals refer to Streeter's horizons (120a,b,c).

b Arabic numerals refer to stages of Hamburger and Hamilton (34a).

c Arabic numerals refer to stages of Shumway (115a).

Dots (...) indicate that landmark is not present in particular species during embryonic life. Blank spaces indicate that information was not available. The symbol ± indicates developmental times for the rat taken from Wilson and Warkany (135a); these values were consistently approximately 1 day older than those presented by other observers for comparable landmarks.

Lengths in millimeters represent, in all cases, greatest or crown–rump measurements.

and 7). The subepicardial space serves as connective tissue supporting the growth of the coronary vessels.

MYOCARDIAL NUTRITION—CORONARY VESSELS

Presumably during early stages of development the nutrition of the myocardium is carried out by diffusion through the cardiac jelly. Little is known of the composition and function of the pericardial fluid, but a possible role in the nutrition of the myocardium and/or the regulation of interstitial pressure of the heart tube cannot be ruled out. The formation of myocardial trabeculae may provide a way for increased metabolic interchange in the thickened ventricular wall. The metabolic interchange in the thinner atrial wall is probably carried out through the apposed endocardium.

After formation of the subepicardial layer, the avascular myocardium develops the intramural vascular pattern of the adult heart (96). The main trunks of the coronary arteries develop as vascular sprouts from the wall of the aorta, at the level of the right and left Valsalva sinuses. The arterial primordia branch out into the subepicardial space, forming a vascular network. These subepicardial vessels send out vascular sprouts toward the underlying myocardium which grow deep into the myocardial wall, forming a rich vascular plexus. The venous blood is received by the coronary veins, which in the meantime have developed as vascular sprouts from the dorsal wall of the sinus venosus (4). Mesenchymal cells penetrate the myocardium accompanying the vascular sprouts and presumably develop into the smooth muscle cells which form the tunica media of the coronary vessels (72).

While the coronary vascular pattern is being formed, the ventricular wall is undergoing a process of compaction. The myocardial trabeculae become apposed and enclose the endocardial outpocketings, which are transformed into slender vascular channels termed sinusoids (82). The blood is still squeezing in and out of the sinusoids, which presumably carry on most of the metabolic interchange. A few connections are established between the developing coronary vessels and the sinusoids (4,72,96). When the coronary vascular bed is well established, the myocardial wall finishes the process of compaction. Then the sinusoids and most of their connections with the coronary vessels are occluded. Some of these connections remain in the adult heart as the thebesian vessels.

The development of the coronary vascular bed is a complex process, and the interrelations between the different vascular channels and the myocardium are not yet clear. Development of the capillary vessels directly from evaginations of the ventricular endocardium (39,132) and from the endocardium of both the sinus venosus and the ventricle (131) has also been described.

CONDUCTION SYSTEM—INNERVATION OF THE HEART

The establishment of the conduction system adds another cellular type to the developing myocardium. It is difficult to say exactly when this system develops, but experimental studies (52,61,93) indicate that a functional conduction system is already present during the final stages of cardiac loop formation. With electron microscopy the cells of the chick conduction system cannot be recognized until about the seventh day of incubation (70). They are found mostly in the vicinity of arterioles and appear to differentiate from the surrounding working cells. They acquire a paler cytoplasm and a lesser amount of myofibrils (130). The cells of the conduction system probably develop from the bulk of myocardial cells. Some of these cells follow a specialized divergent way of differentiation and are transformed into the Purkinje fibers (27,70).

The final organization of the conduction system is similar in most birds and mammals. However, that of the avian heart is a bit more complicated (37,124). It possesses a ring of Purkinje fibers embedded in the connective tissue of the right atrioventricular valve and a more complicated network of subendocardial Purkinje fibers (16). The complexity of the conduction system in birds relative to mammals has been classically related to the maintenance of a faster rhythm of contraction (105).

Sympathetic and parasympathetic (vagal) elements of the autonomic system reach the base of the heart where they form an intricate network of ganglia and nerve fibers. Nerve trunks from this cardiac plexus extend and ramify into the subendocardial space or accompany the right and left coronary arteries embedded in their adventitial tissue. From the subepicardial plexus fine nerve fibers enter into the myocardial tissue either directly or accompanying branches of the coronary arteries (42). Sympathetic (accelerator) and vagal (depressor) afferents control the rate of contraction of the heart. The depressor effect of the vagal afferents is much less intense in the avian than in the human heart.

CONCLUDING REMARKS

The establishment of the form and function of any organ is the result of complex interactions at several levels of biological organization. The diverse cellular activities which result in organ shape are carried on in a strictly regulated microenvironment. The adequate integration of these activities is regulated at both genetic and epigenetic levels.

The heart is a special organ in several ways. Heart development begins at very early embryonic stages, and it is one of the first organs that can be morphologically recognized. (Tables 1 and 2 outline the chronological relationships of the main events of cardiac morphogenesis in various species.) The heart develops at first as a vascular channel, but it soon acquires a muscular wall that is able to contract in the absence of external stimuli. On the other hand, most of the basic heart functions develop well before its morphological development is achieved. Studies on heart development have been limited for many years to simple morphological descriptions. The recent development of structural, biochemical, and immunological techniques has provided new tools for understanding the complex interactions that take place at cellular and subcellular levels during heart morphogenesis. Some of these new approaches have been outlined in the present chapter. Others have been omitted because of lack of space, information, or both. The main aim of this work has been to provide a structural framework on which to place our increasing knowledge of the biochemical and molecular mechanisms of heart development and growth.

ACKNOWLEDGMENTS

The author is indebted to Dr. F. J. Manasek for his invaluable criticism and support. Thanks are also due to N. J. Sissman for kindly permitting reproduction of Tables 1 and 2, and to Dr. K. Hoshino who made available the embryos of the Kyoto Collection to Dr. F. J. Manasek, who photographed the specimens. The author is presently at the Department of Pediatrics, The University of Chicago, under a Fulbright-MUI grant. The use of the scanning electron microscope was supported by grant CA 14599. The work was supported by grant HL 13831.

REFERENCES

1. Arguello, C., De La Cruz, M. V., and Sanchez, C. (1978): Ultrastructural and experimental evidence of myocardial cell differentiation into connective tissue cells in embryonic chick heart. *J. Mol. Cell. Cardiol.*, 10:307–315.
2. Barry, A. (1942): The intrinsic pulsation rates of fragments of the embryonic chick heart. *J. Exp. Zool.*, 91:119–130.
3. Barthel, H. (1960): *Missbildungen des Menschieblen Herzens.* Thieme, Stuttgart.
4. Bennett, H. S. (1936): The development of the blood supply to the heart in the embryo pig. *Am. J. Anat.*, 60:27–53.
5. Born, G. (1889): Beitrage zur Entwicklungsgeschichte des Saugebierherzens. *Arch. Mikr. Anat.*, 33:284–377.
6. Bremer, J. L. (1932): The presence and influence of two spiral streams in the heart of the chick embryo. *Am. J. Anat.*, 49:409–440.
7. Burrows, M. T. (1912): Rhythimische Kontraktionen der isoloierten Herz muskelzelle ausserhalb des Organismus. *Munch. Med. Wochenschr.*, 27:1473–1475.
8. Butler, J. K. (1952): An Experimental Analysis of Cardiac Loop Formation in the Chick. M.A. thesis, University of Texas.
9. Challice, C. E., and Edwards, G. A. (1961): The micromorphology of the developing ventricular muscle. In: *The Specialized Tissues of the Heart*, edited by A. Paes de Carvalho, W. Carlos de Mello, and B. Hoffman, pp. 44–75. Elsevier North-Holland, Amsterdam.
10. Chang, C. (1932): On the reaction of the endocardium to the blood stream in the embryonic heart with special reference to the endocardial thickenings in the atrioventricular canal and bulbus cordis. *Anat. Rec.*, 51:253–265.
11. Clark, A. J. (1927): *Comparative Physiology of the Heart.* Macmillan, New York.
12. Clark, E. B. (1969): Effect of inflow stream alteration on the morphogenesis of the chick heart. *Anat. Rec.*, 163:170–176.
13. Colvee, E., and Hurle, J. M. (1981): Maturation of the extracellular material of the semilunar heart valves in the mouse: a histochemical analysis of collagen and mucopolysaccharides. *Anat. Embryol.*, 162:343–352.
14. Cooper, G., IV, and Tomanek, R. J. (1982): Load regulation of the structure, composition, and function of mammalian myocardium. *Circ. Res.*, 50:788–798.
15. Cooper, T., Napolitano, L. M., Fitzgerald, M. J. T., Moore, K. E., Daggett, W. M., Willman, V. L., Sonnenblick, E. H., and Hanlon, C. R. (1966): Structural basis of cardiac valvular function. *Arch. Surg.*, 93:767–771.
16. Davies, F. (1930): The conduction system of the bird's heart. *J. Anat.*, 64:129–146.
17. Davis, C. L. (1924): The cardiac jelly of the chick embryo. *Anat. Rec.*, 27:201–202.
18. Dehaan, R. L. (1959): Cardia bifida and the development of pacemaker function in the early chick heart. *Dev. Biol.*, 1:586–602.
19. Dehaan, R. L. (1963): Migration patterns of the precardiac mesoderm in the early chick embryo. *Exp. Cell. Res.*, 29:544–560.
20. Dehaan, R. L. (1965): Morphogenesis of the vertebrate heart. In: *Organogenesis*, edited by R. L. DeHaan and H. Ursprung, pp. 377–419. Holt, Rinehart and Winston, New York.
21. De La Cruz, M. V., and Da Rocha, J. P. (1956): An ontogenic theory for the explanation of congenital malformations involving truncus and conus. *Am. Heart J.*, 51:782–805.
22. De La Cruz, M. V., Sanchez Gomez, C., Arteaga, M. M., and Arguello, C. (1977): Experimental

study of the development of the truncus and the conus in the chick embryo. *J. Anat.*, 123:661–686.

23. De Vries, P. A., and Saunders, J. B. de C. M. (1962): Development of the ventricles and spiral outflow tract in the human heart. *Carnegie Inst. Wash. Contrib. Embryol.*, 37:87–114.

24. Dowell, R. T., and McManus, R. E., III (1978): Pressure-induced cardiac enlargement in neonatal and adult rats: left ventricular functional characteristics and evidence of cardiac muscle cell proliferation in the neonate. *Circ. Res.*, 42:303–310.

25. Ellison, J. P., and Hibbs, R. G. (1973): The atrioventricular valves of the guinea pig. I. A light microscopic study. *Am. J. Anat.*, 138:331–346.

26. Flink, I. L., and Morkin, E. (1977): Evidence for a new cardiac myosin species in thyrotoxic rabbit. *FEBS Lett.*, 81:391–394.

27. Forsgren, S., Thornell, L. E., and Eriksson, A. (1980): The development of the Purkinje fibre system in the bovine fetal heart. *Anat. Embryol.*, 159:125–135.

28. Garfield, R. E., Chacko, S., and Blose, S. (1975): Phagocytosis by muscle cells. *Lab. Invest.*, 33:418–427.

29. Girard, H. (1973): Arterial pressure in the chick embryo. *Am. J. Physiol.*, 224:454–460.

30. Goertler, K. (1957): Die Stoffwechseltopographie des embryonalen Huhnerherzens und ihre Bedeutung fur die Entstehung angeborener Herzfehler. *Verh. Dtsch. Ges. Pathol.*, 40:181–185.

31. Goldstein, M. A., Claycomb, W. C., and Schwartz, A. (1974): DNA synthesis and mitosis in well-differentiated mammalian myocytes. *Science*, 183:212–213.

32. Goss, C. M. (1935): Double hearts produced experimentally in rat embyros. *J. Exp. Zool.*, 72:33–45.

33. Goss, R. J. (1964): *Adaptive Growth*. Academic Press, New York.

34. Grant, R. P. (1962): The embryology of ventricular flow pathways in man. *Circulation*, 35:756–779.

34a. Hamburger, W., and Hamilton, H. L. (1951): A series of normal stages in the development of the chick embryo. *J. Morphol.*, 88:49–52.

35. Hay, D. A. (1978): Development and fusion of the endocardial cushions. In: *Morphogenesis and Malformations of the Cardiovascular System*, edited by G. C. Rosenquist and D. Bergsma, pp. 69–90. Alan R. Liss, New York.

36. Hay, D. A., and Low, F. N. (1972): The fusion of dorsal and ventral endocardial cushions in the embryonic chick heart: a study in fine structure. *Am. J. Anat.*, 133:1–24.

37. Hecht, H. H. (1965): Comparative physiological and morphological aspects of pacemaker tissues. *Ann. N.Y. Acad. Sci.*, 127:49–83.

38. Hendrix, M. J. C., and Morse, D. E. (1977): Atrial septation. I. Scanning electron microscopy in the chick. *Dev. Biol.*, 57:345–363.

39. Henningsen, B., and Schiebler, T. H. (1970): Zur Fruhentwicklung der herzeigenen Strombahn: Elektronenmikroskopische Untersuchung an der Ratte. *Z. Anat. Entwick. Gesch.*, 130:101–114.

40. Hibbs, R. G. (1956): Electron microscopy of developing cardiac muscle in chick embryos. *Am. J. Anat.*, 99:17–35.

41. Hibbs, R. G., and Ellison, J. P. (1973): The atrioventricular valves of the guinea pig. II. An ultrastructural study. *Am. J. Anat.*, 138:347–370.

42. Hirsch, E. F. (1970): *The Innervation of the Vertebrate Heart*. Charles C Thomas, Springfield, Illinois.

43. Hurle, J. M., and Ojeda, J. L. (1977): Cardiac jelly arrangement during the formation of the tubular heart of the chick embryo. *Acta Anat. (Basel)*, 98:444–455.

44. Hurle, J. M., Colvee, E., and Blanco, A. M. (1980): Development of mouse semilunar valves. *Anat. Embryol.*, 160:83–91.

45. Hurle, J. M., Icardo, J. M., and Ojeda, J. L. (1980): Compositional and structural heterogenicity of the cardiac jelly of the chick embryo tubular heart: a TEM, SEM and histochemical study. *J. Embryol. Exp. Morphol.*, 56:211–223.

46. Hurle, J. M., Lafarga, M., and Ojeda, J. L. (1977): Cytological and cytochemical studies of the necrotic area of the bulbus of the chick embryo heart: phagocytosis by developing myocardial cells. *J. Embryol. Exp. Morphol.*, 41:161–173.

47. Hurle, J. M., Lafarga, M., and Ojeda, J. L. (1978): In vivo phagocytosis by developing myocardial cells: an ultrastructural study. *J. Cell Sci.*, 33:363–369.

48. Icardo, J. M. (1982): Ultrastructure and function of the cardiac jelly: a review. *Morfol. Norm. Pathol. A-Histol.*, 7:43–58.

49. Icardo, J. M., Ojeda, J. L., and Hurle, J. M. (1982): Endocardial cell polarity during the looping of the heart in the chick embryo. *Dev. Biol.*, 90:203–209.
50. Jaffee, O. C. (1962): Hemodynamics and cardiogenesis. 1. The effects of altered vascular patterns in cardiac development. *J. Morphol.*, 110:217–226.
51. Jeter, J. R., and Cameron, T. L. (1971): Cell proliferation patterns during cytodifferentiation in embryonic chick tissue, liver, heart and erythrocytes. *J. Embryol. Exp. Morphol.*, 25:405–442.
52. Johnston, P. N. (1924): Studies on the physiological anatomy of the embryonic heart. I. The demonstration of complete heart block in chick embryos during the 2nd, 3rd, and 4th days of incubation. *Bull. Johns Hopkins Hosp.*, 35:87–90.
53. Katzberg, A. A., Farmer, B. B., and Harris, R. A. (1977): The predominance of binucleation in isolated rat heart myocytes. *Am. J. Anat.*, 149:489–500.
54. Kinsella, M. G., and Fitzharris, T. P. (1980): Origin of cushion tissue in the developing chick heart: cinematographic recordings of in situ formation. *Science*, 207:1359–1360.
55. Kramer, T. C. (1942): The partitioning of the truncus and conus and the formation of the membranous portion of the interventricular septum in the human heart. *Am. J. Anat.*, 71:343–370.
56. Kurkiewicz, T. O. (1909): O histogenezie miesnia sarcowego zwierzat kregowych. *Bull. Acad. Sci. Cracovie*, 148–191.
57. Laane, H. M. (1979): The septation of the arterial pole of the heart in the chick embryo. IV. Discussion. *Acta Morphol. Neerl. Scand.*, 17:21–32.
58. Lacktis, J. W. (1981): An Experimental and Descriptive Study of Heart Morphogenesis in the Chick. Ph.D. thesis, University of Chicago.
59. Langman, J., and Van Mierop, L. H. S. (1968): Development of the cardiovascular system. In: *Heart Disease in Infants, Children and Adolescents*, edited by A. J. Moss and F. H. Adams, pp. 3–25. Williams & Wilkins, Baltimore.
60. Lewis, M. R. (1920): Muscular contractions in tissue-cultures. *Carnegie Inst. Wash. Contrib. Embryol.*, 9:191–212.
61. Lieberman, M., and Paes de Carvalho, A. (1965): The electrophysiological organization of the embryonic chick heart. *J. Gen. Physiol.*, 49:351–363.
62. Lillie, F. R. (1908): *The Development of the Chick*, 3rd ed., 1965, revised by H. L. Hamilton. Holt, Rinehart and Winston, New York.
63. Lindner, E. (1960): Myofibrils in the early development of the chick embryo hearts as observed with the electron microscope. *Anat. Rec.*, 136:234–235.
64. Lompre, A. M., Mercadier, J. J., Wisnewsky, C., Bouveret, P., Pantaloni, C., D'Albis, A., and Schwartz, K. (1981): Species- and age-dependent changes in the relative amounts of cardiac myosin isoenzymes in mammals. *Dev. Biol.*, 84:286–290.
65. Los, J. A. (1978): Cardiac septation and development of the aorta, pulmonary trunk, and pulmonary veins: previous work in the light of recent observations. In: *Morphogenesis and Malformations of the Cardiovascular System*, edited by G. C. Rosenquist and D. Bergsma, pp. 109–138. Alan R. Liss, New York.
66. Los, J. A., and Van Eijndthoven, E. (1973): The fusion of the endocardial cushions in the heart of the chick embryo: a light-microscopical and electron-microscopical study. *Z. Anat. Entwickl. Gesch.*, 141:55–75.
67. Manasek, F. J. (1968): Embryonic development of the heart. I. A light and electron microscopic study of myocardial development in the early chick embryo. *J. Morphol.*, 125:329–366.
68. Manasek, F. J. (1968): Mitosis in developing cardiac muscle. *J. Cell Biol.*, 37:191–196.
69. Manasek, F. J. (1969): Embryonic development of the heart. II. Formation of the epicardium. *J. Embryol. Exp. Morphol.*, 22:333–348.
70. Manasek, F. J. (1970): Electron microscopic contributions to conduction development. In: *Proceedings of the Conduction Development Conference*, pp. 3–27. National Institutes of Health, Bethesda.
71. Manasek, F. J. (1970): Histogenesis of the embryonic myocardium. *Am. J. Cardiol.*, 25:149–168.
72. Manasek, F. J. (1971): The ultrastructure of embryonic myocardial blood vessels. *Dev. Biol.*, 26:42–54.
73. Manasek, F. J. (1975): The extracellular matrix: a dynamic component of the developing embryo. *Curr. Top. Dev. Biol.*, 10:35–102.
74. Manasek, F. J. (1976): Macromolecules of the extracellular compartment of embryonic and mature heart. *Circ. Res.*, 38:331–337.
75. Manasek, F. J. (1979): Organization, interactions, and environment of heart cells during myocardial

ontogeny. In: *Handbook of Physiology, Vol. 1: The Cardiovascular System*, edited by R. M. Berne, N. Speralakis, and S. R. Geiger, pp. 29–42. American Physiological Society, Bethesda.

76. Manasek, F. J., and Monroe, R. G. (1972): Early cardiac morphogenesis is independent of function. *Dev. Biol.*, 27:584–588.

77. Markwald, R. R., and Adams Smith, W. N. (1972): Distribution of mucosubstances in the developing rat heart. *J. Histochem. Cytochem.*, 29:896–907.

78. Markwald, R. R., Fitzharris, T. P., and Manasek, F. J. (1977): Structural development of endocardial cushions. *Am. J. Anat.*, 148:85–120.

79. Markwald, R. R., Fitzharris, T. P., Bank, H., and Bernanke, D. H. (1978): Structural analysis on the matrical organization of glycosaminoglycans in developing endocardial cushions. *Dev. Biol.*, 62:292–316.

80. Markwald, R. R., Fitzharris, T. P., Bolender, D. L., and Bernanke, D. H. (1979): Structural analysis of cell:matrix interaction during morphogenesis of atrioventricular cushion tissue. *Dev. Biol.*, 69:634–654.

81. Masaki, T., and Yoshizaki, C. (1974): Differentiation of myosin in chick embryos. *J. Biochem.*, 76:123–131.

82. Minot, C. S. (1900): On a hitherto unrecognized form of blood circulation without capillaries in the organs of vertebrata. *Proc. Boston Soc. Nat. Hist.*, 29:185–215.

83. Nakamura, A. (1980): Cardiac hyaluronidase activity of chick embryos at the time of endocardial cushion formation. *J. Mol. Cell. Cardiol.*, 12:1239–1248.

84. Nakamura, A., and Manasek, F. J. (1978): Cardiac jelly fibrils: the distribution and organization. In: *Morphogenesis and Malformations of the Cardiovascular System*, edited by G. C. Rosenquist and D. Bergsma, pp. 229–250. Alan R. Liss, New York.

85. Neffgen, J. F., and Korecky, B. (1972): Cellular hyperplasia and hypertrophy in cardiomegalies induced by anemia in young and adult rats. *Circ. Res.*, 30:104–113.

86. Odgers, P. N. B. (1938): The development of the atrioventricular valves in man. *J. Anat.*, 73:643–657.

87. Ojeda, J. L., and Hurle, J. M. (1981): Establishment of the tubular heart: role of cell death. In: *Mechanisms of Cardiac Morphogenesis and Teratogenesis*, edited by T. Pexieder, pp. 101–113. Raven Press, New York.

88. Okamoto, N., Akimoto, N., Satow, Y., Hidaka, N., and Miyabara, S. (1981): Role of cell death in conal ridges of developing human heart. In: *Mechanisms of Cardiac Morphogenesis and Teratogenesis*, edited by T. Pexieder, pp. 127–137. Raven Press, New York.

89. Orkin, R. W., and Toole, B. P. (1978): Hyaluronidase activity and hyaluronate content of the developing chick embryo heart. *Dev. Biol.*, 66:308–320.

90. Orts Llorca, F., and Jimenez Collado, J. (1968): A radioautographic analysis of the prospective cardiac area in the chick blastoderm by means of labeled grafts. *Wilhelm Roux' Arch.*, 160:298–312.

91. Paff, G. H. (1935): Conclusive evidence for sino-atrial dominance in isolated 48-hour embryonic chick hearts cultivated in vitro. *Anat. Rec.*, 63:203–210.

92. Paff, G. H., Boucek, R. J., and Gutten, G. S. (1965): Ventricular blood pressure and competency of valves in the early embryonic chick heart. *Anat. Rec.*, 151:119–124.

93. Paff, G. H., Boucek, R. J., and Klopfenstein, H. S. (1964): Experimental heart-block in the chick embryo. *Anat. Rec.*, 149:217–224.

94. Patten, B. M. (1922): The formation of the cardiac loop in the chick. *Am. J. Anat.*, 30:373–397.

95. Patten, B. M. (1925): The interatrial septum of the chick heart. *Anat. Rec.*, 30:53–60.

96. Patten, B. M. (1970): The development of the ventricular wall and its blood supply. In: *Cardiac Development with Special Reference to Congenital Heart Disease*, edited by O. C. Jaffee, pp. 1–19. University of Dayton Press, Dayton, Ohio.

97. Patten, B. M., and Kramer, T. C. (1933): The initiation of contraction in the embryonic chick heart. *Am. J. Anat.*, 53:349–375.

98. Patten, B. M., Kramer, T. C., and Barry, A. (1948): Valvular action in the embryonic chick heart by localized apposition of endocardial masses. *Anat. Rec.*, 102:299–311.

99. Pernokopf, E., and Wirtinger, W. (1933): Die Transposition der Herzostienein Versuch der Erklarung dieser Erscheinung: die Phoromonie der Herzentwicklung als morphogenetische Grundlange der Erklarung. I. Teil: die Phoromonie der Herzentwicklung. *Z. Anat. Entwickl. Gesch.*, 100:563–711.

100. Pexieder, T. (1975): Cell death in the morphogenesis and teratogenesis of the heart. *Adv. Anat. Embryol. Cell Biol.*, 51:1–100.

101. Pexieder, T. (1978): Development of the outflow tract of the embryonic heart. In: *Morphogenesis and Malformations of the Cardiovascular System*, edited by G. C. Rosenquist and D. Bergsma, pp. 29–68. Alan R. Liss, New York.

102. Quiring, D. P. (1933): The development of the sino-atrial region of the chick heart. *J. Morphol.*, 55:81–118.

103. Rawles, M. E. (1943): The heart-forming areas of the early chick blastoderm. *Physiol. Zool.*, 16:22–42.

104. Roest-Wagenaar, J. A. (1975): An electronmicroscopic study of the truncus ridges in chick embryos. *Acta Morphol. Neerl. Scand.*, 13:187–200.

105. Romanoff, A. L. (1960): *The Avian Embryo*. Macmillan, New York.

106. Rosenquist, G. C. (1970): Cardiac bifida in chick embryos: anterior and posterior defects produced by transplanting tritiated thymidine-labeled grafts medial to the heart-forming regions. *Teratology*, 3:135–142.

107. Rosenquist, G. C., and Dehaan, R. L. (1966): Migration of precardiac cells in the chick embryo: a radioautographic study. *Carnegie Inst. Wash. Contrib. Embryol.*, 38:111–121.

108. Ruckman, R. N., Cassling, R. J., Clark, E. B., and Rosenquist, G. C. (1981): Cardiac function in the embryonic chick. In: *Mechanisms of Cardiac Morphogenesis and Teratogenesis*, edited by T. Pexieder, pp. 407–418. Raven Press, New York.

109. Rumyantsev, P. P., and Snigirevskaya, E. S. (1968): The ultrastructure of differentiating cells of the heart muscle in the state of mitotic division. *Acta Morphol. Acad. Sci. Hung.*, 16:271–283.

110. Rychter, Z. (1962): Experimental morphology of the aortic arches and the heart loop in chick embryos. *Adv. Morphol.*, 2:333–371.

111. Rychter, Z., and Lemez, L. (1965): Markierung morphogenetischer Bewegungen wahrend der Truncusscheidewandbildung des Herzens beim Huhnerembryo. In: *VIII Internat. Anatomenkongress Wiesbaden*, p. 104.

112. Rychter, Z., and Rychterova, V. (1981): Angio- and myoarchitecture of the heart wall under normal and experimentally changed morphogenesis. In: *Mechanisms of Cardiac Morphogenesis and Teratogenesis*, edited by T. Pexieder, pp. 431–452. Raven Press, New York.

113. Rychter, Z., Kopecky, M., and Lemez, L. (1955): A micromethod for determination of the circulating blood volume in chick embryos. *Nature*, 175:1126–1127.

114. Satow, Y., Okamoto, N., Akimoto, N., Hidaka, N., Miyabara, S., and Pexieder, T. (1981): Comparative and morphometric study on genetically programmed cell death in rat and chick embryo heart. In: *Mechanisms of Cardiac Morphogenesis and Teratogenesis*, edited by T. Pexieder, pp. 115–126. Raven Press, New York.

115. Shimada, Y., and Ho, E. (1980): Scanning electron microscopy of the embryonic chick heart: formation of the epicardium and surface structure of the four heterotypic cells that constitute the embryonic heart. In: *Etiology and Morphogenesis of Congenital Heart Disease*, edited by R. Van Praagh and A. Takao, pp. 63–80. Futura Publishing Co., New York.

115a. Shumway, W. Cited in *Growth, Including Reproduction and Morphologic Development*. Biological data compiled and edited by P. L. Altman and D. S. Dittmer (1962). Federation of American Societies for Experimental Biology, Washington, D.C.

116. Sissman, N. J. (1970): Developmental landmarks in cardiac morphogenesis: comparative chronology. *Am. J. Cardiol.*, 25:141–148.

117. Spratt, N. T. (1942): Location of organ-specific regions and their relationship to the development of the primitive streak in the early chick blastoderm. *J. Exp. Zool.*, 89:69–101.

118. Steding, G., and Seidl, E. (1980): Contribution to the development of the heart. I. Normal development. *Thorac. Cardiovasc. Surg.*, 28:386–409.

119. Stockard, C. R. (1915): An experimental analysis of the origin and relationship of blood corpuscles and the lining cells of vessels. *Proc. Natl. Acad. Sci. USA*, 1:556–562.

120. Streeter, G. L. (1942): Developmental horizons in human embryos. *Carnegie Inst. Wash. Contrib. Embryol.*, 30:211–245.

120a. Streeter, G. L. (1942): Developmental horizons in human embryos. Description of age group XI, 13 to 20 somites, and age group XII, 21 to 29 somites. *Carnegie Inst. Wash. Contrib. Embryol.*, 30:211–245.

120b. Streeter, G. L. (1945): Developmental horizons in human embryos. Description of age group XIII, embryos about 4 or 5 millimetres long, and age group XIV, period of indentation of lens vesicle. *Carnegie Inst. Wash. Contrib. Embryol.*, 31:27–63.

120c. Streeter, G. L. (1948): Developmental horizons in human embryos. Description of age groups XV, XVI, XVII, and XVIII. *Carnegie Inst. Wash. Contrib. Embryol.*, 32:133–203.

121. Tandler, J. (1912): The development of the heart. In: *Manual of Human Embryology*, edited by F. Keibel and F. P. Mall, Vol. 2, pp. 534–570. Lippincott, Philadelphia.

122. Thompson, R. P., and Fitzharris, T. P. (1979): Morphogenesis of the truncus arteriosus of the chick embryo heart: the formation and migration of mesenchymal tissue. *Am. J. Anat.*, 154:545–556.

123. Tonge, M. (1869): Observation of the development of the semilunar valves of the aorta and pulmonary artery of the heart of the chick. *Philos. Trans. R. Soc. (Lond.)*, 159:387–411.

124. Truex, R. C., and Smythe, M. Q. (1965): Comparative morphology of the cardiac conduction tissue in animals. *Ann. N.Y. Acad. Sci.*, 127:18–33.

125. Van Mierop, L. H. S., and Bertuch, J., Jr. (1967): Development of arterial blood pressure in the chick embryo. *Am. J. Physiol.*, 212:43–48.

126. Van Mierop, L. H. S., and Netter, F. H. (1969): Embryology. In: *CIBA Journal, Vol. 5: The Heart*, pp. 112–130. Ciba, Summit, N.J.

127. Van Mierop, L. H. S., Alley, R. D., Kausel, H. W., and Stranahan, A. (1962): The anatomy and embryology of endocardial cushion defects. *J. Thorac. Cardiovasc. Surg.*, 43:71–83.

128. Van Mierop, L. H. S., Alley, R. D., Kausel, H. W., and Stranahan, A. (1963): Pathogenesis of transposition complexes. I. Embryology of the ventricles and great arteries. *Am. J. Cardiol.*, 12:216–225.

129. Viragh, S., and Challice, C. E. (1973): Origin and differentiation of cardiac muscle cells in the mouse. *J. Ultrastruct. Res.*, 42:1–24.

130. Viragh, S., and Challice, C. E. (1973): The impulse generation and conduction system of the heart. In: *Ultrastructure of the Mammalian Heart*, edited by C. E. Challice and S. Viragh, pp. 43–89. Academic Press, New York.

131. Viragh, S., and Challice, C. E. (1981): The origin of the epicardium and the embryonic myocardial circulation in the mouse. *Anat. Rec.*, 201:157–168.

132. Voboril, Z., and Schiebler, T. H. (1969): Uber die Entwicklung der GefaBversorgung der Rattenherzens. *Z. Anat. Entwickl. Gesch.*, 129:24–40.

133. Weinstein, R. B., and Hay, E. D. (1970): Deoxyribonucleic acid synthesis and mitosis in differentiated cardiac muscle cells of chick embryos. *J. Cell Biol.*, 47:310–316.

134. Whalen, R. G., Sell, S. M., Eriksson, A., and Thornell, L.-E. (1982): Myosin subunit types in skeletal and cardiac tissues and their developmental distribution. *Dev. Biol.*, 91:478–484.

135. Willier, B. H., and Rawles, M. E. (1931): Developmental relations of the heart and liver in chorioallantoic grafts of whole chick blastoderms. *Anat. Rec.*, 48:277–301.

135a. Wilson, J. G., and Warkany, J. (1949): Aortic arch and cardiac anomalies in the offspring of vitamin A deficient rats. *Am. J. Anat.*, 85:113–155.

136. Zak, R. (1974): Development and proliferative capacity of cardiac muscle cells. *Circ. Res.*, 34–35(Suppl. II):17–26.

137. Zak, R. (1981): Contractile function as a determinant of muscle growth. In: *Cell and Muscle Motility*, edited by R. M. Dowben and J. W. Shay, Vol. 1, pp. 1–33. Plenum, New York.

138. Zak, R., Kizu, A., and Bugaisky, L. (1979): Cardiac hypertrophy: its characteristics as a growth process. *Am. J. Cardiol.*, 44:941–946.

Growth of the Heart in Health and Disease, edited by Radovan Zak. Raven Press, New York © 1984.

Functional Aspects of Cardiac Development

Edward B. Clark

Department of Pediatric Cardiology, University of Iowa, Hospital and Clinic, Iowa City, Iowa 52242

Studies on the development of the heart have a long history. In part this may be because of the interest one has when viewing an early embryo. In the chick, upon opening the shell, one's attention is drawn to the red pulsating embryonic heart. Aristotle wrote about his observations (96), and generations of students since have been struck by the fact that the heart is functional long before other parts of the embryo are discernible.

During the late nineteenth and early twentieth centuries, detailed investigation of human and mammalian embryos established the structural changes which occur during cardiac morphogenesis. [For a historical perspective see VanMierop (96), DeVries and Saunders (12), and Grant (33).] From the traditional structural studies that used gross dissection, wax plate reconstruction, and light microscopy, investigators devised theories about the mechanisms involved in development.

With the development of surgical techniques for the repair of heart defects, there was a renewed interest in the problem of normal and abnormal cardiac morphogenesis. Many of the theories have been based on deductive analysis of normal and abnormal hearts (98). Although this approach is valuable in establishing hypotheses for testing, experimental studies are still required for verification. The established traditional techniques of embryo studies do not take into account the functional role of the heart during development—which is to provide circulatory support for the embryo. From the early developmental stages of the pulsatile tube, the embryonic heart circulates blood in order to transport nutrients, deliver oxygen, and remove cellular waste products. Many investigators have speculated on the interrelationship of function and form in development (9–11,33), but definition of the mechanisms involved in cardiac development has not progressed as rapidly as research in other areas.

Studies in cardiac development are drawn from material of many species, in particular the chick, rat, mouse, and human embryos. Morphologic analysis of human material has been performed on serial sections and embryo reconstructions, the best known material being from the Carnegie collection originally described by Streeter (89–92). Recently scanning electron microscopy studies have been performed on human embryos, but this technique is limited by the availability of the later stages of heart development (73). The chick embryo is the model most often used for studies in cardiac development because of the ease of access to the embryo and the ability to accurately determine the stage of development (36). Experimental studies are almost all limited to analysis of chick material. The comparison of interspecies stages of development is facilitated by the data of Sissman (88) and Schneider and Norton (84).

In this chapter, I outline the morphologic steps in cardiac development and review the evidence of various developmental mechanisms which participate in morphogenesis. I pay particular attention to the intriguing hypothesis of flow molding, which has somewhat less than full scientific support. Finally, I review studies that characterize the functional aspects of the cardiovascular system during development.

TERMINOLOGY

One of the problems when reviewing the literature on cardiac development is the multitude of names given to the same structure. This confusion in terminology is a severe limiting factor when comparing previous studies. Some of the anatomic terms have their roots in antiquity, wherein others are used by investigators with allegiance to particular developmental theories. I use the terminology adopted by VanMierop because it is concise and widely accepted (95,96). Investigators have agreed on terminology for the proximal three portions of the heart: sinus venosus, primitive atrium, and primitive ventricle. It is naming the distal pole of the heart which causes the controversy (Fig. 1) (1,30,72,88). VanMierop, following Streeter (89), Kramer (50), and Shaner (86), referred to the pole between the primitive

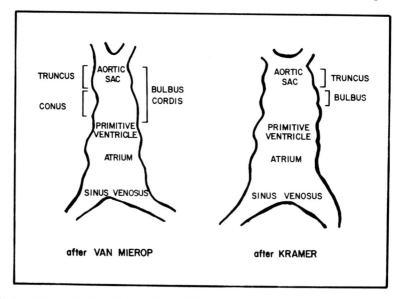

FIG. 1. The primitive heart tube, with the different terminology used for its components. (After Anderson et al., ref. 1.)

ventricle and aortic sac as the bulbus cordis. He subdivided the bulbus cordis into a proximal conus cordis and a distal truncus arteriosus. The latter is not to be confused with the congenital cardiac lesion with the same name which arises from a failure of division of the aortic sac and not of the truncus itself. Keith (48), as followed by Los (54), considered the outflow tract of the heart to be the bulbus and the truncus. A major problem in defining these areas is the fact that the heart tube never exists as it is shown in Fig. 1. As is mentioned later, the heart tube draws mesenchymal tissue from the distal end and incorporates it at the proximal end.

DESCRIPTIVE EMBRYOLOGY OF CARDIAC SEPTATION

The morphologic changes and probable mechanisms responsible for looping of the heart tube were described in a preceding chapter. In this section I briefly review the subsequent events in the partitioning of the heart tube to form the four-chambered adult structure found in birds and mammals. There are several excellent descriptions of the morphologic development of the heart. VanMierop's descriptions (95,96) are perhaps the clearest because of the detailed reconstruction drawings, but the contributions of Los (54) and DeVries and Saunders (12) and the original descriptions by Streeter (89–92) are also valuable. The reader is referred to these works for more detailed descriptions.

Aortic Arch Selections

There are six pairs of aortic arches in mammals and birds, only two or three of which are present at any one time. The first, second, and third pairs participate in the formation of the carotid artery system. In mammals the right fourth aortic arch involutes. The left fourth aortic arch persists as the transverse portion of the definitive aortic arch located between the left carotid and the left subclavian artery. In the chick the opposite occurs: The left fourth aortic arch involutes, and the right fourth aortic arch remains as the definitive aortic arch. From the mid-point of the bilateral sixth aortic arches, the pulmonary arteries grow toward the developing lung buds. In mammals the distal part of the left sixth aortic arch remains patent as the ductus arteriosus, and the right distal sixth aortic arch disappears.

Plastic casts of the aortic arch system of the chick embryo can be used to illustrate the development of the aortic arch system (Fig. 2). The casts are made by injecting an activated monomer into the vascular system of the chick embryo, allowing it to harden, and then digesting the tissue (7). At stage 18, the second and third aortic arches course from the ventral aorta sac to the dorsal aorta. By stage 28, the left fourth aortic arch has involuted and the right persists as the definitive aorta (Fig. 2 **bottom**). From the mid-point of the sixth arches, the true pulmonary arteries course caudally, adjacent to the lung bud. The mechanism responsible for determining which aortic arches remain patent and which involute appears to be related to the volume of flow through the vessels.

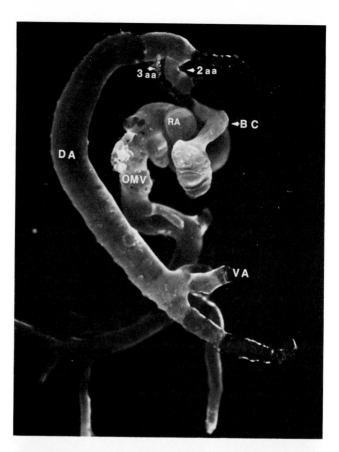

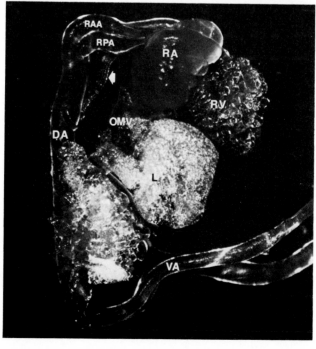

Partitioning of the Bulbus Cordis and Septation of the Ventricle

Septation of the arterial pole of the heart begins at the aortic sac and proceeds toward the ventricle. At the same time, the muscular interventricular septum develops to separate the right and left ventricular cordis. These processes are described in Chapter 30.

MECHANISMS OF CARDIAC DEVELOPMENT

Among the mechanisms often cited in cardiac development are: differential cell growth, cell death, cell migration, extracellular matrix production, and hemodynamic molding. Although traditionally studied individually, these factors are interrelated.

Differential Cell Growth

Classic studies on the rate of cellular replication in the heart involve calculation of a mitotic cell index (75). This index is the number of cells with active mitoses per 100 cells counted. The initial studies performed by Olivio and Slavich (65) reported the mitotic index to be highest during the cardiac loop stage of development and to gradually decrease during morphogenesis. Those studies, however, were not of tissue-specific mitotic indexes. Grohmann (34) studied the mitotic index of three tissue-specific areas: ventricular myocardium, interventricular septum, and atrial myocardium. He noted that the number of cells actively dividing differed from area to area, peaking on the fourth incubation day in the ventricle and 1 day later at the atrial level. Paschoud and Pexieder (68) undertook a more extensive analysis of the rate of cell turnover using a tritiated thymidine marker. With radioautographic techniques, these investigators studied the rate of cellular proliferation in the outflow tract of the chick embryo. They observed that the highest rates were in the endocardium and mesenchymal tissue within the confines of the bulbar cushions. The rate of marker incorporation paralleled the appearance of the proximal and distal cushions of the outflow tract. Although these studies identified areas of high proliferative activity which correlates with cushion growth, it is not clear how cell division is related to morphologic change. Manasek (57) emphasized that this technique does not identify subpopulations of cells which may have different division rates. In addition, some of the cellular material may be moving into the developing heart from adjacent mesenchymal areas in the aortic arch so that incorporation rates and mitotic indexes may reflect division of the migrating tissue as well as the inherent cell population.

─────

FIG. 2. **Top:** Plastic cast of the cardiovascular system from a stage 18 chick embryo viewed from the right. **Bottom:** Plastic cast of the cardiovascular system from a stage 28 chick embryo viewed from the right. True pulmonary artery courses to the lung bud *(arrow)*. *(DA)* dorsal aorta. *(BC)* bulbus cordis region. *(OMV)* omphalomesenteric vein. *(RA)* right atrium. *(2aa)* right second aortic arch. *(3aa)* right third aortic arch. *(VA)* vitelline artery. *(RAA)* right aortic arch. *(RPA)* right pulmonary artery. *(L)* liver. *(RV)* right ventricle. *(RA)* right aorta.

Cell Death

Cell death is a widely occurring process in cardiac development and is observed during primitive endocardial tube fusion, myocardial wall formation, and in the pulmonary artery and aorta and associated semilunar valves. Pexieder (71) systematically studied the location of cell death foci in the endocardial surface of the chick embryo heart and compared these areas in rat and human embryos. He also analyzed the effect of hemodynamics and teratogenic agents on the site and intensity of cell death in hearts *in ovo* and in organ culture. Cell death foci are located in the endothelium of the cushions which divide the atrioventricular (AV) canal, the bulbus cordis, and the walls of the pulmonary artery and aorta. Pexieder observed a change in the loci of cell death in chick hearts grown in culture. He suggested that intracardiac blood flow may have a modulating effect on the position of dead and dying cells, although extraneous effects including the artificial nature of the culture system may be present. He noted that teratogenic agents (dexamethasone and cyclophosphamide) markedly alter the number of stained phagocytes, which he used as an index of cell death.

Satow et al. (83) studied the site of cell death in the bulbar cushions of rat and chick embryos. They defined the pattern of cell death in normal embryos and the change in the pattern of cell death following teratogenic doses of ionizing radiation (64). These investigators described physiological cell death foci in the conal ridge of the embryo rat heart. They treated pregnant rats with a dose of neutron radiation that resulted in an 85% incidence of fetuses with a spectrum of conotruncal defects, including a double-outlet right ventricle and transposition of the great vessels. Analysis of the neutron-treated embryos showed a delay in the onset of cell death and a decrease in the intensity of death in the regions of the bulbar cushions. These investigators have proposed that altering the cell death patterns results in abnormal cushion tissue growth, which leads to morphologic abnormalities.

Although cell death is a well-recognized mechanism for morphologic change in other organ systems (82a), it is still not clear how this phenomenon is related to cardiac morphogenesis. A central issue is whether cell death is genetically controlled. Some investigators (83) have suggested that the death of some cells may be controlled by genetic mechanisms, whereas other cells may be affected by epigenetic or physiological phenomena. The experiments of Pexieder suggest that cell death may result from the hemodynamic forces present within the heart. However, the balance between "programmed" and epigenetically determined cell death is unresolved.

Mesenchymal Tissue Migration

An early event in cardiac development is the migration of precardiac mesoderm through the primitive streak to form the bilateral cardiac tubes (76,77). Cell migration is important in at least two other areas: septation of the arterial pole of the heart and the origin of cellular constituents of the endocardial cushions.

Rychter (79) observed that the rate of cell proliferation in the outflow tract is low at the time that there is a twofold increase in the length of this region. This suggests that cellular proliferation alone does not account for all the material accumulated during the growth of the outflow tract. Rychter (81) tentatively identified the source of this additional material as the prebranchial mesenchyme, which migrates from the aortic arch region to participate in aortic pulmonary septal formation.

Histologically, the aortic arch vessels are composed of hollow cords of dense mesenchyme rather than the three layers found in mature blood vessels. It is particularly interesting that this material seems to be asymmetrically arranged. Rychter placed carbon particles in the mesenchymal tissue along the inferior margin of the fourth and sixth aortic arches (85). Embryos were reincubated, harvested, and serially sectioned. The marks were noted to have migrated into the aortico-pulmonary septum. Carbon particles placed in the right sixth aortic arch mesenchyme appeared in the aorticopulmonary septum, whereas marks positioned in the left sixth aortic arch mesenchyme were located in the anterior portion of the truncus (Fig. 3). Thompson and Fitzharris (94) have also documented the movement of mesenchymal tissue from the branchial arch region into the developing heart. This asymmetrical contribution of material may be important in the partitioning of the outflow tract. VanMierop et al. (99) suggested that the pathogenesis of abnormalities of great vessel assignment, including transposition of the great vessels, results from abnormal septal positioning.

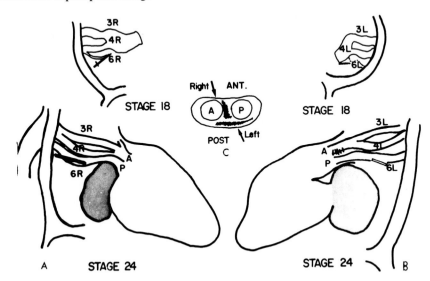

FIG. 3. Fate of carbon particles placed at stage 18 of incubation in the mesenchymal tissue adjacent to the **(A)** right *(R)* and **(B)** left *(L)* sixth aortic arches at stage 24. **C:** Coronal section through the divided outflow tract showing the asymmetrical position of the marks. (After Rychter, ref. 81.)

The other regions of the heart where cell migration is known to take place are the endocardial and bulbar cushions. Patten et al. (69) originally suggested that mesenchymal cells present in cardiac cushions are derived from the endothelial layer of the developing heart. Markwald et al. (60) confirmed these findings in the chick and rat. The cushion mesenchymal cells arise from the endocardial cells which line the atrioventricular canal and bulbus cordis. These cells are activated, develop motile apparatus, migrate into the cardiac jelly, and are transformed into cushion mesenchymal cells.

Kinsella and Fitzharris (49) have shown by cinephotography techniques that these cells break away from the endothelium and move into the extracellular matrix. The fate of these cells is unclear, but they probably participate in the formation of the atrioventricular valves, semilunar valves, and partitioning of the truncal and bulbar regions of the heart.

Extracellular Matrix: Cardiac Jelly

The extracellular matrix, which is the medium for cell migration in the endo-cardial cushions, is composed of glycoaminoglycans and collagen. This material, called cardiac jelly, is secreted primarily by the myocardial cells, although some of the material may be produced by the endocardium (56). The basic hypothesis is that the interaction of glycoaminoglycans and endocardium is important in the process of cellular seeding (59). There is a delay in the seeding of cells from the endothelium into the AV cushions in embryos treated with an agent which decreases the synthesis of glycoaminoglycans. Thus Markwald's experiments support a causal relationship between glycoaminoglycan composition and cell migration. Cardiac jelly and the extracellular matrix have other functions in cardiac development, as noted in Manasek's contribution to this volume. Important from the point of view of our discussion is the plastic nature of cardiac jelly and its response to a deforming force. Other aspects of the extracellular matrix are beyond the scope of this chapter, and the reader is referred to the reviews by Manasek and Markwald for further information.

Hemodynamic Molding

The heart provides circulatory support for the embryo during cardiac morpho-genesis. Thus investigators have speculated on some role of hemodynamic function in structural heart development. Spitzer was perhaps the most enthusiastic in his hypotheses, speculating that blood flow through the heart eroded and molded the cardiac chambers (52). However, defining and testing the relationship of hemody-namic function and form has been a difficult process. Although the theories for a hemodynamic role in heart development are intrinsically attractive, experimental studies provide only inferential support. The role of hemodynamic function seems to be operative at stages following formation of the cardiac loop, as Manasek and Monroe (58) have shown that blood flow is not necessary for loop formation.

Two bloodstreams which spiral around each other exist in the heart during development (Fig. 4). These streams arise from the confluence of blood entering the heart from the sinus venosus and the omphalomesenteric veins. The left stream crosses the boundary of the atrial septum, curves in the primitive ventricle (future area of the true left ventricle), courses in the right posterior lateral aspect to the bulbus cordis, and selectively flows to the fourth aortic arches (future aorta). The right stream courses through the right atrium and the right portion of the primitive ventricle, and spirals anteriorly through the left lateral aspect of the bulbus cordis to perfuse the sixth aortic arches (future pulmonary artery). These streams occupy the areas which will later form the ventricular cavities and coincide with the spiral course of the aorta and pulmonary artery.

How do these streams affect cardiac morphogenesis? Spitzer speculated that the bloodstream pattern had an eroding effect which can be likened to the forces at work in the hydraulic erosion of a meandering river. This is probably not accurate because material is not picked up and deposited as it is in other hydraulic systems (4a). Bremer (3) observed that the cushion tissue which participates in the septation appears to form in the region between the two streams. The current extended hypothesis states that hemodynamic forces mold the plastic cardiac jelly. Thus the diameter of the outflow tract would be determined by the relative dimension diameters of the two streams (43–45,53). With the processes of matrix elaboration and cellular seeding, the cushions bridge the cardiac lumen and fuse, dividing the outflow tract into the aorta and the pulmonary artery.

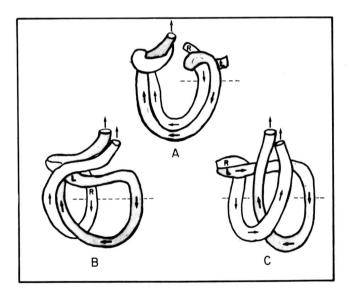

FIG. 4. Spiral bloodstreams in the chick embryo heart at 3 days of incubation. *Dashed line* represents the plane of the AV orifice. **A:** Stage 18. **B:** Stage 21. **C:** Stage 24. (After Bremer, ref. 3.)

The physiological separation of blood flow occurs early in phylogeny and appears to be an antecedent to anatomic septation. One question relates to the phylogenetic occurrence of these streams. Several investigators (20,21,35,47) demonstrated by selective stream labeling that saturated and desaturated blood remain separated in incompletely septated adult frog and toad ventricles. VanMierop (96) noted that physiological separation first occurs in the unseptated hearts of air-breathing fish. Separation of saturated and desaturated blood most likely precedes septation in the fetal lamb (13,14) and presumably in the human fetus.

Why do the streams form? They may do so because of the inherent configuration of the heart tube prior to looping. Goerttler (29) demonstrated streaming in rigid glass models based on early embryonic human hearts. He also showed that a plastic base substance lining the models was shifted to form ridges in the region between the two streams. He noted that the position and spiral course of the streams depended on the inflow angle of the venous fluid. Critical studies of these factors have not been performed in a biologic system.

Experiments designed to test the flow molding hypothesis are difficult to execute and interpret. Studies that have been performed involved the determination of ventricular chamber size, completion of ventricular septation, and selection of the aortic arches. These experiments fall into two broad groups: mechanical interference with developing vessels and teratogenic effects of cardiovascular pharmacologic agents. Some supporting data have also been obtained from analyses of human cardiac specimens with congenital defects. It must be stressed that in no case have investigations involved a controlled alteration of intracardiac blood flow. Rather, the experimental results have been related to manipulations that could be reasonably expected to alter flow patterns.

The two intracardiac streams are assumed to follow the hemodynamic principles of a parallel circuit. Thus an increase in resistance to right stream flow reduces the flow volume of the right stream and concomitantly increases the flow volume of the left stream. Partial occlusion of an atrium would be expected to reduce the compliance and volume of the chamber and subsequently reduce the volume of flow through that atrium. Rychter (80) applied metal clips to the left atrium for 24 to 48 hr and observed a reduction in left ventricular size and narrowing of the aortic outflow tract in surviving embryos. Harh et al. (38) placed nylon fibers through the left side of the atrioventricular canal and observed a decrease in left ventricular cavity size presumably secondary to a decrease in the left stream flow. Sweeney et al. (93), in an extensive series of experiments, excluded approximately two-thirds of the left atrium in embryos at 4 days of incubation, the mid-point of the active septation process. They observed a spectrum of abnormalities: a decrease in mitral valve orifice area, left ventricular volume, and aortic root diameter. They also noted aortic arch selection defects, including an absent fourth aortic arch, aortic coarctation, and hypoplasia of the ascending aorta. The right-sided structures, tricuspid valve area, right ventricular cavity volume, and pulmonary artery diameter were reciprocally enlarged. These experiments were interpreted to indicate that the volume of blood flowing through developing chambers at least in part determines the final cavity volume and orifice area.

Atkins et al. (2) observed in human heart specimens that the area ratio of the foramen ovale and atrial septum was a marker for the volume of transatrial blood flow *in utero*. They noted that the foramen ovale/atrial septal area in a group of defects with obligatory right-to-left atrial shunting (pulmonary atresia, tricuspid atresia) was markedly greater than that observed in normal specimens. Conversely, the area ratio was lower than normal in left-sided obstructive defects, including coarctation of the aorta and aortic valve stenosis.

Another group of experiments involved the outflow pole of the heart. Rychter (80) studied aortic arch selection by mechanically occluding aortic arch vessels individually and in combination. He noted that occlusion of the right fourth aortic arch resulted in the absence of the right aortic arch and persistence of a left aortic arch. He also observed that bilateral sixth aortic arch occlusion resulted in defects of the bulbar portion of the interventricular septum. Using peripheral vitelline vein injections of ink, he showed that the right stream was displaced from its normal position and joined the left stream in the outflow region of the heart. He concluded that blood flow was an important factor in the selection of aortic arches, and that the alteration of flow in the outflow region of the heart interfered with completion of bulbar septation.

Mechanical constriction or manipulation of the conotruncus also results in a change in pattern of the aortic arches. Gessner (24) observed abnormalities in aortic arch selection following elevation of the chick embryo bulbus cordis on a wire ramp. He concluded that the alteration in flow was responsible for the arch selection defects, although mechanical tension on the outflow tract may also have a teratogenic effect. Clark et al. (6) modified the outflow tract in chick embryos by constricting the mid-point of the bulbus cordis to one-half its normal diameter with a 10–0 nylon suture. This alteration in diameter produced an unpredictable change in laminar flow beyond the point of constriction and a spectrum of arch defects.

Analysis of human cardiac specimens provides some evidence to support an effect of hemodynamic molding. Hutchins (42) developed a hypothesis to explain the pathogenesis of coarctation of the aorta. He proposed that this defect represents a branch point in streaming of ductal blood flow. He noted histologic similarities between coarctation and the normal branch point at the bifurcation of the internal iliac arteries. Rudolph et al. (78) and Shinebourne and Elseed (87) supported a hemodynamic explanation for coarctation based on altered fetal blood flow patterns. Moulaert et al. (62) studied human cardiac specimens with aortic arch anomalies and calculated cross-sectional arch areas which correlated with a proposed decrease in fetal blood flow.

It is important to stress, however, that at no time has there been a quantification of alteration in blood flow in either experimental studies or the postmortem analysis of human congenital cardiac defects. The mechanical manipulations have been assumed to alter flow. Neither the total flow nor, perhaps even more importantly, the vector of flow has been measured. This represents a serious deficiency in these studies.

The second area of experimentation has involved studies of the teratogenic action of cardiovascular pharmacologic agents. In a series of papers, Gilbert and colleagues demonstrated that the administration of beta-adrenergic drugs results in anomalies of the outflow tract of the chick embryo heart (39). They also have noted that this teratogenic effect can be inhibited by beta-blocking drugs (26). The authors hypothesized that the teratogenic action of beta-adrenergic drugs is through an alteration of hemodynamic function which changes the intracardiac streams. They reported a decrease in cardiac output in isoproterenol-treated embryos (27). However, the techniques they used to quantify cardiac output—cardiac volume calculations from cinephotographs and cardiac impedance—have been neither validated nor demonstrated to have the precision needed in young embryos. In addition, Jaffee (46) and Gilani and Silvestri (25) reported a teratogenic action of beta-blocking drug alone. The causal relationship between these drugs and cardiac malformations is unclear.

Other problems common to pharmacologic studies in the chick embryo are the route of drug administration and the dose. In all the mentioned studies, the drug was administered by application to the vascular extraembryonic membrane. As a consequence, it is uncertain how much drug was absorbed into the circulatory system. The second problem relates to the quantity of drug required for a teratogenic effect. In the studies of Gilbert et al. (27), chick embryos received a dose of isoproterenol which if completely absorbed would have resulted in an approximately 1,000-fold greater drug concentration (based on a normalized milligram per kilogram embryo weight) than the accepted toxic range in older fetuses. The fact that the dose administered was outside the physiological range raises questions about the hemodynamic versus the toxic effects.

The action of any pharmacologic agent may not be limited to a single site. In the case of isoproterenol, the drug may have a negative inotropic effect on the myocardium and cause vasodilation in the extraembryonic circulation. Multiple drug actions may have a cumulative effect, but these would be difficult to analyze. Although it is important to demonstrate the potential teratogenicity of drugs on cardiac development, drugs with multiple actions may not be helpful in clarifying the question of hemodynamic effects on cardiac morphogenesis.

If one accepts that intracardiac blood flow has an effect on cardiac septation and chamber growth, the mechanisms of such effect are unclear. Several possibilities exist. Cardiac jelly, the extracellular material of the endocardial cushions, may be deformed by the bloodstreams similar to any other plastic substance. The rate and loci of endothelial cell death and proliferation may be modulated by hemodynamic forces. Pexieder (71) presented data to show that the loci of cell death in the bulbar cushions of the chick embryo heart change in location and intensity after a presumed change in endocardiac hemodynamics. He used the technique of Rychter (80) to occlude the bilateral sixth aortic arches. This alteration increased the number of dead and dying cells in the proximal bulbar cushions and was associated with an increased incidence of ventricular septal defects.

In adult vascular endothelium, stress from a jet lesion results in cellular changes and accumulation of extracellular material (23). It is reasonable to speculate that a similar response may occur in the embryonic endothelial cells and subsequently affect the cardiac jelly. Stress may also alter the motile characteristics of the endothelial cells which seed the cushions, leading to subsequent structural changes.

A change in bloodstreaming also changes the volume of blood passing through the region of the developing heart. This change in flow would change the pressure and stress applied to the heart and vessel walls. Fishman et al. (18) observed a marked alteration of left ventricular (LV) morphology in fetal lambs after obstruction to LV outflow presumably secondary to increased intracavitary pressure. Pexieder (70) measured mean blood pressure in the aortic arches. He noted that the blood pressure decreased as arch vessels began to involute, presumably because of a decrease in blood flow. The factors responsible for the decrease in aortic arch vessel blood flow were not defined but may include dilatation of the other paired arch vessels, active constriction of the involuting vessel, or a change in vectorial flow from the ventricle. The first two proposed mechanisms are unlikely because the arch vessels are devoid of muscle at these stages. At present it is not possible to quantitate vectorial flow. Therefore these possibilities remain within the realm of speculation until investigators measure the effect of the interaction of hemodynamic forces and the cell surface of the embryonic heart.

HEMODYNAMIC CHARACTERISTICS OF THE DEVELOPING EMBRYONIC CARDIOVASCULAR SYSTEM

From the previous discussion it is clear that progress in understanding the interrelationship of function and form in cardiac development depends on measuring the hemodynamic characteristics of the embryonic heart. This area has been largely neglected in part because of the lack of technical equipment for measuring pressure and flow in microsystems. In this section I review the studies on cardiac function and report the data from our laboratory. All of these studies have been done in the chick because of the ease of access to the embryo and the anatomic similarities to the mammalian heart. I do not propose, however, that the functional characteristics of the chick cardiovascular system are necessarily similar in every respect to that of the mammal.

Heart Rate

Heart rate is the most extensively studied characteristic of cardiac function. The embryonic heart rate is determined by a group of pacemaker cells located in the region of the sinus venosus (61). These cells are presumably the precursors to the sinus node, although conclusive proof for this is lacking. The remainder of the embryonic myocardium is capable of spontaneous depolarization (9). When separated, the ventricle and bulbus cordis have a slower rate of contraction than the atria. The faster-rate cells determine the rate for the whole system following reaggregation.

The embryonic chick heart begins to contract at 36 hr of incubation, and the rate accelerates rapidly throughout the first 3 days of incubation (75). We (5) studied the increase in rate from the third to the fifth incubation day, stages 18 to 27, and observed a gradual linear increase in rate similar to that observed by others (Fig. 5). The heart rate remains relatively consistent from incubation days 8 to 21 and increases only slightly just prior to hatching, presumably as a result of functional autonomic innervation (67).

The heart rate observed during development may not be that present during undisturbed incubation. These data were obtained by direct observation of embryos through an opening in the shell. The trauma of shell opening may affect the heart rate. In addition, the heart rate of the chick embryo is markedly susceptible to changes in environmental temperature. Studies both *in ovo* and *in vitro* demonstrated a linear relationship between heart rate and temperature (4,8,63,75). We speculated that this may be a protective mechanism, as the embryo is at risk for temperature fluctuation when the hen leaves the nest (100). Thus it is particularly important to control the environmental temperature because of the potential for change in heart rate. Experimental studies in which a change in heart rate alone is measured may be adversely affected by temperature fluctuation, whereas other parameters of myocardial contractility remain unaffected.

Blood Pressure

The initial blood pressure measurements in the chick embryo were made with a modified Landis apparatus (51). This technique uses the observation of the interface

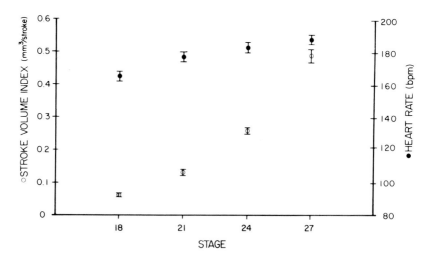

FIG. 5. Heart rate *(right ordinate)* and stroke volume index *(left ordinate)* in the chick embryo from stage 18 to 27 ($\bar{X} \pm$ SEM).

between blood and clear fluid in a capillary tube connected to a water column. When the height of the water column is such that the blood-fluid interface moves toward the embryo, the pressure exceeds the systolic pressure. Conversely, when the interface moves away from the embryo, the column height is less than the embryo's diastolic pressure. Although this technique is applicable for the estimation of pressures, reliance on visual perception of the fluid interface introduces a potential for error. Systolic and diastolic pressures are difficult to determine, and only the mean blood pressure can be accurately measured. Hughes (40) and Paff et al. (66) measured systolic, mean, and diastolic ventricular pressures by direct puncture of the ventricular cavity. Pexieder (70) used this technique to measure the blood pressure in aortic arches, and other investigators have used it to assess the effects of drugs (74) and hypoxia on the embryonic cardiovascular system (32).

With the development of the small volume displacement pressure transducer, it was possible to directly measure intravascular pressures. VanMierop and Bertuch (97) and Girard (28) have reported arterial pressures in chick embryos from 2 days of incubation to hatching. VanMierop and Bertuch used analog processing to correct for signal damping, which occurs in a small-lumen pipette. Girard used a large-diameter pipette inserted in the first branch vitelline arteries. Faber (15) measured intraventricular pressures by direct puncture. The data reported by these investigators vary somewhat. Some of the differences may be related to the degree of embryo development, which may vary considerably if determined only by incubation day instead of developmental stage. Only the data of VanMierop and Bertuch were reported by Hamburger-Hamilton stage.

We recently completed studies of normal intravascular pressures in chick embryos during the phase of rapid cardiac morphogenesis, stages 18 to 27 (5). We used a servo-null pressure measurement system originally developed by Falchuk and Berliner (17) and commercially available from WP Instruments (New Haven, CT). This system uses a 5 μm diameter pipette and has a 10 to 90% response time of approximately 20 msec. Thus pressure can be measured from the proximal extraembryonic arteries with little mechanical interference to blood flow and with excellent frequency response. We observed a gradual rise in systolic, diastolic, and mean arterial pressures during this phase of cardiac development (Fig. 6).

Patten et al. (69) first suggested that the endocardial cushions have a valvular action based on cinephotographs of the beating chick heart. Paff et al. (66), using the Landis blood pressure measurement technique, observed zero blood pressure in the ventricular cavity at 6 days of incubation, which they concluded was evidence for valve-like action by the cushions. We noted that there were distinct systolic and diastolic pressures as early as stage 18 (Fig. 7). This indicates that the outflow tract cushions have a valve-like action that maintains a diastolic pressure before there is significant progress in septation. We agree with VanMierop and Bertuch (97) that the valve-like action is present very early in development and continues through the formation of valve structures.

This valve-like action has important implications on cavitary pressures during development. If the ventricular diastolic pressure falls to zero with each cardiac

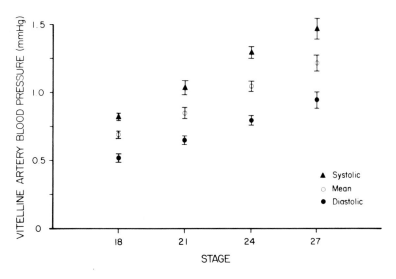

FIG. 6. Systolic, mean, and diastolic vitelline artery blood pressures in the chick embryo from stage 18 to 27 ($\overline{X} \pm$ SEM).

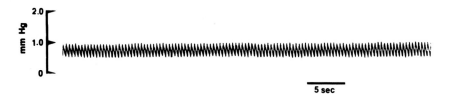

FIG. 7. Vitelline artery blood pressure recording from a stage 18 chick embryo. Note the distinct diastolic pressure indicating a valve-like action by the bulbar cushions.

cycle, the myocardial wall stress is much greater than if blood circulation was by peristaltic motion. Zak et al. (101) speculated that wall stress may have an important effect on myocardial formation.

Cardiac Output

Blood flow, or cardiac output, has been the most elusive of cardiac functional parameters to measure in the embryonic heart. Hughes (41) measured cardiac output from cinephotographic images of the heart. Faber et al. (16) analyzed a larger group of embryos using the same technique. They planimetered a single plane projection of the heart during end-systole and diastole, and calculated the difference in volume using the equation for a sphere. They observed a wide variability in cardiac output using this technique which they suspected was due to experimental "inaccuracies." Included in these inaccuracies is the fact that the heart at these stages is not a proloid ellipse or sphere but, rather, a bent tube. In addition, this technique measures the combined volume of blood, cardiac jelly, and myocardium because the ventricle is trabeculated and it is not possible to define the endocardial-blood margin.

We used a pulsed Doppler technique to measure dorsal aortic blood velocity (5). We calculated dorsal aortic blood flow from measurements of mean dorsal aortic blood velocity and dorsal aortic diameter. However, this technique underestimates cardiac output because blood flow to the head and myocardium originates before the point of measurement. We observed a progressive increase in dorsal aortic blood flow with increasing development (Fig. 8). Dorsal aortic blood flow remained surprisingly constant when corrected for embryo weight (Fig. 8). This suggests that there may be a metabolic control factor for cardiac output rather than simply an increase in circulatory blood volume, as proposed by Rychter et al. (82) and Faber et al. (16).

We also calculated a stroke volume index by dividing the dorsal aortic blood flow by the heart rate (Fig. 5). The doubling of the stroke volume index with embryo growth indicates that an enlargement in chamber size accounts for the majority of the increase in cardiac output, with a smaller component being the increase in heart rate.

Vascular Resistance

Using mean arterial pressure and mean dorsal aortic blood flow, we calculated an index of vascular resistance. Not surprisingly, we observed a progressive decrease in vascular resistance (Fig. 9). The factors responsible for the fall in vascular resistance are unclear, but at least three are possible: an increase in aortic size, the

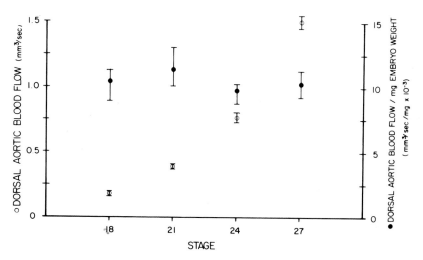

FIG. 8. Dorsal aortic blood flow *(left ordinate)* and blood flow normalized for embryo weight *(right ordinate)* in the chick embryo stage 18 to 27. Normalized blood flow is shown as the mean and 95 percentile confidence limits; it demonstrates little change with embryo growth.

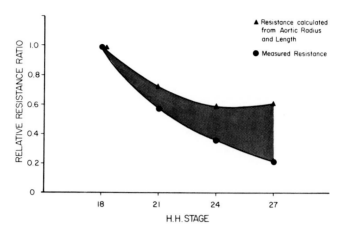

FIG. 9. Ratio of measured vascular resistance and the vascular resistance calculated from aortic diameter and length. The ratio at stage 18 is 1.0.

addition of new resistance vessels, and the development of vascular reactivity in existing vessels. As the embryo grows, the dorsal aorta increases in both diameter and length. We calculated the resistance attributed to the configurational changes in the aorta, assuming that resistance in a biologic system is proportional to the third power of the radius (Fig. 9) (31). The predicted decrease in resistance accounts for only one-half of the resistance drop measured. Therefore the other two factors—the addition of new resistance units, particularly in the extraembryonic bed, and the development of vascular reactivity—are also important.

DIRECTIONS FOR FURTHER RESEARCH

Progress in cardiac morphogenesis must proceed in several areas. The interrelationship of biomechanical stress and biochemical and morphologic changes in the myocardium has been studied in fetal and neonatal animals (22). Similar investigations need to be carried out on the embryonic heart. From our initial studies of the functional characteristics of the chick embryo, we speculate that there is a direct relationship between contractile mass and ventricular function during myocardial formation. Abnormalities of myocardial architecture, e.g., asymmetrical septal hypertrophy, may be disorders of early myocardial formation.

An additional area which has had little attention is the relationship between anatomic innervation of the heart and morphogenesis. Anatomic parasympathetic innervation occurs in the chick at about the time of the onset of the active septation process (67). However, functional innervation does not occur until the latter third of the incubation period. There is also a delay between anatomic and functional innervation of the sympathetic system. The extensive time period between the appearance of the autonomic nerves in the myocardium and their functioning is unexplained. The presence of nerves may alter the functional characteristics of the myocardium as well as serve as inducers of cardiac structures, e.g., atrioventricular valves.

Although there have been extensive studies of the fetal circulation, little is known about the embryonic vascular bed. During early development the extraembryonic vascular system appears to be larger than the embryonic vascular bed. The response of the beds needs to be determined. For example, does the extraembryonic vascular system respond to vasodilators whether hormonal or neural? Do changes in the vascular bed alter the volume and trajectory of the intracardiac streams? We speculate that some teratogenic agents exert their influence on the extraembryonic vascular system and, as a secondary manifestation, alter cardiac morphogenesis. Thus hemodynamic alterations during critical periods of development may be responsible for a proportion of the spectrum of human congenital cardiac defects.

Basic questions must also be answered relating biomechanical force to cell behavior. There is a need for well-controlled experiments studying the effect of changes in pressure and flow on cell proliferation, cell death, migration of mesenchymal tissue, and the elaboration and configuration of extracellular matrix. The techniques necessary to answer these and other questions related to cardiac morphology are available. The only element lacking is the interested investigator.

ACKNOWLEDGMENTS

The author wishes to thank Carleen Clark for her patience in compiling and checking the references and Sue Kucera for her skillful work with the manuscript. Dr. Clark is the recipient of NIH Research Career Development Award HD 00376.

REFERENCES

1. Anderson, R. H., Wilkinson, J. L., and Becker, A. E. (1978): The bulbus cordis and its derivatives. In: *Morphogenesis and Malformation of the Cardiovascular System*, edited by G. Rosenquist and D. Bergsma, pp. 1–28. Alan R. Liss, New York.
2. Atkins, D. L., Clark, E. B., and Marvin, W. J. (1982): Foramen ovale/atrial septum ratio: a marker of transatrial blood flow. *Circulation*, 66:281–283.
3. Bremer, J. L. (1932): The presence and influence of two spiral streams in the heart of the chick embryo. *Am. J. Anat.*, 49:409–440.
4. Cain, J. R., Abbott, U. K., and Rogallo, V. L. (1967): Heart rate of the developing chick embryo. *Proc. Soc. Exp. Biol. Med.*, 126:507–510.
4a. Callander, R. A. (1978): River meandering. *Annu. Rev. Fluid Mech.*, 10:129–158.
5. Clark, E. B., and Hu, N. (1982): Developmental hemodynamic changes in the chick embryo from stage 18 to 27. *Circ. Res.*, 51:810–815.
6. Clark, E. B., and Rosenquist, G. C. (1978): Spectrum of cardiovascular anomalies following cardiac loop constriction in the chick embryo. In: *Morphogenesis and Malformation of the Cardiovascular System*, edited by G. C. Rosenquist and D. Bergsma, pp. 431–442. Alan R. Liss, New York.
7. Clark, E. B., Rooney, P. R., Martini, D. R., and Rosenquist, G. C. (1979): Plastic casts of embyronic respiratory and cardiovascular system: a technique. *Teratology*, 19:357–360.
8. Cohn, A. E. (1927): Physiological ontogeny: A. Chicken Embryos. XIII. The temperature characteristic for the contraction rate of the whole heart. *J. Gen. Physiol.*, 10:369–375.
9. DeHaan, R. L. (1965): Morphogenesis of the vertebrate heart. In: *Organogenesis*, edited by R. DeHaan and H. Ursprung, pp. 377–419. Holt, Rinehart and Winston, New York.
10. DeHaan, R. L. (1967): Development of form in the embryonic heart. *Circulation*, 35:821–833.

11. DeHaan, R. L. (1970): Cardiac development: a problem in need of synthesis. *Am. J. Cardiol.*, 25:139–140.

12. DeVries, P. A., and Saunders, J. B. de C. M. (1962): Development of the ventricles and spiral outflow tract in the human heart. *Carnegie Inst. Contrib. Embryol.*, 37:87–114.

13. Edelstone, D. I., and Rudolph, A. M. (1979): Preferential streaming of ductus venosus blood to the brain and heart in fetal lambs. *Am. J. Physiol.*, 237:724–729.

14. Edelstone, D. I., Rudolph, A. M., and Heymann, M. A. (1978): Liver and ductus venous blood flows in fetal lambs in utero. *Circ. Res.*, 42:426–433.

15. Faber, J. J. (1968): Mechanical function of the septating embryonic heart. *Am. J. Physiol.*, 214:475–481.

16. Faber, J. J., Green, T. J., and Thornburg, K. L. (1974): Embryonic stroke volume and cardiac output in the chick. *Dev. Biol.*, 41:14–21.

17. Falchuk, K. H., and Berliner, R. W. (1971): Hydrostatic pressures in peritubular capillaries and tubules in the rat. *Am. J. Physiol.*, 220:1422–1426.

18. Fishman, N. H., Hof, R. B., Rudolph, A. M., and Heymann, M. A. (1978): Models of congenital heart disease in fetal lambs. *Circulation*, 58:354–364.

19. Deleted in proof.

20. Foxon, G. E. H. (1951): A radiographic study of the passage of the blood through the heart in the frog and toad. *Proc. Zool. Soc. (Lond.)*, 121:529–538.

21. Foxon, G. E. H. (1955): Problems of the double circulation in vertebrates. *Biol. Rev.*, 30:196–228.

22. Friedman, W. F. (1972): The intrinsic physiologic properties of the developing heart. In: *Neonatal Heart Disease*, edited by W. F. Friedman, M. Lesch, and E. H. Sonnenblick, pp. 21–50. Grune & Stratton, New York.

23. Fry, D. L. (1968): Acute vascular endothelial changes associated with increased blood velocity gradients. *Circ. Res.*, 22:165–197.

24. Gessner, I. H. (1966): Spectrum of congenital cardiac anomalies produced in chick embryo by mechanical interference with cardiogenesis. *Circ. Res.*, 18:625–663.

25. Gilani, S. H., and Silvestri, A. (1977): The effect of propranolol upon chick embryo cardiogenesis. *Exp. Cell. Biol.*, 45:158–166.

26. Gilbert, E. F., Bruyere, H. J., Ishikawa, S., Cheung, M. D., and Hodach, R. J. (1977): The effect of practolol and butoxamine on aortic arch malformation in beta adrenoreceptor stimulated chick embryos. *Teratology*, 15:317–324.

27. Gilbert, E. F., Bruyere, H. J., Ishikawa, S., Foulke, L. M., and Heimann, S. R. (1980): Role of decreased cardiac output in isoproterenol-induced cardiovascular teratogenesis in chick embryos. *Teratology*, 21:299–307.

28. Girard, H. (1973): Arterial pressure in the chick embryo. *Am. J. Physiol.*, 224:454–460.

29. Goerttler, K. (1968): Glass model experiments of embryonic human hearts. In: *Cardiac Development with Special Reference to Congenital Heart Disease*, edited by O. C. Jaffee. University of Dayton Press, Dayton, Ohio.

30. Goor, D. A., and Lillehei, C. W. (1976): *Congenital Malformations of the Heart: Embryology, Anatomy and Operative Considerations*. Grune & Stratton, New York.

31. Gow, B. S. (1980): Circulatory correlates: vascular impedance resistance and capacity. In: *Handbook of Physiology, The Cardiovascular System, Vol. II: Vascular Smooth Muscle*, edited by D. F. Bohr, A. P. Somlyo, and H. V. Sparks. American Physiological Society, Bethesda.

32. Grabowski, C. T., Tsai, E. N. C., and Toben, H. R. (1969): The effects of teratogenic doses of hypoxia on the blood pressure of chick embryos. *Teratology*, 2:67–76.

33. Grant, R. P. (1962): The embryology of the ventricular flow pathways in man. *Circulation*, 25:756–779.

34. Grohmann, D. (1961): Mitotische Wachstumintesitat des Embryonalen und Fetalen Hunchenherzens und ihre Bedeutung fur Entstehung Von Herzmissbildung. *Z. Zellforsch.*, 55:104–122 [cited by DeHaan (9)].

35. Haberich, F. J. (1965): The functional separation of venous and arterial blood in the univentricular frog heart. *Ann. N.Y. Acad. Sci.*, 127:459–476.

36. Hamburger, V., and Hamilton, H. L. (1951): A series of normal stages in the development of the chick embryo. *J. Morphol.*, 88:49–92.

37. Deleted in proof.

38. Harh, J. Y., Paul, M. H., Gallen, W. J., Friedberg, D. Z., and Kaplan, S. (1973): Experimental production of hypoplastic left heart syndrome in the chick embryo. *Am. J. Cardiol.*, 31:51–56.

39. Hodach, R. J., Hodach, A. E., Fallon, J. F., Folts, J. D., Bruyere, H. J., and Gilbert, E. F. (1975): The role of beta-adrenergic activity in the production of cardiac and aortic arch anomalies in chick embryos. *Teratology*, 12:33–45.

40. Hughes, A. F. W. (1942): The blood pressure of the chick embryo during development. *J. Exp. Biol.*, 19:232–237.

41. Hughes, A. F. W. (1949): The heart output of the chick embryo. *J. R. Microsc. Soc.*, 69:145–152.

42. Hutchins, G. M. (1971): Coarctation of the aorta explained as a branch-point of the ductus arteriosus. *Am. J. Pathol.*, 62:203–207.

43. Jaffee, O. C. (1962): Hemodynamics and cardiogenesis: the effects of altered vascular patterns on cardiac development. *J. Morphol.*, 110:217–221.

44. Jaffee, O. C. (1965): Hemodynamic factors in the development of the chick embryo heart. *Anat. Rec.*, 151:69–74.

45. Jaffee, O. C. (1967): The development of the arterial outflow tract in the chick embryo heart. *Anat. Rec.*, 158:35–42.

46. Jaffee, O. C. (1972): Effects of propranolol on the chick embryo heart. *Teratology*, 5:153–158.

47. Johnsen, K. (1965): Cardiovascular dynamics in fishes, amphibians and reptiles. *Ann. N.Y. Acad. Sci.*, 127:414–442.

48. Keith, A. (1924): Schorstein lecture on the fate of the bulbus cordis in the human heart. *Lancet*, 2:1267–1273.

49. Kinsella, M. G., and Fitzharris, T. P. (1980): Origin of cushion tissue in the developing chick embryo: cinematographic recordings of in-situ formation. *Science*, 207:1359–1360.

50. Kramer, T. C. (1942): The partitioning of the truncus and conus and the formation of the membranous portion of the ventricular septum in the human heart. *Am. J. Anat.*, 71:343–370.

51. Landis, E. M. (1926): The capillary pressure in frog mesentery as determined by micro injection methods. *Am. J. Physiol.*, 75:548–571.

52. Lev, M., and Vass, A. (1951): *Spitzer's Architecture of Normal and Malformed Hearts*. Charles C Thomas, Springfield, Illinois.

53. Leyhane, J. C. (1969): Visualization of blood streams in the developing chick heart. *Anat. Rec.*, 163:312–313.

54. Los, J. A. (1969): Embryology. In: *Watson's Paediatric Cardiology*. L. Luc, London.

55. Deleted in proof.

56. Manasek, F. J. (1975): The extracellular matrix of the early embryonic heart. In: *Developmental and Physiological Correlates of Cardiac Muscle*, edited by M. Lieberman and T. Sano, pp. 1–20. Raven Press, New York.

57. Manasek, F. J. (1979): Organization interactions and environment of heart cells during myocardial ontogeny. In: *Handbook of Physiology*, Sect. 2 Vol. I, edited by R. M. Berne, pp. 29–42. American Physiological Society, Bethesda.

58. Manasek, F. J., and Monroe, R. G. (1972): Early cardiac morphogenesis is independent of function. *Dev. Biol.*, 27:584–588.

59. Markwald, R. R. (1979): The role of extracellular matrix in cardiogenesis. *Tex. Rep. Biol. Med.*, 39:249–333.

60. Markwald, R. R., Fitzharris, T. P., and Manasek, F. J. (1977): Structural development of endocardial cushions. *Am. J. Anat.*, 148:85–120.

61. Mitchell, S. (1969): *Proceedings of the Conduction Development Conference*, May 27–28. National Heart Lung Institute, Bethesda.

62. Moulaert, A. J., Bruins, C. C., and Oppenheimer-Dekker, A. (1976): Anomalies of the aortic arch and ventricular septal defects. *Circulation*, 53:1011–1015.

63. Murray, H. A. (1925): Physiological ontogeny: A. Chicken embryos. X. The temperature characteristic for the contraction rate of isolated fragments of embryonic muscle. *J. Gen. Physiol.*, 9:781–803.

64. Okamoto, N., Satow, Y., Hidaka, N., and Akimoto, N. (1980): Anomalous development of the conotruncus in neutron-irradiated rats. In: *Etiology and Morphogenesis of Congenital Heart Disease*, edited by R. VanPraagh and A. Takao, pp. 195–214. Futura Publishing Co., Mt. Kisco, New York.

65. Olivo, O. M., and Slavich, E. (1930): Ricerche sulla velocita dell' accrescimento delle cellule e degli organi. *Arch. Entwicklungsmech.*, 121:96–110 [cited by DeHaan (9)].

66. Paff, G. H., Boucek, R. J., and Gutten, G. S. (1965): Ventricular blood pressures and competency of valves in the early embryonic chick heart. *Anat. Rec.*, 151:119–123.

67. Pappano, A. J. (1977): Ontogenic development of autonomic neuroeffector transmission and transmitter reactivity in embryonic and fetal hearts. *Pharmacol. Rev.*, 29:3–33.

68. Paschoud, N., and Pexieder, T. (1981): Patterns of proliferation during the organogenetic phase of heart development. In: *Mechanisms of Cardiac Morphogenesis and Teratogenesis*, edited by T. Pexieder, pp. 73–88. Raven Press, New York.

69. Patten, B. M., Krammer, T. C., and Barry, A. (1948): Vascular action in the embryonic chick heart by localized apposition of endocardial masses. *Anat. Rec.*, 102:299–312.

70. Pexieder, T. (1969): Blood pressure in the third and fourth aortic arches and morphologic influence of laminar blood streams in the development of the vascular system of the chick embryo. *Folia Morphol. (Praha)*, 17:273–290.

71. Pexieder, T. (1975): Cell death in the morphogenesis and teratogenesis of the heart. *Adv. Anat. Embryol. Cell Biol.*, 51(Fasc.3):1–100.

72. Pexieder, T. (1978): Development of the outflow tract of the embryonic heart. In: *Morphogenesis and Malformation of the Cardiovascular System*, edited by G. Rosenquist and D. Bergsma, pp. 29–68. Alan R. Liss, New York.

73. Pexieder, T. (1982): Personal communication.

74. Rajala, G. M., and Kaplan, S. (1980): Abnormally elevated blood pressure in the trypan blue treated chick embryo during early morphogenesis. *Teratology*, 21:247–251.

75. Romanoff, A. L. (1960): *The Avian Embryo: Structure and Functional Development*. Macmillan, New York.

76. Rosenquist, G. C. (1970): Location and movements of cardiogenic cells in the chick embryo: the heart forming portion of the primitive streak. *Dev. Biol.*, 22:461–475.

77. Rosenquist, G. C., and DeHaan, R. L. (1966): Migration of precardiac cells in the chick embryo: a radio autographic study. *Carnegie Inst. Wash. Publ. 625 Contrib. Embryol.*, 38:111–121.

78. Rudolph, A. M., Heymann, M. A., and Spitznas, U. (1972): Hemodynamic considerations in the development of narrowing of the aorta. *Am. J. Cardiol.*, 30:514–524.

79. Rychter, Z. (1959): The vascular system of the chick embryo. III. On the problem of septation of the heart bulb and trunk in chick embryos. *Cesk. Morfol.*, 7:1–20.

80. Rychter, Z. (1962): Experimental morphology of the aortic arches and the heart loop in chick embryo. *Adv. Morphogen.*, 2:333–371.

81. Rychter, Z. (1978): Analysis of relations between aortic arches and aorticopulmonary septation. In: *Morphogenesis and Malformation of the Cardiovascular System*, edited by G. Rosenquist and D. Bergsma, pp. 443–448. Alan R. Liss, New York.

82. Rychter, Z., Kopecky, M., and Lemez, L. (1955): The blood of chick embryos. IV. On the circulating blood volume from the 2nd day of incubation till hatching. *Cesk. Morfol.*, 3:11–25.

82a. Saunders, J. W. (1966): Death in embryonic systems. *Science*, 154:604–612.

83. Satow, Y., Okamoto, N., Akimoto, N., Hidaka, N., Miyabara, S., and Pexieder, T. (1981): Comparative and morphometric study on genetically programmed cell death in rat and chick embryonic heart. In: *Mechanisms of Cardiac Morphogenesis and Teratogenesis*, edited by T. Pexieder, pp. 115–126. Raven Press, New York.

84. Schneider, B. F., and Norton, S. (1979): Equivalent ages in rat, mouse, and chick embryos. *Teratology*, 19:273–278.

85. Seichert, V. (1965): Study of the tissue and organ anlage shifts by the method of plastic linear marking. *Folia Morphol. (Praha)*, 12:228–238.

86. Shaner, R. F. (1962): Comparative development of bulbus and ventricles of vertebrate heart with special reference to Spitzer's theory of heart malformations. *Anat. Rec.*, 142:519–529.

87. Shinebourne, E. A., and Elseed, A. M. (1974): Relation between fetal flow patterns, coarctation of the aorta and pulmonary blood flow. *Br. Heart J.*, 36:492–498.

88. Sissman, N. J. (1970): Developmental landmarks in cardiac morphogenesis: comparative chronology. *Am. J. Cardiol.*, 25:141–146.

89. Streeter, G. L. (1942): Developmental horizons in human embryos: description of age groups XI 13–20 somites and age group XXII 21–29 somites. *Contrib. Embryol.*, 30:211–245.

90. Streeter, G. L. (1945): Development horizons in human embryos: description of age group XIII, embryos about 4–5 mm long, and age group XIV, period of indention of the lens vesicle. *Contrib. Embryol.*, 31:27–63.

91. Streeter, G. L. (1948): Developmental horizons in human embryos: description of age group XV, XVI, XVII, XVIII. *Contrib. Embryol.*, 32:113–203.
92. Streeter, G. L. (1951): Developmental horizons in human embryos: description of age group XIX, XX, XXI, XXII, XXIII. *Contrib. Embryol.*, 34:165–196.
93. Sweeney, L. J. (1981): Morphometric analysis of an experimental model of left heart hypoplasia in the chick. Ph.D. thesis, University of Nebraska Medical Center, Omaha, Nebraska.
94. Thompson, R. D., and Fitzharris, T. P. (1979): Morphogenesis of the truncus arteriosus of the chick embryo heart: the formation and migration of mesenchymal tissue. *Am. J. Anat.*, 154:545–556.
95. VanMierop, L. H. S. (1969): Embryology of the heart. In: *The Ciba Collection of Medical Illustrations: The Heart*, edited by F. H. Netter, pp. 112–130. Ciba, Summit, New Jersey.
96. VanMierop, L. H. S. (1979): Morphological development of the heart. In: *Hand Book of Physiology*, Sect. 2, Vol. I, edited by R. M. Berne, pp. 1–28. American Physiological Society, Bethesda.
97. VanMierop, L. H. S., and Bertuch, C. J. (1971): Development of arterial blood pressure in the chick embryo. *Am. J. Physiol.*, 212:43–48.
98. VanMierop, L. H. S., and Gessner, I. H. (1972): Pathogenic mechanisms in congenital cardiovascular malformations. *Prog. Cardiovasc. Dis.*, 15:67–85.
99. VanMierop, L. H. S., Alley, R. D., Kausel, H. W., and Stranahan, A. (1963): Pathogenesis of transposition complexes: embryology of the ventricles and great arteries. *Am. J. Cardiol.*, 12:216–225.
100. Wispé, J., Hu, N., and Clark, E. B. (1983): Response of the chick cardiovascular system to hypothermia. *Pediatr. Res.*, 17:945–948.
101. Zak, R., Kizu, A., and Bugaisky, L. (1979): Cardiac hypertrophy: its characteristics as a growth process. *Am. J. Cardiol.*, 44:941–947.

Growth of the Heart in Health and Disease,
edited by Radovan Zak. Raven Press,
New York © 1984.

Early Heart Development:
A New Model of Cardiac Morphogenesis

*,**Francis J. Manasek, †Robert R. Kulikowski, *Atsuyo
Nakamura, **Quynhchi Nguyenphuc, and *Joan W. Lacktis

*Departments of *Anatomy and **Pediatrics, University of Chicago, Chicago, Illinois
60637; †Departments of Anatomy and Physiology, Milton S. Hershey Medical Center,
Hershey, Pennsylvania 17033*

Cardiac embryology has traditionally been a descriptive science. It has produced a large body of accurate, detailed studies of heart development which have yielded a significant understanding of the structural chronology of the developing heart at levels of resolution ranging from the ultrastructural to the gross anatomic. From data such as these, attempts have been made to discern mechanisms involved in the formation and malformation of adult structures. For example, it was observed that endocardial cushions swell, fuse, and are remodeled to develop into structures such as the membranous portions of the interventricular septum and valves. Clearly, membranous septum development is regulated by certain tissue properties. In order to understand development at this level we must understand the basic cell biology of the constituent cells, but it is necessary to view cell activities in an integrated context if we are to discern their relationships to tissue shape. It is at this point where attempts to discern morphogenic mechanisms become very difficult. Experimental work is needed to determine causal relationships between cell properties and organ shape. However, the size of the catalogue of known cell activities is so large that it is impossible to test each cell activity for its morphogenetic functions.

In the case of heart development it is most likely that mechanisms controlling shape are not unique to the cardiac structures but that they represent variants of general morphogenic mechanisms operative throughout the embryo. Thus we need not look for special "heart shape factors" but, rather, should place the problem of cardiac development into a broader biological context.

In this chapter we consider one of the most important aspects of the early embryonic growth of the heart, i.e., the mechanisms which effect and regulate its changing shape. We present a model of heart looping which is based largely on a series of experimental and descriptive studies done in this laboratory over the past 15 years. This model provided the basis for a mechanical analog of the looping heart that mimics normal biological shape changes. We propose that the model presented here represents a specialized case of a general morphogenic mechanism operative during early development.

The chapter is divided into three main parts. We first consider the salient aspects of the morphology of the developing heart rudiment and then the possible basis for shape change; finally, we construct our model for looping.

MORPHOLOGICAL CONSIDERATIONS

Looping, we will try to demonstrate, is the morphological consequence of a coordinated series of biochemical events occurring in a developing organ with a unique shape. These biochemical events appear to produce forces that act in a mechanical way to deform the preexisting shape (14). Biological form is therefore viewed not only as an endpoint but as a regulator that dictates and to some degree limits the next possible sequence of shapes. In this section we consider the shape transformations exhibited by the looping heart.

Looping does not "begin" at any specific stage but, rather, represents two components (bending and rotation) of a developmental continuum. It is convenient, however, to distinguish operationally between a "prelooped" and a "looped" heart. The former is more or less bilaterally symmetrical, whereas the latter is distinctly C-shaped. It is germane to point out, in this context, that there is a large morphological variation in hearts at the time of looping (26). Morphological categories are therefore subjective to a large degree, and there is to date no good quantitative method for describing the changing heart shape and defining the morphologic limits of normal development.

Formation of the Tubular Heart

The early chick heart is an epithelial organ that is completely lacking in mesenchymal cells (10). The organ is formed in vertebrates by fusion of bilateral epithelial sheets of splanchnic mesoderm. This fusion has been described in detail (for review see ref. 4). In general, fusion begins at the anterior end and progresses caudad, but there is some evidence that the outflow tract region (variously called conus, bulbus, etc.) is formed after the rest of the tubular structure has fused (3).

The early partially fused primordia appear as raised elevations of the splanchnic mesoderm (Fig. 1). The raised portion of splanchnic mesoderm is destined to become the myocardium, and at this time its cells are all premyocardial cells, or myoblasts. The ultrastructure of these cells does not provide any clues to their myogenic potential. No morphologically recognizable myofilaments can be seen in their cytoplasm (10,25). As myofibrillogenesis begins at a later stage, it is not possible to unequivocally distinguish between precardiac cells and nonmyogenic mesodermal cells on the basis of their ultrastructure alone.

The scanning electron microscope shows that the nascent myocardial surface has a flabby appearance with marked folds and wrinkles (Figs. 1 and 2). There is no noticeable difference between the right and left sides that can be observed consistently. On either side of the myocardial bulges there is a relatively flat zone of splanchnic mesoderm (Fig. 2) that does not become incorporated into the heart. The lateral boundary of the splanchnic mesoderm, where it is continuous with

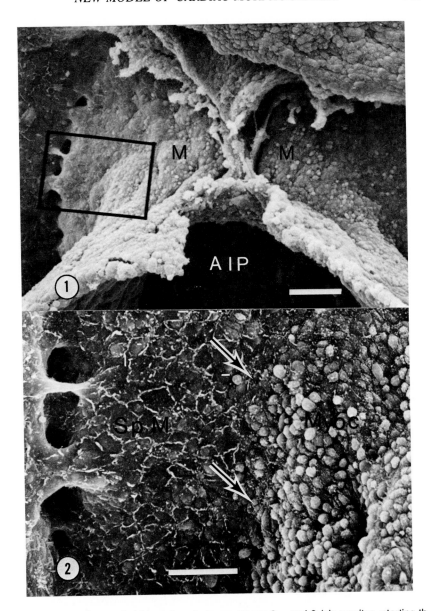

FIG. 1. Heart rudiment of chick embryo between stages 9− and 9 (six somites, starting the seventh). The presumptive myocardium *(M)* appears as a swelling on either side of the ventral mesocardium. The splanchnic mesoderm, continuous with the developing myocardium, is a flattened shield. Buttress-like cellular configurations are seen at its interface with the somatic mesoderm. *(AIP)* anterior intestinal portal. **Inset:** See Fig. 2. Scale: 0.05 mm.

FIG. 2. Higher magnification of the area in Fig. 1. Note the general "flabby" appearance of the myocardium *(Myoc)*, with the folds and wrinkles in the surface. There is a relatively sharp boundary *(arrows)* between the myocardium and the splanchnic mesoderm *(SpM)*, the latter of which appears taut. There are no wrinkles or folds, and the cells appear flattened. The buttresses between splanchnic and somatic mesoderm are seen at the left. Scale: 25 μm.

somatic mesoderm, is a clearly demarcated zone. There are buttress-like groups of cells that bridge the zone between the splanchnic and the somatic mesoderm (Figs. 1 and 2).

The precardiac mesodermal cells (myoblasts) have bulging apical surfaces that are characterized by extensive microplicae (Fig. 3). In contrast, the splanchnic mesoderm on either side of the heart consists of more flattened cells that have reduced apical bulges and lack extensive microplicae (Fig. 4).

The Tubular Heart

Increased outward bulging of the primitive myocardial wall produces a more readily apparent heart rudiment (compare Figs. 1 and 5). At stage 9+ (Fig. 5) the ventral mesocardium is beginning to rupture, marking the essentially complete fusion of right and left rudiments. At this stage the forming heart still has the appearance of being a swollen region of mesoderm. The remainder of the splanchnic mesoderm on either side of the heart is still relatively flat (Figs. 5 and 6), in contrast to the myocardial wall, which remains folded and convoluted (Fig. 6). Closer examination of myocardial cells demonstrates the continued presence of extensive microplicae on their apical surfaces (Figs. 7 and 8).

Continued fusion and bulging of the cardiac regions produce a more clearly defined, elongated heart whose diameter is unequal along its length (Figs. 9 and 10). The ventral mesocardium has ruptured and the ventral surface of the heart is no longer attached (Fig. 9). There is still, however, a remnant of the fusion furrow visible on the ventral surface (Fig. 10). This anatomic landmark demarcates the contributions of the right-sided from the left-sided precardiac mesoderm. The entire heart is more clearly separated from the splanchnic mesoderm (Fig. 10) and no longer appears as a simple bulge. Rather, the dorsal mesocardium appears pinched in, with the lateral sides of the heart overhanging it to a considerable extent. The splanchnic mesoderm is still a flattened layer, and its interface with the somatic mesoderm is characterized by the continued presence of the buttress-like cell formations (Figs. 7 and 8).

Bending and Rotation

The heart, viewed from the ventral aspect, now has a clearly tubular shape and has lost all traces of a fusion furrow (Fig. 11). A prominent sulcus, representing a fold or kink in the myocardial epithelium, has developed in the left side, and the entire structure is bending to the embryonic right side.

Marking experiments (16,30) have shown clearly that the tube is also rotating to the right. In these experiments, the myocardial surface was exposed by removing the pericardial membranes. Particles of iron oxide were placed on the heart surface, and the preparations were examined by means of light microscopy. Over a period of a few hours the particles, representing discrete myocardial loci, were seen to move to the right side. As the particles were firmly adherent to the myocardium, their movement reflected myocardial movement, i.e., rotation. Rotation was greater

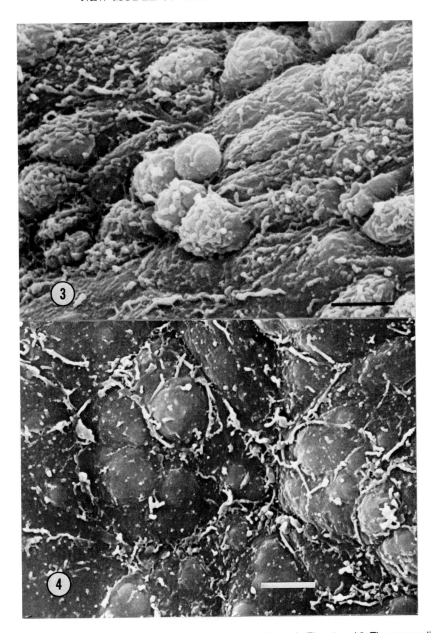

FIG. 3. Higher magnification of the myocardial surface shown in Figs. 1 and 2. The myocardial cells bulge outward and are covered by numerous microridges (microplicae). Scale: 5 μm.

FIG. 4. Higher magnification of the surface of splanchnic mesoderm (Fig. 2) shows the more flattened characteristics. The surface is not covered with microridges, but there are prominent marginal lamellae. Scale: 5 μm.

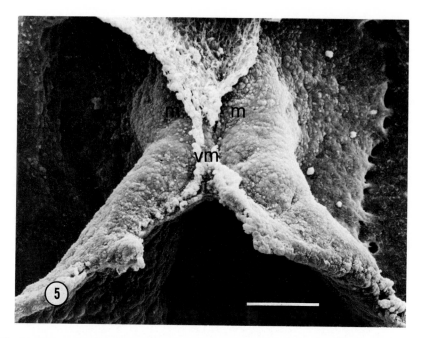

FIG. 5. Stage 9+ chick embryo (eight somites). The myocardium *(m)* appears more elevated than is seen in Fig. 1. The ventral mesocardium *(vm)* is still present, although it is beginning to rupture. Scale: 0.1 mm.

at the latitude of the developing ventricular bulge. Because rotation is not equal along the length of the tube and the ends are fixed, rotational shear is introduced. Such shear must be presumed to have morphological consequences.

Myocardial Cell Surface Topology

Early myocardial cells (to stage 9+) were seen to have extensive microplicae as part of their apical surfaces (Figs. 3, 7, and 8). By the time the heart is looped (Fig. 11), distinct changes have taken place in cell surface topography. The conotruncal region consists largely of flattened cells with marginal lamellopodia (Fig. 12), whereas the rest of the myocardial surface consists of cells with bulging apical surfaces (Fig. 13). There is a wide range in the apical surface areas of these cells (16), and in general the cells with the larger apical areas have fewer microplicae (Fig. 13).

Dorsal Mesocardium

The dorsal mesocardium is more persistent than the ventral mesocardium, and the tubular heart remains attached along its dorsal surface until after bending and rotation are well advanced.

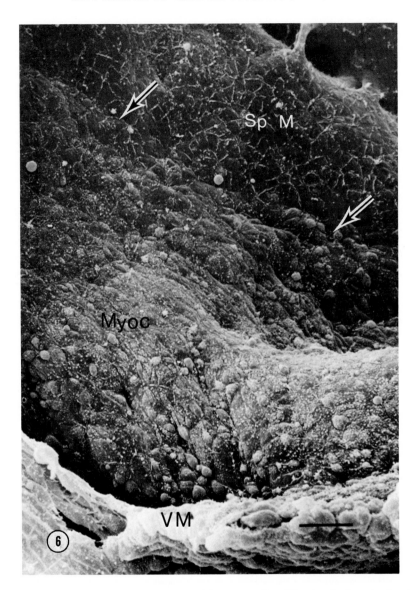

FIG. 6. A higher magnification of a portion of the myocardium *(Myoc)* and adjacent splanchnic mesoderm *(SpM)* of a stage 9+ embryo. The boundary between myocardium and splanchnic mesoderm can be determined by surface features; it is quite distinct *(arrows)*. The myocardium is still characterized by infoldings and has a wrinkled appearance compared to the splanchnic mesoderm. *(VM)* ventral mesocardium. Scale: 20 μm.

The dorsal mesocardium is initially (prior to about stage 10−) a broad area which defines the rather wide, incomplete dorsum of the fusing cardiac troughs. Although at these stages it is probably not quite accurate to call it a mesocardium,

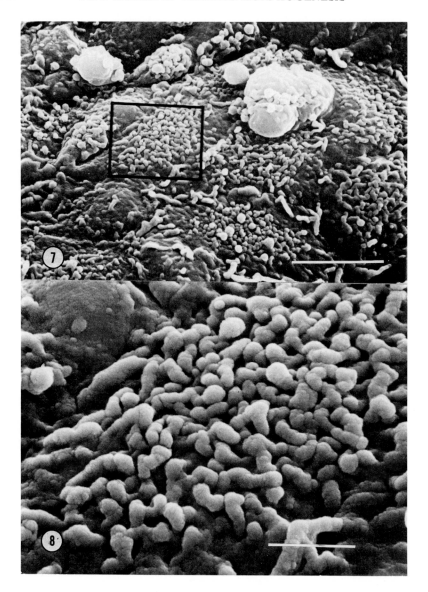

FIG. 7. Higher magnification of the myocardial surface from a stage 9+ embryo reveals the continued presence of extensive surface folds.   **Inset:** See Fig. 8. Scale: 5 μm.
FIG. 8. Higher magnification of the region marked in Fig. 7. The outer membrane of the developing myocardial cells (myoblasts) are extremely folded and tortuous. It is proposed that this provides "spare" membrane for future cell shape changes, resulting in cells that have more surface area. Scale: 1 μm.

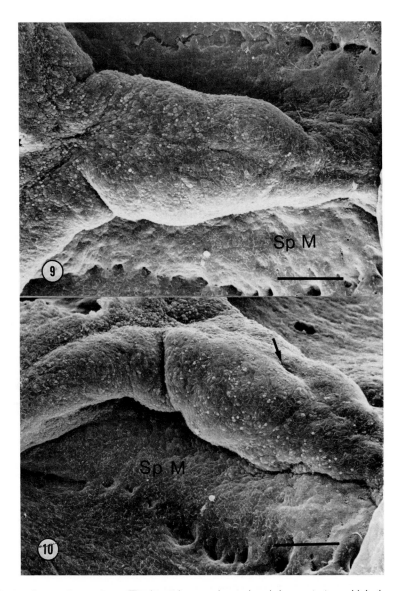

FIG. 9. Stage 10 – embryo. The heart is now elevated and demonstrates a high degree of bilateral symmetry. The paired vitelline veins are to the left. *(SpM)* splanchnic mesoderm. Scale 0.1 mm.

FIG. 10. Oblique view of the heart shown in Fig. 9. Although the ventral mesocardium has disappeared, the fusion furrow *(arrow)* is still visible. The heart appears to be more turgid than in Fig. 5. *(SpM)* splanchnic mesoderm. Scale: 0.1 mm.

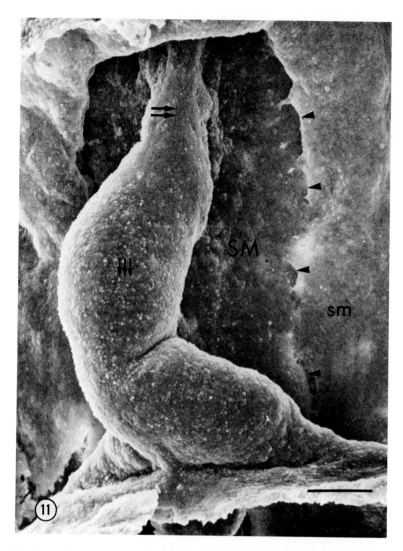

FIG. 11. Stage 11 – (12 somites). Bending to the right has begun, and the typical C-shape of the looped heart is developing. The distinction between the splanchnic mesoderm *(SM)* and the somatic mesoderm *(sm)* is still clear *(arrowheads)*. There is no longer a residual fusion furrow, and the presumptive ventricular region has rotated to the right and is bulging prominently. *Double* and *triple arrows:* refer to Figs. 12 and 13. Scale: 0.1 mm.

we continue to do so to avoid introducing new terminology. In the region where the cardiac jelly is in direct continuity with the extracellular space of the rest of the embryo, there are many specialized matrix features. There is a large concentration of an electron-dense material that morphologically resembles detached basal lamina (5–7,11,12). This material, only weakly anionic, is fucosylated (11,12) and

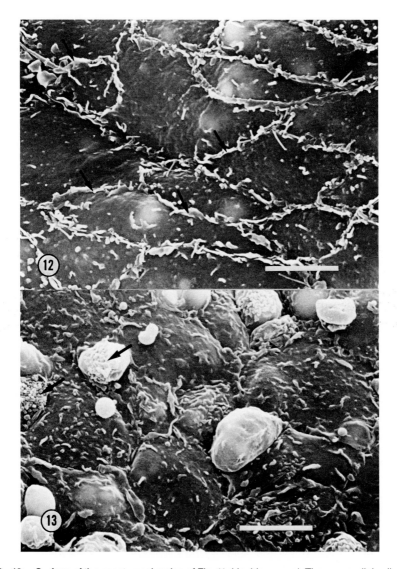

FIG. 12. Surface of the conotruncal region of Fig. 11 *(double arrows)*. The myocardial cells are flattened and have relatively few microplicae, but they do have prominent marginal lamellopodia *(arrows)*. Scale: 10 μm.
FIG. 13. Surface of the ventricular region of the heart shown in Fig. 11 *(triple arrows)*. Myocytes bulge outward and have a markedly lower density of microplicae than earlier (compare with Fig. 7). More rounded cells, presumably with a smaller surface area, have dense accumulations of microplicae *(arrows)*, whereas more flattened cells do not. Scale: 10 μm.

exists in the same location as fibronectin, recently demonstrated immunochemically (33). Initially wide, the dorsal mesocardium narrows as the heart bends. As the structure narrows, the dense matrix inclusions become more concentrated. The cells on either side of the thinning mesocardium come close together and the structure then ruptures (9). Holes appear within the mesocardium, and these holes enlarge rapidly, freeing the tubular heart from its dorsal attachments.

POSSIBLE MECHANISMS OF CARDIAC MORPHOGENESIS

Despite the apparent simplicity of heart looping, no model yet proposed (29) has been adequate to predict mechanisms which might be instrumental in regulating bending and rotation. Some hypotheses, e.g., the differential cell division hypothesis, have proved untenable, whereas others, e.g., "differential adhesivity," are sufficiently vague that they have little predictive value. In this section we review possible mechanisms of morphogenesis and try to relate these to early heart development. We deal entirely with ways in which a hypothetical epithelial organ can undergo shape change. Restricting our consideration to the epithelial phase of cardiogenesis eases our task somewhat, and we need not consider here the much more complicated issues of mesenchyme migration that are involved in later events of heart growth. This restriction makes it possible to begin to analyze the origin of physical forces and their contribution to the shaping of the early heart.

In Fig. 14 we consider possible mechanisms by which epithelial structure (a) can change shape to become (b). This simple and highly schematic shape change can theoretically occur by a number of biological mechanisms, and it is not difficult to see how these mechanisms could be related to other, more complex types of shape transformation. Shape (a) represents an epithelial structure with a central core of extracellular matrix. The elongate transformation to (b) can be effected by remodeling, as in Fig. 14A. Appositional growth followed by removal of the internal mass can transform (a) to (b). The apposition could result from regional hyperplasia, and the removal could be the result of regional cell death or localized proteolysis. Differential growth of any region would also deform the structure. Different shapes result from different patterns of differential epithelial growth. In Fig. 14B, differential growth of the shaded region (a) results in form (b).

So far we have been considering morphogenic mechanisms that involve increases in cell mass, either by hyperplasia or hypertrophy. Next we explore morphogenesis resulting from the redistribution of existing cell volume or from physical forces exerted by extracellular materials. If cells within a given region alter their shape but remain isovolumic, the entire structure changes shape (Fig. 14C). In this example the changing cells flatten, increasing the total amount of epithelial wall surface area and resulting in an overall shape change. In this instance there is thinning of the wall because there is no net increase of tissue mass. If the contents of the circular structure depicted in Fig. 14 increase to create a sufficiently high internal pressure, the internal pressure will deform the container, resulting in a larger one but one with thinner walls. Such a geometrically symmetrical increase would occur only if the elastic modulus of the epithelial wall was the same around the entire perimeter. An increase in internal, or luminal, content could occur if

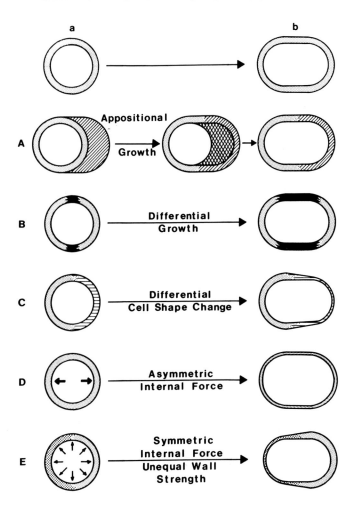

FIG. 14. Possible biological mechanisms involved in transforming shape (a) to shape (b). Shapes (a) and (b) are idealized forms and could represent sections through either a tubular or a closed structure. In sequence **A**, additional material is deposited *(lined area)* creating an intermediate form. Selective removal of the cross-hatched area results in the shape at the right. In sequence **B**, differential growth of the dark regions effects the shape change. Sequences **C**, **D**, and **E** demonstrate deformations rather than growth. In sequence **C**, flattening of the lined region increases its surface area at the expense of wall thickness. An asymmetrical internal force thins the wall uniformly during deformation, whereas in sequence **E** a symmetrical force results in non-uniform shape transition if the elastic modulus of the wall is not uniform.

the cells of the wall either secreted more luminal contents or caused an increase in hydration of the contents by some mechanism (e.g., regulating ion transport). If the contents were isotropic, the pressure would be equal in all directions. Anisotropy of the contents (Fig. 15D) would direct forces and result in an asymmetrical deformation even if the retaining wall of the container had a uniform elastic modulus.

An alternative mechanism to that of Fig. 14D is shown in Fig. 14E. An asymmetry can be generated even if the internal forces are symmetrical. If the wall is not of uniform distensibility, those regions least resistant will deform preferentially. In essence, the "weaker" regions (those with the lowest elastic modulus) will balloon outward. In the example shown in Fig. 15G, the right-hand part of the wall has a higher elastic modulus than the remainder and hence is relatively unchanged when the internal pressure rises, whereas the weaker portion deforms. Differences in the elastic modulus of different portions of the wall could be effected by several mechanisms. Regional increases in rigidity could be induced if the cells in one area differentiate preferentially and acquire internal structures, e.g., cytoskeletal elements or myofibrils, that would make them less deformable. Alternatively, the geometry of a particular structure may dictate which regions can be deformed. For example, a longitudinal structure such as the dorsal mesocardium would be expected to stiffen the dorsum of the tubular heart simply on the basis of architectural considerations.

The various models of shape change illustrated in Fig. 14 are all testable in terms of the looping heart. We next explore the shape change of heart looping in terms of these models in an attempt to identify the mechanisms that are most likely responsible for looping.

MORPHOGENIC MODELS VERSUS REALITY

Any model of heart looping must take into account the fact that the isolated heart is capable of generating its own bend completely independent of surrounding tissue (1). The possible involvement of extracardiac regulators may provide fine tuning to the final shape of the bend, but they are not essential to its generation. Thus we can rule out Patten's suggestion (26) that looping is the result of the heart tube growing too long for the pericardial cavity. Extracardiac factors may indeed influence the *direction* in which the loop is permitted to rotate, but they do not provide the force required for bending.

There is no evidence whatsoever to suggest that significant tissue remodeling occurs to alter heart shape during looping. There is cell death in the endocardium (24) which can be considered part of internal remodeling, but this is probably not related directly to looping. Differential growth has remained a most attractive hypothesis, possibly because it appears to be so logical and simple. However, there does not seem to be any evidence to support the idea that there are significant regional differences in cell division (4,28). Unpublished studies from this laboratory suggest that looping can occur in the presence of vinca alkaloids in concentrations high enough to inhibit cytokinesis.

Differential myocardial cell shape change does occur in the looping heart and has been quantitated (16). The myocardial cells of the bulging convex side of the heart flatten, resulting in a thinning of that region of the myocardium. This is effectively a redistribution of cell volume, and the flattening cells appear to remain isovolumic. As the increase in free or apical cell surface area accounts entirely for the increased surface area of the bulging myocardium, it was proposed that active flattening of the cells in the region of the bulge could actually be the cause of the bulge. These observations are consistent with models C, D, and E in Fig. 14. We constructed a plasticene model of the heart tube and manually thinned one region to mimic the cellular events in this region of the actual heart. When the wall was thinned sufficiently, such plasticene cylinders did indeed bulge (Fig. 15). Such modeling suggests that myocardial wall thinning in the region of the presumptive bulge is sufficient to produce the bulge. Note that this shape change can occur in the absence of any increase in myocardial cell volume. This model does not require either myocardial cell division or hypertrophy. It does require, however, a stimulus or signal that results in a shape change in a relatively small number of cells in a circumscribed area. Thus a single event involving a relatively small group of cells could produce the anatomical changes associated with bending in the heart. These considerations do not, however, prove that this is the mechanism of bending. The observed wall thinning in the region of the bulge could simply be the *result* of bulging and not its cause. Testing this hypothesis by experimental means has proved elusive. However, a recent study (15) has provided indirect evidence that the myocardium may have a greater compliance in the region where cells preferentially flatten out than in other areas of the developing ventricle. This supports the possibility that the observed cell flattening is the result, and not the cause, of bulging. We also consider it highly unlikely that there is a signal as topologically restricted as would be required to initiate cell flattening in this region alone. Thus although the mechanism shown in Fig. 14C remains a possibility, it appears to be less consistent with emerging data.

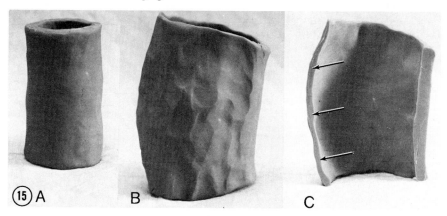

FIG. 15. Isovolumic shape change in one region of a cylinder can change the shape of the entire structure. In this plasticene model, a symmetrical cylinder of equal wall thickness **(A)** was made to "loop" **(B)** by thinning one side (*arrows,* **C**). Thinning of the wall **(C)** was accomplished by deforming the plasticene wall manually. No material was removed or added.

Hydraulic Considerations and the Generation of Force

Anatomically, we can think of the early heart as consisting of a sleeve of tissue surrounding a layer of extracellular matrix, the cardiac jelly. A series of experiments on native isolated cardiac jelly (20,21) demonstrated that this matrix can swell reversibly. One might hypothesize that the myocardium, which is histologically true epithelium, can regulate matrix swelling directly by regulating synthesis or indirectly by regulating cation transport or matrix pH. In any event, it appears that there is an outward pressure from within the tubular heart. Evidence for this is indirect. The heart appears to undergo a transition from a structure that is wrinkled to one that appears to have a taut surface (Figs. 2 and 11). There is also a progressive loss of myocardial microplicae. These surface protrusions may represent spare cell surface that can be mobilized (31). Finally, injection of hyaluronidase directly into the cardiac jelly results in a wrinkled, flaccid myocardium (22). Collectively these observations indicate that the tubular heart is a turgid structure at the time it bends and rotates. The observed reduction of myocardial "wrinkles" with a concomitant increase in the "plump" appearance of the heart surface is shown in Fig. 16.

Clearly any such internal pressure must be contained or the heart would explode. The container wall in this case is the myocardium, which probably acts in concert with a system of radial matrix fibers (6,20,21) that traverse the matrix and insert into the myocardial basal surface. Evidence that containment is not simple was obtained by measuring experimental deformations of the tubular heart (8). The hearts could be deformed to about 150% of their size by application of light pressure, but they were not readily deformable any more. The observed leveling of

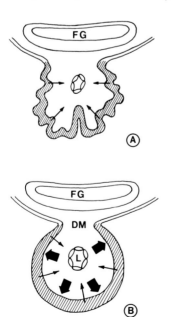

FIG. 16. The heart rudiment is shown schematically. **A:** The myocardium *(shaded)* is wrinkled and folded, as it appears in Figs. 2 and 6. The internal matrix volume is increasing as a result of myocardial activity *(arrows)*. **B:** This volume increase, in turn, exerts an outward pressure *(bold arrows)* which is resisted by the myocardium. The convolutions in **A** make the myocardium more compliant. FG: foregut; DM: dorsal mesocardium; L: lumen.

the stress-strain curve was attributed to the presence of the radial fiber system within the matrix; when these fibers reached their elastic limit, further deformation was inhibited. Thus the mechanics of internal pressure containment in the heart are not as simple as they appear initially. It is extremely difficult to model stress if the radial fiber system, as well as the myocardium, is stressed. Nonetheless, we can make some generalizations about wall stress in the tubular heart. In any cylindrical structure with an internal pressure there are two basic components of wall stress: longitudinal and circumferential (hoop) stress. Hoop stress is always twice the longitudinal stress; hence the wall must be more rigid circumferentially than longitudinally to contain a given pressure. In man-made objects such as tires and hoses a fiber system is incorporated into the wall to counteract the stress, whereas biological systems employ fibrous tissue components. Hydrostatically supported tubular structures are actually quite common in nature, and our evidence that embryonic structures may be also supported in this way can be placed in a biologically larger context. Many tubular organisms (e.g., caterpillars, annelids) have a high internal hydrostatic pressure contained within a fiber-reenforced body. Thus the "skeleton" of fibers is actually under tension. Marine organisms (e.g., coral hydra) are similarly supported, and even more complex organisms (e.g., sharks) have a higher internal pressure and a subdermal winding of fibers. The angle of fiber winding in these organisms is extremely important in regulating such bodily movements as bending, extension, and thickening. See Wainwright et al. (32) for a discussion of biological fiber systems. In the embryonic heart there is no such wound fiber system. Collagen is present but in very low amounts, and fibrillar collagen is extremely rare at the time of looping (7). The few nascent collagen fibrils that are present have no readily apparent order to their orientation. There is no evidence to support the idea that the radial fiber system (20,21) is composed of collagen.

The absence of a wound fiber system in the matrix of the developing tubular heart suggests that the internal pressure must be contained by the myocardium. If the myocardial wall is sufficiently stiff to resist the outward pressure, no size change will occur. If the pressure is great enough, however, the heart will deform. Because hoop (circumferential) stress exceeds longitudinal stress by a factor of 2, the heart diameter will increase preferentially. However, the heart does not simply swell; rather, it undergoes the coordinated series of shape transformations seen in Figs. 1 through 13. If, as is likely (because of hydraulic considerations), the internal pressure is uniform throughout the heart, differential deformation must result from differential myocardial compliance. We have seen that the morphology of the developing heart at different stages suggests that its compliance changes. The myocardium is initially folded and wrinkled. As the heart diameter increases these folds disappear, suggesting that the increase in diameter reflects, in effect, inflation of the structure. The initial inflation would be relatively easy because a folded or wrinkled sheet has a high compliance. When the larger folds have disappeared, the individual myocardial cells are still seen to have wrinkles, or microplicae, on their apical surfaces. With continued "inflation" these too disappear. We view this hierarchical system of wrinkles as a possible way the compliance of the myocardial wall is regulated. Recently Trinkaus (31) proposed that cell surface wrinkles might provide a reserve of surface which could be mobilized when the cell flattens. Thus there would be no need for de novo synthesis of a new surface. Indeed, during epiboly in *Fundulus* eggs, flattening cells lose their surface wrinkles much as the myocardium does as the heart becomes "inflated." This model predicts that once all the available excess surface has been mobilized the cells become less deformable.

Differential shape change would occur if the elastic modulus of the myocardium differed in different regions. Alternatively, the geometry of the tube itself could account for regional bulging as well as bending, and we need make no assumptions that there are, initially, intrinsically different elastic moduli in the cells of different areas of the myocardium. In particular, the dorsal mesocardium provides two longitudinal structures that run the length of the heart. Hence the geometry of the dorsal surface is such that it provides architectural stiffness to that region. We examined what effect such a relatively stiff structure would have on heart looping by using a rubber balloon as a model. Application of a narrow strip of relatively inelastic tape to one side of a partially inflated balloon followed by continued inflation resulted in the balloon bending (Fig. 17). Bending invariably occurred with the lesser curvature of the bend at the side of the strip. The decreased elastic modulus of the strip did not prevent an increase in diameter but did introduce differential longitudinal strain which resulted in a bend. One of the unexpected findings was that the bent structure is stable. If the tape was removed the balloon did not straighten out (Fig. 17D), indicating that the stresses induced in the balloon wall by bending it were relieved. Stress relief probably involved realignment of the rubber polymers of the wall, producing the pattern seen in Fig. 17. This may well be analogous to the heart rudiment *in situ*: When the dorsal mesocardium ruptures, the heart remains bent.

This model suggests a mechanism for the bending component of heart looping. There are two minimal requirements: (a) an internal pressure; and (b) a higher elastic modulus along the dorsum (i.e., dorsal mesocardium). The balloon used air as the distending medium. We propose that the heart uses cardiac jelly. The glycosaminoglycans of cardiac jelly, synthesized largely by the myocardium (18), are produced throughout development of the tubular heart and are not broken down by endogenous hyaluronidases to any great extent (19). Thus there is continued net accumulation which in effect could "overstuff" the heart, producing outward pressure. It is interesting to note that, as far as we can discern, bending of the myocardium depends on a myocardial product, the cardiac jelly. It appears that the secretory activities of the embryonic myocardium are extremely important in heart morphogenesis, and any abnormality of this function could be expected to lead to malformation.

Rotation

The above model for heart bending does not deal with heart rotation. We have seen that a balloon with a relatively inelastic strip on an otherwise isotropic wall

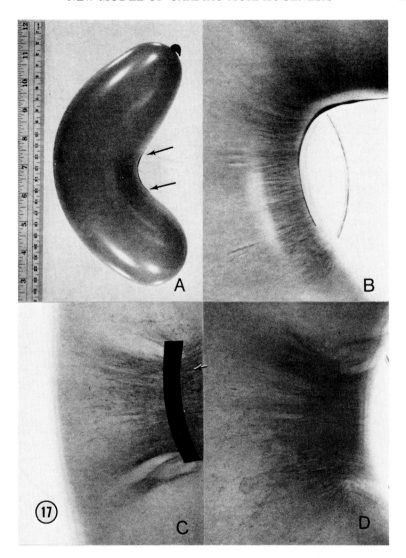

FIG. 17. A thin strip of tape was placed longitudinally along a partially inflated balloon. Further inflation induced bending **(A)** with the tape on the concave side. This is an example of how an isotropic internal pressure (air) deforms a structure if the wall has different physical properties. Close examination of the lesser curvature **(B,C)** reveals that the rubber polymer of the balloon wall is realigned to create linear circumferential arrays. Rubber polymers are asymmetrical and appear to align along the lines of hoop stress. The deformation and the polymeric alignment are permanent and are not reversed when the tape is removed **(D)**.

bends but does not rotate. The force responsible for heart rotation could either be separate from the force responsible for bending the heart or identical to it. In any event, simple mechanical considerations make it obvious that the force must be directed in some way to produce a rotational moment, and such direction absolutely requires the presence of some anisotropic structure. We have seen that extracellular matrix anisotropy is principally radial, resulting from the radial orientation of the matrix filaments. Radial anisotropy would not be able to direct a force to cause rotation unless there was a helical stacking of the radial fibers. With a helical configuration, rotation would result from an increase in distance between filaments (increase in heart length) but not from an increase in heart diameter.

We next examined the myocardium to try to detect any intramyocardial structures that could direct rotation. We concluded that myofibrils are most likely responsible for directing the forces to produce rotation (14,23). Myofibrillogenesis normally occurs in the myocardium during the time the heart loops (10,25). Thus, myocardial cytodifferentiation is temporarily coupled very closely with looping. Experiments suggest that cytodifferentiation (myofibrillogenesis) is obligatory for normal cardiac morphogenesis. General inhibition of protein synthesis prevents looping (12). If myofibril synthesis is inhibited by bromodeoxyuridine, hearts are abnormal (2). If myofibril assembly is blocked by cytochalasin B, looping is prevented even though protein synthesis is normal (12). Thus assembly of myofibrils appears to be crucial to normal looping (17). This idea has received further substantiation in experiments where myosin heavy-chain synthesis was blocked with the drug diazepam (27). Myofibril formation was inhibited in the presence of diazepam, and myocardia of treated embryos did not differentiate normally. Looping was interfered with, and a spectrum of abnormalities ranging from an absence of looping to abnormal looping resulted. Clearly, if myofibrils have a role in directing force in an orderly manner, they must be oriented with respect to the developing organ and exhibit suitable anisotropy. We ascertained that the first myofibrils are oriented in what appears to be largely a circumferential orientation (23). Because there appears to be an obligatory relationship between myofibrillogenesis and heart rotation, we tested experimentally the possibility that the existence of a pitch or helical arrangement to myofibrils could regulate rotation by directing the force derived from the expanding cardiac jelly.

A Model of the Looping Heart

In an attempt to elucidate the morphogenetic consequences of an expanding tubular structure that was encircled by linear elements of a higher elastic modulus (i.e., myofibrils), we constructed a mechanical analog of the tubular heart by using a thin-walled latex cylinder mounted in such a way as to permit controlled inflation. The device is shown in Fig. 18. Myofibrils were mimicked by applying thin lines of a mixture of latex suspension and rayon flock (Fig. 19). The latex suspension alone did not have a significantly greater resistance to deformation than did the cylinder wall. Addition of rayon flock provided the necessary difference in elastic modulus. Application of a helix of latex flock to a partially inflated cylinder resulted in a dramatic rotation as the model was inflated further (Fig. 19). The left or right direction of the helix determined the direction of rotation. In the example shown here the helix is a left-handed one; consequently, rotation is toward the right. This

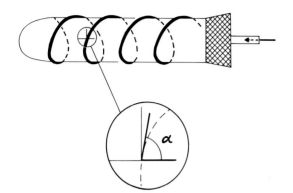

FIG. 18. Latex analog of the tubular heart. A closed latex cylinder was attached to a rubber stopper *(hatched)*. Inflation could be controlled by regulating air flow *(arrow)*. Wall anisotropy was introduced by applying a helix of stiffer material. In this diagram the helix (left-handed) is shown as a single continuous winding, but discontinuous and multiple helices were also used. By convention, the angle (α) of the helix is defined as the angle of the horizontal with a tangent to the helix *(inset)*.

model demonstrated that, if helically oriented, linear structures having a higher elastic modulus than the adjacent wall convert an increase in diameter to rotation. Particularly surprising was the large angular rotation that resulted from a relatively small increase in diameter. Typically, diameter increases in the range of 20 to 30% resulted in rotations of 50° to 70°.

A combination of helices and a tape "dorsal mesocardium" (as used in Fig. 17) results in combined rotation and bending (Fig. 19E). These phenomena do not require that both ends of the cylinder be fixed. Rotation and bending occur equally well if the distal end is free. Our measurements were all made with a fixed end (unchanging total length) for the sake of simplicity.

We investigated the inflation/rotation relationship for a number of parameters. In a continuous winding the angle of the fiber in relation to the long axis of the tube is important. Fiber angle is determined by measuring the angle between a tangent to the helix and the long axis of the cylinder. Thus as angles approach 90° the windings are more circumferential: the smaller the angle the greater the rotation (Table 1) per given increase in cylinder diameter. Diameter increase was also translated into rotation if the fiber winding was discontinuous. Rotations were similar to those obtained with continuous windings (Table 1).

The effect of fiber density was also examined. In these experiments a discontinuous fiber pattern was applied to the cylinder and its inflation/rotation relationship determined. The cylinder was deflated to its starting diameter and a second set of fibers applied, doubling the original number. The inflation/rotation relation was again determined. Increasing the number of fibers resulted in a greater rotation for the same diameter increase (Table 2).

These experiments demonstrate that rotation of a tubular or cylindrical structure can be accomplished by an internal force that is directed by anisotropy within the wall of the structure. We propose that variations in the wall anisotropy (fiber density, angle) can act to regulate the rotation of local regions of the heart tube. Thus depending on the myofibrillar presence (level of differentiation) in different areas of the myocardium, different amounts of rotation for a given expansion would be expected. It is important to emphasize that we have not unequivocally demon-

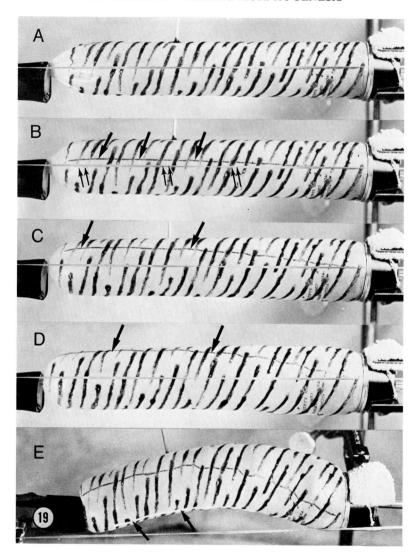

FIG. 19. This figure shows the morphological consequence of inflating a cylindrical structure if it contains a helical pattern of linear elements that are relatively less deformable. **B,C,D** are progressively more inflated. The cylinder rotates markedly, as shown by the movement of the longitudinal line painted on it *(single heavy arrows)* compared to the fixed horizontal line *(thin double arrows)*. In this model the helical lines are analogs of myofibrils. If we combined the helical winding with a tape "dorsal mesocardium," the model both rotated and bent **(E)**.

strated the presence of a helical order to the myofibrilar arrangement in the early tubular heart. In all probability the sense of the helix, if present, is not readily demonstrable, as the myofibrillar arrangement is far more complex than a simple helical winding. We predict, however, that there are overall patterns to the myofi-

TABLE 1. *Relationship between increased diameter and rotation as a function of fiber angle*

Aver. fiber angle	Diam. (cm)	% Increase	Rotation (degrees)
Continuous winding			
82°	3.5	0	0
	4.0	14	8
	4.2	20	20
72°	3.5	0	0
	4.0	14	15
	4.2	20	37
	4.3	23	52
60°	3.2	0	0
	3.3	3	15
	3.5	9	25
	4.0	25	45
	4.2	31	70
Discontinuous winding			
82°	3.5	0	0
	4.0	14	8
	4.2	20	17
72°	3.5	0	0
	4.0	14	15
	4.2	20	32
	4.3	23	49
Mixed	3.5	0	0
	4.0	14	20
	4.2	20	28
	4.5	29	35

brillar order that have the net equivalent effect of a helical order. We have ascertained that there is a sufficient degree of apparent disorder to the packing of myofibrils in the myocardium to preclude easy detection of any statistical alignment. However, such "disorder" may not be random noise but could be a mechanism to regulate small regional deformations. We are currently exploring the possibility of quantitating the myofibrillar pattern to test this hypothesis.

Genetic Control of Morphogenesis

The model proposed here enables us to make predictions about mechanisms underlying morphogenesis. These predictions are testable and should help determine the continued usefulness of the general model. Moreover, testing these hypotheses may clarify our understanding of genetic regulation of morphogenesis. All biological shape is controlled genetically to some extent if for no other reason than it is gene products that are assembled into much of the tissue mass. The principal issue is, we argue, how gene products assemble into organs and how they determine the emerging shape of organs during ontogeny. Are shapes and shape changes dependent on gene products alone, or is there a hierarchical assembly process that removes a complex morphogenic event some distance from gene expression per se?

TABLE 2. *Inflation rotation relationship as a function of fiber density at different angles (discontinuous winding)*

Aver. fiber angle	Diam. (cm)	% Increase	Rotation (degrees)
84°	3.5	0	0
	4.0	14	15
	4.5	29	25
84° (2× density)	3.5	0	0
	4.0	14	20
	4.5	29	30
70°	3.5	0	0
	4.0	14	20
	4.5	29	50
70° (2× density)	3.5	0	0
	4.0	14	30
	4.5	29	55

A number of independently regulated cellular events must occur for normal shape to result. For example, it seems that myocardial cytodifferentiation with the assembly of myofibrils must take place. Morever, there must be either continued elaboration of cardiac jelly matrix or regulated hydration of the existing extracellular mass. If the matrix increased without concurrent myocardial myofibrillogenesis, bending and rotation would not occur. This is seen in embryos where myofibrillogenesis has been experimentally disrupted or inhibited. Rotation of the bend to the right or left requires, according to our model, hydrostatic force, cytodifferentiation, and an overall order to myofibrillar orientation at the tissue level. The sense of overall rotation (right or left) is viewed as a result of the angle of the myofibrils with respect to the long axis of the heart.

Interference with any of these events would be expected to yield a range of anomalous morphologies. An insufficient matrix volume would be expected to produce inadequate force for either bending or rotation. Abnormal expression of the myogenic phenotype or a temporal retardation in fibrillogenesis relative to matrix expansion would result in an uncontrolled shape change. Most intriguing is the possibility that right or left rotation (*d*- or *l*-looping) is mediated by myofibrillar orientation. In this case the mechanism that controls organ asymmetry would be the same subcellular mechanism that regulates myofibrillar orientation.

This model is particularly appealing to us because it does not require any unique set of cell activities whose sole function is to control organ shape. In this context, morphogenesis is viewed as a necessary and inevitable consequence of rather general cellular activities. Looping is clearly under genetic regulation in the sense that gene expression is required, but we have no evidence to support the idea that specific genes or sets of genes have exclusively morphoregulatory activity. Nonetheless, it is clear that a genetic defect which altered one or more of the normal cell activities that contribute to shape determination (e.g., myofibril alignment) would be evidenced by an alteration of gross anatomical form.

Finally, we have attempted to show that more traditional "textbook" ways of viewing early heart morphogenesis no longer bear critical scrutiny. The most reasonable alternatives, from the standpoint of contemporary knowledge of cardiogenesis, have been explored, and in qualitative terms a testable hypothesis has been constructed.

ACKNOWLEDGMENT

Original research presented was supported by USPHS grant HL 13831.

REFERENCES

1. Butler, J. K. (1952): An experimental analysis of cardiac loop formation in the chick. M.A. thesis, University of Texas, Austin, Texas.
2. Chacko, S., and Joseph, X. (1974): The effect of 5-bromodeoxyruidine (BrdU) on cardiac muscle differentiation. *Dev. Biol.*, 40:340.
3. De la Cruz, M. V., Gomez, C. S., Artaege, M. M., and Argüello, C. (1977): Experimental study of the development of the truncus and conus in the chick embryo. *J. Anat.*, 123:661.
4. De Haan, R. L. (1965): Morphogenesis of the vertebrate heart. In: *Organogenesis*, edited by R. De Haan and H. Ursprung, pp. 197–211. Holt, Rinehart and Winston, New York.
5. Hay, D. A., and Markwald, R. R. (1981): Localization of focuse-containing substances in developing atrioventricular cushion tissue. In: *Perspectives in Cardiovascular Research, Vol. 5: Mechanisms of Cardiac Morphogenesis and Teratogenesis*, edited by T. Pexieder, pp. 197–211. Raven Press, New York.
6. Hurle, J. M., Icardo, J. M., and Ojeda, J. L. (1980): Compositional and structural heterogenicity of the cardiac jelly of the chick embryo tubular heart: a TEM, SEM and histochemical study. *J. Embryol. Exp. Morphol.*, 56:211.
7. Johnson, R. C., Manasek, F. J., Vinson, W. C., and Seyer, J. (1974): The biochemical and ultrastructural demonstration of collagen during early heart development. *Dev. Biol.*, 36:252.
8. Lacktis, J. W., and Manasek, F. J. (1978): An analysis of deformation during a normal morphogenetic event. In: *Morphogenesis and Malformation of the Cardiovascular System*, edited by G. C. Rosenquist and D. Bergsma, pp. 205–227. Alan R. Liss, New York.
9. Litke, L. L., and Johnson, R. C. (1980): Rupture of the dorsal mesocardium in the developing chick heart as observed by light and electron microscopy. *Anat. Rec.*, 196:114A.
10. Manasek, F. J. (1968): Embryonic development of the heart. I. A light and electron microscopic study of myocardial development in the early chick embryo. *J. Morphol.*, 125:329.
11. Manasek, F. J. (1976): Glycoprotein synthesis and tissue interaction during establishment of the functional embryonic chick heart. *J. Mol. Cell. Cardiol.*, 8:389.
12. Manasek, F. J. (1976): Heart development: interactions involved in cardiac morphogenesis. In: *The Cell Surface in Animal Embryogenesis and Development*, Vol. 1, edited by G. Poste and G. L. Nicolson, pp. 545–598. North Holland, Amsterdam.
13. Manasek, F. J. (1977): Structural glycoprotein of the embryonic cardiac extracellular matrix. *J. Mol. Cell. Cardiol.*, 9:425–439.
14. Manasek, F. J. (1981): Determinants of heart shape in early embryos. *Fed. Proc.*, 40:2011.
15. Manasek, F. J., and Kulikowski, R. R. (1981): Myocardial filopodia during early heart development. *Scan. Electron Microsc.*, 11:281.
16. Manasek, F. J., Burnside, M. B., and Waterman, R. L. (1972): Myocardial cell shape changes as a mechanism of embryonic heart looping. *Dev. Biol.*, 29:349.
17. Manasek, F. J., Kulikowski, R. R., and Fitzpatrick, L. (1978): Cytodifferentiaton: a causal antecedent of looping? In: *Morphogenesis and Malformation of the Cardiovascular System*, edited by G. C. Rosenquist and D. Bergsma, pp. 161–178. Alan R. Liss, New York.
18. Manasek, F. J., Reid, M., Vinson, W., Seyer, J., and Johnson, R. (1973): Glycosaminoglycan synthesis by the early embryonic chick heart. *Dev. Biol.*, 35:332.

19. Nakamura, A. (1980): Cardiac hyaluronidase activity of chick embryos at the time of endocardial cushion formation. *J. Mol. Cell Cardiol.*, 12:1239.
20. Nakamura, A., and Manasek, F. J. (1978): Cardiac jelly fibrils: their distribution and organization. In: *Morphogenesis and Malformation of the Cardiovascular System*, edited by G. C. Rosenquist and D. Bergsma, pp. 229–250. Alan R. Liss, New York.
21. Nakamura, A., and Manasek, F. J. (1978): Experimental studies of the shape and structure of isolated cardiac jelly. *J. Embryol. Exp. Morphol.*, 43:167.
22. Nakamura, A., and Manasek, F. J. (1981): An experimental study of the relation of cardiac jelly to the shape of the early chick embryonic heart. *J. Embryol. Exp. Morphol.*, 65:235.
23. Nakamura, A., Kulikowski, R. R., Lacktis, J. W., and Manasek, F. J. (1980): Heart looping: a regulated response to deforming forces. In: *Etiology and Morphogenesis of Congenital Heart Disease*, edited by R. Van Praagh and A. Takao, pp. 81–98. Futura, New York.
24. Ojeda, J. L., and Hurle, J. M. (1975): Cell death during the formation of the tubular heart of the chick embryo. *J. Embryol. Exp. Morphol.*, 33:523.
25. Orts Llorca, F., and Gonzalez-Santander, R. (1969): Estudio electromicroscopica de la primera aparicion y desairollo de los miofilamentos cardiacos (miofibrillogenesis) en el embrion de pollo. *Rev. Esp. Cardiol.*, 4:537.
26. Patten, B. M. (1922): The formation of the cardiac loop in the chick. *Am. J. Anat.*, 30:373.
27. Renehan, W. E., and Kulikowski, R. R. (1981): Abnormal development in Valium treated embryos. *Biophys. J.*, 33:244a.
28. Sissman, N. J. (1966): Cell multiplication rates during development of the primitive cardiac tube in the chick embryo. *Nature*, 210:504.
29. Stalsberg, H. (1970): Mechanism of dextral looping of the embryonic heart. *Am. J. Cardiol.*, 25:265.
30. Stalsberg, H., and De Haan, R. L. (1969): The precardiac areas and formation of the tubular heart in the chick embryo. *Dev. Biol.*, 19:128.
31. Trinkaus, J. P. (1980): Formation of protrusions of the cell surface during tissue cell movement. In: *Tumor Cell Surfaces and Malignancy*, pp. 887–906. Alan R. Liss, New York.
32. Wainwright, S. A., Biggs, W. D., Currey, J. D., and Gosline, J. M. (1976): *Mechanical Design in Organisms*. Wiley, New York.
33. Waterman, R. W., and Balian, G. (1980): Indirect immunofluorescent staining of fibronectin associated with the floor of the foregut during formation and rupture of the oral membrane in the chick embryo. *Anat. Rec.*, 198:619–635.

Growth of the Heart in Health and Disease,
edited by Radovan Zak. Raven Press,
New York © 1984.

Cardiac Growth, Maturation, and Aging

Karel Rakusan

*Department of Physiology, University of Ottawa, School of Medicine,
Ottawa, Ontario, Canada*

In my recent review on postnatal development of the heart (138) I pointed out that developmental aspects are often a neglected dimension in medical and biological research. However, during the last few years, we have witnessed a considerable expansion of both original papers and review articles on various aspects of cardiac growth, development, and aging. Developmental and aging processes are similar in many ways, and it is often difficult to identify a given process as being one or the other. Although *aging* in the strict sense of the word means changes with age, i.e., with any age, it is commonly associated with changes accompanying senescence. Similarly, *developmental changes* have a relatively wide connotation, but they are usually related to maturation, which evidently lasts until the organism reaches maturity, which is often described in mammals as the age at which growth of the long bones stops. *Growth* may be defined as an increase in volume and/or mass of the organism or its part. Even this definition, however, may be disputed. For instance, an increase in volume and mass due to an increase in water content in a case of edema can hardly be described as biological growth. An alternative definition of growth may be an increase in volume or mass of living tissue resulting from assimilation (17,105).

The aim of this chapter is to present a concise description of changes associated with growth, maturation, and aging in the normal mammalian heart. A hierarchical framework has been employed to present the data which corresponds to the arrangement in our survey of methods available for the assessment of cardiac growth (Chapter 2). First, we describe changes at the organ level, i.e., the macrostructure. This section includes a description of postnatal changes in cardiac mass and shape as well as changes in the coronary vascular bed and in cardiac innervation. This is followed by a description at the tissue level, which concerns microstructure as usually examined with light microscopy. The description concentrates mainly on two major components of cardiac tissue, i.e., coronary capillaries and myocardial muscle cells. The review is concluded by a section dealing with the cellular level, i.e., the microstructure, as is usually examined with electron microscopy. In this section we summarize the development of subcellular compartments from both qualitative and quantitative points of view.

In order to keep the review concise, the metabolic and mechanical aspects with their many ramifications are only briefly outlined. Similarly, no pathological alterations are included, notwithstanding the fact that cardiac pathology and aging are closely related (107). Special attention is paid to data obtained from studies of human growth and development, and these are compared with those from commonly utilized laboratory mammals and are occasionally complemented with data from other mammalian species.

Important questions are how to arrange the data within the life span of the species, and how to relate the measurements obtained from one species to that of another. Cardiac growth and development is a four-dimensional phenomenon, and therefore the first approach is to arrange the data with respect to the time axis (i.e., the age of the subjects or animals). Fetal and early postnatal changes are more pronounced and accelerated than those during later life. Consequently, quite often in such studies it is more practical to express age on a logarithmic scale. When comparing the data from one species to another it is not appropriate to simply take an average life span and compare different ages as a calculated fraction of an average life span due to different rates of growth and development in each species. An alternative approach is to divide the whole life span into periods delineated by developmental landmarks, e.g., birth, weaning, onset of puberty. Even this approach, however, is of limited usefulness, as the degree of maturity at birth varies by a sizable margin among mammalian species. Therefore birth is not a directly comparable point of development in different species. The same applies to the remaining developmental landmarks. For instance, the time period between the weaning and the onset of puberty is much shorter in the rat than in man even on a relative chronological scale.

There is no doubt that the trends in many postnatal changes of various parameters are similar in various mammalian species as is demonstrated later in this chapter. The rate of these changes may vary, however, and therefore it is doubtful that we will ever end up with a uniform formula for comparing the different age scales. Only a detailed description of these individual changes may lead to the establishment of relative time scales for each parameter. We hope that our review will contribute to such a process.

For the reasons described above, it is also advisable to distinguish between the relative contributions of growth and age, which are closely related under normal conditions. In the early stages of postnatal development of some experimental animals, the method of choice for distinguishing these two aspects is the use of fast- and slow-growing animals resulting from the adjustment of the number of animals per litter. As a result, animals from small litters grow faster than animals from large litters, and we obtain animals of different body weights but of the same age. The effect of age and growth may thus be studied separately. Later in life, pair feeding or establishing separate age and weight controls might help in dissociating the effects of age and growth.

In addition to chronological age, a concept of biological age should be introduced. This concept is very important for gerontological research as it allows evaluation of the success of attempts to alter the rate of aging. To accomplish this, a verifiable difference between the chronological age and biological age must be found. Biological age is based on the assumption that in the course of normal aging several biological parameters change in a predictable fashion. Recently several authors attempted to define the biological age and to outline methods for its measurement (38,71,109,169). These authors used multiple regression analysis of various vital functions as a model for predictions of the biological age of the whole organism. Several cardiac parameters included in the model have a relatively high predictive value (e.g., heart rate, heart weight, myocardial concentration of collagen, hexosamine, lipofuscin). We are not aware of any attempt to define separately the biological age of a single organ, e.g., the heart.

MACROSTRUCTURE—ORGAN LEVEL

Cardiac Size and Shape

The values of the external dimensions of the human heart have been reported extensively in the older morphological literature; some of these data are given in biological tables (6). The major feature of the postnatal changes in the human heart is the more spherical appearance of the adult heart than that of the newborn. For instance, the length and breadth of the heart are almost the same in the adult heart, whereas the length of the heart at birth is only 75% of its breadth (Fig. 1).

Postnatal changes of the internal cardiac dimensions as defined and described by Lev and co-workers (98) have been studied thoroughly by several authors (35,39,151). These studies also include data on the circumference of the atrioventricular orifices and the orifices of the major vessels, as well as some estimates of the ventricular volumes. For example, a graphic display of postnatal changes of

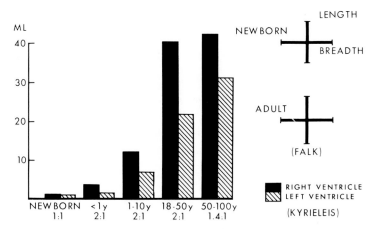

FIG. 1. Age-related changes in the capacity of the cardiac ventricles. Data are from Kyrieleis (92). The relative proportion of external cardiac dimensions of length and breadth are as reported by Falk (45).

one- and three-dimensional cardiac parameters is presented in Fig. 2. The graph is constructed using the data supplied by Eckner and co-workers (39), and the data are expressed as a percentage of the values in newborns. As may be seen in Fig. 2, the relative increase in ventricular volumes exceeds the increase in cardiac mass. The fastest growing one-dimensional parameters are the pulmonary and aortic valve circumferences, whereas the smallest relative increase was noted in the left ventricular outflow tract.

The right ventricular wall is usually found to be thinner than the left ventricular wall, and this difference increases with age. Rowlatt and co-workers (151) recorded no changes in the thickness of the right ventricular wall at three well-defined points in the hearts of children from birth to 15 years of age. Similarly, no changes during the postnatal period were found in a longitudinal echocardiographic study by Oberhänsli and co-workers (123). Kyrieleis (92) described a significant decrease in the average thickness of the right ventricular wall during the first postnatal year. On the other hand, De la Cruz and co-workers (35) and Eckner and co-workers (39) reported a modest increase in the right ventricular wall thickness combined with a marked increase in the left ventricular wall thickness during postnatal growth. The thickness of the left ventricular wall in the human heart as measured by echocardiography increases with age from the second to the eighth decade (53,93,168). Echocardiographic measurements of the cardiac growth pattern between infancy and early adulthood were described by Henry and co-workers (64) and Rogé and co-workers (149).

Kyrieleis (92) measured ventricular volumes directly in human hearts obtained from section material. He found the volumes of the right and left ventricular cavities to be approximately the same at birth. In the infant group, the right ventricular volume was double that for newborns, whereas the left ventricular volume did not change. Later the ratio of both volumes became established at 2:1 and did not change with age, indicating a similar increase in both ventricular volumes. In the old age group, a greater increase in the left ventricular volume was observed, suggesting relative left ventricular dilatation (Fig. 1).

The age-related changes in several ventricular dimensions in dogs are described by House and Ederstrom (77). Grimm and co-workers (59) reported no change in

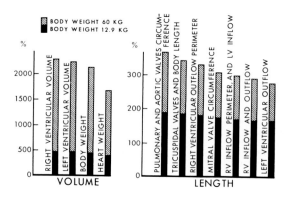

FIG. 2. Relative changes in the internal dimensions of the human heart expressed as the percentage of newborn values and calculated from the equations proposed by Eckner and co-workers (39).

the basic geometry of the left ventricle in rats during postnatal development. On the other hand, Shreiner and co-workers (167) found a relative left ventricular dilatation in old male rats and ex-breeder female rats.

Finally, Lee and co-workers (95) compared ventricular weights and their geometry in newborn, young, and adult animals of seven mammalian species. According to these authors, the basic geometry of the heart does not change with age in the cat, rabbit, and guinea pig. In the remaining four species (sheep, swine, dog, and rat) the left ventricles from adult animals are more spherical than those in newborns.

Cardiac Mass

The first record of cardiac weight can be found in *Natural History* by Pliny the Elder (A.D. 23–79). This author described the practice of ancient Egyptian embalmers who recorded the weight of various internal organs including the heart. The heart was the most important for the following reasons: They believed that the human heart grows larger every year, reaching its heaviest weight at the age of 50, and from that point on it loses weight at the same rate. Consequently, cardiac weight is decreased to its minimal values by the age of 100 years, and the resulting atrophy of the senile heart was held responsible for the accepted life span of 100 years. It is of interest that if one uses a more detailed report of the same findings by Censorinus, a Roman astrologer of the third century, the predicted cardiac weight for age groups 30 to 70 years is well within the accepted limits of the human cardiac weight as we know it in modern times: 192 g for decades 30 and 70, 256 g for decades 40 and 60, and a peak value of 320 g at age 50 years (23).

The oldest reference to postnatal development of heart weight in man still commonly quoted, though rarely directly from the source, is an 1883 book by Müller (117). Other early measurements are included in a book by Boyd (22) and in biological tables in Altman and Dittmer's work (6).

The rate of cardiac growth with respect to body growth is given by the index α, which is an exponent from the allometric formula. Consequently, values of α close to 1 indicate growth of the organ proportional to the growth of the total body, whereas values smaller than 1 reflect an organ growth rate slower than that of the total body, and vice versa. (For more details see Chapter 2). Reported values of α for different species are summarized in Fig. 3. As may be seen, the rate of cardiac growth varies from as low as two-thirds the rate of body growth in sheep up to equal rates in several other species including man. The highest allometric growth constant of 1.1 was reported by Papritz and co-workers (129) for growing beagles.

It is of interest that a comparison of heart weight and body weight in adult specimens of more than 100 mammalian species yields α values close to 1, independent of the sex of the animals and their natural habitat (terrestrial versus aquatic mammals) (135).

The linear relationship between the logarithm of organ weight and body weight accentuates the importance of early stages of growth, which occupy a relatively large proportion of the logarithmic scale. As early as 1901, Falk (45) found the

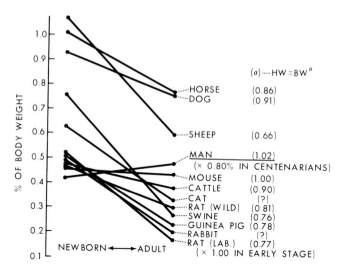

FIG. 3. Comparison of newborn and adult values of relative heart weight in several mammalian species. The rate of growth, expressed as α, is in parentheses. (HW) heart weight. *(BW)* body weight. (α) exponent from the allometric equation. Data were obtained from the following studies: man: Mühlmann (116) and Linzbach and Akuomoa-Boateng (106); cat and rabbit: Lee and co-workers (95); guinea pig: Webster and Liljegren (191); laboratory rat: Rakusan and co-workers (144); wild rat: Wachtlova and co-workers (188).

greatest rate of increase of human cardiac weight during the first postnatal year; the heart doubled its birth weight by 6 months of age and tripled by 1 year. Thereafter, the cardiac growth was more gradual. Similarly, Keen (82) reported that the growth rate of human hearts is faster during the first two postnatal months than later in life. Hirokawa (69) also found faster cardiac growth in a group of young infants, with a slope of 1.19, later decreasing to 0.89. A parallel course was found in rats by Rakusan and co-workers (142). According to these authors, the rat heart grows proportionally to the weight of the body (α = 1.01) during the early postnatal period (first month of age), whereas later the cardiac growth rate is slower than that of the organism as a whole (α = 0.70).

The relative cardiac weight is usually highest in newborn animals and decreases with age (Fig. 3). Consequently, α is smaller than 1 in allometric formulas for postnatal cardiac growth in most mammalian species. An important exception is the case of the human heart, where the relative weight remains at values close to 0.5% of the body weight during the first 30 years of life but increases up to 0.8% in centenarians (106). This increase in relative heart weight, which starts earlier in males than in females, is probably due to a concomitant age-related increase in the mean arterial blood pressure.

At birth, weights of the right and left ventricles are similar (45,69,82,116,117), or the right ventricular weight is even greater than the left ventricular weight (24, 43,146). During early postnatal development, the left ventricular preponderance is well established either by the postnatal atrophy of the right ventricle or by its slower rate of growth. Consequently, the contribution of the right ventricle to the total cardiac weight is higher at birth than later in life in various experimental animals, as documented in Fig. 4.

The greatest collection of data on the weight of human hearts was published by Linzbach and Akuamoa-Boateng (106). It is based on the analysis of 7,112 human hearts collected from 63 places around the world. Their age range is from birth to 110 years. According to these authors, the absolute cardiac weight increases continually up to the ninth decade of life, with only a slight reduction during the 10th and 11th decades. The annual increase in cardiac weight from 30 years on was 1 g in men and 1.5 g in women. These values are close to the annual rate of increase of 1.1 g reported by Rosahn (150). Similar results were also obtained by Meyer and co-workers (114), who analyzed 927 autopsies from patients in the older age groups. These authors, however, reported a higher rate of increase in the weight of male hearts than of female hearts.

Postnatal changes in the weight of the human heart can be summarized as follows: After a brief spurt during the early postnatal period, the increase in cardiac weight is proportional to the increase in body weight, resulting in a constant relative cardiac weight throughout the first half of life. Therefore the growth of the cardiac mass during this period follows directly the growth of the total body and is relatively independent of age. During the second half of life, the effect of age is apparent, resulting in a moderate increase in cardiac weight irrespective of body weight changes. Similar but not identical trends may be detected in experimental animals. The most detailed description is available for the changes in the rat heart. After a brief, relatively high rate of growth immediately after birth, cardiac growth follows the growth in the total body albeit with a somewhat slower rate resulting in a gradual decrease in relative cardiac weight (1,144,190). Nevertheless, heart weight is closely related to body weight, and it is relatively independent of the animal's age. For instance, when the heart weight from fast- and slow-growing rats killed at 21 days of age is measured, the relationship between heart weight and body weight is the same as that of animals of differing ages but with similar body weights

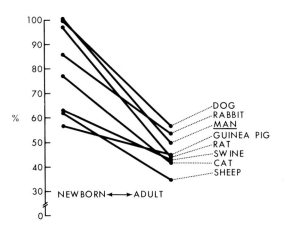

FIG. 4. Comparison of newborn and adult values of right ventricular weight expressed as a percentage of left ventricular weight. Data for man are averaged from various reports cited in the text, and for experimental animals from Lee and co-workers (95).

(137). Another example is the observation of Walter and Addis (190) on fasting rats. In animals with decreased body weight due to fasting, the heart weight is the same as that of normal younger animals of similar body weight. Although body weight is the most important determinant of cardiac weight throughout most of life, the effect of age is more pronounced in senescent animals. An increase in the cardiac weight of senescent rats has been reported (16), particularly when expressed as relative heart weight. Senescence, however, is characterized by a variable body weight, and the body weight is therefore not an ideal reference parameter at this period of life. If the tibial length was used as a reference parameter, a modest yet significant increase in heart weight was found in senescent rats (195).

The interspecies variability of relative heart weight is rather small in newborns; it is more pronounced later in life, perhaps as a consequence of differences in life-style and environment (Fig. 3). On the other hand, the variability of heart weight within the same species is highest in the newborn group and decreases with age. For instance, the cardiac weight of small children or infants of the same body weight varies sometimes by a factor of two (24). Subsequently, variability of the cardiac weight decreases with age up to senescence (106). According to Gewert (54), heart weights are more variable in women than in men.

Coronary Vascular Bed

In this section we concentrate on the coronary arteries only, as age-related changes of the coronary capillaries are discussed in a section dealing with cardiac growth, maturation, and aging at the tissue level. The coronary vascular bed in man is established well before birth. The number of small branches of the coronary arteries increases continually from birth to the seventh decade, with the greatest changes taking place during the first two decades (41). The growth of the coronary ostia was studied by Vogelberg (187). In newborns the areas of the left and right coronary ostia are approximately the same. Afterward, the area increases with the growth of the heart up to the age of 35, at which time growth stops. The postnatal increase in the area of the left coronary ostium is greater than of the right one. If one calculates the combined coronary artery cross section as a percentage of the aortic cross section, a continuous decrease is found from 9% in newborns to 4% in the oldest age group (80 to 90 years). No changes in the size of the coronary ostia after 30 years of age were found by Paulsen and co-workers (130).

The caliber of the human coronary arteries has been investigated by several authors with conflicting results. According to Rabe (136), both coronary arteries increase in size up to the age of 30 years. Beyond this age, the diameters of the coronary arteries remain unchanged, irrespective of age and cardiac weight (Fig. 5). On the other hand, Ehrich and co-workers (41) and Arai and co-workers (12) described the growth of the coronary lumen as proportional to the growth of the ventricular mass. Finally, Hutchins and co-workers (78) found a direct linear relationship between the cardiac mass and the coronary artery caliber raised to the third power. In addition, these authors also studied the tortuosity of the coronary

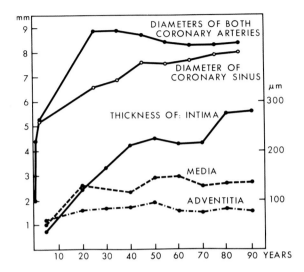

FIG. 5. Age-related changes of coronary artery diameters (136), the diameter of the coronary sinus (187), and the thickness of the individual layers of the coronary arteries (127).

arteries, defined as length related to distance traveled. Tortuosity was predicted by an equation combining age positively and heart weight negatively. Therefore tortuosity increases with age and cardiac shrinking but decreases with cardiac enlargement.

The average caliber of the coronary sinus varies to a considerable degree. There is a moderate increase with age and no definite relationship between the cross section of the coronary sinus and the cross section of coronary arteries (136).

Age-related changes in the thickness of individual layers of the left coronary artery are also depicted in Fig. 5. The data are based on the measurements of Papacharalampous (127). According to this author, the thickness of the intima increases continuously with age in both coronary arteries, and it is 10 times thicker in the oldest group (90 years) than in the youngest group (first decade). The thickness of the media in the left coronary artery reaches its maximum at 30 years of age, whereas in the right coronary artery the increase is less steep and the highest values are found at the age of 50. The thickness of the adventitia in both coronary arteries does not change with age. Similar results were obtained by Weiler (193).

In contrast to the situation in the human heart, the coronary vascular bed in the rat heart at birth is less mature and continues to develop postnatally (33a,186). The stems of both coronary arteries together with their septal and parietal branches are already present at birth. Postnatal development usually concerns the formation of the coronary artery branches which supply the atria and the establishment of intercoronary anastomoses. The definite pattern is established around the 12th postnatal day; no new arterial stems or anastomoses are built after this date, and the vascular system already formed only adapts itself to the growing heart.

Cardiac Innervation

Autonomic innervation of the heart is both morphologically and functionally immature at birth. For instance, it has been known for more than a century that stimulation of the vagus nerve has much less effect on the heart in newborns than in adult animals (8). There are, however, relatively important differences between adrenergic and cholinergic innervation as well as large differences among various mammalian species. The differentiation is usually more pronounced in the case of adrenergic innervation.

In the rat heart at birth, mainly the atria and the pericardium of the ventricles contain adrenergic fibers detectable by a fluorescence method (125). Adrenergic innervation patterns of adult animals were observed at the end of the third postnatal week, whereas the thickness of the nerve fibers and the density of their network reached adult values by the end of the fifth postnatal week (34,160). A similar trend was observed in several species with differing time sequences; for example, the development of the adrenergic innervation of the guinea pig is more advanced than in the rat heart (34,48–50,108,128). The adrenergic response to transmural stimulation is already functionally mature in 7-day-old rats according to Vlk and Vincenzi (184). Recently, Mackenzie and Standen (110) reported the presence of fully developed positive inotropic responses to exogenous norepinephrine or iso-prenaline in preparations from newborn rats, thus revealing the presence of already functioning β-receptors at this age. The inotropic response to sympathetic nerve stimulation did not develop until 2 to 3 weeks of age. Similarly, Friedman (48) reported the presence of receptor sites before the development of the extrinsic nerve supply in the rabbit heart.

The maturation of the cholinergic supply was investigated by histochemical determination of cholinesterase activity within the cardiac ganglia and nerves by Navaratnam (121). True cholinesterase appears in the cytoplasm of the cardiac nerve cells well before birth in human, rabbit, and guinea pig hearts. In rat hearts the first appearance in the cardiac ganglia was recorded on the fourth day of postnatal life. Earlier development in the rat heart was described by Taylor (174), who used electron microscopy. Finally, Vlk and Vincenzi (184) reported that parasympathetic innervation of the rat heart is quite immature during the perinatal period, and several weeks of postnatal life are required for its maturation. This contrasts with the situation in the guinea pig and the rabbit, whose hearts are functionally mature shortly after birth. Vlk (182) studied the postnatal development of postganglionic parasympathetic neurons in the rat sinoatrial node. These neurons matured functionally in the relatively short period between the 10th and 20th day of postnatal life. Maturation of the neurons in this case was defined as the ability to release acetylcholine in response to electrical stimuli.

The structural and functional changes are closely related to biochemical changes. The concentration of endogenous norepinephrine (NE) is very low at birth and increases rapidly during the first postnatal weeks in the hearts from several species [sheep (49); swine (49,172); rabbit (50); rat (34,62,80,153,185); hamster (170)].

On the other hand, in hearts from old rats, the endogenous concentration of NE is lower than in the samples from young adult rats (26,52,55,94,99). This difference, however, was found only in male hearts by Martinez et al. (111), whereas no changes were found in female rats. The ability to accumulate exogenous NE increases with age. The uptake is very low at birth, but it increases rapidly with age under both *in vivo* and *in vitro* conditions (56,80,153,179).

In aging rats the reports on myocardial uptake and storage of exogenous NE are controversial. Both increased and decreased as well as unchanged handling has been reported (51,55,70,99).

The rate of NE formation is determined by tyrosine hydroxylase, whose activity increases with age (49,172). Moreover, the activity of monoamine oxidase, which catalyzes the oxidative deamination of NE, increases several-fold during the life span (27,36,49,51,134). On the other hand, the activity of the second enzyme involved in the destruction of NE, catechol-O-methyltransferase, is not influenced by age (55,172).

Postnatal changes concerning the biochemistry of the cholinergic system in the heart can be summarized as follows: The activity of nonspecific cholinesterase is histochemically identifiable within the human and rat heart before birth (7,46). The amount of acetylcholine in atrial tissue increases after birth in both growing puppies (183) and rats (90) concomitant with an increase in choline acetyltransferase activity (178). Acetylcholine synthesis is diminished in atria from senescent rats when compared to their adult counterparts, probably due to decreased activity in choline acetyltransferase in the atria of old rats (181).

MICROSTRUCTURE—TISSUE LEVEL

The most prominent tissue components are coronary capillaries and cardiac myocytes. Methods available for their quantitative evaluation were analyzed previously (Chapter 2); age-related changes in these two components are described in the subsections which follow. The rest of the tissue has seldom been analyzed to any great extent. The tissue volume occupied by the cardiac myocytes remains relatively constant (close to 80%) in both the right and left ventricles of the canine myocardium (96), whereas a significant decrease from the birth value of 86% to 75% at the age of 11 days has been noted in the rat heart (9). Consequently, the extracellular compartment in the canine myocardium remains unchanged throughout the postnatal period, whereas its fraction increases in the early postnatal period of the rat heart. In contrast, Sheridan and co-workers (165) reported a decrease in the extracellular fraction, from 22% in neonatal cat myocardium to 13% in adult hearts. The extracellular compartment contains capillaries and larger vessels which were analyzed separately. The remainder is composed mainly of the collagen matrix. In quantitative terms, several authors have attempted to estimate the total number of "nonmuscle" cells in the heart, i.e., mainly fibrocytes and endothelial cells. These numbers and their age-related changes are described in conjunction with a description of the corresponding changes in the population of cardiac myocytes.

Myocardial Capillary Supply

Man

The only systematic description of changes in the capillary supply of the human heart is that of Roberts and Wearn (148). These authors described a rapid decrease of the fiber/capillary ratio from 6 in newborns to 1 in adults (Fig. 6). They also reported no change in the capillary density during normal heart development. In their own material, however, on the average 4,100 capillaries/mm² were found in hearts from infants compared to 3,342 capillaries/mm² in adult hearts. Similarly, Hort and Severidt (76) found 2,689 capillaries/mm² in the papillary muscles from infant hearts, although the same authors previously described 1,965 capillaries/mm² in normal adult hearts and 1,834 capillaries/mm² in hearts from patients older than 80 years (74,75). Finally, Arai and co-workers (12) described a decrease in the total length of capillaries per unit muscle volume with increasing weight and age in human hearts.

Experimental Animals

A qualitative description of the early postnatal development of the terminal vascular bed in canine myocardium was published by Legato (96). Capillaries have much thicker walls during this period than later in life. The walls themselves are remarkable for their abundance of micropinocytic vesicles. Also, rough endoplasmic reticulum and free ribosomes are abundant in the newborn capillary wall in contrast to the situation later in life. In the rat myocardium, the final architecture of the terminal vascular bed is developed only during the first postnatal weeks (33a,186).

A quantitative description of age-related changes in the capillary supply of the rabbit heart was published by Shipley and co-workers (166). They found a decrease

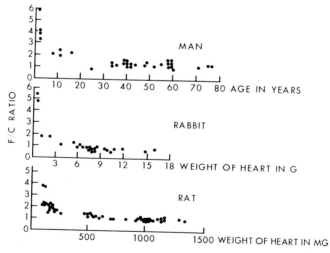

FIG. 6. Development of the fiber/capillary ratio in various mammalian species: man: Roberts and Wearn (148); rabbit: Shipley and co-workers (166); rat: Rakusan and Poupa (139).

of the fiber/capillary ratio from 6 in newborns to 1 in adult animals, similar to the changes of the same index in the human heart (Fig. 6). On the other hand, they reported no age-related changes in capillary density. In contrast, Rakusan and co-workers (141) found a rapid proliferation of the capillaries in the rabbit heart during the first postnatal weeks; it later diminished, and no growth was detected in adult animals.

The early stages of cardiac development of the rat were studied quantitatively by Olivetti and co-workers (124). These authors analyzed the hearts from rats at 1, 5, and 11 days of age. They found a general decline in the average luminal area of capillary profiles with age. The total area of capillary cross sections more than doubled in both ventricles during this age period, however, which is consistent with proliferation of capillaries and their change in shape to a longer and narrower configuration. The faster proliferation of capillaries relative to myocytes is apparent also from the rapid decline of the myocyte/capillary ratio during this period. The average number of capillaries across the left ventricular wall increases from 16 to 79, whereas the similar increase in the right ventricle is only from 14 to 22. The average intercapillary distance, which is more or less the same in both ventricles, decreases from 31 to 18 μm at the age of 11 days. This study may be complemented by observations of Rakusan and Poupa (139,140), who also described noticeable capillary proliferation during the early postnatal period. The fiber/capillary ratio in the left ventricle decreases from 4 in 5-day-old rats to approximately 1 in adult animals. Hence similar age-related changes may be found in human, rabbit, and rat hearts (Fig. 6). The capillary density reaches its peak in 4-week-old rats, resulting in an intercapillary distance of approximately 16 μm. Afterward, the intercapillary distance gradually increases to approximately 19 μm in adult rats and 21 μm in old rats (Fig. 7). A similar trend in the age-related changes in the capillary density in the hearts of older animals was found by Tomanek (175).

Finally, changes in the intercapillary distance during normal growth of the rat were measured *in vivo* on the surface of the beating left ventricle by Henquell and

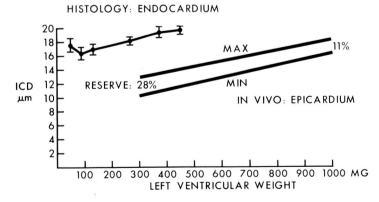

FIG. 7. Comparison of the postnatal development of the intercapillary distance in the rat heart as measured by the histological method (139) and the *in vivo* method (63).

co-workers (63). Their results are similar to those obtained from morphological measurements (Fig. 7). Between 40 and 400 days of age the average intercapillary distance increased from 12.5 μm to 19.5 μm. These values may be decreased by 2 μm in hypoxia in all ages studied. The decrease of the average intercapillary distance is the result of recruitment of additional capillaries. The capillary reserve contains about 1,280 capillaries/mm^2 in a 40-day-old rat, and it declines to only 280 capillaries/mm^2 in 400-day-old animals. This corresponds to 28% of all capillaries in the heart of a 40-day-old rat and 13% of all coronary capillaries in a 400-day-old rat. Similar results were also obtained by Korecky and co-workers (86).

Cardiac Myocytes

Man

The average diameter of cardiac myocytes was measured in human hearts by Ashley (13). He reported that during the early postnatal period the diameter is smaller in the ventricular wall than in the papillary muscle, but no differences were found between the left and right ventricles (10.8 and 9.5 μm, respectively, for papillary muscles and 8.4 and 8.0 μm for the ventricular walls). In adult and old subjects the average diameter increased up to 20 μm in the left ventricular wall compared to 16 to 17 μm in the right ventricle (Fig. 8). Similar values for papillary muscles were slightly lower. The average cell diameter in the left ventricles from subjects ranging in age from 2 months to 75 years was also estimated by Arai and co-workers (12). Their data were not tabulated, but their figures showed an increase in the diameter of cardiac myocytes from approximately 5 μm in infants to 14 μm in adults. If one plots the average cell diameter versus muscle volume of the left ventricle on a double-logarithmic scale, a linear relationship is obtained with a regression coefficient of 0.34. Assuming no changes in the length/width ratio, this is indirect support for the premise that the postnatal growth of the muscle mass is

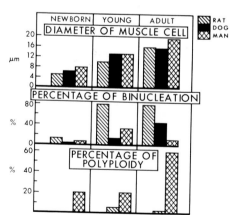

FIG. 8. Age-related changes in the diameter of the muscle cell, the percentage of binucleation, and the percentage of polyploidy in man, dog, and rat. The data cited are from the following references: man: Ashley (13), Schneider and Pfitzer (162), and Adler and Costabel (3); dog: Munnell and Getty (118) and Korecky et al. (87); rat: Rakusan and Poupa (139), Korecky et al. (87), and Grove et al. (60).

due to an increase in the volume of cardiac myocytes without changes in their number.

Estimation of the total number of cardiac myocytes is closely related to investigation of the DNA content and counts of the number of nuclei. Therefore age-related changes of these parameters are described in a single section. According to most authors, cardiac myocytes divide by mitosis. However, observations of mitotic figures in human hearts after birth are rare (113). Information about the results of mitotic divisions, i.e., cell counts, may be obtained by various methods described in Chapter 2. The early postnatal period is also characterized by a division of some cell nuclei without being followed by a division of cells, i.e., karyokinesis without subsequent cytokinesis. Hence the number of nuclei per myocyte varies with age. In some of these bi- and polynucleated myocytes the nuclei subsequently fuse, resulting in an increased amount of DNA per nucleus (polyploidy). This is a typical feature of the development of human hearts, although in many experimental animals the percentage of bi- and polynucleated cells remains high throughout the rest of life. Data on DNA concentration and content should also be adjusted for the contribution of the "nonmuscle" cells. Therefore the estimates of the total number of myocytes is usually accompanied by the simultaneous estimation of the counts of the remaining cells as well.

DNA concentration and content in growing human hearts were determined by Adler (2) and Adler and Costabel (4). DNA concentration is highest at birth and decreases exponentially with the growth of the heart. The total amount of myocardial DNA increases from approximately 10 mg at birth to 80 to 100 mg in the normal adult heart. It is composed of material originating from muscle cell nuclei as well as fibroendothelial cell nuclei. At birth these two types of nuclei are present in approximately the same numbers, but by childhood the number of fibroendothelial cell nuclei is already higher by about 50%, and in adults the number is more than double the number of muscle cell nuclei (3). The amount of DNA in the nuclei of human cardiac myocytes also increases with age. The same authors investigated the varying degree of ploidy by cytophotometry. In the hearts of children up to age 7 years, 80 to 90% of the cell nuclei are diploid. Afterward, a polyploidization begins with augmentation of the percentage of tetraploid nuclei, which become the most common class of cell ploidy in adult hearts (60 to 79%). The same process of polyploidization takes place in the right ventricle, but approximately 4 years later. Similarly, Eisenstein and Wied (42) described a decreasing frequency of diploid nuclei. In their material, all muscle cell nuclei in hearts from infants were diploid compared to only 60% in the samples from adult hearts. The polyploidization of heart muscle nuclei is probably irreversible: no decrease of the nuclear DNA content was observed in atrophic hearts (156).

The amount of DNA material per cardiac myocyte depends not only on the amount of DNA per nucleus but also on the number of nuclei per cell. At birth, the majority of cardiac myocytes are mononucleated: only 8% of the cells are binucleated in the left ventricle and 14% in the right ventricle (162). The percentage of binucleated cells increases postnatally up to 33% during late infancy or early childhood with a subsequent decrease to adult values—to 5 to 13% in the left ventricle and 7% in the right ventricle (14,73,162).

The first indirect observations concerning the total number of myocardial muscle cells in human heart based on quantitative morphology date back to the investigations of Linzbach (102–104) and Hort (73). According to these authors, shortly after birth the number of muscle cell nuclei doubles in the left ventricle; the same occurs in the right ventricle but with a slight delay. Afterward, the number of cardiac muscle nuclei remains constant as does the number of cardiac muscle cells. Similar indirect observations concerning the "cell constancy" of human hearts during normal growth and development were reported by Black-Schaffer and Turner (20) and Arai and Machida (11).

The total number of myocytes in the human left ventricle was estimated by Sandritter and Adler (155) to be 2×10^9. The changes in the cell populations with age and cardiac growth were studied by Adler and Costabel (3,4). According to these authors, the amount of cardiac myocytes at birth is 0.7 to 0.9×10^9; this figure varies between 1×10^9 and 2×10^9 later on, being more dependent on cardiac weight than on age. The number of connective tissue cells at birth is similar to the number of myocytes, but their final adult values are much higher (4×10^9 to 6×10^9). On the other hand, Arai and Machida (11) reported a constant number of myocytes in the left ventricle in those 5 months to 90 years of age. Their estimates of the total number of cells were quite variable ranging from 4×10^9 to 10×10^9.

Quantitative studies on changes in specialized conduction tissue have described the decreasing amount of conducting muscle accompanied by a relative increase in connective tissue. This applies to both the sinoatrial node (33) and the bundle of His (61).

Experimental Animals

The early stages of postnatal development of canine cardiac muscle were described by Legato (96,97). Immediately after birth, myocardial tissue has a heterogeneous pattern. Rarely (more commonly in the right ventricle than in the left) are there areas where cells look like those of the adult heart. Most of the cells, however, show considerable disorganization of their geometric arrangement and their interior architecture. Mitotic nuclei are seen occasionally at this age. The definite development of intercellular connections in the form of intercalated discs is achieved by about 2 weeks of age. The estimates of cell diameter, based on a relatively small number of measurements, revealed that they increased in the left ventricle from 4 μm at birth to 6 μm in 5-month-old puppies, whereas in the right ventricle they varied without any distinct pattern.

The diameter of muscle cells in the canine myocardium was also measured by Munnell and Getty (118) in dogs ranging from 2 days to 19 years of age. According to these authors, the average diameter of cardiac myocytes is about 6 μm; this remains rather constant during the first 3 months of life and later increases continually with age. The rate of increase is rapid at the beginning: By 6 months of age the diameter is already double the value at birth and then increases slowly to 14.5 μm in old dogs (Fig. 8). The same authors also comment on the appearance of binucleated cells in the hearts of older dogs. Unfortunately, no quantitative data are provided.

The neonatal growth of canine heart was also studied by Bishop and Hine (19) using the method of isolated cells. Although left ventricular weight increased considerably from birth, there was no increase in the size of the individual myocytes until 4 to 6 weeks of age, indicating proliferation of cardiac myocytes during the early postnatal period. At birth almost all myocytes were mononucleated, whereas in the adult animals myocytes with a single nucleus constituted only about half of the cell population.

The number of nuclei in isolated myocytes from porcine hearts were studied by Grabner and Pfitzer (57). At birth, 39% of the myocytes contained only one nucleus, 55% were binucleated, and the rest were polynucleated. With increasing age there was a shift to cell classes with more nuclei. The percentage of mononucleated cells decreased to only 13% at the age of 30 days and was less than 10% in older animals. Most of these nuclei were diploid, but polyploidy was also present.

In the cat myocardium, Sheridan and co-workers (165) described an increase in the diameter of myocytes from 7.1 μm in neonatal hearts, to 9.3 μm in infant cats (16 to 18 days old) to 18.9 μm in adult animals.

Quantitative aspects of the early postnatal growth of the rat heart were investigated by Anversa and co-workers (9). The dimensions of the average myocyte in both left and right ventricles increased steadily during the first 11 postnatal days. The average length of myocytes in both ventricles doubled from 22 μm to 44 μm, and the average cell volume almost tripled during this period. No differences were observed in the characteristics of epicardial and endocardial myocytes in either ventricle during this period. The percentage of binucleated myocytes increased in both ventricles from 3% at birth to values close to 50% at 11 days of age. The total number of myocytes doubled in the left ventricle from 7×10^6 at birth to 14×10^6 at 11 days of age. In contrast, only a 24% increase in the number of myocytes was detected in the right ventricle (from 6.3×10^6 to 7.8×10^6).

The average diameter of the myocytes as measured in histological sections of the left ventricle increased from 5 μm at birth to 16 μm in adult rats (Fig. 8) (139). Comparable data for the early period were also reported by Hirakow and Gotoh (66) and Nakata (120). Hirakow and co-workers (68) reported an increase in average cell diameter from 6 μm at day 1 to 14 μm in 2-month-old rats. The size of the cell during this age period was the same in both ventricles. The atrial cells, which were of similar size at birth, increased only slightly during this period. Similar development was found in guinea pig heart (67). The rate of growth of cardiac myocytes during the early postnatal period of the rat is more dependent on the rate of growth of the heart than on the age of the animal (145). Measurements of cardiac dimensions on isolated cells revealed the same trend of changes in the dimensions of cardiac myocytes as in histological measurements. Their absolute values, however, were higher. For instance, Korecky and Rakusan (85) described an increase in cell width from 15 μm in a group of young rats (body weight 81 g) to 25 μm in adult rats (body weight 650 g). Corresponding changes were also noted in the average cell length as the length/width ratio remained constant. The rates of increase in the volume of an average myocyte and in the left ventricular mass were found to be similar, indicating that normal cardiac growth during this period could be explained by an increase in the size of existing myocytes, and so no proliferation is required. Similar results were also found by Katzberg and co-workers (81).

The method of isolated myocytes also enables counting the number of nuclei per myocyte. The hearts of newborn rats are composed mainly of mononucleated cells, but during the early postnatal period the percentage of binucleated cells increases rapidly and reaches its adult values of 80 to 94%. When heart growth is either accelerated or slowed down, the rate of appearance of binucleation correlates with the organ size rather than with the age of the animal (81,87).

Most of the muscle cell nuclei are diploid in the rat heart. In contrast to the situation in human hearts, the frequency of polyploidy, which is rather low at birth, even decreases slightly with age in these hearts (60,115). The DNA synthesis in the nuclei can be examined by autoradiography. Rumyantsev (152) described a rapid decrease in the percentage of labeled nuclei from 20% at birth to very low values 2 weeks later. The percentage of nuclei in mitosis was approximately 10 times smaller. Kunz and co-workers (91) reported that 1.6% of muscle nuclei and 3.6% of nuclei from fibroblasts are still labeled in 15-day-old rats, but their fraction rapidly decreases with age and was very low in rats older than 2 months.

This is related to the *in vitro* studies of Claycomb (28), who reported a rapid decline of the incorporation of radioactive thymidine into cardiac DNA. The incorporation was essentially "turned off" in hearts from 17-day-old rats in conjunction with a disappearance of the activity of soluble cardiac DNA polymerase.

According to Sasaki et al. (157–159), the percentage of rat cardiac myocytes with mitotic activity decreases from 2% on the first day of life to 0.1% at 4 weeks of age and to zero thereafter. The mitotic rate of interstitial cells at birth is approximately the same as that of cardiac myocytes, but its postnatal decline is much slower. Similar results were also described by Rumyantsev (15) and Klinge (83).

DNA concentration and total DNA content of the rat heart or its parts have been investigated by several authors (37,44,58,72,143,158). They found that the DNA concentration decreased rapidly during the early postnatal period and more slowly later on, resulting in a continually increasing total DNA content. Most of these studies, however, did not distinguish between the contribution of nuclei from cardiac myocytes and nuclei from the remaining cell population. The percentage of "non-muscle" nuclei in the total population increases with advancing age.

Finally, the first attempt to estimate the total number of myocytes in adult rat heart was by Black-Schaffer and co-workers in 1965 (21). These authors used the nuclear counting method and estimated the total number of myocytes to be 90×10^6. A similar method was used by Sasaki and co-workers (157), who reported an increase in the total number of myocytes in the rat heart from 5×10^6 at birth to 19×10^6 during the first month of life with a subsequent small increase to 20×10^6 by the age of 2 years. Corresponding data for the interstitital cells were 3.5×10^6, 28×10^6, and 72×10^6, respectively. These authors, however, did not take into account the binuclearity of the majority of rat myocytes. Anversa and co-workers (9) found 7×10^6 myocytes in the left ventricle of rats at birth, and 14×10^6 at the age of 11 days. Rakusan and co-workers (143) examined 1-month-old rats and found similar results—the average number of cardiac myocytes per left ventricle was between 15 million and 20 million, depending on the method of estimation, and insignificantly increased in older animals. The final number of cardiac myocytes also depends on the rate of cardiac growth during the early postnatal period. Accelerated growth of the heart during the early postnatal period is associated with increased proliferation of myocytes (143,145).

According to Petersen and Baserga (131), DNA content in the mouse heart increases rapidly during the first postnatal month and slowly later on. These authors found no significant polyploidy in myocytes from murine hearts of different ages. The percentage of labeled heart muscle nuclei determined by autoradiography was rather high in 8-day-old mice (9.4%), decreased to 2.2% on day 32, and was absent in older mice. A lower percentage of labeled nuclei and an earlier disappearance of labeling was reported in murine hearts by Walker and Adrian (189) and Kranz and co-workers (88). Brodsky and co-workers (25) described an increase in binucleated cells from 25% at birth to 70 to 80% in older mice. Binucleated cells were rarely polyploid. On the other hand, 30 to 40% of mononucleated cells were polyploid. Changes in the volume of isolated cardiac myocytes and their total number during the first year of postnatal life in mice were investigated by Belov and co-workers (15). According to these authors, the absolute number of cardiac myocytes is about one million at birth and doubles during postnatal life; the percentage of binucleated cells increases to the adult values of approximately 80%. Cell proliferation stops completely only during the third month of postnatal life.

Conclusion

Early postnatal growth of the mammalian heart is realized by an increasing volume of the individual myocytes as well as their increasing number. The cell diameter, which appears to be similar in hearts from all mammalian species, increases during the life span to two to three times its value at birth. In contrast to older concepts of the heart as a "cell-constant" organ, it seems evident from the presented material that proliferation of muscle cells takes place in newborn hearts. It is not clear, however, when or why the proliferation stops. Linzbach (103) and Hort (74) were the first to suggest that hearts from newborns contain only half the total number of myocytes present in the adult human heart at autopsy. Adult values, however, are reached rapidly during the first few postnatal months by the final amitotic division of the cell population. Postnatal proliferation of normal myocytes is at present widely accepted, but not necessarily their amitotic character (132).

Proliferation of the cardiac myocytes in normal-growing canine hearts was suggested by the indirect evidence of Bishop and Hine in 1975 (19). The same was advanced for rat myocardium by several authors. Rakusan and co-workers (142,144) proposed that cardiac myocytes cease proliferation at the time of weaning (i.e., during the fourth postnatal week); Sasaki and co-workers (159) and Dowell and McManus (37) placed this date later; and Claycomb (28,29) proposed the 17th postnatal day as a "cut-off" date.

There is no agreement as to what causes the cardiac myocytes to cease proliferation. Linzbach (103) and Hort (73) assumed that cardiac myocytes are simply programmed for a finite number of nuclear and cellular divisions. At the present time, however, it seems to be accepted that the final number of cardiac myocytes can be increased by increasing the rate of early postnatal growth of the heart, whether the character of stimuli is physiological (72,145) or pathological (37,122,133,192). These results also refute the explanation proposed by Bischoff and Holtzer (18) for skeletal muscle based on mutual exclusiveness between DNA replication and synthesis of myofibrillar proteins. On the other hand, gradually accumulating cell-specific structures could present a progressive hindrance to mitotic divisions (196). Other suggested mechanisms are the loss of activity of DNA polymerase (28), contact inhibition of myocyte proliferation (47), a decline of nuclear phosphokinase activities, or an absence of regulatory cytoplasmic factors which are not yet identified (100,101). It has been suggested that either an increased workload associated with increasing peripheral resistance and blood pressure (142) or the completion of adrenergic innervation (29,30,89) provides physiological signals for the change in growth pattern.

An increasing volume of the individual cell is also accompanied by an increase in the amount of DNA per cell, thus preventing an excessive rise in the volume of protoplasm governed by a unit of DNA. In human and monkey hearts, the predominant mode of this increase is polyploidy, i.e., the increase of DNA material per single nucleus, whereas the number of cells containing two or more nuclei is relatively low. In contrast, rat and mouse hearts react to this challenge by increasing the number of nuclei per cell, although the incidence of polyploidy remains low, mainly confined to mononucleated cells which have also a smaller size. The canine myocardium occupies a middle position between these two types of reaction to the increasing volume of individual myocytes.

MICROSTRUCTURE—CELL LEVEL

Qualitative Changes

Descriptions of the age-related changes in the cellular structures and subcellular organelles of human myocytes are rare. Adler and co-workers (5) studied the form and structure of cell nuclei in growing human hearts. These authors described the transformation of the rounded nuclei in newborn hearts to the rectangular nuclei of normal adult hearts. The internal structure of myocardial nuclei is granular during the perinatal period, net-like during childhood, and coarsely granular in the adult heart. The average nuclear length in fetal, children's, and normal adult heart is constant, close to 10 μm. Similarly, the length of the nuclei does not change with age in the guinea pig (67) and rat (68) heart. In addition, Strehler and co-workers (173) examined lipofuscin accumulation by means of fluorescence micros-copy in a large number of human hearts of various age. Pigment was absent in the children's heart, whereas later the average concentration increased linearly as a function of age. The fraction of the myocardium occupied by this pigment increased by 0.66% per decade.

The postnatal development of subcellular structures in the canine heart was described by several authors. According to Legato (96,97), myocytes during the neonatal period are often round with a relatively large nucleus, sparse myofibrils running in all directions, and abundant rough endoplasmic reticulum. The sarcom-eric Z-bands of young myocytes tend to be more irregular in shape. There is no transverse tubular system in the myocytes of either ventricle in the newborn puppy. The T-system starts to develop only at 2 months of age in the left ventricle and even later in the right ventricle. Similar descriptions can be found in an article by Schulze (163), who also reported the formation of H- and M-bands of the myofibrils only after 1 month of age. The sarcomere length does not change with the age of animals, even though its variability is much larger in puppies than in adult dogs (171,180). The rate of accumulation of cardiac lipofuscin in dogs of different ages has been studied by Munnell and Getty (118,119). No pigment was observed in any dog under 6 months of age, and only traces and small amounts were found in those up to 3.5 years of age. From this age on, it appeared to increase linearly with age.

The ultrastructural maturation of cat myocardium was studied by Sheridan and co-workers (165). They described changes similar to those discussed in the section on canine myocardium. Neonatal myocytes are not only smaller but also rounder in transverse sections and consequently are packed less tightly together than adult myocytes. Rough endoplasmic reticulum is a prominent feature in neonatal my-ocytes. Myofibrils tend to be arranged around the periphery of the cell, whereas mitochondria at this stage frequently occupy the center of the cell. Myofibrils are less regularly aligned; they are thinner, and often one can see them branching. Transverse tubules are absent in the neonatal cat heart.

Early stages of the postnatal development of the hamster heart has been studied by Colgan and co-workers (31), and changes in the myocardial ultrastructure associated with aging were described by Sachs and co-workers (154). Myocytes from the neonatal heart differ from adult myocytes in many respects: The nucleus still occupies a large portion of the cell, the myofibrils are not well organized in space, and the intercalated discs are poorly developed. There is no evidence of transverse tubule formation at this time. At 30 days of age, the heart already closely resembles the adult myocardium, with well-developed sarcomeres as well as junc-tional complexes and T-tubules. The main feature of cells from senescent hearts is the presence of a large number of lipid droplets and aggregations of dense bodies (lysosomes), which are often found in the vicinity of the nucleus. The majority of nuclei from aging cells have rough or even highly indented surfaces. No differences in the number of nucleoli or chromatin distribution were apparent when comparing the young adult heart with the aging heart.

Schiebler and Wolf (161) studied cardiac development of rats during the late embryonic period and for the first postnatal month. During this period, they found continuous changes uninterrupted by birth itself. The final differentiation of the subcellular structures occurs postnatally. The earliest maturation was found in mitochondria, which reach their final appearance by the age of 16 days and complete their distribution by the 24th day of life. At this time the differentiation and orientation of myofibrils is also completed. The longest differentiation was found in the sarcoplasmic reticulum and the T-system. Early postnatal development of cardiac myofibrils in the rat heart was studied by Anversa and co-workers (10). They described an absence of the M-band in 1-day-old animals. The M-band is a distinctive structural feature of mature myofibrils. It is rarely detected in 5-day-old hearts, but it is present in the majority of hearts from 11-day-old rats.

The myocardial ultrastructure of senescent rats has been studied by several authors (147,176,177). Cardiac myocytes of senescent rats are characterized by increased amounts of lipofuscin pigment, primary lysosomes, and lipid droplets. Golgi structures are numerous, and myofibrils are often in disarray. Foci of small, densely packed mitochondria and dilated vesicles in the intercalated disc region are common features.

Differentiation of murine myocytes follows a pattern similar to that in the rat myocardium. Detailed descriptions can be found in the studies of Edwards and Chalice (40) and Ishikawa and Yamada (79).

Quantitative Changes

Age-related changes in volume densities of the major cellular compartments are summarized in Table 1. As may be seen from this table, the composition of mammalian cardiac myocytes is rather uniform. As a matter of fact, the results of various authors who studied the same species often varied more than the results from different species. The composition of the cardiac myocytes seems to be similar in both ventricles. On the other hand, atrial myocytes probably have a lower mitochondrial fraction than myocytes from cardiac ventricles. Not only does the composition of cardiac myocytes seem to be similar in all mammalian species, but their postnatal changes also seem to follow the same pattern. The early postnatal development is characterized by a significant increase in the mitochondrial fraction, accompanied by a more moderate increase in the myofibrillar fraction. Similarly, the contribution of the sarcoplasmic reticulum to the cell volume increases with the age of the animals. On the other hand, the percentage of cell volume occupied by the nucleus decreases considerably with increasing age of the animal. Most of the above changes take place shortly after birth, and thereafter the volume densities of the major cellular compartments are relatively stable and not influenced either

TABLE 1. *Age-related changes in major subcellular fractions of cardiac myocytes[a]*

Age	Mitochondrial	Myofibrillar	Nuclear	Sarcoplasmic reticulum	Remarks
Dog					
24 hr	20 and 20	—	8 and 8	—	(97)
3 mon	35 and 29	—	2 and 4	—	Right and left ventricle
5 mon	31 and 28	—	3 and 2	—	
Cat					
72 hr	16	34	11	0.7	(164)
16 days	21	40	10	0.6	Right ventricular
Adult	22	48	5	0.4	papillary muscle
Guinea pig					
0 day	29 and 28	53 and 53	—	—	(68)
7 days	33 and 33	53 and 56	—	—	Right and left ventricle
14 days	36 and 37	53 and 57	—	—	Percentage of cell volume minus nuclear volume
0 day	13 and 14	64 and 62	—	—	Right and left atrium
7 days	13 and 13	66 and 61	—	—	
14 days	18 and 19	65 and 65	—	—	
Hamster					
1 day	16	31	12	1.0	(31, 154)
16 days	35	36	4	1.5	Left ventricle
30 days	32	37	3	2.0	
250–300 days	28	46	1	3.0	
555 days	33	45	1	2.0	
Rat					
0 day	25 and 23	44 and 46	—	—	(120)
7 days	31 and 30	48 and 49	—	—	Right and left ventricle
90 days	36 and 35	53 and 57	—	—	
0 day	27 and 23	47 and 48	—	—	Right and left atrium
7 days	31 and 31	47 and 48	—	—	
90 days	32 and 32	58 and 57	—	—	
1 day	20 and 18	33 and 37	9 and 10	1.1 and 1.0	(124)
5 days	33 and 26	36 and 40	10 and 10	1.1 and 1.6	Right and left ventricle
11 days	35 and 34	44 and 44	8 and 8	2.1 and 2.5	
0 day	16	52	—	—	(32)
7 days	19	44	—	—	Left ventricle
14 days	26	55	—	—	
21 days	24	43	—	—	
1 mon	32	55	—	—	
6 mon	33	56	—	—	
1	19 and 17	55 and 58	—	—	(67)
10	29 and 31	59 and 57	—	—	Right and left ventricle
20	37 and 38	57 and 54	—	—	Percentage of cell volume minus nuclear volume
30	37 and 34	53 and 56	—	—	
60	36 and 34	59 and 61	—	—	
1	23 and 18	39 and 48	—	—	Right and left atrium
10	22 and 20	53 and 60	—	—	
20	26 and 27	54 and 59	—	—	
30	23 and 26	53 and 50	—	—	
60	24 and 29	61 and 58	—	—	
Body weight					
36 g	35	49	7	—	(126)
120 g	35	48	4.5	—	Left ventricle
227 g	35	47	2	—	

[a]Percentage of cell volume.

by the growth of the cell and the heart or by the age of the animal. The only possible exceptions are changes associated with aging. Kment and co-workers (84) found no differences in the mitochondrial fraction of cardiac myocytes from 5- and 21-month-old rats. However, the size of individual mitochondria was smaller in the senescent heart, and therefore the total number per unit of cell section was higher. On the other hand, Herbener (65) reported a decrease in the mitochondrial fraction of myocytes from old mice which was associated with unchanged mitochondrial size and surface density.

In addition to volume densities, several authors measured surface densities as well. For instance, in the hamster heart the relative area of sarcoplasmic reticulum increases after birth, whereas a decline of this parameter has been noted in senescent hearts. The area of the outer mitochondrial membrane expressed per mitochondrial volume does not change during the life span. On the other hand, the ratio of inner membrane plus cristae per mitochondrial volume rises significantly during the first postnatal month but decreases with aging (31,154).

Olivetti and co-workers (124) analyzed the early postnatal development of the rat heart (1 to 11 days of age). They reported a decreasing surface/volume ratio of mitochondria consistent with an increased average size of mitochondria during this period. The surface/volume ratio of smooth endoplasmic reticulum was constant, suggesting that the geometric configuration of these tubular elements underwent little change other than an increase in length. Finally, Page and co-workers (126), in their studies of older rats, reported a decrease in the classic surface/volume ratio of cells, reflecting the growth of cell size. However, the so-called composite surface/volume ratio, which included sarcolemmal and T-tubular area expressed per unit cell volume, remained almost constant as a result of compensatory accumulation of the T-tubular membrane.

SUMMARY AND CONCLUSIONS

It is not an easy task to summarize succinctly the vast amount of material presented in this chapter. Unfortunately, in the field of cardiac growth and development, we are still at the stage of data collection, and a synthetic approach has yet to be developed. Even with the data collection, however, there are some surprising gaps in our knowledge. A striking example of this is our lack of information on age-related changes in subcellular compartments of human cardiac myocytes. As we mentioned at the beginning of the chapter, there are significant species differences, mainly related to various rates of development in individual mammalian species, commencing by various degrees of maturity at birth. On the other hand, it is even more interesting to observe very similar patterns in the postnatal growth and development of human hearts and the hearts of other mammals. An example is the almost identical postnatal evolution of the ratio of myocardial muscle cells per capillary in hearts from such different species as man, rabbit, and rat (Fig. 6).

Postnatal growth and development of the mammalian heart can be divided into three stages:

1. *Early postnatal stage*—characterized by profound qualitative and quantitative changes. The interspecies differences are most clearly manifested here, and the variation within individual species is considerable.

2. *Adult stage*—where the qualitative changes more or less disappear and the only changes are of a quantitative nature. This stage encompasses most of the chronological life span.

3. *Senescent stage*—which includes the reappearance of new qualitative changes. These "normal" changes associated with late aging are sometimes difficult to separate from underlying pathological processes. In addition, the trend of several quantitative changes is reversed.

Early Postnatal Stage

The duration of the early postnatal period is variable and depends on the species analyzed and the parameter measured. For instance, most of the changes described below take place during the first postnatal year in man and the first postnatal month in the rat. At the organ level, this stage is characterized by an increase in cardiac mass which is similar to the increase in body mass in most mammalian species ($\alpha = 1$). At the same time, the left ventricular mass increases more than the right ventricular mass, and therefore the left ventricular preponderance is firmly established. On the other hand, the intraventricular volume of the right ventricle increases more than the left one, leading to a significant difference in the thickness of the right and left ventricular walls. The development of the coronary vascular bed and cardiac innervation vary by a large margin, depending on the degree of maturity of the species at birth.

At the tissue level, growth is due to an increase in both the volume of individual myocytes and their number (cell proliferation). An increasing volume of the individual cells is also accompanied by an increase in the amount of DNA per cell. Whereas cardiac myocytes at birth contain one diploid nucleus, the number of binucleated cells increases rapidly during the early postnatal stage. In human cardiac myocytes, the majority of these nuclei subsequently fuse, leading to an increasing degree of polyploidy (increased DNA per nucleus). In rat and mouse hearts, binucleated cells remain the predominant type throughout the rest of life, and the incidence of polyploidy is low. Hearts from the remaining species contain both binucleated and polyploid cells, and they therefore lie somewhere between these two types of nuclear reactions to the increasing volume of individual myocytes. This period is also characterized by a rapid proliferation of capillaries, as illustrated by a decrease in the number of myocytes supplied by a capillary from values of four to six myocytes per capillary at birth to 1:1 ratio in adult animals.

At the cell level, the final differentiation of the cell structure takes place. The major quantitative change is an increase in mitochondrial and possibly myofibrillar fractions, mainly at the expense of cell volume previously occupied by the nucleus.

Adult Stage

As mentioned above, the adult stage encompasses most of the chronological life span of the animal. It is characterized mainly by quantitative changes, whereas the composition of the structures does not change appreciably.

Cardiac mass continues to grow at rates which vary from as low as two-thirds of the rate of body growth in sheep to equal rates in man. Consequently, relative heart weight decreases with age in most experimental animals. In contrast, the relative heart weight in man does not change considerably from birth to adulthood, and it increases from 0.55% of the body weight during middle age to 0.80% in centenarians. This increase in relative heart weight is probably due to a concomitant age-related increase in blood pressure.

At the tissue and cell levels, the adult stage is the most stable period. The number of capillaries and myocytes per heart is constant, and growth of the heart is characterized by an increase in the size of individual myocytes. The cell diameter, which appears to be similar in hearts from all mammalian species, increases during the life span to two to three times its value at birth. As a consequence, the intercapillary distance increases with age and cardiac weight. The composition of cardiac myocytes is also stable, and the volume densities of the major cellular compartments do not change with age during this period.

Senescent Stage

At present, research is concentrating on the senescent stage, and the reader is referred to recent monographs by Weisfeldt (194) and Masoro (112) for more information on this topic. At this point, it is difficult to distinguish between signs of "normal aging" and signs that reflect associated pathological processes in senescence.

The cardiac mass continues to increase moderately in aging animals with the possible exception of man, where a slight reduction of cardiac mass was noted at extreme age (10th and 11th decades). Relative left ventricular dilatation in senescent hearts has been described in both human subjects and experimental animals.

At the tissue level, a moderate increase in the size of cardiac myocytes and decreased capillarity probably reflect a modest increase in cardiac mass. The ultrastructure of the cardiac myocytes undergoes typical changes during senescence, the most apparent being the increasing concentration of lipofuscin.

CONCLUSION

The major purpose of this review was to summarize our current knowledge concerning cardiac growth, development, and aging. It has become obvious that in spite of a vast amount of data collected, several areas remain to be mapped. In addition, there is little information on sex differences in cardiac growth and development. Even less well known are the mechanisms behind the developmental changes. For instance, why do the cardiac myocytes and coronary capillaries cease to proliferate at a certain stage of heart development? Is it possible to influence this phenomenon? What is its relation to cardiac function and pathology? Finally, there is a need for a synthesis of the discussed data. In the introduction, we briefly mentioned attempts to define and measure the biological age of the organism. A common approach in this case is the use of multiple regression analysis of various vital functions for predictions of biological age. It is of interest that among the parameters having the highest predictive values are several cardiovascular measurements, e.g., heart rate, heart weight, myocardial concentration of lipofuscin. It may be possible to define and measure the biological age of the heart separately and use it for subsequent evaluation of attempts to influence the aging of this important organ.

REFERENCES

1. Addis, T., and Gray, H. (1950): Body size and organ weight. *Growth*, 14:49–80.
2. Adler, C.-P. (1976): DNS in Kinderherzen: biochemische und zytophotometrische Untersuchungen. *Beitr. Pathol.*, 158:173–202.
3. Adler, C.-P., and Costabel, U. (1975): Cell number in human heart in atrophy, hypertrophy, and under the influence of cytostatics. *Recent Adv. Stud. Cardiol. Struct. Metab.*, 6:343–355.
4. Adler, C.-P., and Costabel, U. (1980): Myocardial DNA and cell number under the influence of cytostatics. I. Post-mortem investigations of human hearts. *Virchows Arch. [Cell Pathol.]*, 32:109–125.
5. Adler, C.-P., Hartz, A., and Sandritter, W. (1977): Form and structure of cell nuclei in growing and hypertrophied human hearts. *Beitr. Pathol.*, 161:342–362.
6. Altman, P. L., and Dittmer, D. S. (1962): *Biological Handbooks: Growth.* Federation of the American Society of Experimental Biology, Bethesda.
7. Anderson, R. H., and Taylor, I. M. (1972): Development of atrioventricular specialized tissue in human heart. *Br. Heart J.*, 34:1205–1214.
8. Anrep, B. V. (1880): Ueber die Entwicklung der hemmenden Funktionen bei Neugeborenen. *Pfluegers Arch.*, 21:78–106.
9. Anversa, P., Olivetti, G., and Loud, A. V. (1980): Morphometric study of early postnatal development in the left and right ventricular myocardium of the rat. I. Hypertrophy, hyperplasia and binucleation of myocytes. *Circ. Res.*, 46:495–502.
10. Anversa, P., Olivetti, G., Bracchi, P.-G., and Loud, A. V. (1981): Postnatal development of the M-band in rat cardiac myofibres. *Circ. Res.*, 48:561–568.
11. Arai, S., and Machida, A. (1972): Myocardial cell in left ventricular hypertrophy. *Tohoku J. Exp. Med.*, 108:361–367.
12. Arai, S., Machida, A., and Nakamura, T. (1968): Myocardial structure and vascularization of hypertrophied hearts. *Tohoku J. Exp. Med.*, 95:35–54.
13. Ashley, L. M. (1945): A determination of the diameters of myocardial fibers in man and other mammals. *J. Anat.*, 77:325–347.
14. Baroldi, G., Falzi, G., and Lampertico, P. (1967): The nuclear patterns of the cardiac muscle fiber. *Cardiologia*, 51:109–123.
15. Belov, L. N., Leontjeva, T. A., and Kogan, M. E. (1977): Quantitative estimate of the muscle cell proliferation during postnatal cardiogenesis in mice. [in Russian]. *Ontogenesis*, 8:442–450.
16. Berg, B. N., and Harmison, C. R. (1955): Blood pressure and heart size in aging rats. *J. Gerontol.*, 10:416–419.
17. Bertalanffy, L.v. (1951): *Theoretische Biologie, Bd. 2: Stoffwechsel, Wachstum.* Karger, Basel.
18. Bischoff, R., and Holtzer, H. (1969): Mitosis and the process of differentiation of myogenic cells in vitro. *J. Cell Biol.*, 41:188–201.
19. Bishop, S. P., and Hine, P. (1975): Cardiac muscle cytoplasmic and nuclear development during canine neonatal growth. *Recent Adv. Stud. Cardiol. Struct. Metab.*, 8:77–98.
20. Black-Schaffer, B., and Turner, M. E. (1958): Hyperplastic infantile cardiomegaly. *Am. J. Pathol.*, 34:745–765.

21. Black-Schaffer, B., Grinstead, C. E., and Braunstein, J. N. (1965): Endocardial fibroelastosis of large mammals. *Circ. Res.*, 16:385–390.
22. Boyd, E. (1952): *An Introduction to Human Biology and Anatomy for First Year Medical Students.* Child Research Council, Denver.
23. Boyd, E. (1980): *Origins of the Study of Human Growth.* University of Oregon, Health Sciences Center, Portland.
24. Breining, H. (1968): Massenverhältnisse und Gewichtsrelationen des Herzens von der Frühgeborenperiode bis zum Erwachsenalter. *Virchows Arch. [Pathol. Anat.]*, 345:15–22.
25. Brodsky, W. Y., Arefyeva, A. M., and Uryvaeva, I. V. (1980): Mitotic polyploidization of mouse heart myocytes during the first postnatal week. *Cell Tissue Res.*, 210:133–144.
26. Burkard, W. P., Gey, K. F., and Pletscher, A. (1966): Alterations of the catecholamine metabolism of the rat heart in old age. In: *Proceedings of the 7th International Congress of Gerontology*, pp. 237–239.
27. Callingham, B. A., and Della Corte, L. (1972): The influence of growth and adrenalectomy upon some rat heart enzymes. *Br. J. Pharmacol.*, 46:530–531.
28. Claycomb, W. C. (1973): DNA synthesis and DNA polymerase activity in differentiating cardiac muscle. *Biochem. Biophys. Res. Commun.*, 54:715–720.
29. Claycomb, W. C. (1976): Biochemical aspects of cardiac muscle differentiation. *J. Biol. Chem.*, 251:6082–6089.
30. Claycomb, W. C. (1977): Cardiac muscle hypertrophy: differentiation and growth of the heart cell during development. *Biochem. J.*, 168:599–601.
31. Colgan, J. A., Lazarus, M. L., and Sachs, H. G. (1978): Post-natal development of the normal and cardiomyopathic Syrian hamster: a quantitative electron microscopic study. *J. Mol. Cell Cardiol.*, 10:43–54.
32. David, H., Myer, R., Marx, I., Guski, H., and Wenzelides, K. (1979): Morphometric characterization of left ventricular myocardial cells of male rats during postnatal development. *J. Mol. Cell Cardiol.*, 11:631–638.
33. Davies, M. J., and Pomerance, A. (1972): Quantitative study of ageing changes in the human sinoatriad node and internodal tracts. *Br. Heart J.*, 34:150–152.
33a. Dbaly, J. (1973): Postnatal development of coronary arteries in the rat. *Z. Anat. Entwickl. Gesch.*, 141:89–101.
34. DeChamplain, J., Malmfors, T., Olson, L., and Sachs, C. (1970): Ontogenesis of peripheral adrenergic neurons in the rat: pre- and postnatal observations. *Acta Physiol. Scand.*, 80:276–288.
35. DeLa Cruz, M. V., Anselmi, G., Pomero, A., and Monroy, G. (1960): A qualitative and quantitative study of the ventricles and great vessels of normal children. *Am. Heart J.*, 60:675–690.
36. Della Corte, L., and Callingham, B. A. (1977): The influence of age and adrenalectomy on rat heart monoamine oxidase. *Biochem. Pharmacol.*, 26:407–415.
37. Dowell, R. T., and McManus, R. E., III (1978): Pressure induced cardiac enlargement in neonatal and adult rats. *Circ. Res.*, 42:303–310.
38. Dyundikova, V. A., Silvon, Z. K.., and Dubina, T. L. (1981): Biological age and its estimation. I. Studies of some physiological parameters in albino rats and their validity as biological age tests. *Exp. Gerontol.*, 16:13–24.
39. Eckner, F. A. O., Brown, B. W., Davidson, D. L., and Glagov, S. (1969): Dimensions of normal human hearts. *Arch. Pathol.*, 88:497–507.
40. Edwards, G. A., and Challice, C. E. (1958): The fine structure of cardiac muscle cells of newborn and suckling mice. *Exp. Cell. Res.*, 15:247–250.
41. Ehrich, W., De La Chapelle, C., and Cohn, A. E. (1931–1932): Anatomical ontogeny. B. Man (a study of the coronary arteries). *Am. J. Anat.*, 49:241–282.
42. Eisenstein, R., and Wied, G. L. (1970): Myocardial DNA and protein in maturity and hypertrophied hearts. *Proc. Soc. Exp. Biol. Med.*, 133:176–179.
43. Emery, J. L., and Mithal, A. (1961): Weight of cardiac ventricles at and after birth. *Br. Heart J.*, 23:313–316.
44. Enesco, M., and Leblond, C. P. (1962): Increase in cell number as a factor in the growth of the organs and tissues of the young male rat. *J. Embryol. Exp. Morphol.*, 10:530–562.
45. Falk, A. (1901): The growth of the child's heart related to age. Dissertation, St. Petersburg. Cited in Altman and Dittmer (6) and Rowlatt et al. (151).
46. Finlay, M., and Anderson, R. H. (1974): The development of cholinesterase activity in the rat heart. *J. Anat.*, 117:239–298.

47. Fishman, D. A., Doyle, C. M., and Zak, R. (1976): DNA synthesis in chick cardiac muscle: comparative observations of in vivo and in vitro growth. In: *Developmental and Physiological Correlates of Cardiac Muscle*, edited by M. Lieberman and T. Sand, pp. 67–79. Raven Press, New York.

48. Friedman, W. F. (1972): Neuropharmacologic studies of perinatal myocardium. *Cardiovasc. Clin.*, 4:44–57.

49. Friedman, W. F. (1972): The intrinsic properties of the developing heart. *Prog. Cardiovasc. Dis.*, 15:87–111.

50. Friedman, W. F., Pool, P. E., Jacobowitz, D., Seagren, S. C., and Braunwald, E. (1968): Sympathetic innervation of the developing rabbit heart: biochemical and histochemical comparisons of fetal, neonatal and adult myocardium. *Circ. Res.*, 23:25–32.

51. Frolkis, V. V., and Bogatskaya, L. N. (1968): The energy metabolism of myocardium and its regulation in animals of various age. *Exp. Gerontol.*, 3:199–210.

52. Frolkis, V. V., Berzukov, V. V., Bogatskaya, L. N., Verkhratsky, N. S., Zamostian, V. P., Shevtchuk, V. G., and Shtchegoleva, I. V. (1970): Catecholamines in the metabolism and function regulation in aging. *Gerontologia*, 16:129–135.

53. Gerstenblith, G., Frederiksen, J., Yin, F. C., Fortuin, N. J., Lakatta, E. G., and Weisfeldt, M. L. (1977): Echocardiographic assessment of a normal adult aging population. *Circulation*, 56:273–278.

54. Gewert, M. (1929): Ueber die Schwankungen des Herzgewichts in dem verschiedenen Lebensaltern unter der normalen und pathologischen Verhaltnissen. Cited in Boyd (23).

55. Gey, K. F., Burkard, W. P., and Pletscher, A. (1965): Variation of the norepinephrine metabolism of the rat heart with age. *Gerontology*, 11:1–11.

56. Glowinski, J., Axelrod, U., Kopin, I. J., and Wurtman, R. J. (1964): Physiological disposition of H^3-norepinephrine in tissues of the developing rat. *J. Pharmacol. Exp. Ther.*, 146:48–53.

57. Grabner, W., and Pfitzer, P. (1974): Number of nuclei in isolated myocardial cells of pigs. *Virchows Arch. [Cell Pathol.]*, 15:279–294.

58. Grimm, A. F., De La Torre, L., and La Porta, M. (1970): Ventricular nuclei-DNA relationship with myocardial growth and hypertrophy in the rat. *Circ. Res.*, 26:45–52.

59. Grimm, A. F., Katele, K. V., Klein, S. A., and Lin, H. L. (1973): Growth of the rat heart: left ventricular morphology and sarcomere lengths. *Growth*, 37:189–201.

60. Grove, D., Nair, K. G., and Zak, R. (1969): Biochemical correlates of cardiac hypertrophy. III. Changes in DNA content; the relative contributions of polyploidy and mitotic activity. *Circ. Res.*, 25:463–471.

61. Hecht, F. M. (1980): Studie über quantitative Altersveränderungen am Hisschen Bündel des Menschen. *Virchows Arch. [Pathol. Anat.]*, 386:343–365.

62. Heggenes, F. W., Diliberto, J., and Distefano, V. (1970): Effect of growth velocity on cardiac norepinephrine content in infant rats. *Proc. Soc. Exp. Biol. Med.*, 133:1413–1416.

63. Henquell, L., Odoroff, C. L., and Honig, C. R. (1976): Coronary intercapillary distance during growth: relation to PCO_2 and aerobic capacity. *Am. J. Physiol.*, 231:1852–1859.

64. Henry, W. L., Ware, J., Gardin, J. M., Hepner, S. I., McKay, J., and Weiner, H. (1978): Echocardiographic measurements in normal subjects: growth-related changes that occur between infancy and early adulthood. *Circulation*, 57:278–285.

65. Herbener, G. H. (1976): A morphometric study of age-dependent changes in mitochondrial populations of mouse liver and heart. *J. Gerontol.*, 31:8–12.

66. Hirakow, R., and Gotoh, T. (1976): A quantitative ultrastructural study on the developing rat heart. In: *Developmental and Physiological Correlates of Cardiac Muscle*, edited by M. Lieberman and T. Sand. Raven Press, New York.

67. Hirakow, R., and Gotoh, T. (1980): Quantitative studies on the ultrastructural differentiation and growth of mammalian cardiac muscle cells. II. The atria and ventricles of the guinea pig. *Acta Anat. (Basel)*, 108:230–237.

68. Hirakow, R., Gotoh, T., and Watanabe, T. (1980): Quantitative studies on the ultrastructural differentiation and growth of mammalian muscle cells. I. The atria and ventricles of the rat. *Acta Anat. (Basel)*, 108:144–152.

69. Hirokawa, K. (1972): A quantitative study on pre- and postnatal growth of human heart. *Acta Pathol. Jpn.*, 22:613–624.

70. Hody, G., Jonec, W., Morton-Smith, W., and Finch, C. E. (1975): NE uptake by the myocardium of the senescent mouse in vitro. *J. Gerontol.*, 30:275–278.

71. Hofecker, G., Skalicky, M., Kment, A., and Niedermüller, H. (1980): Models of the biological age of the rat. I. A factor model of age parameters. *Mech. Ageing Dev.*, 14:345–359.
72. Hollenberg, M., Honbo, N., and Samorodin, A. J. (1977): Cardiac cellular responses to altered nutrition in the neonatal rat. *Am. J. Physiol.*, 233:H356–H360.
73. Hort, W. (1953): Quantitative Histologische Untersuchungen an Wachsenden Herzen. *Virchows Arch. [Pathol. Anat.]*, 323:223–242.
74. Hort, W. (1955): Morphologische Untersuchungen an Herzen vor, während und nach der postnatalen Kreislaufumschaltung. *Virchows Arch. [Pathol. Anat.]*, 326:458–484.
75. Hort, W. (1955): Quantitative Untersuchungen über die Kapillarisierung des Herzmuskels im Erwachsenen-und Greisenalter, bei Hypertrophie und Hyperplasie. *Virchows Arch. [Pathol. Anat.]*, 327:560–576.
76. Hort, W., and Severidt, H.-J. (1966): Kapillarisierung und mikroskopische Veränderungen im Myokard bei angeborenen Herzfehlern. *Virchows Arch. [Pathol. Anat.]*, 341:192–203.
77. House, E. W., and Ederstrom, H. E. (1968): Anatomical changes with age in the heart and ductus arteriosus in the dog after birth. *Anat. Rec.*, 160:289–296.
78. Hutchins, G. M., Bulkley, B. H., Miner, M. M., and Boitnott, J. K. (1977): Correlation of age and heart weight with tortuosity and caliber of normal human coronary arteries. *Am. Heart J.*, 94:196–202.
79. Ishikawa, H., and Yamada, E. (1976): Differentiation of the sarcoplasmic reticulum and T-system in developing mouse cardiac muscle. In: *Developmental and Physiological Correlates of Cardiac Muscle*, edited by M. Lieberman and T. Sano, pp. 21–36. Raven Press, New York.
80. Iversen, L. L., De Champlain, J., Glowinski, J., and Axelrod, J. (1967): Uptake, storage and metabolism of norepinephrine in tissues of the developing rat. *J. Pharmacol. Exp. Ther.*, 157:509–516.
81. Katzberg, A. A., Farmer, B. B., and Harris, R. (1977): The predominance of binucleation in isolated rat myocytes. *Am. J. Anat.*, 149:489–500.
82. Keen, E. N. (1955): The postnatal development of the human cardiac ventricles. *J. Anat.*, 89:484–502.
83. Klinge, O. (1967): Proliferation und Regeneration am Myokard. *Z. Zellforsch. Mikrosk. Anat.*, 80:488–517.
84. Kment, A., Leibetseder, J., and Burger, H. (1966): Gerontologische Untersuchungen an Rattenherzmitochondrien. *Gerontologia*, 12:193–199.
85. Korecky, B., and Rakusan, K. (1978): Normal and hypertrophic growth of the rat heart: changes in cell dimensions and number. *Am. J. Physiol.*, 234:H123–H128.
86. Korecky, B., Hai, C. M., and Rakusan, K. (1982): Functional capillary density in normal and transplanted rat hearts. *Can. J. Physiol. Pharmacol.*, 60:23–32.
87. Korecky, B., Sweet, S., and Rakusan, K. (1979): Number of nuclei in mammalian cardiac myocytes. *Can. J. Physiol. Pharmacol.*, 57:1122–1129.
88. Kranz, D., Fuhrmann, I., and Keim, U. (1975): Ein Beitrag zum physiologischen Herzwachstum. *Z. Mikrosk. Anat. Forsch.*, 89:207–218.
89. Kugler, J. D., Gillette, P. C., Graham, S. P., Garson, A., Goldstein, M. A., and Thompson, H. K. (1980): Effect of chemical sympathectomy on myocardial cell division in the newborn rat. *Pediatr. Res.*, 14:881–884.
90. Kuntscherová, J., and Vlk, J. (1979): Postnatal changes in the amount of acetylcholine in the atrial tissue of the albino rat heart. *Physiol. Bohemoslov.*, 28:569–572.
91. Kunz, J., Keim, V., and Fuhrmann, I. (1972): Die Proliferation von Muskelzellen und Bindegewebszellen des Rattenherzens während des postnatalen Wachstums. *Exp. Pathol.*, 6:270–277.
92. Kyrieleis, C. (1963): Die Formveränderungen des menschlichen Herzens nach der Geburt. *Virchows Arch. [Pathol. Anat.]*, 337:142–163.
93. Lakatta, E. G. (1979): Alterations in the cardiovascular system that occur in advanced age. *Fed. Proc.*, 38:163–167.
94. Lakatta, E. G., Gerstenblith, G., Angell, C. S., Shock, N. W., and Weisfeldt, M. L. (1975): Prolonged contraction duration in aged myocardium. *J. Clin. Invest.*, 55:61–68.
95. Lee, J. C., Taylor, J. F. N., and Downing, S. E. (1975): A comparison of ventricular weights and geometry in newborn, young and adult mammals. *J. Appl. Physiol.*, 38:147–150.
96. Legato, M. J. (1979): Cellular mechanisms of normal growth in the mammalian heart. I. Qualitative and quantitative features of ventricular architecture in the dog from birth to five months of age. *Circ. Res.*, 44:250–262.

97. Legato, M. J. (1979): Cellular mechanisms of normal growth in the mammalian heart. II. A quantitative and qualitative comparison between the right and left ventricular myocytes in the dog from birth to five months of age. *Circ. Res.*, 44:263–279.

98. Lev, M., Rowlatt, U. F., and Rimoldi, H. J. A. (1961): Pathologic methods for the study of congenitally malformed hearts. *Arch. Pathol.*, 72:491–511.

99. Limas, C. J. (1975): Comparison of the handling of norepinephrine in the myocardium of adult and old rats. *Cardiovasc. Res.*, 9:664–668.

100. Limas, C. J. (1978): Myocardial nuclear protein kinases during postnatal development. *Am. J. Physiol.*, 235:H338–H344.

101. Limas, C. J. (1980): Cytoplasmic control of DNA synthesis by myocardial nuclei. *Am. J. Physiol.*, 238:H66–H72.

102. Linzbach, A. J. (1947): Mikrometrische und Histologische Analyse hypertropher menschlicher Herzen. *Virchows Arch. [Pathol. Anat.]*, 314:534–592.

103. Linzbach, A. J. (1950): Die Muskelfaserkonstante und das Wachstumgesetz der menschlichen Herzkammer. *Virchows Arch. [Pathol. Anat.]*, 318:575–618.

104. Linzbach, A. J. (1952): Die Anzahl der Herzmuskelkerne in normalen, überlasteten, atrophen und Corhormon behandelten Herzkammer. *Z. Kreislaufforsch.*, 41:641–658.

105. Linzbach, A. J. (1955): Quantitative Biologie und Morphologie des Wachstums einschliesslich Hypertrophie und Riesenzellen. In: *Handbuch der Algemeinen Pathologie*, Band 6, Teil 1. Springer, Berlin.

106. Linzbach, A. J., and Akuamoa-Boateng, E. (1973): Die Alternsveränderungen des menschlichen Herzens. I. Das Herzgewicht im Alter. *Klin. Wochenschr.*, 51:156–163.

107. Linzbach, A. J., and Akuamoa-Boateng, E. (1973): Die Alternsveränderungen des menschlichen Herzens. II. Die Polypathie des Herzens im Alter. *Klin. Wochenschr.*, 51:164–175.

108. Lipp, J. M., and Rudolph, A. M. (1972): Sympathetic nerve development in the rat and guinea pig heart. *Biol. Neonate*, 21:76–82.

109. Ludwig, F. C., and Smoke, M. E. (1980): The measurement of biological age. *Exp. Aging Res.*, 6:497–522.

110. Mackenzie, E., and Standen, N. B. (1980): The postnatal development of adrenoreceptor responses in isolated papillary muscles from rat. *Pfluegers Arch.*, 383:185–187.

111. Martinez, J. L., Vasquez, B. J., Messing, R. B., Jensen, R. A., Liang, K. C., and McGaugh, J. L. (1981): Age-related changes in the catecholamine content of peripheral organs in male and female F344 rats. *J. Gerontol.*, 36:280–284.

112. Masoro, J. (1981): *Handbook of Physiology in Aging.* CRC Press, Boca Raton, Florida.

113. McMahon, H. E. (1938): Hypertrophy of the heart in infants. *Am. J. Dis. Child.*, 55:93–97.

114. Meyer, W. W., Peter, I., and Solth, K. (1964): Die Organgewichte in den höheren Alterstufen (70-92 Jahre) in ihrer Beziehung zum Alter und Korpergewicht. *Virchows Arch. [Pathol. Anat.]*, 337:17–32.

115. Mirakayan, V. O., and Rumyantsev, P. P. (1968): DNA synthesis in postnatal histogenesis of myocardium and under its infarction, hypertrophy and regeneration. *Proc. Acad. Sci. USSR*, 10:964–980.

116. Mühlmann, M. (1927): Wachstum, Altern und Tod. *Ergeb. Anat. Entwickl.*, 27:1–245.

117. Müller, W. (1883): *Die Massenverhältnisse des menschlichen Herzens.* Voss, Hamburg.

118. Munnell, J. F., and Getty, R. (1968): Nuclear lobulation and amitotic division associated with increasing cell size in the aging canine myocardium. *J. Gerontol.*, 23:363–369.

119. Munnell, J. F., and Getty, R. (1968): Rate of accumulation of cardiac lipofuscin in the aging canine. *J. Gerontol.*, 23:154–158.

120. Nakata, K. (1977): Quantitative analysis of ultrastructural changes in developing rat cardiac muscle during normal growth and during acute volume overload. *Jpn. Circ. J.*, 41:1237–1256.

121. Navaratnam, V. (1965): The ontogenesis of cholinesterase activity within heart and cardiac ganglia in man, rat, rabbit and guinea pig. *J. Anat.*, 99:467–469.

122. Neffgen, J. F., and Korecky, B. (1972): Cellular hyperplasia and hypertrophy in cardiomegalies induced by anemia in young and adult rats. *Circ. Res.*, 30:104–113.

123. Oberhänsli, I., Brandon, G., Lacourt, G., and Friedli, B. (1980): Growth patterns of cardiac structures and changes in systolic time intervals in the newborn and infant. *Acta Paediatr. Scand.*, 69:239–247.

124. Olivetti, G., Anversa, P., and Loud, A. V. (1980): Morphometric study of early postnatal devel-

opment in the left and right ventricular myocardium of the rat. II. Tissue composition, capillary growth and sarcoplasmic alterations. *Circ. Res.*, 46:503–512.

125. Owman, C., Sjoberg, N. O., and Swedin, G. (1971): Histochemical and chemical studies on pre-natal and post-natal development of the different systems of short and long adrenergic neurons in peripheral organs of the rat. *Z. Zellforsch. Mikrosk. Anat.*, 116:319–341.

126. Page, E., Earley, J., and Power, B. (1974): Normal growth of ultrastructures in rat ventricular myocardial cells. *Circ. Res. [Suppl. 11]*, 34-35:11–16.

127. Papacharalampous, N. X. (1964): Altersbedigte histologische und histochemische Veränderungen der Coronargeffässe. *Virchows Arch. [Pathol. Anat.]*, 338:187–193.

128. Papka, R. E. (1981): Development of innervation to the ventricular myocardium of the rabbit. *J. Mol. Cell. Cardiol.*, 13:217–228.

129. Pappritz, G., Schneider, P., and Trieb, G. (1977): Allometric analysis of the atrioventricular heart-valve weights in beagle dogs. *Basic Res. Cardiol.*, 72:628–635.

130. Paulsen, S., Vetner, M., and Hagerup, L. M. (1975): Relationship between heart weight and the cross sectional area of the coronary ostia. *Acta Pathol. Microbiol. Scand.*, 83A:429–432.

131. Petersen, R. O., and Baserga, R. (1965): Nucleic acid and protein synthesis in cardiac muscle of growing and adult mice. *Exp. Cell Res.*, 40:340–352.

132. Pfitzer, P. (1980): Amitosis: a historical misinterpretation? *Pathol. Res. Pract.*, 167:292–300.

133. Poupa, O., Korecky, B., Krofta, K., Rakusan, K., and Prochazka, J. (1964): Effect of anemia during early post-natal period on vascularization of the myocardium and its resistance to anoxia. *Physiol. Bohemoslov.*, 13:281–287.

134. Prange, A. J., White, J. E., Lipton, M. A., and Kinkead, A. M. (1967): Influence of age on monoamine oxidase and catechol-O-methyl-transferase in rat tissue. *Life Sci.*, 6:581–586.

135. Prothero, J. (1979): Heart weight as a function of body weight in mammals. *Growth*, 43:139–150.

136. Rabe, D. (1973): Kalibermessungen an den Herzkranzarterien und dem Sinus coronarius. *Basic Res. Cardiol.*, 68:356–379.

137. Rakusan, K. (1975): Hemoglobin values and organ weights in fast and slow growing rats at the time of weaning. *Growth*, 39:463–473.

138. Rakusan, K. (1980): Postnatal development of the heart. In: *Hearts and Heart-Like Organs*, edited by E. Bourne, Vol. 1, pp. 301–348. Academic, New York, London, Toronto.

139. Rakusan, K., and Poupa, O. (1963): Changes in the diffusion distance in the rat heart muscle during development. *Physiol. Bohemoslov.*, 12:220–227.

140. Rakusan, K., and Poupa, O. (1964): Capillaries and muscle fibres in the heart of old rats. *Gerontologia*, 9:107–112.

141. Rakusan, K., Du Mesnil De Rochemont, W., Braasch, W., Tschopp, H., and Bing, R. J. (1967): Capacity of the terminal vascular bed during normal growth, in cardiomegaly and in cardiac atrophy. *Circ. Res.*, 21:209–214.

142. Rakusan, K., Jelinek, J., Soukupova, M., Korecky, B., and Poupa, O. (1965): Postnatal development of muscle fibers and capillaries in the rat heart. *Physiol. Bohemoslov.*, 14:32–37.

143. Rakusan, K., Korecky, B., and Mezl, V. (1982): Cardiac hypertrophy and/or hyperplasia? In: *Biology of Myocardial Hypertrophy and Failure*, edited by N. Alpert. Raven Press, New York.

144. Rakusan, K., Korecky, B., Roth, Z., and Poupa, O. (1963): Development of the ventricular weight of the rat heart with special reference to the early phases of postnatal ontogenesis. *Physiol. Bohemoslov.*, 12:518–525.

145. Rakusan, K., Raman, S., Layberry, R., and Korecky, B. (1978): The influence of aging and growth on the postnatal development of cardiac muscle in rats. *Circ. Res.*, 42:212–218.

146. Recavaren, S., and Arias-Stella, J. (1964): Growth and development of the ventricular myocardium from birth to adult life. *Br. Heart J.*, 26:187–192.

147. Reichel, W. (1968): Lipofuscin pigment accumulation and distribution in five rat organs as a function of age. *J. Gerontol.*, 23:145–153.

148. Roberts, J. T., and Wearn, J. T. (1941): Quantitative changes in the capillary-muscle relationship in human hearts during normal growth and hypertrophy. *Am. Heart J.*, 21:617–633.

149. Rogé, C. L. L., Silverman, N. M., Hart, P. A., and Ray, R. M. (1978): Cardiac structure growth pattern determined by echocardiography. *Circulation*, 57:285–290.

150. Rosahn, P. D. (1941): The weight of the normal heart in adult males. *Yale J. Biol. Med.*, 14:209–233.

151. Rowlatt, U. F., Rimoldi, H. J. A., and Lev, M. (1963): The quantitative morphology of the normal child's heart. *Pediatr. Clin. North Am.*, 10:499–588.
152. Rumyantsev, P. P. (1965): DNA synthesis and nuclear division in embryonal and postnatal histogenesis of myocardium (autoradiographic study). *Fed. Proc.*, 24:899–902.
153. Sachs, C., De Champlain, J., Halmfors, T., and Olson, L. (1970): The postnatal development of noradrenaline uptake in the adrenergic nerves of different tissues from the rat. *Eur. J. Pharmacol.*, 9:67–79.
154. Sachs, H. G., Colgan, J., and Lazarus, M. L. (1978): Ultrastructure of the aging myocardium: a morphometric approach. *Am. J. Anat.*, 150:63–72.
155. Sandritter, W., and Adler, C. P. (1971): Numerical hyperplasia in human heart hypertrophy. *Experientia*, 27:1435–1437.
156. Sandritter, W., and Adler, C. P. (1978): Polyploidization of heart muscle nuclei as a prerequisite for heart growth and numerical hyperplasia in heart hypertrophy. *Rec. Adv. Stud. Cardiol. Struct. Metab.*, 12:115–127.
157. Sasaki, R., Morishita, T., and Yamagata, S. (1968): Mitosis of heart muscle cells in normal rats. *Tohoku J. Exp. Med.*, 96:405–411.
158. Sasaki, R., Watanabe, Y., Morishita, T., and Yamagata, S. (1968): Determination of deoxyribonucleic acid content of heart muscle and myocardial growth in normal rats. *Tohoku J. Exp. Med.*, 95:185–192.
159. Sasaki, R., Watanabe, Y., Morishita, T., and Yamagata, S. (1968): Estimation of the cell number of heart muscles in normal rats. *Tohoku J. Exp. Med.*, 95:177–184.
160. Schiebler, T. H., and Heene, R. (1968): Nachweis von Katecholaminen in Rattenherzen während die Entwicklung. *Histochemie*, 14:328–334.
161. Schiebler, T. H., and Wolff, H. H. (1966): Elektronenmikroskopische Untersuchungen am Herzmuskel der Ratte während der Entwicklung. *Z. Zellforsch. Mikrosk. Anat.*, 69:22–40.
162. Schneider, R., and Pfitzer, P. (1973): Die Zahl der Kerne in isolierten Zellen des menschlichen Myokards. *Virchows Arch. [Pathol. Anat.]*, 12:238–258.
163. Schulze, W. (1961): Elektronenmikroskopische und histometrische Untersuchungen des Herzmuskelgewebes vom Hund während des postnatalen Wachstums. *Acta Biol. Med. Germ.*, 7:24–31.
164. Sheridan, D. J., Cullen, M. J., and Tynan, M. J. (1977): Postnatal ultrastructural changes in the cat myocardium: a morphometric study. *Cardiovasc. Res.*, 11:536–540.
165. Sheridan, D. J., Cullen, M. J., and Tynan, M. J. (1979): Qualitative and quantitative observations on ultrastructural changes during postnatal development in the cat myocardium. *J. Mol. Cell. Cardiol.*, 11:1173–1181.
166. Shipley, R. A., Shipley, L. J., and Wearn, J. T. (1937): The capillary supply in normal and hypertrophied hearts of rabbits. *J. Exp. Med.*, 65:29–44.
167. Shreiner, T. P., Weisfeldt, M. L., and Shock, N. W. (1969): Effects of age, sex and breeding status on the rat heart. *Am. J. Physiol.*, 217:176–180.
168. Sjögren, A. L. (1971): Left ventricular wall thickness determined by ultrasound in 100 subjects without heart disease. *Chest*, 60:341–346.
169. Skalicky, M., Hofecker, G., Kment, A., and Niedermüller, M. (1980): Models of the biological age of the rat. II. Multiple regression models in the study on influencing aging. *Mech. Ageing Dev.*, 14:361–377.
170. Sole, M. J., Lo, C. M., Laird, C. W., Sonnenblick, E. H., and Wurtman, R. J. (1975): Norepinephrine turnover in the heart and spleen of the cardiomyopathic Syrian hamster. *Circ. Res.*, 37:855–862.
171. Spotnitz, W. D., Spotnitz, H. M., Truccone, N. J., Cottrell, T. S., Gersony, W., Malm, J. R., and Sonnenblick, E. H. (1979): Relations of ultrastructure and function: sarcomere dimensions, pressure-volume curves, and geometry of the intact left ventricle of the immature canine heart. *Circ. Res.*, 44:679–691.
172. Stanton, H. C., and Mueller, R. L. (1975): Ontogenesis of catecholamines and some related enzymes in heart and spleen of swine (Sus domesticus). *Comp. Biochem. Physiol.*, 50C:171–176.
173. Strehler, B. L., Mark, D. D., Mildvan, A. S., and Gee, M. V. (1959): Rate and magnitude of age pigment accumulation in the human myocardium. *J. Gerontol.*, 14:430–435.
174. Taylor, I. M. (1977): The development of innervation in the rat atrioventricular node. *Cell Tissue Res.*, 178:73–82.
175. Tomanek, R. J. (1970): Effects of age and exercise on the extent of the myocardial capillary bed. *Anat. Rec.*, 167:55–62.

176. Tomanek, R. J., and Karlsson, U. L. (1973): Myocardial ultrastructure of young and senescent rats. *J. Ultrastruct. Res.*, 42:201–220.
177. Travis, D. F., and Travis, A. (1972): Ultrastructural changes in the left ventricular rat myocardial cells with age. *J. Ultrastruct. Res.*, 39:124–148.
178. Tucek, S. (1965): Changes in choline acetyltransferase activity in the cardiac auricles of dogs during postnatal development. *Physiol. Bohemoslov.*, 14:530–535.
179. Tynan, M., Davies, P., and Sheridan, D. (1977): Postnatal maturation of noradrenaline uptake and release in cat papillary muscle. *Cardiovasc. Res.*, 11:206–299.
180. Urthaler, F., Walker, A. A., Kawamura, K., Hefner, L. L., and James, T. N. (1978): Canine atrial and ventricular muscle mechanics studied as a function of age. *Circ. Res.*, 42:703–713.
181. Verkhratsky, N. W. (1970): Acetylcholine metabolism peculiarities in aging. *Exp. Gerontol.*, 5:49–56.
182. Vlk, J. (1979): Postnatal development of postganglionic parasympathetic neurones in the heart of the albino rat. *Physiol. Bohemoslov.*, 28:561–568.
183. Vlk, J., and Tucek, S. (1962): Changes in the acetylcholine content and cholinesterase activity in dog atria during the early postnatal period. *Physiol. Bohemoslov.*, 11:53–58.
184. Vlk, J., and Vincenzi, F. F. (1977): Functional autonomic innervation of mammalian cardiac pacemaker during the perinatal period. *Biol. Neonate*, 31:19–26.
185. Vlk, J., and Volin, M. (1980): Specific characteristics of sympathetic fibres innervating the heart of young rats. *Physiol. Bohemoslov.*, 29:201–208.
186. Vořil, Z., and Schiebler, T. H. (1969): Uber die Entwicklung der Gefässversorgung des Rattenherzens. *Z. Anat. Entwickl. Gesch.*, 129:24–40.
187. Vogelberg, K. (1957): Die Lichtungsweite der Koronarostien an normalen und hypertrophen Herzen. *Z. Kreislaufforsch.*, 46:101–115.
188. Wachtlova, M., Rakusan, K., Roth, Z., and Poupa, O. (1967): The terminal vascular bed of the myocardium in the wild rat and in the laboratory rat. *Physiol. Bohemoslov.*, 16:548–556.
189. Walker, B. E., and Adrian, E. K. (1966): DNA synthesis in the myocardium of growing mature, senescent and dystrophic mice. *Cardiologia*, 49:319–328.
190. Walter, F., and Addis, T. (1939): Organ work and organ weight. *J. Exp. Med.*, 69:467–483.
191. Webster, S. H., and Liljegren, E. J. (1949): Organ-body weight ratios for certain organs of laboratory animals. II. Guinea pigs. *Am. J. Anat.*, 85:199–230.
192. Wegner, G., and Mölbert, E. (1966): Das Verhalten des Myokards bei der experimentellen supravalvulären Aortenstenose. *Virchows Arch. [Pathol. Anat.]*, 341:54–63.
193. Weiler, G. (1975): Untersuchungen über die Zahl der Kerne und die Dicke von Media und Intima der Koronararterien bei normalen Herzen der zweiten und dritten Lebensdekade und bei Herzen mit Koronarsklerose und Hypertonie. *Z. Kardiol.*, 64:995–1003.
194. Weisfeldt, M. L., editor (1980): *The Aging Heart. Its Function and Response to Stress.* Raven Press, New York.
195. Yin, F. C. P., Spurgeon, H. A., Rakusan, K., Weisfeldt, M. L., and Lakatta, E. G. (1982): Use of tibial length to quantify cardiac hypertrophy. *Am. J. Physiol.*, 243:H941–H947.
196. Zak, R. (1974): Development and proliferation capacity of cardiac muscle cells. *Circ. Res. [Suppl. II]*, 34-35:17–26.

Growth of the Heart in Health and Disease,
edited by Radovan Zak. Raven Press,
New York © 1984.

Factors Controlling Cardiac Growth

Radovan Zak

*Department of Medicine and Pharmacological and Physiological Sciences, University of
Chicago, Chicago, Illinois 60637*

Cardiac growth can be viewed as a system controlled by two sets of factors. The
first, *intrinsic*, includes those factors that are time-dependent only and are not
related to functional demands such as cardiac morphogenesis, which occurs prior
to the development of the circulatory system. The second, *extrinsic*, involves those
elements that are related to the contractile activity of the heart such as the compensatory hypertrophy, which follows the increase in hemodynamic load. (These
factors are also referred to as epigenetic, a term that applies to all factors and
mechanisms by which genes bring about their phenotypic effect.)

In this chapter we analyze the roles of intrinsic and extrinsic factors in the
development of the heart. More emphasis, however, is placed on the relationship
between functional intensity and rate of growth rather than on the time-dependent
factors, which is reviewed only briefly, because the latter factors are not necessarily
specific for the heart but rather apply to growth regulation of most tissues and
organs. More in-depth analysis can be found in previously published studies on
growth control (27a) and in articles dealing with the rapidly advancing field of cell
differentiation (55).

THEORIES OF GROWTH REGULATION: AN OVERVIEW

Regulation of growth is one of the key topics of biology which has attracted the
attention of investigators for more than a century. Consequently, a large volume of
material has accumulated and many ingenious theories have been proposed. None
of these, however, is generally accepted. In this chapter we center our attention
only on representative examples of current thoughts about growth regulation. A
more systematic and historical approach to this intriguing subject is found in Goss
(27,28).

Time-Dependent Developmental Program

The general nature of time-dependent factors involved in growth regulation is
seen in the decline in mitotic activity of hepatocytes and myocytes of the heart and
skeletal muscle and connective tissue cells (Fig. 1). Although the time characteristics of the mitotic decline vary widely between cell types, the overall trend applies

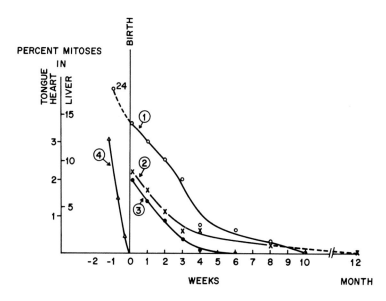

FIG. 1. Mitotic activity of various cell types at different stages of rat growth: (1) hepatocytes, (2) heart connective tissue cells, (3) heart myocytes, and (4) skeletal muscle (tongue).

to cells of any organ whose size approaches a limit, e.g., the liver or heart, in an adult organism. There are, however, cells in the body which are not under such stringent time restraints. The best examples are the cells of tissues like epidermal or intestinal epithelium, which are constantly lost and replaced by proliferation of stem cells that retain mitotic activity throughout the whole lifetime of the animal. However, even these cells do show some decline in proliferation during senescence, although to a much smaller degree than the cell shown in Fig. 1.

Regarding heart growth, there are numerous examples of regulation independent of function (88,89). Perhaps the best example is the cytodifferentiation of cardiac myocytes which occurs prior to development of the circulatory system and, hence, in the absence of any hemodynamic forces. At the very beginning, the development of the heart consists of the proliferation of myogenic cells which, in their structure, are not different from the undifferentiated cells of any tissue. At this stage the myogenic cells are referred to as presumptive myoblasts or premyoblasts by various investigators. As the first sign of overt myogenesis, the premyoblasts become elongated. Next, some cells initiate synthesis of muscle-specific proteins which culminates in thick and thin filaments and, eventually, cross-striated myofibrils. Since the content of muscle-specific structures changes with time, the myogenic cells at this stage are referred to as developing myocytes. The differentiation process in the heart, however, is not synchronized and consequently in the very early developmental phase two cell populations are present at the same time: premyoblast and developing myocytes. Gradually, however, more and more cells accumulate muscle-specific proteins, and eventually all the cells acquire myofibrils and no undifferentiated myogenic cells remain in the heart.

As the myofibrillar mass accumulates within the spindle-shaped developing myocytes, the myocytes are gradually transformed into cylindrical and fully functioning adult myocytes. Mitotic divisions even at this advanced stage of cytodifferentiation still take place, although at a very low rate. Nevertheless, mitosis in adult myocytes have been shown conclusively by electron microscopic examination which detected the simultaneous presence of myofilaments and of nuclei in metaphase (60). Moreover, even in beating myocytes, cellular divisions were also depicted in cinematographic recordings (61).

All the stages of myogenesis described above are governed solely by intrinsic time-dependent factors because the circulatory system has not yet developed. The time-dependent, programmed character of early myogenesis is also evident from experiments demonstrating that the primary cultures derived from embryonic hearts follow the same developmental pattern as the cells within the intact embryo. Additionally, studies of skeletal muscle indicate that all the cells in a clone derived from a myogenic cell eventually express muscle characteristics (52).

The second example of programmed developmental pattern in the cardiac morphogenesis is the transformation referred to as looping. This process coincides with the first contractions, which, in the chick, occur at approximately 30 hr of incubation. The hemodynamic forces, however, do not appear to be the triggering mechanism of looping. When contractions and the heart beat are blocked by placing explanted embryos into a medium containing a high concentration of potassium, the progression of looping is similar to that seen *in vivo*. The possible mechanical factors accompanying looping and responsible for morphological transformation are discussed in detail in Chapter 5.

The role of the endogenous developmental program and the effects of circulatory activity on cardiac morphogenesis in the stages that follow looping are difficult to separate as both heart and circulation develop simultaneously. However, this area holds considerable promise as adult heart cells have been maintained in culture for extended periods of time (e.g., ref. 11). Most interestingly, the adult myocytes in long-term culture undergo morphological and biochemical changes reminiscent of embryonic and neonatal periods. For example, during the first 24 hr of culture the cells lose their cylindrical shape and assume an irregularly round shape. At the same time, the cells cease to contract and myofibrils become disorganized and their content gradually diminished. After several days, however, the cells resume synthesis of DNA, the myofibrils become gradually reorganized into double hexagonal lattice, and eventually the cells resume contractile activity again. The adult myocyte thus undergoes a cycle of morphological dedifferentiation and redifferentiation (e.g., ref. 65). This model will undoubtedly be useful in studies on the role of factors responsible for the time-dependent loss of mitotic activity seen in developing myocytes.

At present the nature of factors that regulate the mitotic activity in myocytes, as well as in other cells, remains largely obscure. Concerning the heart, several hypotheses have been proposed. According to one, the gradually accumulating cell-specific structures present a hindrance to mitotic division of the nucleus (73). There are several lines of evidence to support this hypothesis. First, the duration of cell cycle in developing cardiac myocytes increases as the myofibrils accumulate. Second, those myocytes that contain a smaller fraction of cellular volume occupied by myofibrils, such as amphibian ventricles and mammalian atria, are able to resume DNA synthesis after injury. In contrast, myocytes that contain a larger relative proportion of myofibrils, e.g., mammalian ventricles, never resume DNA synthesis after injury. Third, the myofibrils of cells displaying mitotic activity become dispersed (e.g., ref. 33). After the mitosis is completed a gradual restoration of well-organized myofibrils takes place. Although this theory is consistent with many observations, there are also some exceptions that argue against its general applicability. For example, it was shown that cultured cells derived from the heart of neonatal rats are capable of cytokinesis, even while contracting (48). This can occur in some cases by a cleavage furrow perpendicular to myofibrils which takes place without any disruption of the double hexagonal lattice (49). Similarly, some cells in embryonic hearts whose nuclei were labeled with (^{3}H)thymidine appeared morphologically indistinguishable from unlabeled cells (26).

The second hypothesis postulates that the loss of proliferative capacity is a consequence of a specified mitosis leading to a new phenotype cell: a mitosis of an undifferentiated myogenic cell abruptly produces a daughter cell which differs from its parent cell (42). The daughter cell produced by such a critical mitosis is visualized as withdrawing from the cell cycle by repressing DNA synthesis and initiating synthesis of cell-specific proteins. This hypothesis obtained its support from studies of skeletal muscles in which the synthesis of DNA and of cell-specific proteins, i.e., myosin, do not take place at the same time. In the heart, however, as we have mentioned in the preceding section, these two processes are not mutually exclusive. It can be argued that in the heart more time is required for reprogramming, and consequently the repression of DNA may not become effective until one or two additional mitoses. Evidence against this argument, however, is that the developing myocytes can divide for several generations (82). Also, the fact that adult myocytes resume their mitotic activity after being silent for a long time speaks against this hypothesis. As we have already mentioned, there are two examples of resumed mitotic activity: the morphologically dedifferentiated adult myocytes in long-term culture and the myocytes in injured portions of atria.

Concerning the mechanism that might be common to the regulation of synthetic programs of all differentiating cells, several theories have been proposed recently. According to one theory, the signal that regulates cellular divisions is provided by the spatial arrangement of membrane components (4). The evidence for this theory comes from the demonstration that the capacity of some cells, e.g., lymphocytes, to divide can be influenced by alterations in the mobility of some of its membrane components. Microtobules and microfilaments are the most likely candidates for such a function. For example, bundles of microfilaments have been identified under the membrane of normal cells that are undergoing characteristic changes in their shape, whether dividing or quiescent. This is in contrast to virally transformed cells which do not undergo such a change in shape and contain much smaller amounts of microfilaments.

The second theory proposes that the characteristic decline of proliferation capacity of a given cell type is a part of genetic programming. For example, cultured human fibroblasts double only limited numbers of times before they lose their capacity to divide, deteriorate, and eventually die (33a). The number of divisions in culture is related to the age of the donor and to the life span of its species. In the heart, however, the concept of genetically programmed numbers of cell divisions did not receive support from studies showing that the factors that affect body growth also affect the number of cell divisions. For example, two groups of investigators manipulated the rate of body growth by adjusting the number of newborn animals per litter. The smaller the litter, the greater was the rate of postnatal growth. The proliferative rate of cardiac myocytes in these experiments was derived either from a histometrically determined total number of cells (72) or from the decrease in the density of nuclear labeling with (^{3}H)thymidine (38). Although each method has its own limitations, the data obtained are consistent with the interpretation that the rate of myocyte proliferation can be increased when the body growth is enhanced during the weanling period.

The genetic apparatus, however, might be involved in the regulation of cytodifferentiation other than by determining the total number of mitoses. This view received support from studies of transformed cells. For example, myoblasts derived from skeletal muscles that were transformed either with viruses or with chemical carcinogens remained in a proliferative phase and never initiated expressions of muscle-specific characteristics (12). In contrast, normal cells underwent only a limited number of divisions leading to postmitotic myoblasts. Once quiescent, these cells initiate synthesis of myosin and presumably of other muscle-specific proteins and eventually undergo differentiation to contracting cells. Of great interest is the proposal that there is a specific point (referred to as restriction point) in the G1 phase of mitotic cycle which is involved in the control of cellular proliferation (68). It is visualized that quiescent cells are blocked at the restriction point. Under conditions that favor proliferation, the cells pass this point and become committed to the mitotic cycle. This theory receives support from the isolation of mutants which lack the ability to become quiescent under nutritional deprivation as wild cells do (80). Apparently traversing the restriction point requires the activity of specific gene(s) that is missing in mutants. It is conceivable that, as in the case of hormones (see Chapter 1), the activity of these genes depends on a variety of conditions such as cell size, nutrition, or the presence of soluble growth factors.

Humoral Factors Regulating Growth

The involvement of soluble factors exerting profound effects on cellular growth has been known to students of cultured cells for a long time. A variety of factors have been described in these studies which regulate not only growth, but cytodifferentiation as well. Concerning growth regulation, many normal (i.e., nontransformed) cells grow rapidly when seeded at low densities. Their rate of growth however, gradually declines and eventually, after reaching critical (saturation) density, the cells become quiescent (see ref. 39).

Regarding the effects of soluble factors on cytodifferentiation, several good examples have come from studies on cultured myocytes derived from skeletal muscles (7,15). The transition from undifferentiated myogenic cells to myoblast initiating synthesis of muscle-specific proteins can be modified by manipulation of the growth media. The transition from proliferating to differentiating cells in the above studies was preceded by gradual lengthening of the cell cycle. When the old cultures, i.e., those with relatively long generation times, were readministered fresh medium, the length of their cycles became that of young cultures and vice versa. Thus, it is not the time in the culture but, rather, the change that occurs in the media that determines the stage-specific characteristics of the cell cycle. In support of these experiments, it was also found that cultured myoblasts, which would normally fuse to form multinucleated myotubes after terminal mitosis, can be forced into additional mitosis by manipulating their plating density and cellular environment (67).

Although examples of humoral regulation of cell growth are quite numerous, relatively little is known about the chemical nature of the regulatory factors involved. However, it is known that they may be either macromolecules or substances of low molecular weight. Concerning the first class, it includes various cell-specific growth factors such as fibroblast, epidermal, and nerve growth factors (35), insulin (40), and even proteolytic enzymes (9). As examples of the small molecules, calcium (16), cyclic nucleotides (76), and steroid hormones (57) are a few that can be named.

The action mechanism of humoral factors is even less well known than the chemical nature. Their effects might be similar to that of some hormones, however. Such an analogy might include tropic hormones, some of which induce growth in their target organs. Our best understanding of growth regulation, however, has been gained through studies of small molecular weight substances, namely, the action of steroid hormones (e.g., ref. 45). In several experimental models it was demonstrated that their action involves initial binding of the hormone to the receptor molecule in the cytoplasm of the target cell. Subsequently, the hormone complex migrates into the nucleus where it becomes associated with chromatin. Interaction of the receptor with the nuclear site results in the activation of RNA polymerase and subsequent cellular response. The multiple effects of stimulating substances required for orderly growth can result from the cascade action of integrator genes as postulated in the Britten-Davidson model of gene control (see Chapter 1).

In addition to steroid hormones, gene activation by thyroid hormone, growth hormone, and insulin are also known in some detail. Undoubtedly our understanding of the action of growth factors is contingent on the advancement of knowledge of gene control in general.

The above discussions of growth regulation were centered on stimulatory factors. There are, however, other known factors that have the opposite effect. One of the best examples is suppression of the growth of adrenal tumor cells by adrenocorticotropin (62). The second example of inhibitory factors is the incompletely characterized chalones. These substances are thought to be endogenous mitotic inhibitors specified for the tissue of their origin. The chalone hypothesis postulates that the chalones are produced by dividing cells. Once a critical mass of cells is reached, the concentration of chalones becomes high enough to block DNA synthesis. Chalones are somewhat reminiscent of antitemplates postulated in the self-inhibitory theory of growth proposed by Weiss. It was thought that these hypothetical substances were produced by cells of each organ and passed freely through the cell membrane. Within the cell the antitemplates were postulated to inhibit templates that when free, stimulate growth (84). This general theory of growth regulation has received some support from recent studies on the action of hormones. For example, several models of negative posttranscription control (see Chapter 1) include the action of a repressor that interacts with messenger RNA (mRNA), rendering it either more susceptible to degradation or inactive in the translation processes.

Functional Demand Theory

Long before growth regulation had been analyzed experimentally, many biologists and physicians recognized that the functional load placed on an organ influences its size. Sustained use of an organ results in its enlargement—hypertrophy— whereas disuse results in atrophy. Although this observation is undoubtedly valid, at least for some organs such as muscles or kidney, the signal-linking function—a physical phenomenon—to gene activity remains elusive. Moreover, the function-growth relationship does not apply to all forms of growth. First, there are some parts of the body where growth is not regulated by use, e.g., hair, teeth, etc. Second, it is clear that organs initiate and maintain growth well before they initiate their physiological function (see preceding section on time-dependent developmental program). Finally, the size of most fully functioning organs exceeds certain minimal value needed for survival. In other words, an organ has a reserve which is called upon in emergencies only, and, consequently, its overall size is for the most part independent of use (27,28).

Thus, it is clear that functional demand is not the only growth-regulating mechanism. Rather, it acts as a modifier superimposed on the intrinsic developmental program. Nevertheless, when applied to muscles, the concept of functional demand has received strong support and has led to many important conclusions. For example, it was shown that decreased muscular activity secondary to denervation, tenotomy, or differentiation affects slow muscles more than fast ones (35). This was best documented by measurements of total muscular mass of the slow muscle soleus and the fast muscle extensor digitorium longus (EDL) of the rat (3a). In accordance with these measurements of total muscle mass, the incorporation of tracer amino acid by a cell-free system obtained from denervated muscles detected a decrease in slow muscle only (70). Of great interest is the observation that the difference between slow and fast muscle can be detected not only in the loss of tissue but also in its gain. Following reinnervation, for example, the rate of recovery of muscle weight was about four times higher in the soleus muscle than in the fast EDL muscle (3a). Thus, the difference between these two muscle types can be seen in protein degradation and synthesis, as well.

The effects of disuse stand in contrast to the hormonal and nutritional effects on muscle mass. Starvation, for example, results in a rapid loss of mass in fast glycolytic muscles while relatively lesser wasting occurs in predominantly slow oxidative ones (35,56).

The observed differences between slow and fast muscle in regard to growth response is undoubtedly related to the properties of their neurons. Whereas slow muscle receives a sustained train of electric impulses, fast muscle is recruited only intermittently. Consequently, the state of differentiation in fast muscle is less dependent on neural imput than is the case in slow muscle. However, when the neural import remains intact, slow muscle is relatively resistant to metabolic mobilization. Obviously, the continuously used slow muscle is under more stringent homeostatic control than fast muscle, which is used only intermittently.

Concerning the heart, the function-growth relationship and the search for the signal linking the growth of the heart to its hemodynamic function have attracted more attention than that of skeletal muscle. Therefore, the effect of function on the heart is discussed separately in the following sections.

STIMULUS FOR CARDIAC GROWTH

Adjustment of cardiac mass to hemodynamic load is a fundamental characteristic of the heart. Despite numerous hypotheses, however, the nature of the link between function and cardiac size remains elusive as the factor(s) controlling the growth processes in general.

Contractile Activity as Determinant of Muscle Growth: An Overview

As is described in detail through the following two sections of this book, cardiac mass adjusts to its hemodynamic load as does skeletal muscle. The functional demand—the muscle ultimately reflected in the activity of myosin cross-bridges—provides some kind of signal that modulates the predetermined developmental program. Not only the size of a muscle changes, but the properties of its constituents change as well. Eccles and his associates (8) have demonstrated that in skeletal muscles the contraction speed of a given muscle follows the discharge properties of its innervating motor nerves. In a typical experiment the motoneurons of selected fast and slow muscles were cut and transposed so that the nerve originally innervating the fast muscle reinnervated the slow muscle and vice versa. Within several weeks, the contraction properties of the two cross-innervated muscles reversed.

In later years it was shown that the activity of myosin ATPase of cross-innervated muscles follows the newly acquired speed of shortening. In addition to myosin, changes induced by altered neural input have also been detected in troponin inhibitory subunit, sarcoplasmic and mitochondrial proteins (85). Myosin, however, was studied in the greatest detail. The cross-innervation-induced change in myosin involves not only its enzymatic activity, but the entire molecule. This conclusion was inferred from the analysis of peptide maps (e.g., ref. 83) and from the determination of *N*-methyl-histidine (78), which is present only in myosin of fast glycolytic fibers. The evidence for changes in the expression of myosin genes after cross-innervation received full support from electrophoretic analysis of myosin in native (36) and denatured states (83a). The switch in gene expression, however, appears not to affect all proteins in the same way, at the same time. For example, transformation of myosin light chains lags behind changes in the speed of shortening and ATPase activity, both of which are believed to be determined by heavy chains (83). The reason for this lack of coordination between light and heavy chains is not known at the present time. It is of interest, however, that both classes of myosin chains are coded by different sets of genes, and even in normal muscles they are synthesized and degraded at different rates (87).

Regarding the factors involved in the control of gene expression in skeletal muscles, two kinds of mechanisms are postulated: trophic substances supplied by the nerve and factors related to the pattern of impulse activity. Experimental evidence has shown that the latter is likely the case. For example, when a sustained low-frequency activity typical of "slow" nerves was imposed on the "fast" moto-neurons, the transformation achieved was like that in the cross-innervation exper-iment (74).

The effect of contractile activity on the myocardium is more difficult to study than that in skeletal muscles. The reason is that the heart is an autonomous organ whose function cannot be controlled as easily as the firing frequency of motoneu-rons. Nevertheless, there are numerous examples of the function-dependent nature of cardiac growth both when its hemodynamic load is increased or when it is decreased. The first case leads to hypertrophy; the second to atrophy or to the regression of previously acquired hypertrophy. Of these processes, the first has received most of the attention in both the clinic and the laboratory not only because hypertrophy is clinically more common than atrophy, but also because it is relatively easy to induce experimentally. Nevertheless, with the advent of corrective cardiac surgery, negative cardiac growth gained in importance.

In principle, the functional unloading of the heart can occur in two situations: during chronically decreased hemodynamic activity, such as disease-associated bedrest, and following removal of hemodynamic overload, such as closure of arteriovenous fistula. In the first situation the loss of cardiac mass which occurs in an otherwise healthy heart is usually referred to as atrophy. In contrast, the change in heart size which follows removal of hemodynamic overload is referred to as regression of cardiac hypertrophy. Most of the description of cardiac atrophy comes from clinical studies, such as chronic reduction in the mean arterial pressure,

Addison's disease, and loss of body mass due to starvation (34). A common observation in these studies is that loss of cardiac mass is accompanied by a decrease in the diameter of myocytes. Very little is known about the functional characteristics of atrophic hearts. Moreover, clinical circumstances are difficult to interpret since factors such as hormones undoubtedly come into play, in addition to mechanical unloading.

Experimental studies of mechanical unloading, which can be induced in the absence of additional factors, have been attempted only recently (12a). For example, the right ventricular papillary muscles of a cat were studied after transection of their chordae tendinae. The operation was followed by a rapid decrease in cardiac mass which was accompanied by a decrease in the size of muscle cells. These results are similar to those obtained in studies of the regression of cardiac hypertrophy, such as removal of experimental aortic constriction, cessation of hyperthyroid state, or of high-altitude hypoxia (e.g., ref. 6). The exact time and extent of cardiac regression, however, differ depending on the experimental model. This is undoubtedly related to the various characteristics of hypertrophic heart prior to removal of work overload (13).

In comparison with studies of cardiac size, only recently have changes in the properties of constituting proteins in overloaded hearts been examined. Consequently, less is known about these properties than in comparable studies of skeletal muscles. Nevertheless, transformation in the molecular variants of myosin in overloaded hearts is clearly evident. Generally, hypertrophy characterized by increased shortening of velocity (e.g., hyperthyroidism) is accompanied by accumulation of high ATPase isomyosin V1. In contrast, hypertrophy associated with decreased shortening of velocity (e.g., pressure overload) leads to preferential expression of the low ATPase variant, V3 (2).

Many aspects of cardiac function in overloaded and unloaded hearts still remain to be established. Nevertheless, results obtained so far clearly indicate that the heart has effective mechanisms for adjusting its size to functional demand, as does skeletal muscle.

ATP Depletion Theory

It is well established that increased tension in the ventricular wall correlates with increased metabolic activity in the heart. According to the ATP depletion theory, the increased rate of ATP utilization results in temporal depletion of energy stores. This depletion is, in turn, sensed by a process that determines the mass of cellular components, including both synthetic as well as degradative pathways. As a result, compensatory growth ensues, and the energy stores are eventually restored to normal values.

The basic postulate of this theory has received wide support from numerous investigators who have noted that many, if not all, circumstances leading to cardiac compensatory growth are accompanied by increased oxygen consumption and ATP hydrolysis. Therefore, a drop in the energy potential of the myocardial cell (i.e., the concentration ratio of ATP to its hydrolytic products, ADP and inorganic phosphate) must occur. The magnitude of this drop and, more importantly, its temporal correlation to the induced growth, however, are not altogether clear (23). The increased requirement for ATP during acute work overload of the heart is effectively met by the respiratory control mechanism: the accumulating ADP stimulates oxidative phosphorylation. Thus, under aerobic conditions, the increase in ATP utilization is coupled with the increased rate of its production. The high efficiency of this control mechanism is evident from the fact that no trace of lactic acid production occurs even during strenuous activity.

The dependence of the heart on the oxidative processes is reflected by the high content of mitochondria, which occupy 35% of the cardiac cell volume. Although the heart appears to be well adapted for a wide variation in its workload, mitochondria have been shown to accumulate preferentially to other cell constituents during the earliest stage of pressure-induced hypertrophy. This was demonstrated by both quantitative electron microscopic description and biochemical analysis. For example, a significant increase in mitochondrial cytochrome content and respiratory enzyme activity per gram of tissue was detected 24 hr after constriction of the ascending aorta (1). The preferential accumulation of mitochondrial components, however, is only transient: during the later phases of compensatory growth, myofibrils accumulate more rapidly than mitochondria. Also, in other forms of overload, such as volume overload secondary to an arteriovenous fistula or prolonged forced exercise in rats, the relative mitochondrial mass remains unchanged (71). Thus it appears that work-induced cardiac growth at least in some instances can take place without preferential accumulation of mitochondria.

The second difficulty of the ATP depletion theory is that actual measurements did not provide unequivocal evidence of changes in the energy potential of the overloaded myocardium (71). Some workers have found no detectable changes in ATP or creatine phosphate levels. Some have noted a decrease in creatine phosphate only; whereas others have detected quite a marked decrease in energy potential resulting from a decrease in ATP and an increase in ADP and inorganic phosphate. These different findings are due to the fact that the analyses were carried out at various times during the development of hypertrophy and in hearts overloaded to different severities. Moreover, currently available analytical procedures have severe limitations since energy stores cannot be measured in separate cellular compartments. Even if these difficulties were to be resolved, however, the ATP depletion theory does not provide any hint of how the growth machinery is activated by decreased levels of ATP.

Stretch Theory

This theory of growth regulation has its origin in the classical observations of Feng (19), who demonstrated that passive stretching of isolated skeletal muscle increases its oxygen consumption and heat production. In analogy, the enhanced preload and afterload of the overloaded myocardium result in the stretching of its cells; it is conceivable that this stretch stimulates metabolic pathways which, in turn, lead to compensatory growth as originally proposed by Eyster et al. in 1927 (18).

The most solid support for this theory comes from reports in which muscle enlargement was induced by various forms of passive stretching. The earliest example of such mechanical effects on muscle growth involves studies of the diaphragm following the sectioning of its nerve (77,79). Contrary to other skeletal muscle, the diaphragm muscle undergoes substantial hypertrophy during the first week after the nerve has been severed. For example, the denervated hemidiaphragm weighs approximately 40% more at its maximum weight, which occurs about 6 days after the operation, than the sham-operated contralateral half (86). Following this enlargement, atrophy and eventual degeneration ensue just as is the case of a typical skeletal muscle (e.g., ref. 29).

This puzzling transient growth of the denervated diaphragm was later found to be a consequence of passive stretching by the contralateral functioning half which remained innervated to serve as a control. When this rhythmical stretch was eliminated, the enlargement of the diaphragm was prevented. The stretch exerted on the paralyzed half of the diaphragm was eliminated in two ways. First, the bilateral section of nervus phrenicus was performed so that both hemidiaphragms were paralyzed (20). In a second experiment a "tenotomy" of the diaphragm was attempted by a vertical section of three ribs at the level of the diaphragm attachment. Although this procedure does not completely eliminate the stretch exerted on the denervated diaphragm by its "tenotomized" innervated half, the hypertrophy was completely eliminated (30).

It is of great interest that the stretch affects not all the fibers in the same way. This was shown by measurements of fiber diameter which indicate that hypertrophy occurs only in the oxidative type. In contrast, the fast glycolytic fibers underwent atrophy immediately after the nerve was severed. The conclusion that, indeed, the atrophic process begins immediately after denervation received further support from measurements of catheptic activity in muscle homogenate (30). Thus, it appears that the increased enlargement of denervated diaphragm is the result of the combined hypertrophy of oxidative fibers and the atrophy of glycolytic ones. Since the former constitute approximately 70% of the total, the overall result is an increase in muscle mass.

Another example of stretch-induced growth includes wing-supporting muscles after denervation. The sectioning of nerves innervating the latissimus dorsi (LD) muscles in a chicken led to temporal enlargement of anterior LD (ALD) muscle. Four weeks after the operation the muscle became twice the size of its innervated control. After that time, its weight began to decline, but in the eighth postoperative week it was still slightly above control values. In contrast, the posterior LD (PLD) muscle lost it weight from the very onset of denervation (21,46).

Similarly, as was the case of the diaphragm, stretch was also involved in the induction of ALD enlargement. When the drooping and consequent stretching of the denervated wing was prevented by restraining the wing into a normal position, the enlargement was substantially reduced, although some hypertrophy was still present (21); tenotomy of ALD had similar effects (46). Moreover, the enlargement of fully innervated ALD can be induced by stretching the wing with a weight placed around the humerus (41,54).

The third example of stretch effect on muscle is illustrated in the so-called compensatory hypertrophy induced by the elimination of the synergistic muscle either by extirpation, tenotomy, or denervation. At first, it was believed that this procedure was a model of work hypertrophy because the remaining muscle became functionally overloaded when it compensated for the loss of its synergist. Later, however, it was shown that during the early phase of growth, it is the stretch rather than the work overload that is the growth-inducing factor. When the passive stretching of the experimental muscle was eliminated by removal (31) or concomitant denervation (58) of the antagonist muscle, no enlargement occurred. Moreover, growth can be induced by stretching even in nonworking denervated muscle (25,31).

Comparison of the growth response of different types of muscles is of great interest. It appears that only the slow oxidative (SO), but not the fast glycolytic (FG), muscles respond to stretching. This was shown both in mammals and birds. In the rat, for example, soleus, predominantly SO type, undergoes hypertrophy after tenotomy of its synergist. The extensor digitorum longus, predominantly FG type, remains unaffected (58). (The same preferential response of SO fibers was found in the denervated diaphragm as already mentioned.) The striking difference between the slow and fast muscles can also be seen in the comparison of ALD and PLD muscles of the chicken. Whereas PLD is pure FG muscle with focal innervation typical of twitch muscles, ALD is composed of tonic fibers with diffuse "en grappe" innervation and has contractile properties resembling those of the slow muscles of mammals. It is the ALD muscles that undergo hypertrophy during stretching. Thus, both disuse (see Functional Demand Theory) and stretch (and possible overload) affect primarily the muscle fibers that are in steady use as are the slow muscles with their posture-maintaining and antigravitational function.

The mechanisms of growth-inducing effects of stretching were investigated only recently and, consequently, very little is known. Studies carried out using live animals indicate that both the rates of synthesis and the degradation are increased by stretch, possibly reflecting transformation of molecular variants of muscle proteins. In these studies the synthetic rate was estimated following continuous administration of tracer amino acid. The degradation rate was calculated from the difference between the fractional synthetic and the growth rates (54). While the first procedure is the most reliable of currently available techniques, the latter is rather crude mostly owing to problems in obtaining accurate estimates of growth rates. It is of interest, however, that the same effects of the stretch were found when the rates of synthesis and degradation were measured *in vitro* (24).

In contrast, in several *in vitro* models the rate of degradation was reduced by stretch. For example, the release of tyrosine from intact rat musculi soleus was reduced when the muscle was incubated at a position corresponding to 110% of its resting length (17). Similar results were obtained when myotubes attached to collagen-coated membrane were stretched to a similar degree (81). Also, when the m. soleus (but not m. extensor digitorum longus) was incubated with tension partially reduced by two perpendicular cuts, the rate of protein degradation was decreased when compared with muscles fixed at resting length (75). The effect of stretching, however, is not a simple one, and it appears to depend on the level of intracellular calcium. Thus, the rates of synthesis were increased and the rate of degradation decreased when the tension was applied in the presence of calcium ionophore. No effects were noticed in its absence (17).

From the above brief survey, it is evident that most of the studies on the molecular mechanisms of stretching are rather preliminary; nevertheless, the data are promising and undoubtedly will be subject to further more definitive analysis.

Humoral Growth Factors in the Heart

There are several examples of humoral factors involved in the regulation of cardiac growth. The most dramatic is the cardiac hypertrophy accompanying thyrotoxicosis (64). Although there is no doubt that large doses of thyroid hormone have a profound effect on cardiac growth, it is also clear that the heart can undergo enlargement in the absence of any changes in the level of this hormone (e.g., during pressure overload).

Furthermore, it has also been shown that adrenocortical, thyroid, and growth hormones can affect the compensatory growth response of the hemodynamically overloaded heart (5). This, however, is most likely due to the systemic effects of those hormones, with the possible exception of the adrenal cortex (see below).

In addition to the above examples, moderate cardiac enlargement was detected after chronic infusion of norepinephrine in doses that do not lead to hypertension (Chapter 13). It is also suggested by increased concentration of norepinephrine in the heart following aortic constriction that catecholamines can, indeed, participate in the compensatory response to work overload (10).

Of interest are the recent reports on the presence of substances produced by the overloaded heart which are able to promote protein synthesis. In one such report (32) extracts of the overloaded heart, when included into the perfusion medium, increased cell-free protein synthesis directed by cytoplasmic RNA that had been extracted from perfused, normal hearts. In another study (51) the incorporation of trace amino acid into the sliced normal heart was increased by postribosomal supernatant obtained from hypertrophic hearts.

Very little is known about the chemistry of putative mediators of cardiac hypertrophy. Interestingly, however, is that the currently unknown glucocorticoid, with digitalis-like immunological properties, was detected in the sera of rats with developing hypertrophy (51). In support of the involvement of adrenal cortex in the development of compensatory growth, the same authors report that the gland increases in proportion to the enlarging heart.

Hypoxia as Growth Stimulus

This theory proposes that increased ventricular wall stress will result in oxygen deficiency in overloaded muscle cells and that decreased partial tension of oxygen, in turn, will derepress biosynthetic activities. Two lines of evidence support this theory. First, in a variety of cells oxygen toxicity has been demonstrated *in vitro*. For example, primary cultures of chicken embryonic heart cells incorporated progressively less radiolabeled precursors into proteins and nucleic acids as the partial pressure of oxygen in the gas phase was increased from 5% to 80% (37). The second line of support for the hypoxia theory is derived from the fact that the growth of the heart (as of most other tissues) decreases after birth when the Po_2 in arterial blood increases dramatically relative to values measured *in utero*. Arguing against any simple effect of Po_2 on biosynthetic processes, however, is the fact that the rate of tissue growth declines exponentially during both late embryonic and postnatal periods whereas the values of Po_2 change in stepwise fashion. Also, if indeed oxygen pressure exerts any regulatory function, it has to be topographically specific, since the growth rate of the two ventricles change disproportionately after birth.

Regarding the hypoxia theory, it is of interest that simulated ischemia in the perfused heart is associated with an increased RNA synthesis measured in isolated mitochondria (50). *In vivo*, however, oxygen deprivation has an opposite effect which results in the increased degradation of mitochondria (3).

Growth Control by Cell Degradation Products

According to this theory, increased contractile activity of myocardial cells results in "wear and tear" on its components, and the degradation products serve as activators of the growth process (62a). This theory is inspired by turn-of-the-century views of the growth process (see refs. 27 and 27a) and of protein metabolisms.

The theory of growth regulation by hypothetical degradation products received little experimental support. It is true that tissue damage accompanies many forms of cardiac overload, but this is related to the abruptness of the experimental model of cardiac hypertrophy, rather than to the growth response itself. When a more gradual onset of overload is selected, cardiac enlargement takes place without cellular damage (47). Moreover, no solid data is available to support the belief that increased contractile activity results in the alteration of contractile proteins to make them more susceptible to the degradation process. Folin's (22) concept of tissue "wear and tear" reflecting endogenous metabolism was disproved when it was shown that all body constituents are in a state of flux and therefore constantly being degraded and resynthesized. Moreover, when degradation of cellular constituents takes place, such as in hypoxia, the rate of protein synthesis declines (3).

Growth Stimuli—An Analysis at the Molecular Level

The common denominator for function-related cardiac growth is the extent of the energy utilization during actin-myosin interaction. In this final section we will discuss how the rate of energy utilization can be linked to the expression of specific genes.

As discussed in Chapter 1, loosening of the DNA fiber within the chromatin is a prerequisite for transcription to take place. There are several known instances when nonhistones, a class of chromatin proteins, can be covalently modified. For example, phosphorylation of nonhistone proteins are related to transcriptional activity in various tissues (89). In some instances, the extent of phosphorylation appears to be correlated with the activity of cyclic-AMP-dependent nuclear protein kinase.

The second covalent modification of chromatin proteins which might be involved in the control of gene expression is ADP-ribosylation (Fig. 2). This pathway involves the formation of a conjugate between ADP-ribose, which is enzymatically liberated from poly ADP-ribose, and the ε-amino group of a lysine residue in the target protein. After ADP-ribosylation of specific chromatin protein, the transcription of DNA is postulated to be inhibited. Poly ADP-ribose is formed within the cell by sequential addition of ADP ribose moiety of nicotinamide adenine dinucleotide phosphate (NADP) to the growing polymer.

The fact that NADP and not nicotinamide adenine dinucleotide, (reduced form NADH) is the precursor of the protein-modifying reagent makes this theory particularly attractive. The cellular ratio of NADP/NADH, closely reflecting the state of

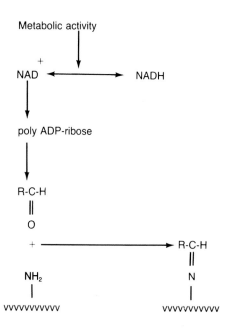

FIG. 2. Scheme of protein ribosylation. NADP, whose level reflects the metabolic activity of a cell, is a precursor of poly ADP-ribose. Enzymatically liberated ADP-ribose (an aldehyde) from its polymere forms a Schiff's base with an amino group of proteins. Polyamines can serve as competitive inhibitors of this reaction. After ADP-ribosylation, the biological activity of protein becomes altered (e.g., repression of transcription).

oxidation, is known to decrease when the workload of the heart increases. Reduced level of NADP, in turn, might result in depletion of poly ADP-ribose, with consequent derepression of transcription.

Several observations support this theory (53,63). First, the turnover of poly ADP-ribose is high, making it a suitable regulatory metabolite. Second, the nonhistone proteins of chromatin appear to be the preferential acceptor of ADP-ribose. And third, an inverse correlation between the level of poly ADP-ribose and the induction of specific enzyme has been found in the heart. However, a correlation is not necessarily proof of a direct regulatory role of poly ADP ribose. Moreover, the chromatin proteins that are covalently modified by ADP-ribosylation remain to be identified. Of additional interest is that polyamines, which are present in elevated amounts in growing organs, have been shown to serve as traps for formaldehydes (e.g., ADP-ribose) and might thus prevent chromatin modification. The growth-stimulating effects of polyamines, however, are contradicted by demonstration that inhibition of ornithin decarboxylase and subsequent depletion of polyamines in the heart do not prevent development of cardiac hypertrophy (69).

As far as other possible regulatory mechanisms of gene expression, several examples are worthy of mentioning. Extracted from a heart was a class of RNA which influences cardiac morphogenesis when added to chick embryo at an early stage of development (14). The exact role of this "cardiogenic" RNA is not known, but it appears that its effect might be coupled to the activity of adenylcyclase, since cyclic AMP mimics its action (2a). It is of interest that extracts obtained from the hearts of weanling rats undergoing cardiac enlargement stimulate synthesis of DNA in heterologous nuclei (88). It remains to be established whether or not this activation has some relationship to the growth-promoting factors mentioned earlier in this chapter.

CONCLUSION

The differentiation and growth of the heart are governed by two sets of factors: those that are time-dependent and those that are function-dependent. The first set is effective during the very first stages of embryonic cardiac development which take place in the absence of hemodynamic function. During most of life, however, the growth of the heart is closely matched to its functional load.

This function-dependent nature of cardiac growth can be seen when the workload is either increased or decreased. In the former, hypertrophy results. In the latter, atrophy or regression of previously induced hypertrophy is the result.

Since the functional load of the heart is ultimately reflected in the rate of ATP hydrolysis during the cross-bridge cycle, it follows that the extent of energy consumption is coupled (in some yet unspecified way) to the genetic activities of the myocardial cell. The growth-regulating signal still remains elusive. Several hypotheses were presented in this chapter, none fully compatible with all the aspects of cardiac growth. It should be kept in mind that the compensatory growth of the heart is not all that eludes our understanding. Theories that attempt to explain the growth process in general are equally vague and incompatible with the established facts. It has been realized only during the last decade that when studying an organ, one has to study specific cells and specific proteins rather then their mixtures. Any meaningful analysis of the mechanisms that regulate growth has to proceed toward the development of probes for specific genes and their products.

REFERENCES

1. Albin, R., Dowell, R. T., Zak, R., and Rabinowitz, M. (1973): Synthesis and degradation of mitochondrial components in hypertrophied rat heart. *Biochem. J.*, 136:629–637.
2. Alpert, N. (1983): *Myocardial Hypertrophy and Failure*. Raven Press, New York.
2a. Arnold, H. H., Innis, M. A., and Siddiqui, M. A. (1978): Control of embryonic development: Effect of an embryonic inducer RNA on *in vitro* translation of mRNA. *Biochemistry*, 17:2050–2054.
3. Aschenbrenner, V., Zak, R., Cutilletta, A. F., and Rabinowitz, M. (1971): Effect of hypoxia on degradation of mitochondrial components in rat cardiac muscle. *Am. J. Physiol.*, 221:1418–1425.
3a. Beranek, R., Hnik, P., Vrbova, G. (1957): Denervation atrophy of various skeletal muscles in rats. *Physiol. Bohemoslov.*, 6:200–212.
4. Berlin, M. D. (1975): *Microtubules and Microtubule Inhibitors*. Edited by M. Borges and M. de Brabander. North-Holland, Amsterdam.
5. Beznak, M. (1952): The effect of the pituitary and growth hormone on the blood pressure and on the ability of the heart to hypertrophy. *J. Physiol.* 116:74–83.
6. Beznak, M., Korecky, B., and Thomas, C. (1969): Regression of cardiac hypertrophies of various origin. *Can. J. Physiol. Pharmacol.*, 47:579–586.
7. Buckley, P. A., and Konigsberg, I. R. (1973): Myogenic fusion and the duration of the postmitotic gap (G_1). *Dev. Biol.*, 37:193–212.
8. Buller, A. J., Eccles, J. C., and Eccles, R. M. (1960): Interaction between motoneurones and muscles in respect of their characteristic speeds of their responses. *J. Physiol. (Lond.)*, 150:417–439.
9. Burger, M. M. (1970): Proteolytic enzymes initiating cell division and escape from contact inhibition of growth. *Nature*, 227:170–171.
10. Caldarera, C. M., Casti, A., Rossoni, C., and Visioli, O. J. (1971): Polyamines and noradrenaline following myocardial hypertrophy. *J. Mol. Cell. Cardiol.*, 3:121–126.
11. Claycomb, W. C., and Palazzo, M. C. (1980): Culture of the terminally differentiated adult cardiac muscle cell: A light and scanning electron microscope study. *Dev. Biol.*, 80:466–482.
12. Cohen, R., Pacifici, M., Rubinstein, N., Biehl, J., and Holtzer, H. (1977): Effect of a tumor promoter on myogenesis. *Nature*, 266:538–540.
12a. Cooper, J., and Tomanek, R. J. (1982): Load structure, composition, and function of mammalian myocardium. *Circ. Res.*, 50:788–798.
13. Cutilletta, A. F., Dowell, R. T., Rudnik, M., Arcilla, A., and Zak, R. (1975): Regression of myocardial hypertrophy. I. Experimental model, changes in heart weight, nucleic acids and collagen. *J. Mol. Cell. Cardiol.*, 7:767–780.
14. Deshpande, A. K., Jakowlew, S. B., and Arnold, H. H., et al. (1977): A novel RNA affecting embryonic gene functions in early chick glastoderm. *J. Biol. Chem.*, 252(18):6521–6527.
15. Doering, M., and Fischman, D. (1974): The in vitro cell fusion of embryonic chick muscle without DNA synthesis. *Dev. Biol.*, 36:225–235.
16. Dulbecco, R., and Elkington, J. (1975): Induction of growth in resting fibroblastic cell cultures by Ca^{++}. (Balb/c 3T3 cells/Ca^{++} ionophore/cell morphology/serum). *Proc. Natl. Acad. Sci. USA*, 72:1584–1588.
17. Etlinger, J. D., Kameyama, T., Toner, K., Van der Westhuyzen, D., and Matsumoto, K. (1980): *Calcium and Stretch-dependent Regulation of Protein Turnover and Myofibrillar Disassembly in Muscle. Plasticity of Muscle*. Edited by Dirk Pette Walter de Gruyter & Co., Berlin, New York.
18. Eyster, J. A. E., Meek, W. J., and Hodges, F. J. (1927): Cardiac changes subsequent to aortic lesions. *Arch. Intern. Med.*, 39:536–549.
19. Feng, T. P. (1932): The effect of length on the resting metabolism of muscle. *J. Physiol.*, 74:441–454.

20. Feng, T. P., Lu, D. X. (1965): New lights on the phenomenon of transient hypertrophy in the denervated hemidiaphragm of the rat. *Sci. Sin. (Peking)*, 14:1772–1784.

21. Feng, T. P., Jung, H. W., and Wu, W. Y. (1962): The contrasting trophic changes of the anterior and posterior latissimus dorsi of the chick following denervation. *Acta Physiol. Sin.*, 25:431–441.

22. Folin, O. (1905): A theory of protein metabolism. *Am. J. Physiol.* 13:117–138.

23. Gevers, W. (1972): The stimulus to hypertrophy in the heart. *J. Mol. Cell. Cardiol.*, 4:537–541.

24. Goldspink, D. F. (1977): The influence of immobilization and stretch on protein turnover of rat skeletal muscle. *J. Physiol.*, 264:267–282.

25. Goldspink, D. F. (1978): The influence of passive stretch on the growth and protein turnover of the denervated extensor digitorum longus muscle. *Biochem. J.*, 174:595–602.

26. Goode, D. (1975): Mitosis of embryonic heart muscle cells in vitro. An immunofluoresence and ultrastructural study. *Cytobiologie*, 11:203–229.

27. Goss, R. J. (1964): *Adaptive Growth*. pp. 9–360. Academic Press, New York.

27a. Goss, R. J. (1967): The strategy of growth. In: *Control of Cellular Growth in Adult Organisms*, edited by H. Teir and T. Rytomaa, pp. 4–27. Academic Press, London.

28. Goss, R. J. (1972): Theories of growth regulation. In: *Regulation of Organ and Tissue Growth*, edited by R. J. Goss, pp. 1–11. Academic Press, New York, London.

29. Gutmann, E., editor (1962): *The Denervated Muscle*. Czechoslovak Academy of Sciences, Prague.

30. Gutmann, E., Hanikova, M., Hajek, I., Klicpera, M., and Syrovy, I. (1966): The postderivation hypertrophy of the diaphragm. *Physiol. Bohemoslov.*, 15:508–521.

31. Gutmann, E., Schaiffino, S., and Hanzlikova, V. (1971): Mechanism of compensatory hypertrophy in skeletal muscle of the rat. *Exp. Neurol.*, 31:451–464.

32. Hammond, G. L., Lai, Y. K., and Market C. L. (1982): The molecules that initiate cardiac hypertrophy are not species specific. *Science*, 216:529–531.

33. Hay, D. A., and Low, F. N. (1972): The fine structure of progressive stages of myocardial mitosis in chick embryos. *Am. J. Anat.*, 134:175–203.

33a. Hayflick, L. (1965): The limited *in vitro* lifetime of human diploid cell strains. *Exp. Cell. Res.*, 37:614–636.

34. Hellerstein, H. K., and Santiago-Stevenson, D. (1950): Atrophy of the heart: A correlative study of eighty-five proved cases. *Circulation*, 1:93–126.

35. Hnik, P. (1962): Rate of denervation muscle atrophy. In: *The Denervated Muscle*, edited by E. Gutmann, pp. 341–371. Publishing House of Czechoslovak Academy of Sciences, Prague.

36. Hoh, J. F. Y., Kwan, B. T. S., Dunlop, C., and Kim, B. H. (1980): Effects of nerve cross-union and cordotomy on myosin isoenzymes in fast-twitch and slow-twitch muscles of the rat. In: *Plasticity of Muscle*, edited by D. Pette. Walter de Gruyter, Berlin.

37. Hollenberg, M. (1971): Effect of oxygen on growth of cultured myocardial cells. *Circ. Res.*, 28:148–157.

38. Hollenberg, M., Honbo, N., and Samorodin, A. J. (1977): Cardiac cellular responses to altered nutrition in the neonatal rat. *Am. J. Physiol.*, 233:H356–H360.

39. Holley, R. W. (1975): Control of growth of mammalian cells in cell culture. *Nature*, 258:487–490.

40. Holley, R. W., and Kiernan, J. A. (1974): Control of the initiation of DNA synthesis in 3T3 cells: Serum factors (fibroblast growth factor/insulin/dexamethasone). *Proc. Natl. Acad. Sci. USA*, 71:2908–2911.

41. Holly, R. G., Barnett, J. G., Ashmore, C. R., Taylor, R. G., and Mole, P. A. (1980): Stretch induced growth in chicken wing muscles: a new model of stretch hypertrophy. *Am. J. Physiol.*, 238 *(Cell Physiol.*, 7):C62–C71.

42. Holtzer, H. (1970): *Myogenesis in Cell Differentiation*, edited by O. Schjeide, pp. 476–503. Van Nostrand Reinhold Co.

43. Houck, J. D. (1976): *Chalones*. North-Holland Publishing Co., Amsterdam.

44. Jean, D. H., Albers, R. W., Guth, L., and Aron, H. J. (1975): Differences between the heavy chains of fast and slow muscle myosin. *Exp. Neurol.*, 49:750–757.

45. Jensen, E. V., and DeSombre, E. R. (1972): Mechanism of action of the female sex hormones. *Annu. Rev. Biochem.*, 41:203–230.

46. Jirmanova, I., and Zelena, J. (1970): Effect of denervation and tenotomy on slow and fast muscles of the chicken. *Z. Zellforsch.*, 106:337–347.

47. Julian, F. J., Morgan, D. L., Moss, R. L., Gonzales, M., and Dwivedi, P. (1981): Myocyte growth

without physiological impairment in gradually induced rat cardiac hypertrophy. *Circ. Res.*, 49:1300–1310.

48. Kasten, F. H. (1972): Rat myocardial cells in vitro: mitosis and differentiated properties. *In Vitro*, 8:128–150.
49. Kelley, A. M., and Chacko, S. (1976): Myofibril organisation and mitosis in cultured cardiac muscle cells. *Dev. Biol.*, 48:421–430.
50. Kleitke, B., and Wollenberger, A. (1978): Accelerated RNA and protein synthesis in mitochondria isolated from unperfused myocardium. Possible involvement of cyclic AMP. *J. Mol. Cell. Cardiol.*, 10:827–845.
51. Kölbel, F., and Schreiber, V. (1983): Biochemical regulators in cardiac hypertrophy. *Basic Res. Cardiol.*, 78:351–363.
52. Konigsberg, I. R. (1963): Clonal analysis of myogenesis. *Science*, 140:1273–1284.
53. Kun, E., Chang, A. C. Y., Sharma, M. L., Ferro, A. M., and Nitecki, D. (1976): Covalent modification of proteins by metabolites of NAD$^+$. *Proc. Natl. Acad. Sci. USA*, 73:3131–3135.
54. Laurent, G. J., Sparrow, M. P., and Millward, D. J. (1978): Turnover of muscle protein in the fowl. Changes in rates of protein synthesis and breakdown during hypertrophy of the anterior and posterior latissimus dorsi muscles. *Biochem. J.*, 176:407–417.
55. Levenson, R., and Housman, D. (1981): Commitment: How do cells make the decision to differentiate? *Cell*, 25:5–6.
56. Li, J. B., and Goldberg, A. L. (1976): Effects of food deprivation on protein synthesis and degradation in rat skeletal muscles. *Am. J. Physiol.*, 231:441–448.
57. Liao, S. (1975): Cellular receptors and mechanism of action of steroid hormones. *Int. Rev. Cytol.*, 41:87–172.
58. Mackova, E., and Hnik, P. (1972): Time course of compensatory hypertrophy of slow and fast rat muscles in relation to age. *Physiol. Bohemoslov.*, 21(1):9–17.
59. Mackova, E., and Hnik, P. (1973): Compensatory muscle hypertrophy induced by tenotomy synergists is not true working hypertrophy. *Physiol. Bohemoslov.*, 22:43–49.
60. Manasek, F. J. (1968): Mitosis in developing cardiac muscle. *J. Cell Biol.*, 37:191–196.
61. Mark, G. E., and Strasser, F. F. (1966): Pacemaker activity and mitosis in cultures of newborn rat heart ventricle cells. *Exp. Cell Res.*, 44:217–233.
62. Masui, H., and Garren, L. D. (1971): Inhibition of replication in functional mouse adrenal tumor cells by adrenocorticotropic hormone mediated by adenosine 3,5 cyclic monophosphate. *Proc. Natl. Acad. Sci. USA*, 68:3206–3210.
62a. Meerson, F. Z. (1969): The myocardium in hyperfunction hypertrophy and heart failure. *Circ. Res.*, 25(Suppl. II):1–163.
63. Minaga, T., Marton, L. J., Piper, W. N., and Kun, E. (1978): Induction of cardiac L-ornithine decarboxylase by nicotinamide and its regulation by putrescine. *Eur. J. Biochem.*, 91(2):577–585.
64. Morkin, E., Flink, I. L., and Goldman, S. (1983): Biochemical and physiological effects of thyroid hormone on cardiac performance. *Prog. Cardiovasc. Dis.*, 25:435–464.
65. Nag, A. C., Cheng, M., Fischman, D. A., and Zak, R. (1983): Long-term culture of adult cell of mammalian cardiac myocytes: Electron microscopic and immunofluorescent analyses of myofibrillar structure. *J. Mol. Cell. Cardiol.*, 15:301–317.
66. Deleted in proof.
67. O'Neil, M. C., and Stockdale, F. E. (1972): Akinetic analyses of myogenesis in vitro. *J. Cell. Biol.*, 52:52–65.
68. Pardee, A. B. (1974): A restriction point for control of normal animal cell proliferation (growth control/cell survival/cancer). *Proc. Natl. Acad. Sci. USA*, 71:1286–1290.
69. Pegg, A. E. (1981): Effect of alpha-difuoromethylortnithine on cardiac polyamine content and hypertrophy. *J. Mol. Cell. Cardiol.*, 1:881–887.
70. Pluskal, M. G., and Pennigton, R. J. (1976): Protein synthesis by ribosomes from normal and denervated red and white muscles. *Exp. Neurol.*, 51:571–578.
71. Rabinowitz, M., and Zak, R. (1975): Mitochondria and cardiac hypertrophy. *Circ. Res.*, 36:367–376.
72. Rakusan, K., Raman, S., Layberry, R., and Korecky, B. (1978): The influence of aging and growth on the postnatal development of cardiac muscle in rats. *Circ. Res.*, 42:212–218.
73. Rumyantsev, P. P. (1977): Interrelations of the proliferation and differentiation processes during cardiac myogenesis and regeneration. *Int. Rev. Cytol.*, 51:187–273.

74. Salmons, S., and Sreter, F. A. (1976): Significance of impulse activity in the transformation of skeletal muscle type. *Nature (Lond.)*, 263:30–34.
75. Seider, M. J., Kapp, R., Chen, Ch. P., and Booth, F. W. (1980): The effects of cutting or of stretching skeletal muscle in vitro on the rates of protein synthesis and degradation. *Biochem. J.*, 188:247–254.
76. Seifert, W. E., and Rudland, P. S. (1974): Possible involvement of cyclic GMP in growth control of cultured mouse cells. *Nature*, 248:138–140.
77. Sola, O. M., Christensen, D. L., and Martin, A. W. (1973): Hypertrophy and hyperplasia of adult chicken anterior latissimus dorsi muscles following stretch with and without denervation. *Exp. Neurol.*, 41:76–100.
78. Sreter, F. A., Elzinga, M., Mabuchi, K., Salmons, S., and Luff, A. (1975): The N-methyl-histidine content of myosin in stimulated and cross reinervated skeletal muscle of the rabbit. *FEBS Letters*, 57:107–114.
79. Stewart, M. D., and Martin, A. W. (1956): Hypertrophy of the denervated hemidiaphragm. *Am. J. Physiol.*, 186:497–500.
80. Sudbery, P. E., Goodey, A. R., and Carter, B. L. A. (1980): Genes which control cell proliferation in the yeast Saccharomyces cerevisiae. *Nature*, 288:401–404.
81. Vanderburgh, H. H., and Kauman, S. (1980): In vitro skeletal muscle hypertrophy and Na pump activity. In: *Plasticity of Muscle*, edited by D. Pette. W. de Gruyter & Co., Berlin, New York.
82. Weinstein, R. B., and Hay, E. D. (1970): DNA synthesis and mitosis in differentiated cardiac muscle cells of chick embryos. *J. Cell Biol.*, 47:310–316.
83. Weeds, A. G., and Burridge, K. (1975): Myosin from cross-reinervated cat muscles. Evidence for reciprocal transformations of heavy chains. *FEBS Letters*, 57:203–208.
83a. Weeds, A. G., Trentham, D. R., Kean, C. J., and Buller, A. J. (1974): Myosin from cross-reinnervated cat muscle. *Nature*, 247:135–139.
84. Weiss, P., and Kavanau, J. L. (1957): A model of growth and growth control in mathematical terms. *J. Gen. Physiol.*, 41:1–47.
85. Zak, R. (1981): Contractile function as a determinant of muscle growth. *Cell Muscle Motility*, 1:1–32.
86. Zak, R., Grove, D., and Rabinowitz, M. (1969): DNA synthesis in the rat diaphragm as an early response to denervation. *Am. J. Physiol.*, 216:647–654.
87. Zak, R., Martin, A. F., Prior, G., and Rabinowitz, M. (1977): Comparison of turnover of several myofibrillar proteins and critical evaluation of double isotope method. *J. Biol. Chem.*, 252:3430–3435.
88. Zak, R., Kizu, A., and Bugaisky, L. (1979): Cardiac hypertrophy: Its characteristics as a growth process. *Amer. J. Cardiol.*, 44:941–946.
89. Zak, R., and Rabinowitz, M. (1979): Molecular aspects of cardiac hypertrophy. *Annu. Rev. Physiol.*, 41:539–552.

Growth of the Heart in Health and Disease,
edited by Radovan Zak. Raven Press,
New York © 1984.

Cardiac Hypertrophy:
Morphological Aspects

Victor J. Ferrans

*Pathology Branch, National Heart, Lung, and Blood Institute, National Institutes of
Health, Bethesda, Maryland 20205*

CARDIAC HYPERTROPHY:
DEFINITION AND CLASSIFICATION

In its simplest definition, cardiac hypertrophy refers to heart weights exceeding the accepted limits of normal for age, sex, and body weight (average, 295 g for adult men and 250 g for adult women). Normal cardiac weight is best estimated on the basis of its relationship to body weight (0.43 per cent in men and 0.40 per cent in women). Hypertrophic human hearts can weigh up to four times as much as normal hearts. Patients with severely narrowed coronary arteries and no evidence of other cardiovascular disease may have hearts weighing up to 500 g. Cardiac weights uncommonly exceed 600 g in isolated mitral stenosis, 800 g in isolated aortic valvular stenosis, or 1,000 g in systemic hypertension. Hearts weighing more than 1,000 g are rare and occur mostly in aortic regurgitation (either isolated or complicated by mitral regurgitation or associated with ventricular septal defect) and in hypertrophic cardiomyopathy (68).

The term hypertrophy traditionally has meant that the increase in the mass of the heart is a consequence of an increase in the size of its constituent cells. Thus, hypertrophy differs from hyperplasia, in which the growth of an organ is mediated by an increase in the number of its cells. Although it has been considered that the increased tissue mass in hypertrophy results from enlargement of individual muscle cells, this is an oversimplification. It is now recognized that cardiac hypertrophy involves (a) increase in size, and in certain instances also in number, of cardiac muscle cells; (b) increase in number of various types of connective tissue cells; and (c) deposition of increased amounts of connective tissue proteins in the interstitial spaces.

Concentric and Eccentric Hypertrophies

Depending on the specific cause, the increase in tissue mass in cardiac hypertrophy produces characteristic alterations in the volume of the cardiac cavities and in the thickness of its chambers (Figs. 1 and 2). These changes provide a basis for

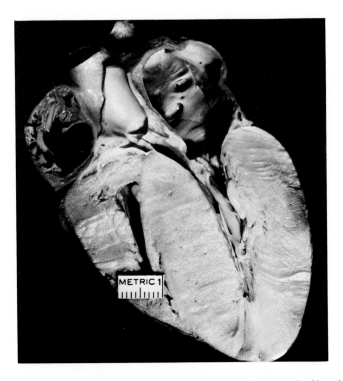

FIG. 1. Gross photograph of heart of child with hypertrophic cardiomyopathy. Note the marked thickening of the ventricular walls, the dilatation of the atria, the small ventricular chambers, and the asymmetric septal hypertrophy.

the classic concept that cardiac hypertrophy can be classified as being either concentric (hearts with small cavities and thick walls) or eccentric (hearts with large, dilated cavities and walls that are relatively thin, although they may be actually thicker than normal). In a normal adult human heart, the right and left atria measure 1 to 2 mm in thickness; the right ventricle, 2 to 3 mm; and the left ventricular free wall and the ventricular septum, 8 to 10 mm. In measuring the thickness of the ventricular walls, care must be taken not to include the thickness of the papillary muscles and the trabeculae carneae. Concentric hypertrophy usually is associated with conditions that cause pressure overloading, e.g., aortic or pulmonic stenosis. Eccentric hypertrophy is associated with congestive cardiomyopathies and with conditions that cause volume overloading, e.g., mitral or tricuspid regurgitation. The distinction between these two types of hypertrophies is not always clear, as the gross anatomic picture of eccentric hypertrophy also may develop as the result of cardiac failure and dilatation in the late, decompensated stages of pressure overloading.

Symmetric and Asymmetric Hypertrophies

Cardiac hypertrophy also may be classified as symmetric or asymmetric, depending on whether or not different regions of a given chamber become hypertro-

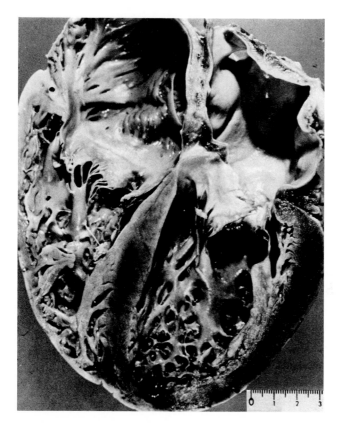

FIG. 2. Heart from patient with Chagas' disease showing marked dilatation of all chambers and thinning of the ventricular walls.

phied to a comparable extent. The term asymmetric hypertrophy usually is employed to designate the bizarre type of hypertrophy that occurs in hypertrophic cardiomyopathy and in association with a few rare disorders. This hypertrophy (Fig. 2) characteristically involves the ventricular septum to a greater extent than the free walls of the ventricles. In contrast, the ventricular septum in the usual types of hypertrophies, i.e., concentric and eccentric, becomes thickened to the same extent as the free walls of the ventricles (69).

Physiological and Pathological Hypertrophies

Cardiac hypertrophy can occur as a consequence of increased physiological activity (physiological hypertrophy) or in association with disease states (pathological hypertrophy). In either of these circumstances, hypertrophy represents a phenomenon of adaptive growth that takes place in response to mechanical or chemical alterations in cardiac function. The exact mechanisms by which such alterations induce an increase in cardiac mass are poorly understood, although it is known that work overload rapidly stimulates the synthesis of RNA and protein in the heart.

It is by no means certain that the mechanisms that activate these synthetic processes are the same in cardiac hypertrophy of different causes. It is clear, however, that the interactions between these growth processes and hemodynamic events result in different geometric configurations in concentric and in eccentric hypertrophy.

The distinction between concentric and eccentric types of hypertrophies can be made not only in hearts undergoing pathological hypertrophy but also in those showing physiological hypertrophy. Morganroth et al. (58) made echocardiograms in 56 athletes involved either in primarily isotonic exercise (swimmers and runners) or in primarily isometric exercise (wrestlers and shot putters). Mean left ventricular end-diastolic volume (181 ml) and mass (308 g were increased in swimmers and runners (160 ml and 302 g) when compared with controls (101 ml, 211 g), whereas wall thickness was normal (<12 mm). In contrast, wrestlers and shot putters had normal mean left ventricular end-diastolic volumes (110 ml and 122 ml, respectively) but increased wall thickness (13–14 mm) and mass (330 g, 348 g, respectively). These data show that athletes participating in strenuous isotonic exercise tend to have increased left ventricular mass with cardiac changes similar to those present in patients with chronic volume overloading, whereas athletes participating in chronic isometric exercise tend to have increased left ventricular mass with cardiac changes similar to those present in patients with chronic pressure overloading.

Finally, a most useful way of classifying hypertrophy relates to the fact that cardiac morphology and function undergo a series of progressive changes during the time course of hypertrophy. Based primarily on observations made in dogs and rabbits with experimentally induced aortic constriction, Meerson et al. (57) formulated the concept that the heart in hypertrophy evolves through three distinct stages: (a) transient breakdown or damage of the muscle cells and rapid increases in energy production and protein synthesis; (b) stable hyperfunction or "compensated hypertrophy"; (c) gradual exhaustion of the heart's ability to synthesize proteins resulting from failure to renew mitochondria and myofibrils and from myofibrillar damage and cellular atrophy. As discussed in detail below, this concept of three stages is also applicable to hypertrophic human hearts.

CELLULAR BASIS OF CARDIAC ENLARGEMENT: HYPERTROPHY VERSUS HYPERPLASIA

Much of our understanding of the cellular basis of cardiac enlargement is based on the results of studies by Linzbach and Hort. Their conclusions (see Linzbach, refs. 43,44, and Hort, ref. 35 for reviews) can be summarized as follows:

1. All normal human hearts have essentially the same number of cardiac muscle cells. At birth this number is essentially the same as at maturity. The muscle cells are considerably thinner in newborns than in adults. During normal postnatal physiologic growth the number of muscle cells remains constant; the cells enlarge, but their length-to-width ratio remains constant.

2. The number of cardiac muscle cell nuclei also is approximately constant in normal adult human hearts. In the newborn the number of cardiac muscle cell nuclei is roughly half as large as in the adult. The number of these nuclei doubles after birth as the result of nuclear division. This division is not accompanied by cytoplasmic division, with the result that many cells become binucleated. The number of cells remains unchanged.

3. The number of myocardial capillaries increases with growth, with one capillary per four muscle cells in the infant and one capillary per each muscle cell in the adult.

4. The number of cells is roughly the same in the left and in the right ventricle. The left ventricle is heavier than the right because its muscle cells have larger transverse diameters and because the layers of individual muscle cells are more numerous in the left than in the right ventricular wall.

5. Through athletic exertion the weight of the heart can increase (physiological hypertrophy) from 300 to 500 g. This increase is due to an extension of physiological growth and occurs without an increase in the number of cardiac muscle cells.

6. In pathological hypertrophy, the "critical" heart weight of 500 g may be exceeded only by an increase in the number of cardiac muscle cells, which show little further increase in size after this weight is exceeded. These observations on the relationships between heart weights and myocyte diameters have been independently confirmed by Astorri et al. (5). Linzbach postulated that this numerical increase is mediated through "amitotic division" of cardiac muscle cells. Capillaries also increase in number, and the one to one ratio of capillaries and muscle cells is maintained.

7. Chronic cardiac dilatation results not from overstretching of sarcomeres, but from preferential longitudinal growth of the muscle cells (i.e., end-to-end addition of sarcomeres) and from rearrangement of the layers of muscle cells.

Mitosis and DNA Synthesis in Myocardium

Both undifferentiated muscle cells and muscle cells containing myofibrillar proteins undergo mitotic division at a relatively rapid rate during embryonic development of the heart (see Zak, ref. 86, and Bugaisky and Zak, ref. 13, for review). This rate decreases rapidly during late embryonic and early postnatal development. The ability to undergo mitosis seems to be irreversibly lost in adult mammalian ventricular myocardium, but persists to a very limited extent in atrial myocardium of mammals and is not lost in ventricular myocardium of certain amphibians. Cellular hyperplasia, as evidenced by increased DNA synthesis and by mitotic figures in ventricular muscle cells, plays a role in the development of pathologic cardiac enlargement in very young rats and dogs. By contrast, DNA synthesis in hypertrophying ventricles of adult rats and dogs is demonstrable only in connective tissue cells. In the human, polyploidization of nuclear DNA of cardiac muscle cells takes place during normal development. This occurs between 5 and 9 years of age.

Between birth and this event, the number of binucleated cells increases but individual nuclei remain diploid. In adult human hearts about two-thirds of the nuclei of muscle cells are polyploid, with a DNA content of 4C, 8C, or 16C (1,2,66). In human cardiac hypertrophy, a further shift to higher degrees of polyploidy occurs (2). It should be noted, however, that extensive polyploidy of cardiac muscle cells has been found to be peculiar to man and the rhesus monkey; other mammals have mostly diploid nuclei, although multinucleated cardiac muscle cells are common in the pig (Fig. 3) (32). This shows that nuclear DNA synthesis can occur normally to a limited extent in cardiac muscle cells during the postnatal period. This synthesis does not lead to cytoplasmic division; in some species it leads mainly to polyploidization, and in others to multinucleation.

Cessation of Mitosis in Cardiac Muscle Cells

The reasons for the cessation of mitotic activity in adult mammalian ventricular muscle cells remain unclear. The three main possibilities that have been considered are:

1. *Critical mitosis theory.* It has been suggested that synthesis of DNA and of cell-specific (i.e., myofibrillar) proteins are mutually exclusive processes. A block of DNA synthesis is thought to occur during differentiation of myoblasts as a consequence of a specific mitosis leading to a new phenotype cell. This appears

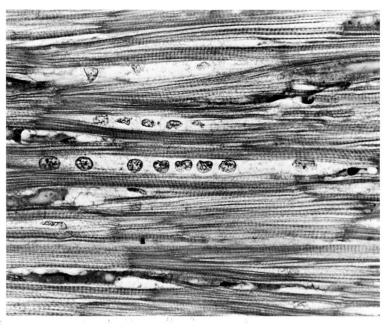

FIG. 3. Multinucleated myocytes in left ventricle of pig. 1-μ-thick section of plastic-embedded tissue. Alkaline toluidine blue stain (×500).

to be the case in skeletal, but not in cardiac muscle cells; the latter can continue to divide after they have well developed myofibrils.

2. *Critical mass theory.* It is postulated that the gradually accumulating cell-specific structures present a hindrance to mitotic division of the nucleus. After a critical mass has been reached, no more mitoses are possible. Of special interest is the observation (62,60) that the Z-bands disappear, at least partially, as cardiac muscle cells undergoing mitosis reach the stage of metaphase. It has been suggested that the presence of large amounts of Z-band material in a cardiac muscle cell may render it incapable of further mitoses.

3. *Repression of DNA synthesis.* Synthesis of DNA in developing myocytes declines with maturation, but under rare conditions it can be reactivated, suggesting that it is repressed rather than irreversibly blocked. This concept received considerable support from the work of Rumyantsev et al. (70–73) and Oberpriller et al. (61), who showed that rat atrial myocytes are capable of synthesizing DNA and undergoing mitotic nuclear division as part of the responses of the heart to ligation of the left coronary artery. The exact mechanism leading to these changes is unknown. Nevertheless, it is clear that up to 70% of left atrial myocytes take up tritiated thymidine within 5 to 10 days after the coronary ligation; mitotic figures also are frequently encountered in left atrial myocytes (Fig. 4). In contrast, only less than 4% of left ventricular myocytes demonstrate uptake of tritiated thymidine, and mitoses in left ventricular myocytes are very uncommon. Recent work by Oberpriller et al. (61) confirms these findings and shows that the DNA content of nuclei of left atrial myocytes tends to rise above 2C values after left ventricular infarction and that the percentage of binucleated left atrial myocytes increases markedly (as demonstrated in preparations of enzymatically dissociated atrial tissue). However, it is not known to what extent the nuclear division observed in these activated cells is capable of continuing to cytoplasmic division and to a true increase in cell number.

Hyperplasia of ventricular muscle cells ceases as the heart grows during the first weeks of postnatal life, after which hypertrophy becomes the mechanism by which adult cardiac size is attained. Hypertrophy also can account for an increase in size of the adult human heart up to the critical weight of 500 g. The critical heart weight theory has not been tested in experimental animals because the degrees of cardiac hypertrophy attained in animal models usually do not result in doubling of the cardiac weight; however, the calculations of Zak (86) suggest that increases in the number of cardiac muscle cells also occur during normal growth in certain animals. It is uncertain if such increases take effect through mitosis. Because of the absence of mitoses in adult ventricular muscle cells, the occurrence of another, qualitatively different process of myocyte division has been postulated to account for the increased number of muscle cells that is thought to be necessary to mediate further increases in the weight of hypertrophied human hearts. Nevertheless, the process of nuclear cleavage and longitudinal splitting of the cytoplasm, as postulated by Linzbach, remains a matter of conjecture. The occurrence of this process has

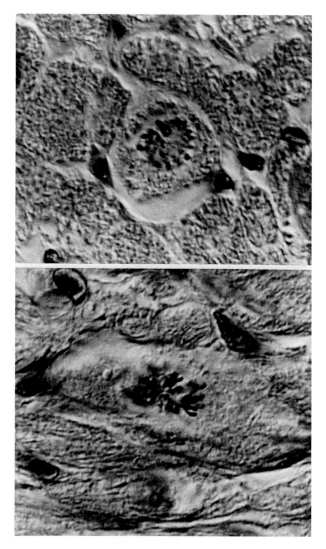

FIG. 4. Two views of mitotic figures in rat left atrial myocytes. 1-μ-thick section of plastic-embedded tissue examined with Nomarski differential interference contrast optics. Alkaline toluidine blue stain. (× 1,200).

not been demonstrated unequivocally, and it is possible that this hyperplasia is mediated by mitoses which occur with a frequency below that detectable by currently used techniques.

GROSS ANATOMIC CHANGES IN CARDIAC HYPERTROPHY

To understand the gross structural changes that the ventricular walls undergo in concentric and eccentric hypertrophies, it should be appreciated that such changes represent exaggerations of the configurations that the heart assumes as a function of different intraventricular volumes and that these changes are given permanence by the development of interstitial fibrosis and endocardial thickening. Alterations occurring in eccentric hypertrophy bear resemblances to configurations imposed by high intraventricular volumes; those in concentric hypertrophy, to configurations resulting from low intraventricular volumes. Alterations in asymmetric cardiac hypertrophy are discussed separately.

Structure of Normal Ventricular Walls

The studies of Streeter et al. (78) demonstrated that more than 60% of muscle cells in the free wall of the left ventricle form a circumferential band in the middle of the wall; the remaining cells are oriented in increasingly oblique spirals toward the endocardial and epicardial surfaces. Other studies (see Spotnitz et al., ref. 77, for review) have shown that in the canine heart a 60% decrease in ventricular volume during systole is associated with a 30% to 50% increase in average thickness of the ventricular wall, but only with a 13% decrease in midwall sarcomere length. It is evident from these data that changes in cell thickness proportionate to a 13% decrease in sarcomere length cannot explain the observed increase in wall thickness unless considerable rearrangement of the muscle cells also occurs.

The mechanisms responsible for internal volume-dependent changes in the thickness of the left ventricular wall were examined in detail by Spotnitz et al. (77), who made detailed morphometric studies of vertical cross sections of the left ventricles of arrested rat hearts that had been fixed at different ventricular volumes. Spotnitz showed that increased ventricular volume was associated with decreases in wall thickness, which followed theoretical predictions for a spherical ventricular model. Their data indicate that acutely induced changes in wall thickness are primarily due to changes in the number of cells aligned across the wall (i.e., along the radius of the ventricle). In hypertrophy-induced changes in wall thickness, additional factors must be taken into account, including changes in length and transverse diameter of the muscle cells and the presence or absence of interstitial fibrosis. Some very heavy and dilated hearts have ventricular walls that actually are thinner than normal. Perhaps the most extreme examples of this are found in Chagas' disease, in which the apical regions of very dilated ventricles are paper-thin and are composed of endocardium and epicardium, which are apposed with few intervening cardiac muscle cells.

The rearrangement in the alignment of the cells composing the ventricular wall is facilitated by cleavage planes that are present between groups of muscle cells in the ventricular wall. The orientation of these planes varies with ventricular volume. In the thick walls of ventricles with low internal volumes, the cleavage planes become oriented more horizontally and follow a straight path across the wall, almost perpendicular to the epicardial and endocardial surfaces. In the thin walls of high-volume ventricles, the planes of cleavage are tilted toward the vertical axis of the heart, run obliquely across the wall, and form acute angles with the endocardium and epicardium. These changes in angle permit the ventricular wall to increase in height (i.e., length from apex to base) and to decrease in thickness. Conversely, the shift from high to low intraventricular volume is accompanied by decreased ventricular height, a change that makes more muscle cells available for increasing the thickness of the wall. The movements just described imply a small shearing motion (about 15 degrees of angular motion during normal systole) between adjacent layers of myocardium abutting on the cleavage planes. Spotnitz et al. (77), point out that this may contribute to the oxygen cost of ventricular contraction and could prove to be a problem in the presence of fibrosis and scarring, which would increase the amount of work required to alter wall thickness. Fibrosis is also likely to result in decreased myocardial compliance. Similarly, fibrosis may reduce or prevent the regression of myocardial dilatation when the cause of hypertrophy is removed.

Anatomic Changes in Concentric and Eccentric Hypertrophies

As mentioned previously, the gross anatomy of the ventricular walls differs in concentric hypertrophy, eccentric hypertrophy, and asymmetric hypertrophy (Figs. 1 and 2). The consistency of the walls also differs: in eccentric hypertrophy the walls generally are more flabby than in concentric hypertrophy. The reason for this difference is not known. The atria can undergo considerable degrees of dilatation, with internal volumes exceeding 1,000 ml. The ventricles show much lesser degrees of dilatation, but greater degrees of hypertrophy and wall thickening. According to Wartman and Hill (82), dilatation of the left ventricle is accompanied by lengthening of the chamber in the apex to base direction. This dilatation involves the apical portion of the left ventricle more than the region in front of the anterior leaflet of the mitral valve; the portion behind the posterior leaflet of the mitral valve is least affected. Because of this involvement, the left ventricle becomes less conical and more hemispherical in shape as the left ventricle dilates, and the papillary muscles appear to originate more cephalad on the wall than is the case in concentric hypertrophy; the trabeculae carneae tend to flatten out. The change in position of the papillary muscles and the change in the angle that they form with the plane of the mitral valve orifice eventually lead to inadequate closure of the mitral valve and to valvular regurgitation. This is often the case in congestive cardiomyopathy.

In right ventricular hypertrophy without dilatation, the trabeculae carneae form a massive, prominent network. This network tends to become attenuated in right ventricular hypertrophy with dilatation. As right ventricular dilatation develops, the free wall of the right ventricle bulges outward. This bulge can extend beyond the area of attachment of the right ventricular walls to the ventricular septum. Near the apex of the right ventricle, this dilatation may carry the free wall down to the level of the left ventricular apex, thus giving the appearance of a double or bifid apex.

Anatomic Changes in Hypertrophic Cardiomyopathy

Definition of the gross anatomic and microscopic changes in the hearts of patients with hypertrophic cardiomyopathy has brought about a new understanding of the unique pathophysiology of this disease. Hypertrophic cardiomyopathy is genetically transmitted as an autosomal dominant trait and encompasses a wide spectrum of anatomic and clinical manifestations.

Hypertrophic cardiomyopathy is characterized morphologically (21,69) by a severe degree of cardiac hypertrophy, with the following characteristics: (a) increased thickness of the free walls of both ventricles; (b) a narrow, abnormally shaped left ventricular cavity; (c) asymmetric hypertrophy of the ventricular septum, the maximal thickness of which exceeds that of the posterobasal left ventricular free wall (measured at the level of the inferior border of the posterior leaflet of the mitral valve) by a factor of 1.3 or greater (normal = 1.0); (d) dilated atria, normal-sized ascending aorta, normal aortic valve, and variably thickened mitral valvular leaflets, especially the anterior leaflet; (e) thickened endocardium in the area of the ventricular septum opposite to the anterior mitral leaflet; (f) foci of bizarre disarray of myocytes (28) (Figs. 5 and 6); and (g) a high incidence of fibromuscular intimal and medial thickening in small, intramural coronary arteries. The latter change can be the cause of myocardial necrosis in patients with normal large extramural coronary arteries (49). The clinical and anatomic features show consid-

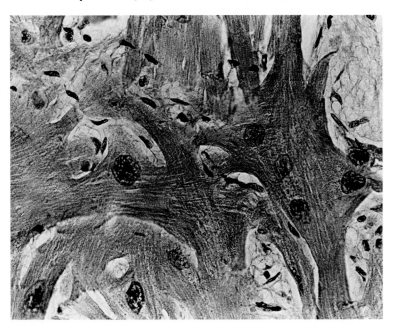

FIG. 5. Histological section of ventricular septal myocardium of patient with hypertrophic cardiomyopathy, showing severe hypertrophy, nuclear enlargement, and myocyte disarray. Hematoxylin-eosin stain (×400).

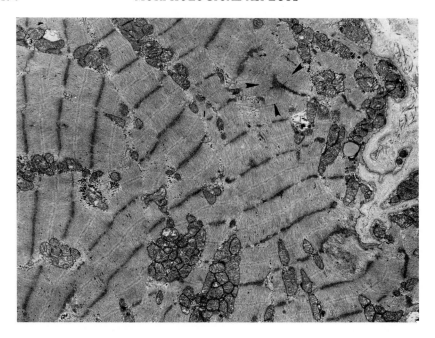

FIG. 6. Electron micrograph of part of ventricular septal muscle cell from patient with hypertrophic cardiomyopathy. Myofibrils course in various directions and show branching *(arrowheads)*. Z-bands are irregularly widened (×8,600).

erable variation from one patient to another, even among members of a given affected family. Accordingly, patients with hypertrophic cardiomyopathy can be classified into the following groups: (a) patients who have obstruction to left ventricular outflow (and, less frequently, also to right ventricular outflow) under basal conditions, (b) patients who do not have obstruction to ventricular outflow under basal conditions but who can develop such an obstruction as a result of physiological maneuvers or pharmacological interventions, and (c) patients in whom obstruction to ventricular outflow is neither present at rest nor provoked by physiological or pharmacological maneuvers (21).

Types of Hypertrophic Obstructive Cardiomyopathy

Patients with the obstructive form of hypertrophic cardiomyopathy can be subdivided into those with the usual form of obstruction to left ventricular outflow; those with midventricular obstruction, also involving the left ventricle; and those with obstruction to right ventricular outflow. Most patients with obstructive disease belong to the first of these groups, in which the mechanism of obstruction to left ventricular outflow is considered to involve an abnormal systolic displacement (in the anterior direction) of some of the components of the mitral valvular apparatus (especially the anterior mitral leaflet), thus narrowing the left ventricular outflow tract. This abnormal motion of the anterior mitral leaflet can lead to actual contact with the ventricular septum, resulting in the development of fibroelastic thickening in the ventricular surface of the anterior mitral leaflet and in the corresponding area of contact in the ventricular septal surface (69). Because of this, the finding of a plaque-like area of endocardial thickening in the septal wall of the left ventricular outflow tract is regarded as evidence of present or previous obstructive disease in patients with hypertrophic cardiomyopathy.

The type of obstruction just described was also observed in a few patients with concentric left ventricular wall thickening not associated with asymmetric hypertrophy of the ventricular septum (54). Symmetric hypertrophic cardiomyopathy is extremely rare.

The second type of mechanism of obstruction to left ventricular outflow is known as midventricular obstruction and is uncommon. The patients have the usual characteristic clinical features of hypertrophic obstructive cardiomyopathy but are found (by angiography and by measurements of pressure at multiple sites in the left ventricular cavity) to have a level of obstruction located lower along the ventricular septum than is usually the case (22,23). It is critical that this type of obstruction be recognized before operation, because its surgical relief may require a technique that differs from the transaortic left ventricular myotomy-myectomy employed in the usual patient with hypertrophic cardiomyopathy and obstruction to left ventricular outflow.

In the majority of patients with hypertrophic cardiomyopathy who have obstruction to right ventricular outflow, this phenomenon occurs only to a minimal extent and is associated with a severe degree of left-sided obstruction (21). In adults, it is extremely rare to find obstruction that is either predominant in, or limited to, the right ventricular outflow tract; however, right-sided obstruction is relatively common in infants and children (6,16). This obstruction is thought to be related to encroachment of a massively hypertrophic ventricular septum on the right ventricular outflow tract, especially in the region of the crista supraventricularis.

Types of Hypertrophic Nonobstructive Cardiomyopathy

Patients with nonobstructive hypertrophic cardiomyopathy can be subdivided into two classes according to their cardiac gross anatomic features. The hearts of patients in the first of these classes differ (21,69) in relatively few respects from those of patients with hypertrophic obstructive cardiomyopathy: The degree of asymmetric hypertrophy of the ventricular septum usually is similar, but the degree of hypertrophy of the posterobasal wall of the left ventricle is less marked, and the endocardial plaque in the upper portion of the left ventricular surface of the ventricular septum usually is not present in patients with nonobstructive disease. Finally, the extent of the thickening that occurs in other areas of the left ventricular free walls of these patients may show considerable regional variations. In patients with obstructive disease, such variations are much less obvious, presumably because they are equalized by the development of more diffuse hypertrophy, induced by pressure overload related to outflow tract obstruction.

In the second group of patients with hypertrophic nonobstructive cardiomyopathy, the mass of asymmetrically hypertrophic muscle is localized in the lower third of the ventricular septum, forming an irregular mass that fills the apical region of the left ventricular cavity, simulating the angiographic appearance of an intracardiac tumor or thrombus (85).

Association of Hypertrophic Cardiomyopathy with Other Diseases

In the majority of patients with hypertrophic cardiomyopathy, the disease occurs without being associated with other cardiac or noncardiac diseases; however, in a sizable minority of adult patients, it is associated with systemic hypertension. A few, rare patients with hypertrophic cardiomyopathy also have been found to have other diseases, among which are lentiginosis, Turner phenotype (Noonan's syndrome), von Recklinghausen's disease, tuberous sclerosis, Friedreich's ataxia, functioning pancreatic islet cell tumors (insulinomas), hyperthyroidism, hypercalcemia, and mitral valvular prolapse (see Perloff, ref. 65, for review). It remains uncertain whether such uncommon associations are simply coincidental or indicative of a true pathogenetic link.

Asymmetric cardiac hypertrophy also has been reported in patients with Pompe's disease or infantile form of type II glycogen storage disease (19,20). In some of these patients, severe degrees of wall thickening are associated with small cardiac cavities and with obstruction to left and/or right ventricular outflow; other patients, however, show cardiac dilatation (9). In 13 patients with Pompe's disease studied by Bloom et al (9), the left ventricular free wall was hypertrophied to a much greater extent than was the ventricular septum; no obstruction to left ventricular outflow was observed in any of these patients either at rest, after isoproterenol infusion, or after ventricular premature contractions. Therefore, these features differ from those in hypertrophic cardiomyopathy.

Hypertrophic cardiomyopathy in infants must be distinguished from a transient, nonfamilial condition that was recently described in infants of diabetic mothers and is manifested by disproportionate thickening of the ventricular septum, systolic anterior motion of the anterior mitral leaflet (associated with a left ventricular outflow gradient), hyperdynamic left ventricular contraction, and signs and symptoms suggestive of congestive heart failure. These changes, which usually regress within the first few months of life, are thought to represent manifestations of the generalized organomegaly present in infants of diabetic mothers rather than of a primary cardiomyopathic process (33).

The diagnosis of hypertrophic cardiomyopathy in infants is complicated by limitations in the use of the septal-free wall thickness ratio of 1.3 or greater as the sole diagnostic criterion (56). This ratio, which was established on the basis of studies in adults, is much less specific for hypertrophic cardiomyopathy in infants. The reason is that this ratio is frequently found (25%) in infants with congenital heart disease unrelated to hypertrophic cardiomyopathy and, less frequently, in normal infants (see Maron and Roberts, ref. 56, for review).

A wide variety of congenital cardiac malformations and acquired heart diseases have been found to coexist with asymmetric septal hypertrophy or with "muscular" obstruction to left ventricular outflow (56). These patients represent only a minority of all patients with such congenital or acquired lesions. The limited data available suggest that the majority of these patients do not have the familial form of hypertrophic cardiomyopathy. The highest incidence of asymmetric septal hypertrophy associated with congenital heart disease has been found in patients with very severe degrees of right ventricular systolic overloading, as manifested in primary pulmonary hypertension, isolated pulmonary stenosis, and after pulmonary arterial banding in ventricular septal defect. In these patients, the asymmetric septal hypertrophy is thought to be caused by the contribution of right ventricular hypertrophy to overall ventricular septal thickness. A high frequency of asymmetric septal hypertrophy also has been found in patients with the parachute mitral valve syndrome and its variant forms (Shone's syndrome) (56).

A few patients with left ventricular hypertrophy due to other types of obstruction to left ventricular outflow, including valvular and subvalvular (fibrous ring type) subaortic stenosis, also have been found to have asymmetric septal hypertrophy. These cases are nonfamilial and can present difficult diagnostic problems. Finally, a few patients with systemic hypertension, coronary artery disease, mitral valvular disease, and combined aortic and mitral valvular disease also have been reported to have asymmetric septal hypertrophy (48).

In the vast majority of 125 infants with congenital heart disease studied by Maron et al (47), the disproportionate septal thickening was considered not to be a manifestation of associated hypertrophic cardiomyopathy because of the absence of other features of the latter disease. As discussed above, hemodynamic alterations related to congenital heart disease constitute a major factor responsible for the occurrence of disproportionate ventricular septal thickening in these infants. In addition, a minor error in the assessment of the small ventricular wall thickness in infants can lead to a large error in the calculation of the septal-free wall ratio. Finally, "abnormal" septal-free wall thickness ratios in some infants with congenital heart disease may be only a manifestation of the usual relation of ventricular septal thickness and left ventricular free wall thickness present in neonatal hearts. A septal-free wall ratio >1.3 was found in more than 90% of human embryos and young fetuses, in 65% of older fetuses, in 25% of live-born infants, and in 12% of those over 2 weeks of age. Disproportionate thickening of the septum is quite marked in young embryos, with septal-free wall ratios of more than 2.0. During the subsequent prenatal and postnatal growth, this ratio gradually diminishes and disproportionate septal thickening progressively becomes less common (56).

The disarray of myocytes in hypertrophic cardiomyopathy involves more than 5% of the cells in the ventricular septum. This differentiates such disarray from that which occurs in other types of heart disease, in which less than 5% of the cells are affected (55,46). Because of the findings just reviewed, the diagnosis of hypertrophic cardiomyopathy in infants requires, in addition to the characteristic clinical and hemodynamic features of the disease and an abnormal septal-free wall ratio, four other criteria: (a) a hypertrophic, nondilated ventricle; (b) a ventricular septum that is clearly thicker than normal in absolute measurements; (c) evidence of genetic transmission of the disproportional septal thickening in first-degree relatives; and (d) marked disorganization of ventricular septal myocardium (if necropsy evaluation is possible).

HISTOLOGICAL AND ULTRASTRUCTURAL ASPECTS OF CARDIAC HYPERTROPHY

This section presents data on (a) the mechanisms by which new contractile elements are formed in cardiac muscle cells, (b) qualitative myocardial structural changes in the different stages of hypertrophy, and (c) quantitative changes in subcellular components of hypertrophic hearts.

Morphogenesis of Sarcomeres in Normal Growth and Hypertrophy

The formation of sarcomeres is a complex event that involves the synthesis of appropriate amounts of a variety of different proteins. These proteins then become aggregated into filaments, which, in turn, are organized into specific tridimensional arrays and aligned with respect to other contractile elements already present in the cell. Most of our knowledge of these events has been obtained from autoradiographic studies of labeled amino acids incorporated into cardiac muscle cells and from studies of ultrastructural images that have been interpreted as representing various stages in the process of sarcomerogenesis.

A continuous process of synthesis and breakdown of proteins goes on in fully developed sarcomeres of normal cardiac muscle, as evidenced by studies showing that the half-life of cardiac myosin and actin is less than 2 weeks (59). It is not clear whether different sarcomeric proteins turn over simultaneously, although this seems unlikely, or whether this turnover occurs evenly throughout different regions of myocardium. In any case, no morphologic evidence of breakdown or new synthesis of contractile filaments is usually seen on ultrastructural examination of normal myocardium of adult animals.

Autoradiographic studies of labeled aminoacids incorporated into myocardium have provided useful information on myofibrillogenesis, even though the conclusions of these investigations are limited by the large size of the developed silver grains with respect to the subcellular structures in question, by the relatively nonspecific nature of the labeling, and by the inability of autoradiographic techniques to distinguish between protein synthesis related to turnover in preexisting myofilaments and that related to the addition of new ones. The localization of newly formed contractile proteins in normal, mature cardiac and skeletal muscle was studied by Morkin (1974) in rabbit right ventricular papillary muscle and rat diaphragm that had been labeled *in vitro* with (^{3}H)leucine and then glycerinated to extract soluble, noncontractile proteins. Electron microscopic study of autoradiographs of these preparations showed that the developed grains occurred with the greatest frequency a short distance from the margins of myofibrils. The pattern of grains observed coincided with that expected to result from multiple-point sources of radioactivity located on the surfaces of the myofibrils. Solubilization of contractile proteins removed most of the radioactivity, thus supporting the idea that the distribution of developed grains represented the location of newly synthesized contractile proteins.

Evidence also implicating peripheral regions of the myofibrils and Z-bands as sites of rapid turnover of contractile proteins in hypertrophied myocardium was obtained by Anversa et al. (4), who made quantitative analyses of the distribution of radioactivity in cardiac muscle cells of rats given (^{3}H)leucine at 8, 13, and 40 days after aortic constriction. Light microscopic examination of autoradiographs showed many silver granules uniformly spread inside the muscle cells, with no predominance of labeling in their peripheral regions. Electron microscopy showed that the silver grains were associated with every organelle of the cardiac muscle cells. However, when the percentage distribution of developed grains associated with specific structures was compared with the percentage of the cell volume occupied by the same structures, it became evident that the periphery of the myofibrils and the Z-bands had a consistently higher concentration of grains than would be expected from a purely random distribution. Although Anversa et al. (4) found the structure of most Z-bands to be the same in normal and hypertrophied muscle, they also observed anomalous Z-bands, with accumulations of dense Z-band material associated with a disordered array of myofilaments, at all three time intervals studied. Areas of Z-substance accumulation also were found at the periphery of the cells, under the sarcolemma and near intercalated discs. The developed grains in these regions were very few and did not show a preferential association with the anomalous Z-band material. Thus, these findings constitute evidence against the concept that accumulations of Z-band material in hypertrophic hearts are sites of selective incorporation of newly synthesized protein into contractile elements.

More direct information concerning mechanisms of sarcomere formation has been obtained from morphological studies of embryonic myocardium (45). In the very early stages of cardiac muscle cells development, both thick and thin myofilaments are free and located predominantly in subsarcolemmal regions. Organization of these filaments proceeds in association with dense, amorphous material that forms either plaques along the inner aspect of the sarcolemma or isolated condensations that are free in the sarcoplasm. These sites are considered organizing centers for myofibrillogenesis because the free filaments of more differentiated muscle cells insert into the material of these loci. The association of filaments with organizing centers produces structures that consist of thin filaments that insert into one or both sides of a centrally located, widened Z-band, and of thick filaments that are loosely associated with thin filaments. Interconnection of these structures has been proposed as the mechanism by which primitive, branched myofibrillar bundles characterized by widened Z-bands and loosely aggregated filaments are formed in later stages. These myofilaments then come into closer contact and into closer registration with one another. This results in the appearance of discrete A- and I-bands. I bands are seen only in those sarcomeres in which the Z-bands have narrowed and the filaments have become more closely packaged. H-bands and M-lines do not appear until sarcomerogenesis is nearly complete. Intercellular junctions develop wherever myofilaments insert perpendicular to sarcolemmal plaques. The lateral connections existing between myofilaments and sarcolemmal plaques at the levels of Z-bands are retained throughout gestation and in the immediate postnatal period, but gradually become inconspicuous and much less numerous as final cardiac size is attained. When myofibrils first develop in cardiac myoblasts, these cells are oval or stellate in shape and have intercellular junctions located randomly along their periphery. As more myofibrils develop they fill the central regions of the cells and become oriented parallel to the longitudinal axis. The cells gradually become cylindrical in shape, and their junctions become preferentially localized at the distal ends of the cells, with only a few side-to-side or lateral junctions remaining. Cell-to-cell interactions, mediated by the mechanical forces exerted on a given cell by its neighbors, are thought to play an important role in establishing the final pattern of orientation of cardiac muscle cells and their contractile components. Such a role is similar to that played by mechanical forces in determining the alignment of other fibrous proteins such as those in bone and tendon.

The preceding observations suggest that (a) sarcomere formation in normal embryonic myocardium occurs primarily at the periphery of the muscle cells, with new sarcomeres being added end-to-end at the free ends of myofibrils and in the vicinity of intercalated discs, and side-to-side in subsarcolemmal areas along the lateral surfaces of the cells; (b) accumulations of electron-dense material, which resembles that in mature Z-bands, play an "organizer" role in which they serve as sites where myofilaments attach and subsequently become oriented into parallel, interdigitating arrays; and (c) mechanical forces influence the alignment of newly formed sarcomeres.

The possible role of Z-band material in the formation of new sarcomeres has received considerable attention in studies on cardiac hypertrophy. As discussed previously, considerable evidence supports the concept that accumulations of Z-band material are associated with the formation of new sarcomeres and that these accumulations serve as templates on which other sarcomeric components are brought into their proper three-dimensional relationships (8,42). Nevertheless, other evidence shows that accumulations of Z-band material also can occur as a result of disruption of myofibrils and reaggregation of their Z-band material as well as in other conditions unrelated to the formation of new sarcomeres. Thus, accumulations of Z-band material should not be regarded as necessarily indicative of a process of continuing synthesis of new sarcomeres (53).

Studies of Z-bands and sarcomere formation in hypertrophying myocardium of newborn dogs (7) are of special interest because they have a bearing on the question of whether or not the mechanisms of sarcomerogenesis differ in normal growth and in hypertrophy. In addition to incompletely organized myofilaments along the periphery of the cells (as in normal newborn dogs), myocardium from newborn dogs with aortic constriction showed increased folding and tortuosity of intercalated discs and various degrees of widening of the Z-bands. The changes in the intercalated discs suggest that the synthesis of new plasma membrane material in cardiac hypertrophy occurs before that of myofibrils. The increased folding of the discs provides space for insertion and alignment of new myofilaments in these areas. The expansions of Z-band material appear to displace adjacent sarcomeres in a longitudinal direction, resulting in a misalignment of these sarcomeres with respect to those of neighboring myofibrils. It should be pointed out that although these structures are referred to as expansions of Z-band material or widened Z-bands, they consist of at least two morphologically distinct components, which are actin filaments and Z-band-like material. Part of the latter material is attached to the actin filaments, and part of it forms a filamentous mat similar to that of normal Z-bands. The Z-band-like material often shows a periodicity of about 200 Å along the longitudinal axis of the actin filaments. The lattice arrangement in these Z-bands has a complex tetragonal substructure (30).

Although accumulations of Z-band material were first regarded as being composed mainly of tropomyosin, more recent studies show that α-actinin is one of their major components (see Maron et al, ref. 53, for review). Immunohistochemical studies have demonstrated that anti-α-actinin antibodies bind selectively to the Z-bands of porcine skeletal muscle, dense bodies or myofilament attachment sites (structures that are considered analogous to Z-bands of striated muscles) of smooth muscle cells, Z-bands and intercalated discs of porcine cardiac muscle cells, and to Z-bands and nemaline rods of skeletal muscle cells of patients with nemaline myopathy (the condition in which large masses of Z-band material were first described).

The anomalous expansions of Z-band material in hypertrophying myocardium were similar in adult dogs with banding of the pulmonary artery (8) and in newborn dogs with aortic constriction (7). In both of these groups these expansions were especially prominent in animals with congestive heart failure, were less frequent in those with hypertrophy without failure, and were either very rare or absent in control animals. These correlations suggest that these Z-band expansions are related to cardiac failure. Other studies have shown, however, that anomalous Z-band material also occurs in circumstances that are unrelated to cardiac failure and that it may be related to a mechanism of sarcomerogenesis that differs from that usually operative in normal myocardium. Also, abnormalities of Z-band material can assume several morphologically different forms. The various alterations of material resembling that in Z-bands of cardiac muscle can be classified (Figs. 7–11) as follows: (a) widening of Z-bands, with or without periodicity, as described above; (b) simple extensions of Z-band material into adjacent regions of the sarcomeres; (c) accumulations of Z-band material, without periodic substructure, in areas adjacent to the sarcolemma and intercalated discs; (d) splitting of Z-bands; (e) focal loss of Z-band material; and (f) clumping of Z-band material, in areas of myofibrillar damage or disorganization, into elongated masses that lack periodicity and are oriented parallel to the longitudinal axis of the cell. Of these six types of Z-band alterations, the first three occur in hypertrophying muscle cells in a variety

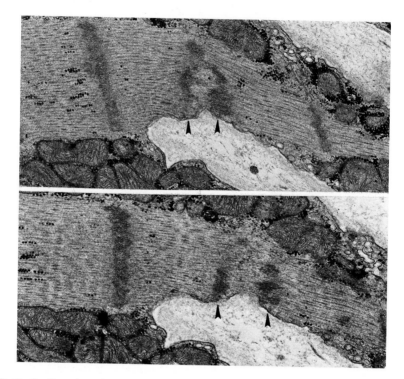

FIG. 7. Sections through two levels of a splitting Z-band in crista supraventricularis muscle from patient with Fallot's tetralogy. In the section shown at **top**, the Z-band *(arrowheads)* appears to be beginning to split asymmetrically, with an area of separation being evident only in its lower portion. At the level of the section shown at the **bottom**, the Z-band splitting *(arrowheads)* appears to have progressed to a greater extent, and short myofilaments are present between the two parts of the splitting Z-band. Note widening of the adjacent Z-band at the left of the picture (×26,500).

of conditions in humans and experimental animals, in normal cells of the atrioventricular conduction system of a variety of species, and in ventricular myocardium of old but apparently healthy cats and dogs. A relation has been found between the occurrence of these three types of changes and the degree of atrial hypertrophy in patients with rheumatic heart disease, and, as mentioned previously, the presence of congestive heart failure in dogs (see Maron et al., ref. 53, and Ferrans and Butany, ref. 25, for reviews). The fourth of these alterations, splitting of Z-bands, represents the most direct evidence of actual replication of sarcomeres and has been observed consistently in hearts undergoing hypertrophy, but only very infrequently in normal hearts or in rapidly growing embryonic muscle. For this reason, it is not certain that this change is related to normal sarcomerogenesis.

We believe that the basic changes in the first four types of Z-band alterations listed above are basically similar and that they relate to an increased ability of actin filaments to associate with Z-band material. This increased association, which may

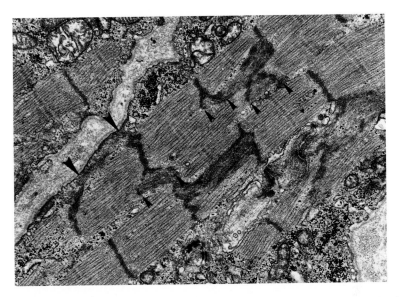

FIG. 8. Subsarcolemmal accumulations of material *(large arrowheads)* resembling that in Z-bands, and Z-bands that show splitting and marked widening *(small arrowheads)* are present near intercellular junction in left atrial muscle cell from patient with mitral valvular disease of rheumatic origin (×20,000).

be a response to excessive stretch, then may lead to interactions with myosin and to eventual completion of formation of the sarcomeres. It is by no means certain that these changes, because of the circumstances in which they occur, progress to actual completion of sarcomere formation, particularly the very large masses of Z-band material with a periodic substructure. The presence of large amounts of Z-band material in some cells suggests that this material may be produced in excessive quantities and that the cells fail to produce corresponding amounts of other sarcomeric components. Perhaps the most convincing evidence that accumulations of Z-band material are not necessarily related to normal sarcomerogenesis has been obtained from studies of skeletal muscle, in which large masses of Z-band material are known to develop in many degenerative diseases, myopathies, and experimentally produced damage (53).

We regard the fifth and sixth of the alterations listed above as degenerative, since we have found them frequently in degenerated left ventricular muscle cells from patients undergoing operation for treatment of aortic regurgitation, combined aortic stenosis and regurgitation, and hypertrophic obstructive cardiomyopathy, and from patients receiving anthracycline drugs for treatment of neoplasms. They also are very common in the dilated left atria of patients with mitral valvular disease (80, 53,25). The elongated streaming masses of Z-band material in cardiac muscle cells of these patients are associated with irregularly arranged actin filaments in a manner reminiscent of that typically seen in smooth muscle cells.

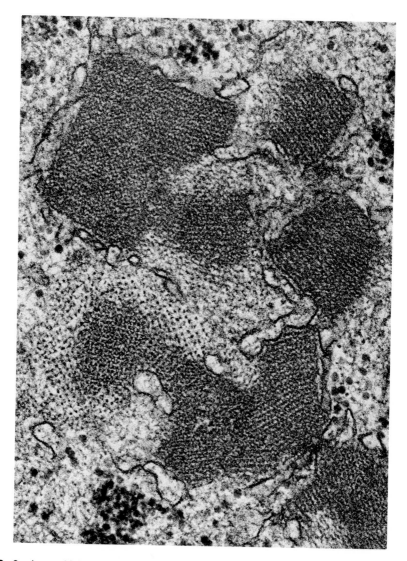

FIG. 9. Large, highly organized expansions of Z-band material are seen in left atrial muscle cell from patient with mitral valvular disease. A square lattice array is evident on study of cross-sections of these widened Z-bands ($\times 70,000$).

The following conclusions may be derived from the preceding considerations:

1. Maintenance of normal mechanical forces in cardiac muscle cells is necessary for the preservation of normal Z-band structure.
2. Disturbances in the equilibrium of these forces may be the basic cause of accumulation of Z-band material.

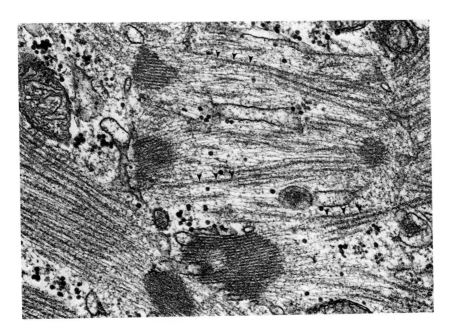

FIG. 10. Accumulations of Z-band material with periodic substructure are present in area of myofibrillar lysis in left atrial muscle cell from patient who had aortic stenosis and regurgitation and mitral stenosis, and who underwent replacement of the mitral and aortic valves. Note that myosin filaments *(small arrowheads)* are reduced in number to a greater extent than are actin filaments; the latter appear thin and thread-like. This preferential loss of myosin filaments is frequently observed in cardiac muscle cells of patients with severe, long-standing hypertrophy (×60,000).

3. Such accumulations may not be accompanied or followed by synthesis of other sarcomeric components, and thus they may lead to the formation of aberrant masses of Z-band material.

4. The ultrastructural images produced by actual proliferation of Z-band material often are difficult to distinguish from those caused by various distortions of Z-band material in myofibrils undergoing lysis, particularly that which occurs in the late stages of hypertrophy.

Histological Changes in Cardiac Hypertrophy

On histological study, the most readily recognizable indications of cardiac hypertrophy are increases in the transverse diameters of the muscle cells and in the size and basophilia of their nuclei (Figs. 5,11, and 12). Myofibrillar changes of the types described in the preceding section of this chapter are very difficult to detect by light microscopy. Normal left ventricular muscle cells range up to 15 μ in diameter. In hypertrophy, the diameters of many of the muscle cells exceed 20 μ, although cells with diameters exceeding 50 μ may be found. Electron microscopic studies of such cells (28,36,37) have confirmed the fact that they are single cells

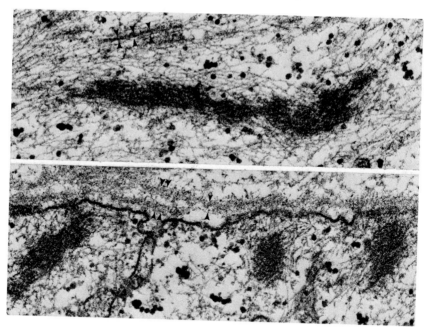

FIG. 11. Two views of accumulations of Z-band material in severely degenerated muscle cell from crista supraventricularis of 43-year-old patient with tetralogy of Fallot. **Top:** Elongated mass of Z-band material without orderly substructure is associated with tangled, disorganized actin filaments. Only one myosin filament *(arrowheads)* is seen in this area. **Bottom:** Three masses of Z-band material, similar to that shown at top, are subjacent to the sarcolemma. The basement membrane of the muscle cell is thickened throughout *(single arrowheads)* and partially reduplicated *(double arrowheads)*. (each, ×75,000).

and not groups of smaller cells with boundaries that are not identifiable by light microscopy. Marked variations in the transverse diameters of immediately adjacent muscle cells are frequently observed in hypertrophied hearts. The reasons for these variations, which occur in cells that presumably are subject to the same stimuli to undergo hypertrophy, are not clear. In histological preparations the cytoplasm of hypertrophied cardiac muscle cells may not show any abnormal features. The orderly arrangement of cardiac muscle cells is maintained in hypertrophy due to either pressure or volume overloading. As mentioned previously, this arrangement is abnormal in hypertrophic cardiomyopathy.

The nuclei of hypertrophic muscle cells usually appear enlarged, hyperchromatic (i.e., intensely basophilic), and vary in shape from oval or rectangular with blunted ends to highly irregular with highly convoluted surfaces. The increase in nuclear basophilia is considered to be related to polyploidy. The nuclei in hearts of patients with hypertrophic cardiomyopathy are the most likely to exhibit bizarre shapes and pronounced degrees of enlargement (24,28).

Hypertrophied cardiac muscle cells tend to become more irregular and less smoothly cylindrical in shape than normal cells (Figs. 13–15). These changes, however, may not be readily evident on histological study. Irregularities of cellular

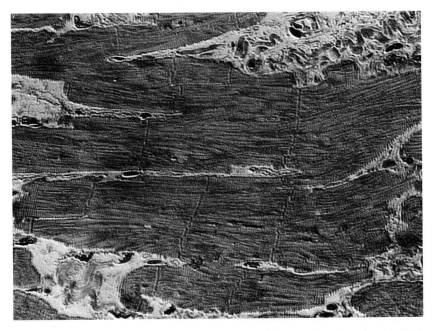

FIG. 12. Severe cellular enlargement (transverse diameters in excess of 50 μ) and mild interstitial fibrosis are evident in light micrograph of crista supraventricularis muscle from 25-year-old-man with atrial septal defect and combined infundibular and valvular pulmonic stenosis. 1-μ-thick section of plastic-embedded tissue photographed using Nomarski interference contrast optics. Toluidine blue stain (×560).

contour in hypertrophied muscle cells (Fig. 15) indicate that selective addition of newly formed sarcomeres can occur in certain sharply localized areas of the muscle cells, which then grow asymmetrically (36,37). Such changes are manifested in the form of (a) increased tortuosity of their intercellular junctions and, to a lesser extent, of nonspecialized regions of their surfaces; and (b) dilatation and tortuosity of their T tubules. Both of these changes frequently can be identified on light microscopic study of semithin (1-μ thick) sections of plastic-embedded tissues. The increased tortuosity of intercellular junctions is of special interest because areas in their vicinity are considered to be loci of preferential addition of new sarcomeres during the process of hypertrophy.

In addition to the changes just described, hearts with long-standing hypertrophy often show atrophy and degeneration of muscle cells (Figs. 16–19), diffuse interstitial fibrosis, and thickening and increased opacity of mural endocardium. Atrophic muscle cells often are isolated from adjacent cells by fibrous connective tissue and may be altered to such an extent that they resemble connective tissue cells. Degenerative changes in the cytoplasm of the muscle cells include loss of myofibrils, intracellular edema, and vacuolization. These changes may be difficult to evaluate in tissues that have undergone postmortem autolysis and are best appreciated on ultrastructural study of biopsied or operatively obtained material. The picture of

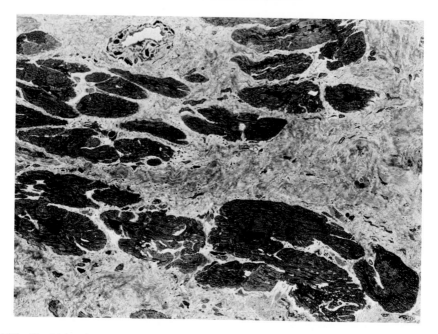

FIG. 13. Light micrograph of area of crista supraventricularis from 41-year-old man with tetralogy of Fallot, showing moderate hypertrophy and marked irregularities of contour of the muscle cells, and severe interstitial fibrosis. 1-μ- section of plastic-embedded tissue. Alkaline toluidine blue stain (×400).

vacuolization in histological sections may be due to dilatation of the sarcoplasmic reticulum or the T system, mitochondrial damage and swelling, or deposition of lipid or glycogen. Histochemical and electron microscopic studies are required to evaluate these changes (25).

Endocardial mural thickening tends to be more pronounced in volume hypertrophy than in pressure hypertrophy. The areas of endocardial thickening contain smooth-muscle cells, fibroblasts, myofibroblasts, collagen fibrils, microfibrils, small elastic fibers, and deposits of acid mucopolysaccharides. Mural thrombosis also is associated with dilatation of the atria (particularly in the presence of atrial fibrillation) or the ventricles and is a common finding in patients with congestive cardiomyopathies. Proliferation of connective tissue cells and increased synthesis of connective tissue proteins have been shown to occur from the early stages of hypertrophy (12). These phenomena are probably responsible, at least in part, for both the endocardial thickening and the diffuse interstitial fibrosis that gradually develop in many hypertrophied hearts. The endocardial thickening also may constitute a response of the endocardial surface to abnormal mechanical forces due to changes in wall tension and intracardiac blood flow in dilated, poorly contracting chambers. Similarly, the occurrence of mural thrombosis in the absence of muscle necrosis is usually regarded as resulting from blood stasis.

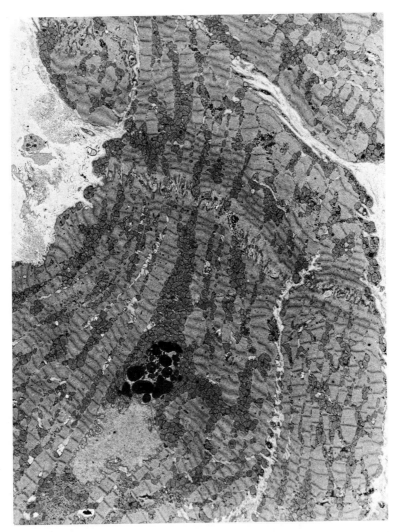

FIG. 14. Low magnification electron micrograph of hypertrophic but normally arranged cardiac muscle cell from patient with tetralogy of Fallot. Note the highly folded intercalated disk (ID), the nucleus (N), and the lipofuscin granules in the perinuclear zone (×3,000).

Ultrastructural Changes in Early Hypertrophy

Numerous ultrastructural studies have been made of hypertrophied myocardium, and the following four generalizations can be drawn from these studies:

1. The hexagonal array of the myofilaments, the dimensions of the sarcomeres, and the diameters of the thick and thin myofilaments are similar in normal and hypertrophied muscle cells (67). Therefore, hypertrophy is not mediated by alterations in the size of the contractile elements.

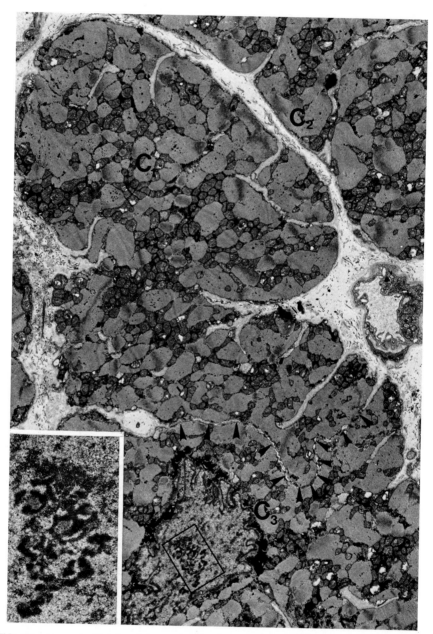

FIG. 15. Low-magnification electron micrograph of section of crista supraventricularis muscle from 36-year-old man with atrial septal defect and infundibular and valvular pulmonic stenosis. A cross-section of a cell (C_1) is shown with parts of two other cells (C_2 and C_3). Note the extremely irregular shape of cell C_1, which is joined to cell C_3 by a tortuous intercellular junction *(arrowheads)*. Prominent T tubules and slit-like invaginations of plasma membrane are seen throughout. A capillary is shown at the right of center, and small numbers of collagenous fibrils are scattered throughout the interstitial space ($\times 6,000$). **Inset** shows higher magnification view of the coiled, ribbon-like nucleolus (enclosed within rectangle in main picture) of cell C_3 ($\times 18,000$).

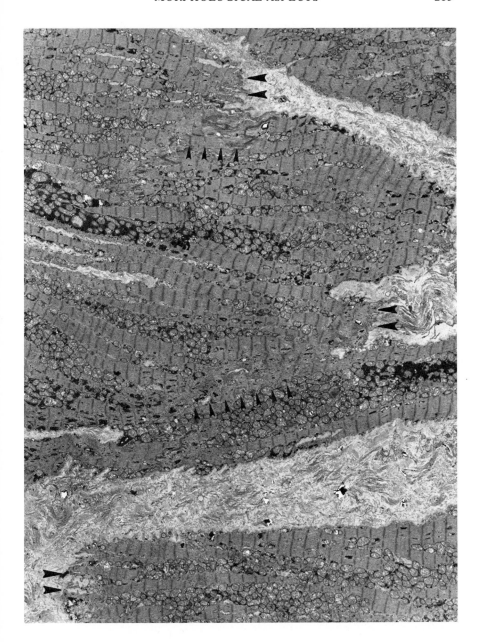

FIG. 16. Electron micrograph of hypertrophied muscle cells from left ventricular apex of patient with hypertrophic obstructive cardiomyopathy. Two foci of myofibrillar damage are indicated by *small arrowheads.* The tips of three muscle cells that appear to have lost their intercellular contacts are indicated by large, paired *arrowheads.* These tips typically appear irregularly shaped or serrated (see Fig. 18 for additional details of this type of alteration). The interstitial space is entirely filled with collagen fibrils ($\times$3,750).

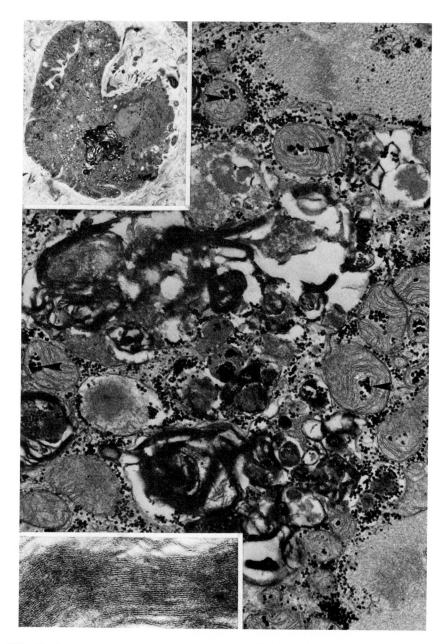

FIG. 17. Degenerated cardiac muscle cell from crista supraventricularis of 41-year-old patient with tetralogy of Fallot contains intramitochondrial glycogen deposits *(arrowheads)*, concentric lamellae, and associated electron-dense residual bodies (×35,000). **Upper inset** shows that concentric lamellae also are evident in light micrograph of a 1-μ-thick section of plastic-embedded tissue. Toluidine blue stain. ×1,200. **Lower inset** shows high magnification view of concentric lamellae, which have a periodic spacing of 40 Å (×126,000).

2. The ultrastructural appearance of hypertrophied cardiac muscle cells varies according to the cause and stage of the hypertrophy.

3. The cardiac muscle cells in hypertrophic cardiomyopathy show distinctive morphological features.

4. Electron microscopic study permits the recognition of a variety of degenerative changes that are not distinguishable by light microscopy.

In Meerson's first stage of hypertrophy, the cardiac muscle cells show evidence of increased synthesis of proteins. They also may show evidence of damage and destruction, involving mainly the myofibrils and mitochondria. The latter changes probably do not constitute a true manifestation of early hypertrophy; instead, they may occur as a consequence of the use of traumatic methods to induce hypertrophy (for example, sudden imposition of severe degrees of aortic constriction or aortic regurgitation). Evidence of increased protein synthesis in the early stages of hypertrophy consists of (a) nuclear and nucleolar alterations, particularly the formation of coiled, ribbon-like nucleoli; (b) increased number of free ribosomes and of cisterns of rough-surfaced endoplasmic reticulum, mainly at the poles of the nuclei; (c) enlargement of the Golgi complexes; (d) increased width and extent of folding of the intercellular junctions; and (e) changes suggestive of the formation of new sarcomeres and mitochondria. The latter changes are characterized by the presence of sarcomeres in various stages of formation and of mitochondria which either differ from normal in size or appear to be budding. These changes are discussed in separate sections of this chapter.

Ultrastructural Changes in the Stable Phase of Hypertrophy

After hypertrophy has developed for a certain time, the rate of cellular enlargement and the rate of formation of new cellular organelles appear to decrease, and the changes described above tend to subside or at least to become less prominent. Thus, in the second stage of hypertrophy (stable hyperfunction), ultrastructural study of myocardium may disclose cells that are larger than normal and contain greater numbers of mitochondria and myofibrils, but show few or no abnormalities in their organelles. Some degree of interstitial fibrosis also may be present. In several animal models of cardiac hypertrophy, morphometric study of electron micrographs has demonstrated that hypertrophied cells differ from normal-sized cells of normal animals in other, more subtle ways. These relate to changes in the volume fractions (i.e., percentages of the total cell volume) occupied by myofibrils, mitochondria, and other organelles. Such data clearly imply that all organelles in hypertrophied cardiac muscle cells do not increase in size or in number in a synchronous manner or to the same ultimate extent and that the relative growth of different organelles is not the same in hypertrophy of different causes.

Ultrastructural abnormalities that may be present in hearts in the stable phase of hypertrophy include intramitochondrial glycogen, large numbers of multiple intercalated discs, and a variety of alterations in the nuclear membranes.

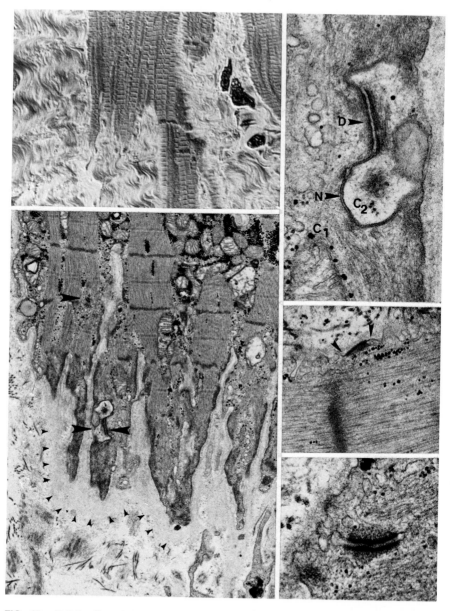

FIG. 18. Cellular dissociation and abnormalities of intercellular contacts in hypertrophy associated with severe interstitial fibrosis. **Upper left:** Light micrograph of tapering end of hypertrophied cardiac muscle cell from same patient as in Fig. 13. Only a small area of contact remains between this cell and an adjacent, slender cell. Dense fibrous tissue surrounds the cells. 1-μ-thick section of plastic-embedded tissue photographed using Nomarski interference contrast optics. Alkaline toluidine blue (× 1,600). **Lower left:** Low magnification electron micrograph of area similar to that shown in upper left panel. Note the accumulations of Z-band material in the tips of the cell, the marked thickening of the basement membrane (the outer boundary of which

Glycogen in cardiac muscle cells is normally present in the form of single particles of β or monoparticulate glycogen that range from 150 to 400 Å in diameter and are free in the cytoplasm (24). In addition to these particles, hypertrophied cardiac muscle cells also may contain a small population of mitochondria within which glycogen particles are present (Fig. 17). These particles are localized within the outer mitochondrial compartment. The number of mitochondria showing this change is usually small (less than 1%). We have found intramitochondrial glycogen deposits (some of the β type, others of the α or rosette type, and others of mixtures of these two types) in left ventricular myocardium of 4 of 16 patients with aortic valvular disease, 5 of 16 patients with hypertrophic cardiomyopathy (52), and in crista supraventricularis muscle of 17 of 59 patients with congenital heart diseases associated with obstruction to right ventricular outflow (37). Thus, intramitochondrial glycogen is a relatively common finding in cardiac hypertrophy. Less commonly observed abnormalities of cardiac glycogen in hypertrophy include glycogen deposits with nuclei (27) and deposits of α-glycogen in the cytoplasm of the muscle cells (51).

Since mitochondria normally do not contain glycogen or the enzymes of glycogen synthesis and breakdown, we have postulated that intramitochondrial glycogen deposits are formed *de novo* within mitochondria as the result of two factors: an increase in the permeability of the outer mitochondrial membrane and penetration of the enzymes of glycogen synthesis (which are too large to diffuse across normal outer mitochondrial membranes) into the outer mitochondrial compartment, where they eventually proceed to synthesize glycogen. The finding of frequent intramitochondrial glycogen deposits in cardiac muscle cells of dogs surviving anoxic, normothermic cardiac arrest (14) supports the concept that ischemia is a factor that can cause an increase in mitochondrial permeability and solubilization of the enzymes of glycogen synthesis. These enzymes normally are bound to the glycogen granules but are released from them as glycogenolysis takes place during ischemia. It is possible, therefore, that intramitochondrial glycogen in hypertrophied myo-

---

is partly outlined by *small arrowheads*), the small area of specialized intercellular junction *(paired large arrowheads)* with another cell, and small intracytoplasmic desmosomes *(single large arrowhead)*. Ventricular septal myocardium from patient with hypertrophic cardiomyopathy and fibrous ring type of subaortic stenosis ($\times$ 11,600). **Upper right:** Higher magnification view of small intercellular junction at one of the tips of the cell shown in the lower left panel. A nexus (N) and a desmosome (D) are present in this small area of specialized intercellular contact between the main cell (C_1) and a cell (C_2), of which only a small process surrounded by C_1 is seen in this section ($\times$ 42,000). **Center right:** Hemidesmosome *(arrowheads)* is located on side of muscle cell in area of fibrosis. Structures of this type presumably are derived from the separation of a desmosome into its two constituent halves (compare with desmosome in **upper right panel**). Left ventricular myocardium from patient with aortic regurgitation ($\times$ 32,000). **Lower right:** Intracytoplasmic desmosome with an attachment plaque on each of its sides is located near the surface of a hypertrophied muscle cell in area of fibrosis. Although this junctional structure resembles an intercellular desmosome, its intracellular localization is shown by the continuity of the membrane forming one side of the desmosome with the membrane on the other side and by the continuity of the cytoplasm on both sides of the junctional structure. This shows that only one membrane, and thus only one cell, is involved in the formation of this junction. Ventricular septal myocardium from patient with hypertrophic cardiomyopathy ($\times$ 54,000).

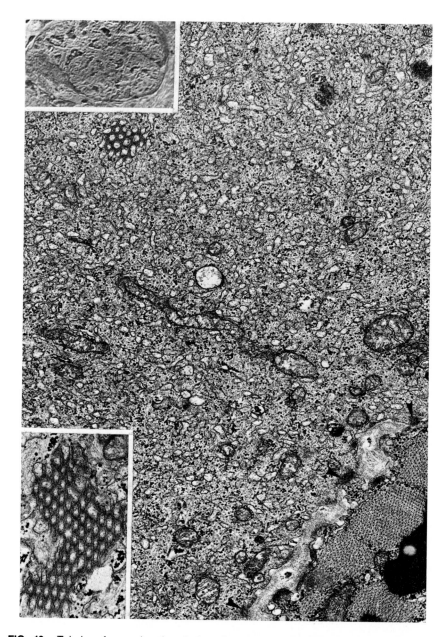

FIG. 19. Tubules of sarcoplasmic reticulum show marked proliferation in cardiac muscle cell that has lost virtually all of its contractile elements. Mitochondria are very sparse, and only a few electron-dense patches of Z-band material *(arrowheads)* remain in this cell located near an intercellular junction that appears to be undergoing dissociation. Contractile elements in the other cell forming this junction **(lower right)** appear normal. Some elements of reticulum form an aggregate of tubules at the **upper left**. Left atrial myocardium from patient with mitral valvular

cardium is a manifestation of focal chronic hypoxia that develops when the work demands on the hypertrophied muscle cells exceed their oxygen supply.

Multiple intercalated discs were first described by Laks and associates (41) in cardiac muscle cells of normal dogs and of dogs with right ventricular hypertrophy induced by banding of the pulmonary artery. These structures consist of two, three, or four transverse segments of intercalated discs lying parallel to each other and perpendicular to the long axis of the myofibrils: Each two of these transverse segments are separated by a maximum of 10 clearly distinguishable and continuous sarcomeres (Fig. 20). Other studies (50,3) show that multiple intercalated discs are the intercellular junctions forming the boundaries of lateral processes of cardiac muscle cells and that these structures occur more frequently in hypertrophic hearts than in normal hearts. We have postulated that lateral cytoplasmic processes develop from remodeling of side-to-side intercellular junctions in association with lateral growth of cardiac muscle cells and that localized mechanical tensions induce their formation. These tensions, which presumably are due to shearing forces exerted at side-to-side junctions when contraction occurs, lead to asymmetric but complementary growth of sarcomeres along the two sides of the side-to-side junctions, to reorientation of these junctions, and to the eventual formation of lateral processes that interlock the cytoplasm of adjacent cardiac muscle cells. Thus, these processes reinforce the connections between adjacent layers of myocardium and tend to limit or prevent their "slippage."

Abnormalities observed by us (26) in nuclear membranes of cardiac muscle cells in 134 patients with cardiac hypertrophy of various causes consisted of increased foldings and convolutions; nuclear pseudoinclusions formed by cytoplasmic organelles protruding into saccular invaginations of the nuclear membranes, and intranuclear tubules (Fig. 21). The increased foldings and convolutions of the nuclear membranes and the nuclear pseudoinclusions appear to result from synthesis of nuclear membranes in excess of that required to accommodate the increase in nuclear volume which occurs in hypertrophy. Intranuclear tubules were present in 6 of 134 patients and consisted of tubular invaginations (400 to 650 Å in diameter) of the inner nuclear membranes into the nucleoplasm. Some of these tubules were straight and cylindrical and were associated with a peripheral layer of marginated chromatin; others were not associated with chromatin, appeared coiled, and followed irregular courses. We consider that intranuclear tubules in cardiac muscle cells probably represent an extreme type of response to the stimulus to hypertrophy (10,26).

---

disease of rheumatic origin ($\times$25,500). **Upper inset** shows the light microscopic appearance, i.e., pale-staining and empty-looking, of a cell such as that shown in the main panel. 1-μ-thick section of plastic-embedded tissue. Toluidine blue stain, Nomarski interference contrast ($\times$1,600). **Lower inset** shows hexagonal arrangement of aggregate of tubules in cardiac muscle cell from patient with hypertrophic cardiomyopathy and pulmonary sarcoidosis. Tubules in aggregates of this type are derived from, and continuous with, tubules of sarcoplasmic reticulum. These aggregates occur mostly in cells that contain few or no myofibrils ($\times$35,000).

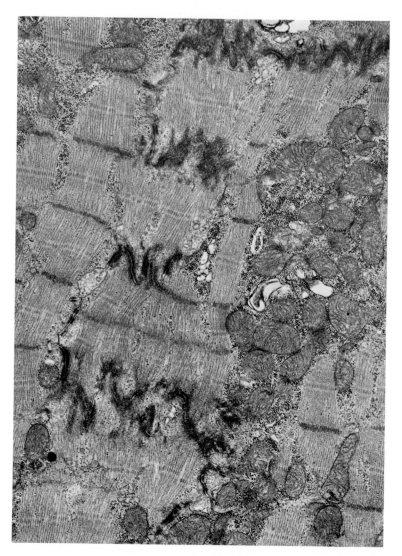

FIG. 20. Multiple intercalated discs are formed by side-to-side interdigitations of two adjacent myocytes in left atrium of patient with mitral valvular disease. (× 16,000).

Ultrastructural Changes in the Late Stage of Hypertrophy

In the third stage (Meerson's stage of cellular exhaustion, ref. 53,57) the morphologic picture is dominated by degenerative changes in the muscle cells and by interstitial fibrosis. Although the exact relationship of these changes to myocardial failure has not been determined, it appears likely that they account for the irreversibility of cardiac failure in certain patients in whom operative correction of the hemodynamic lesion does not result in appreciable clinical improvement.

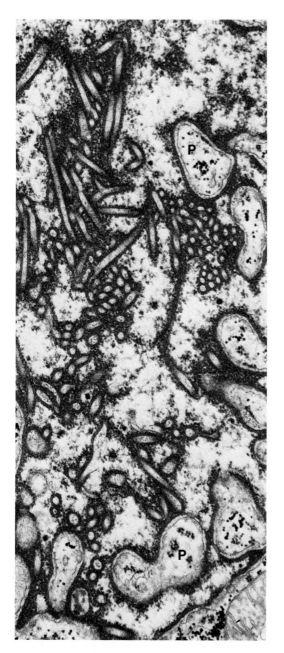

FIG. 21. View of part of nucleus of cardiac muscle cell in ventricular septum of patient with hypertrophic cardiomyopathy. Numerous intranuclear tubules are present which are derived from invaginations of the inner nuclear membranes. Nuclear pseudoinclusions (P), caused by portions of cytoplasm indenting the nuclear membranes, also are shown (×33,000).

Ultrastructural studies have shown that myocardial degenerative changes are frequent in patients with aortic valvular disease, congestive cardiomyopathy, or hypertrophic cardiomyopathy (53), and in older patients with congenital heart diseases associated with obstruction to right ventricular outflow (25,36,37). We have classified (53) cardiac muscle cells with evidence of degeneration as showing mild, moderate, or severe degeneration, according to the nature and extent of their morphologic changes. Although these three categories are described separately below, they represent three stages in a continuum of morphologic changes, and they frequently coexist in a given area of myocardium.

Cardiac muscle cells with evidence of early degeneration are either normal-sized or hypertrophied. By light microscopy these cells cannot be distinguished from hypertrophied, nondegenerated cells. Ultrastructurally, they differ from the latter only in respect to focal alterations in the myofibrils and sarcoplasmic reticulum. Abnormalities of myofibrils in mildly degenerated cells consist of various alterations of Z-band material and of focal loss of myofilaments. The loss of myofilaments is unusual in that it affects the myosin filaments to a much greater extent than the actin filaments. This preferential loss of thick myofilaments results in the presence of disproportionately greater numbers of thin myofilaments in affected cells (Figs. 10 and 11). Z-band changes in mildly or moderately degenerated cells consist of fragmentation of Z-band material and of spreading of Z-band material into adjacent regions of the sarcomeres, often in association with preferential loss of thick myofilaments. Mild, focal thickening of Z-bands and subsarcolemmal accumulations of Z-band material are common in mildly or moderately degenerated cells.

Cardiac muscle cells with advanced degenerative changes usually are either normal-sized or atrophic, usually are present in areas of marked interstitial fibrosis, and often appear to have lost their connections with adjacent cells. They demonstrate marked loss of contractile elements and a spectrum of changes involving virtually every type of organelle. The surfaces of these cells frequently are associated with spherical microparticles and often show marked irregularities of contour and marked thickening of basement membranes. These alterations are associated with prominent changes in the T tubules and intercellular junctions. True T tubules (as opposed to shallow surface invaginations that are not related to Z-bands) are rarely observed in these cells.

Spherical microparticles (Fig. 22) composed of central, dense cores surrounded by single, trilaminar membranes are found in close relationship to the basement membranes and outer surfaces of the plasma membranes of cardiac muscle cells in areas of cellular dissociation and/or interstitial fibrosis (29). These particles are thought to be the result of budding from the plasma membranes. Spherical microparticles occur along the outer surfaces on the sides and free ends of muscle cells in areas of fibrosis, in the widened spaces between membranes of partially dissociated intercellular junctions, and within cytoplasmic vesicles considered to be phagocytic. Spherical microparticles frequently are joined together by minute nexuses that are structurally identical with those forming parts of intercellular junctions of muscle cells. Such a process mediates the shedding of certain areas of plasma membranes, particularly those of junctions, where remodeling of cardiac muscle cell surfaces occurs. Spherical microparticles occur commonly in tissues other than myocardium, particularly in diseased renal glomeruli (29).

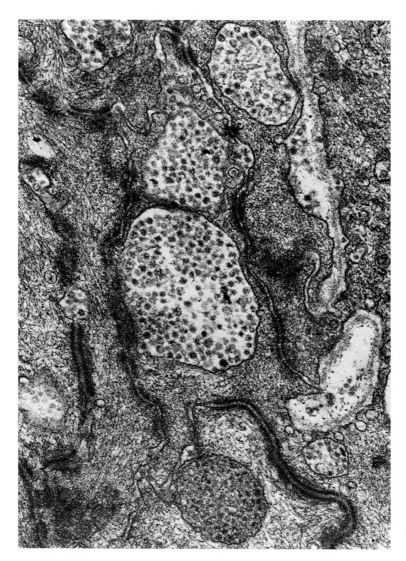

FIG. 22. Spherical microparticles are present in dilated spaces between membranes of an intercalated disc in left atrium of patient with mitral valvular disease (×55,000).

Intercalated discs joining degenerated cells often show various degrees of dissociation, characterized by separation of their apposed membranes (Fig. 18). Some cells contain unusual junctional structures formed by the apposition of two areas of the plasma membrane of the same cell. Some of these structures resemble desmosomes, whereas others are more complex and resemble larger parts of intercalated discs. These junctional structures, usually present in peripheral areas of cytoplasm at the sides or ends of the cells, have been termed intracytoplasmic junctions and probably result from the remodeling of cell surfaces that occurs when degenerated cardiac muscle cells lose their intercellular contacts (15). The structure of myofibrils is markedly altered in cardiac muscle cells with severe degeneration. Myofibrils are almost completely absent in some of these cells and disrupted in others. Masses of Z-band-like material often are scattered randomly throughout these cells. These masses are traversed by thin myofilaments arranged either at random or in parallel, but thick filaments are rare or absent in these areas. Cytoskeletal filaments measuring 100 Å in diameter frequently form tangled masses in these areas of myofibrillar disruption.

Sarcomeric disruption, perhaps the most important alteration in degenerated cells, is apparent by lysis of both thick and thin myofilaments, usually with preferential loss of the thick filaments. Because of this preferential loss, large areas of cells affected by this change appear devoid of myofibrils and contain disorganized tangles of actin filaments and 100 Å filaments. As mentioned previously, lysis of myofibrils is often accompanied by the formation of masses of Z-band-material arranged in clumps or in streaming patterns. Some of these masses of Z-band material have a complex, paracrystalline structure. Cells with loss of contractile elements are distinguishable from necrotic cardiac muscle cells by the preservation of other cellular organelles (mitochondria, glycogen, nuclei, and sarcolemma) which are disrupted in cellular necrosis.

Foci of cellular and myofibrillar disorganization of hypertrophied hearts are manifested by cells that are randomly arranged, stellate in shape, and irregularly connected to each other. These cells, which usually are located in areas of interstitial fibrosis, have myofibrils coursing in several directions rather than in parallel. This disorganization is qualitatively similar to, but much less extensive than, that present in myocardium of patients with hypertrophic cardiomyopathy.

Some hypertrophied cardiac muscle cells contain numerous large, spherical lipid droplets. These cells usually show other morphologic signs of degeneration, such as myofibrillar lysis or proliferation of sarcoplasmic reticulum (SR). Cardiac muscle cells from similar areas contain large numbers of myelin figures composed of electron-dense, concentrically arranged lamellae (Fig. 17). These lamellae may form by the aggregation of phospholipid material derived from the breakdown of mitochondria.

Other cardiac muscle cells, which appear pale and nonstriated by light microscopy, contain increased numbers of tubules or cisterns of SR which almost entirely fill the sarcoplasm (79,80). Tubular and vesicular proliferation of free SR may completely replace other cardiac muscle organelles, forming a network that occupies virtually the entire cytoplasm. Abnormalities observed in the SR of hypertrophic cardiac muscle cells consist of (a) proliferation of tubules of free SR; (b) aggregates of regularly arranged tubules of free SR associated with Z-band material and with actin filaments; (c) aggregates of long, straight, irregularly arranged tubules of free SR; and (d) proliferation and aggregation of cisterns of extended junctional SR.

Proliferation of free SR occurs mainly in cells showing loss of contractile elements and increased numbers of cytoskeletal filaments (Fig. 19). Aggregates of SR tubules associated with Z-band material also are found in cells showing myofibrillar loss. In contrast to this, the aggregates of long, straight tubules of SR occur in less severely altered cells. The SR changes just described have been observed in both atrial and ventricular muscle cells; however, proliferation and aggregation of cisterns of extended junctional SR have been reported only in atrial myocardium, in which this type of SR is normally present. Extended junctional SR is defined as including those SR components that have an electron-dense content (similar to that of junctional SR components) but do not become apposed to either T tubules or to free sarcolemma at the cell surface. It is thought that extended junctional SR is well developed in atrial muscle cells because of the paucity or absence of T tubules in these cells (79,80).

Two different types of complexes of cisterns of extended junctional SR have been found (Fig. 23), in hypertrophic human atrial myocardium (79). The first (type A) of these complexes consists of large, convoluted cisterns that are wide (550–650 Å in thickness) and have an electron-dense content but lack a central lamina; the second is composed of stacks of concentric or parallel (type B) cisterns that are narrower (220–300 Å in thickness), have an electron-dense central lamina, and are separated from one another by layers of glycogen granules. The formation of these complexes of cisterns is regarded as an extreme form of overdevelopment of extended junctional SR. These complexes are very uncommon in ventricular muscle cells.

Some degenerated, but nonatrophic cells (transverse diameters 12–20 μ) contain huge, confluent masses of monoparticulate glycogen (up to 35 μ in length and 9 μ in width) which occupy large, central areas of cytoplasm. These have few peripherally located myofibrils which do not show evidence of lysis. Instead of glycogen, a few cardiac muscle cells have large accumulations of fibrils of the glycogen-related type of basophilic degeneration material (24); other cells contain a particulate material that appears to be intermediate in structure between normal glycogen and basophilic degeneration material. This particulate material may represent an early stage in the development of basophilic degeneration. The nuclei in all types of severely degenerated cells are irregularly shaped and often show marked convolutions of their membranes. Variable numbers of lipofuscin granules usually are present in central areas of the cytoplasm. Capillaries appear to be decreased in number in areas of fibrosis; however, normal-appearing capillaries occasionally are immediately adjacent to degenerated cardiac muscle cells.

The following conclusions can be drawn from the just reviewed studies of degeneration of hypertrophied cardiac muscle cells: (a) Loss of contractile elements and of specialized intercellular contacts are the key morphological features of this degeneration; (b) loss of contractile elements in the late stages of hypertrophy tends to affect preferentially the thick, myosin filaments; (c) the overall appearance of degenerated cells depends on the alterations that other cytoplasmic organelles

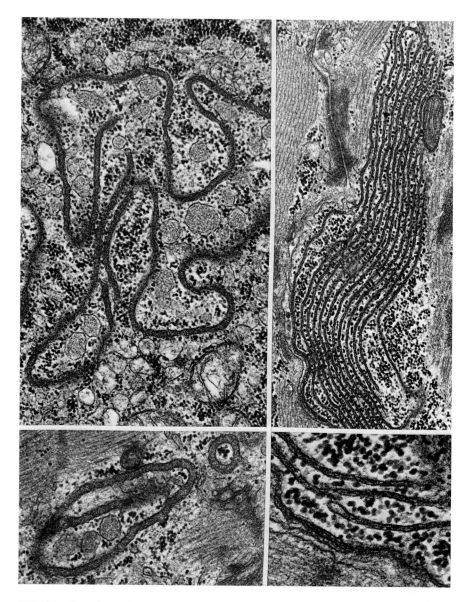

FIG. 23. Complexes of type A (upper and lower left) and type B (upper and lower right) cisterns of sarcoplasmic reticulum in hypertrophic myocytes. **Upper left:** Convoluted type-A cisterns filled with finely granular, electron-dense material. These cisterns are associated with vesicles that contain a similar material ($\times 40,900$). **Lower left:** View of small type-A cisterns similar to those in the **upper panel** ($\times 40,900$). **Upper right:** Complex array of type-B cisterns of sarcoplasmic reticulum. These cisterns are separated by layers of glycogen granules ($\times 35,500$). **Lower right:** High magnification view of type B-cisterns, showing an electron-dense central line in their lumina ($\times 90,000$).

undergo in association with myofibrillar loss; and (d) these changes are associated with interstitial fibrosis.

Myofibrillar loss in degenerated cardiac muscle cells may result from any of the following three types of alterations in contractile proteins: (a) inhibition of synthesis or perhaps even synthesis of abnormal proteins, (b) acceleration of breakdown, and (c) disaggregation. The relative importance of each of these mechanisms in the myofibrillar loss in late stages of hypertrophy is uncertain. Furthermore, it is unclear to what extent the disappearance of myosin and actin filaments represents actual physical loss of protein from muscle cells or simply a phenomenon of disaggregation, so that myosin and actin are still present within the cell but not in the form of filaments. The loss of myofibrils which occurs in degeneration of hypertrophied cardiac muscle is associated with survival of other organelles, including the nuclei and mitochondria. These features distinguish this type of degeneration from a true phenomenon of necrosis. The degenerative alterations in hypertrophied cardiac muscle cells constitute part of the spectrum of changes described as myocytolysis by light microscopists. Both these degenerated cardiac muscle cells and other cells described as showing myocytolysis are characterized by loss of myofibrils. Degenerated cardiac muscle cells undergo preferential loss of thick filaments and myofibrillar lysis unassociated with contraction bands. These alterations differ from those in the usual type of myocytolysis in which selective lysis of thick filaments does not occur and formation of contraction bands is a prominent phenomenon (contraction band necrosis).

The ultrastructural features of moderately or severely degenerated cardiac muscle cells suggest that they are manifestations of the end stages of cellular hypertrophy. This concept is supported by the fact that cells with advanced degeneration often have few or no normal myofibrils or T tubules and have marked alterations in the sarcoplasmic reticulum. Furthermore, some degenerated cells have lost their connections with adjacent cells and, therefore, do not have the capacity to directly transmit electrical activation to other muscle cells or to contribute effectively to myocardial contractility. Therefore, it is reasonable to conclude that these cardiac muscle cells are not capable of normal contractile function and correspond to cells in the third stage of hypertrophy as described by Meerson and co-workers. The finding of cardiac muscle cells with similar degenerative features in a wide variety of conditions suggests that these morphological alterations represent a final common pathway of cell injury (25).

Quantitative Ultrastructural Changes in Cardiac Hypertrophy

The application of techniques of stereological analysis has provided useful information about the quantitative composition of normal myocardium and about the role of subcellular organelles in hypertrophy of cardiac muscle cells. Page and McCallister (63) found normal rat ventricular muscle cells to have the following quantitative composition (in volume fractions, expressed as mean percentages of total cell volume $\pm$ SE): myofibrils, 47.6 ± 0.7; mitochondria, 35.8 ± 0.6; sarcoplasmic reticulum, 3.5 ± 0.02, of which 0.35 was contributed by the terminal cisterns and 3.15 by the remainder of the reticulum; T system, 1 ± 0.1; and sarcoplasm and nuclei, 12.1. The area of plasma membrane per unit of cell volume was calculated to be $0.39 \pm 0.02 \ \mu^2/\mu^3$, of which 0.30 consisted of membranes of "external" sarcolemma and 0.09 of membranes of T tubules. Thus, the T tubules account for 25% of the surface area of a ventricular myocyte. The ratio of the fractional volumes of mitochondria and myofibrils, hereafter referred to as mitochondria/myofibril ratio, was 0.752. The type of hypertrophy that has been investigated most extensively by morphometric techniques is that produced experimentally by constriction of the aorta, either by various methods of banding or by the use of Ameroid constrictors. The latter have the advantage of producing gradual constriction not associated with acute myocardial damage. The first study of this model, by Wollenberger and Schulze (84), disclosed that the mitochondria/myofibril ratio underwent a marked, progressive decrease with increasing duration of the hypertrophy. Meerson et al (57) obtained data indicating that the mitochondria/myofibril ratio increased during the first stage of hypertrophy induced by aortic constriction and then decreased as mentioned above. Page and McCallister (63) further showed that the altered mitochondria/myofibril ratio in hypertrophy induced by aortic constriction results from an increase in the volume fraction of myofibrils and from a decrease in the volume fraction of mitochondria. The increase in the volume fraction of myofibrils occurs partially at the expense of mitochondrial volume and partially by encroachment on the volume fraction occupied by sarcoplasm. During the second (stable hyperfunction) stage of cardiac hypertrophy, these changes are not accompanied by alterations in internal structure of mitochondria and do not seem to depend on a reduction in the numbers of mitochondria. They are associated with increased pleomorphism of mitochondria and with a significant increase in their surface-to-volume ratio. Since this ratio is inversely related to mitochondrial size, these data indicate that the cardiac muscle mitochondria in pressure hypertrophy are smaller than normal. This is also evident from the qualitative study of electron micrographs. As discussed below, the volume fraction of the myofibrils decreases in the late stages of human cardiac hypertrophy.

Studies of quantitative changes in other subcellular organelles of cardiac muscle cells undergoing hypertrophy due to pressure overloading have shown that the volume fraction of the sarcoplasmic reticulum remains unchanged, while that of the T system increases; the thickness of Z-bands and the width of intercalated discs also increase. It would appear that the sarcoplasmic reticulum is synthesized in the same proportion as the cell volume as a whole. The area of sarcoplasmic reticulum membrane per unit of cell volume increases during hypertrophy, and such an increase is proportional to that in myofibrillar volume. As the cell increases in size, the volume fraction of the T system increases, and the ratio of external sarcolemmal membrane per unit of cell volume decreases. The increase in membrane area and in volume fraction of the T system compensates for the relative decrease in external sarcolemmal area, so that the overall surface-to-volume ratio of the hypertrophying muscle cell remains constant (63). These changes are manifested by enlargement and dilatation of T tubules. It should be emphasized, however, that these generalizations about possible compensatory mechanisms to maintain harmonious growth are based on study of hypertrophy of brief duration and of minimal-to-moderate severity. It is not known whether they are applicable to human cardiac muscle cells in severe, long-standing hypertrophy.

Detailed review of the morphometric changes found in hypertrophic animal hearts is beyond the scope of this communication. However, the study of Wiener et al. on normal and hypertensive rat hearts is of particular interest in that it illustrates a number of general differences between epicardial and endocardial myocytes. Wiener et al. (83) applied a method of determining the mean volume of cells within a tissue to the measurement of endocardial and epicardial myocytes in the left ventricle of normal and hypertensive rats. Compared with the epicardial regions, the normal endocardial regions contained 30% more myocytes, 27% less interstitial space, 48% less capillary volume, 17% less capillary surface, and the same capillary length per unit of tissue volume. In terms of both relative and absolute volumes and surface areas of their organelles, the cytoplasmic composition of normal epicardial and endocardial myocytes was nearly identical. After 4 weeks of hypertension induced by renal artery constriction, endocardial myocytes enlarged from $10,370 \pm 410$ to $12,520 \pm 490$ μm^3, whereas epicardial myocytes enlarged from $12,600 \pm 1,600$ to $17,300 \pm 1,100$ μm^3. The number of myocytes and the total length of capillaries remained constant. The epicardial region enlarged 37% with proportional increases of myocyte and interstitial volumes. In contrast, the endocardial enlargement was only 26%, consisting of 21% hypertrophy of myocytes and a 55% increase in interstitial components. Expansion of capillary lumina accounted for much of the interstitial enlargement throughout the myocardium. Hypertrophy of myocytes in the epicardial region was accompanied by a reduced mitochondria-to-myofibril ratio and disproportionately large increases (two- to threefold) in both sarcoplasmic reticulum and T system volume and surface area. The morphometric characteristics of myocytes from hypertensive rats differed significantly from normal, and significant differences occurred between the inner and outer layers of myocardium for practically every cytoplasmic component.

Less extensive morphometric data are available on other animal models of cardiac hypertrophy than on the pressure-overloading models mentioned above. In hypertrophy due to aortic regurgitation, Hatt et al. (34) found an increase, but only a modest one, in the mitochondria/myofibril ratio. This increase was more pronounced in animals with overt cardiac failure than in those with dubious failure. In contrast to these findings, in another study of hypertrophy induced by volume overloading (aortocaval fistula), Papadimitriou et al. (64) found a decrease in the mitochondria/myofibril ratio. This ratio reverted to close to normal (as did the width of the intercalated discs and the number of mitochondria, which had been increased) 6 months after closure of the fistula. Thus, the data of Papadimitriou et al. indicate that their model of hypertrophy behaves similarly to the aortic constriction model. The reason for the differences between these two models and that involving aortic regurgitation is not clear.

In contrast to the relatively small differences found in the studies reviewed above, remarkable increases in the mitochondria/myofibril ratio in cardiac muscle cells have been observed in forced exercise, thiamine deficiency, copper deficiency, and iron deficiency. In exercise experiments, an increase in the mitochondria/myofibril ratio occurred after only half an hour of swimming; after 13 hr of forced swimming this ratio became more than twice normal, and in animals subjected to repeated episodes of forced swimming this ratio eventually (43 days) tended to normalize, apparently because of the increased synthesis of new contractile elements (11). Laguens et al. (40) showed that the increase in the mitochondria/myofibril ratio was accompanied by an increase in the volume fraction of mitochondria and that the occurrence of these increases was prevented by pretreatment of the animals with acriflavine, a drug that binds to mitochondrial DNA and prevents its replication. Laguens and Gómez-Dunn (39) had previously shown that the very early changes induced in mitochondria by exercise were mediated by increase in size, rather than in number, and that reproduction of mitochondria subsequently took over as the primary mechanism responsible for later increases. In deficiency of copper, iron (17,31), or thiamine (11), significant cardiomegaly develops in association with marked increases in mitochondrial size and mitochondria/myofibril ratios. In fact, Goodman et al. (31) calculated that 75% of the increase in cardiac weight in rats with iron deficiency was due to mitochondrial mass. The changes in the deficiency states just described are reversible, at least when they are of short duration, and reversion is accomplished more rapidly (within 16 days of iron replacement therapy) than in hypertrophy due to aortocaval fistula. In thiamine deficiency, regression of mitochondrial changes begins to be evident within a few hours after administration of a single dose of thiamine. Mitochondria in cardiac muscle cells of hypothyroid rats given thyroxin show responses similar to those in the deficiency states listed above (63). It appears, therefore, that the relative contributions of mitochondria and myofibrils to the cardiac enlargement occurring in these metabolic deficiencies differ clearly from those in hypertrophy due to pressure overloading.

The observations just reviewed serve as useful reminders of two facts concerning the genetic control of growth of subcellular organelles: (a) that control of the growth of new mitochondria is mediated through poorly understood interactions between mitochondrial and nuclear DNA and (b) that control of growth of the sarcoplasmic reticulum, the myofibrils, the T system, and the "external" sarcolemma appears to be mediated only through nuclear DNA. These differences in mechanisms of growth control seem to be responsible for the discrepancies noted above in the relative contributions of mitochondria and other cellular organelles to the enlargement of cardiac muscle cells.

Little is known of the mechanisms controlling mitochondrial size and mitochondrial reproduction, although it is now known that mitochondrial DNA is a small molecule with a very limited coding capacity and that the majority of mitochondrial components are synthesized in extramitochondrial locations (81). It is also evident that there can be great variability in the size that mitochondria ultimately attain in cardiac muscle cells; some mitochondria can fuse, resulting in extremely elongated or giant forms (Fig. 24), and others have small surface projections suggestive of budding. The significance of these changes has not been determined. Elucidation of nuclear-mitochondrial relationships in cardiac muscle cells appears of great importance for understanding mechanisms of hypertrophy.

During the past few years several morphometric studies have been made of human cardiac hypertrophy, mainly on patients with aortic valvular disease. Although these studies have been somewhat limited, they represent the auspicious beginning for the application of cardiac morphometric techniques to clinical medicine.

In 21 patients with aortic valvular disease studied by Schwarz et al. (74), the percentage of fibrosis, determined by morphometry in biopsies obtained at the time

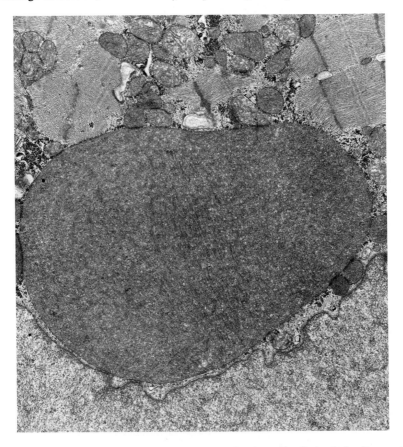

FIG. 24. Giant mitochondrion in left atrial myocyte of patient with mitral valvular disease. Note part of the nucleus **(bottom)** and cytoplasm **(top)**, with normal-sized mitochondria (× 14,000).

of operation, was significantly higher in the endocardium than in the subepicardium (19% vs 13%) of pressure-overloaded hearts (predominant stenosis), but was equal in both layers of volume-overloaded hearts (predominant regurgitation) (19% vs 18%). All but two of the patients had significant cardiac ultrastructural alterations. When all patients, regardless of the type of aortic valvular lesion, were considered, there was no significant correlation between percentage of fibrosis and preoperatively obtained values for ejection fraction or mean normalized systolic ejection rate. But there was a significant inverse relation between left ventricular mass and ejection fraction and mean normalized systolic ejection rate. These data were interpreted as suggesting that (a) depressed left ventricular function in aortic valvular disease is associated with ultrastructural degenerative changes, but complete recovery of cardiac function after successful operation is not prevented by these changes, and that (b) interstitial myocardial fibrosis is not a primary determinant of depressed cardiac function in aortic valvular disease. The latter conclusion is somewhat at variance with that of Donaldson (18), who obtained left ventricular biopsies before and 1 year after aortic valvular replacement in 12 patients; five of these had normal end-diastolic dimensions postoperatively, and seven had persistent postoperative dilatation. Increased fibrous tissue and loss of myofibrillar components from hypertrophic myocardial cells correlated with persistent dilatation and hypertrophy. In another study, Schwarz et al. (75) determined the relation between quantitative ultrastructural changes of left ventricular myocardium and contractile function in two groups of patients with aortic stenosis. Group I consisted of seven patients with ejection fractions greater than 55% and mean left atrial pressures less than 15 mm Hg; Group II consisted of 12 patients with ejection fractions less than 55% and left atrial pressures exceeding 15 mm Hg. Patients in Group I had lower left ventricular end-diastolic volume (91.9 vs 145.3 ml/m²) than did patients in Group II. The volume fraction of myofibrils was higher in Group I than in Group II patients (48.4 vs 42.1%, $p<0.05$), whereas volume fractions of sarcoplasm (31.7 vs 36.0%, $p>0.05$) and mitochondria (20.9 vs 22.0%, $p>0.05$) were comparable. Interstitial myocardial fibrosis did not differ between groups (16.3 vs 14.7%, $p>0.05$). No significant differences were found in the ultrastructural data obtained from patients in Group I and control patients with moderate degrees of coronary artery disease and normal wall motion in the areas biopsied. The volume fraction of myofibrils was lower in Group II patients than in controls (42.1 vs 52.9% $p<0.001$), and the volume fraction of sarcoplasm was higher (36.0 vs 21.1%, $p<0.001$). The extent of interstitial fibrosis and the volume fraction of mitochondria did not differ in Group II and control patients. Thus, a reduction in the volume fraction of myofibrils was the major morphologic finding in left ventricular biopsy samples from patients with decompensated pressure overload.

The findings just cited were basically similar to those in a group of nine patients with severe aortic regurgitation who also were studied by Schwarz et al. (76). These patients had a high end-diastolic volume (180 vs 77 ml/m²) and a lower ejection fraction (51 vs 69%) than control patients. The volume fraction of myofibrils was lower than in controls (44 vs 53%, $p<0.001$), and the volume fraction of sarcoplasm was higher (33 vs 21%, $p<0.01$); however, mitochondria and interstitial fibrosis did not differ significantly in the two groups. Thus, reduction in the volume fraction of myofibrils also was the major structural finding in left ventricular myocardium of patients with decompensated volume overload.

In contrast to the studies just reviewed, the importance of myocardial fibrosis with respect to myocardial function in patients with aortic valvular disease was emphasized by Krayenbühl et al. (38), who performed left ventricular cineangiography, micromanometry, and endomyocardial biopsies in 13 patients with aortic valve disease before and 12 to 28 months after successful valvular replacement. In nine patients (Group I) the postoperative left ventricular ejection fraction and V_{max} were depressed. Preoperatively, mean muscle fiber diameter was 32 μ in Group I and 38 μ in Group II ($p<0.01$). After operation, muscle fiber diameter decreased to 27 μ in Group I and 28 μ in Group II ($p<0.02$). In biopsies taken prior to operation, the left ventricular connective tissue content showed no significant correlation with the ejection fraction or V_{max}; however, in biopsies taken after operation, the fibrous tissue content was inversely related to the ejection fraction and to V_{max}. From these observations, Krayenbühl et al. (38) concluded that (a) in aortic valvular disease massive preoperative fiber hypertrophy heralds impaired postoperative left ventricular function, (b) fiber hypertrophy regresses after aortic valvular replacement regardless of the functional state of the left ventricle, and (c) the content of fibrous tissue appears to be a determinant of postoperative left ventricular function.

REFERENCES

1. Adler, C. P. (1976): DNS in Kinderherzen. Biochemische und Zytophotometrische Untersuchungen. *Beitr. Pathol.*, 158:173–202.
2. Adler, C. P., and Sandritter, W. (1971): Numerische Hyperplasie der Herzmuskelzellen bei Herzhypertrophie. *Dtsch. Med. Wochenschr.*, 96:1895–1897.
3. Adomian, G. E., Laks, M. M., Morady, F., and Swan, H. J. C. (1974): Significance of the multiple intercalated disc in the hypertrophied canine heart. *J. Mol. Cell. Cardiol.*, 6:105–109.
4. Anversa, P., Hagopian, M., and Loud, A. V. (1973): Quantitative radioautographic localization of protein synthesis in experimental cardiac hypertrophy. *Lab. Invest.*, 29:282–292.
5. Astorri, E., Bolognesi, E., Colla, B., Chizzola, A., and Visioli, O. (1977): Left ventricular hypertrophy: A cytometric study on 42 human hearts. *J. Mol. Cell. Cardiol.*, 9:763–775.
6. Barr, P. A., Celermajer, J. M., Bowdler, J. D., and Cartmill, T. B. (1973): Idiopathic hypertrophic obstructive cardiomyopathy causing severe right ventricular outflow tract obstruction in infancy. *Br. Heart J.*, 35:1109–1115.
7. Bishop, S. P. (1973): Effect of aortic stenosis on myocardial cell growth, hyperplasia, and ultrastructure in neonatal dogs. In: *Recent Advances in Studies on Cardiac Structure and Metabolism, Vol. 3, Myocardial Metabolism*, edited by N. S. Dhalla, pp. 637–656. University Park Press, Baltimore.
8. Bishop, S. P., and Cole, C. R. (1969): Ultrastructural changes in the canine myocardium with right ventricular hypertrophy and congestive heart failure. *Lab. Invest.*, 20:219–229.
9. Bloom, K. R., Hug, G., Schubert, W. K., and Kaplan, S. (1974): Pompe's disease and the heart. *Circulation*, 49, 50 *[Suppl.]*:III-56.
10. Boor, P. J., Ferrans, V. J., Jones, M., Kawanami, O., Thiedemann, K.-U., Herman, E. H., and Roberts, W. C. (1979): Tubuloreticular structures in myocardium: an ultrastructural study. *J. Mol. Cell. Cardiol.*, 11:967–979.
11. Bózner, A., Knieriem, H. J., Meesen, H., and Reinauer, H. (1969): Die Ultrastruktur und

Biochemie des Herzmuskels der Ratte im Thiaminmangel und nach einer Gabe von Thiamin. *Virchows Arch. Zellpathol.*, 2:125–143.

12. Buccino, R. A., Harris, E., Spann, J. F., and Sonnenblick, E. H. (1969): Response of myocardial connective tissue to development of experimental hypertrophy. *Am. J. Physiol.*, 216:425–428.

13. Bugaisky, L., and Zak, R. (1979): Cellular growth of cardiac muscle after birth. *Tex. Rep. Biol. Med.*, 39:123–135.

14. Buja, L. M., Ferrans, V. J., and Levitsky, S. (1972): Occurrence of intramitochondrial glycogen in canine myocardium after prolonged anoxic cardiac arrest. *J. Mol. Cell. Cardiol.*, 4:237–254.

15. Buja, L. M., Ferrans, V. J., and Maron, B. J. (1974): Intracytoplasmic junctions in cardiac muscle cells. *Am. J. Pathol.*, 74:613–648.

16. Casanova, M., Gamallo, C., Quero-Jiménez, M., García-Aguada, A., Burgueros, M., García, S., and Suárez, A. (1979): Familial hypertrophic cardiomyopathy with unusual involvement of the right ventricle. *Eur. J. Cardiol.*, 9:145–159.

17. Datta, B. N., and Silver, M. D. (1975): Cardiomegaly in chronic anemia in rats. An experimental study including ultrastructural, histometric, and stereologic observations. *Lab. Invest.*, 32:503–514.

18. Donaldson, R. M. (1982): Left ventricular hypertrophy in aortic valve disease. Regression of ventricular mass and volume following surgery for chronic volume overload. *Eur. Heart J.*, 3:179–186.

19. Ehlers, K. H., and Engle, M. A. (1963): Glycogen storage disease of myocardium. *Am. Heart J.*, 65:145–147.

20. Ehlers, K. H., Hagstrom, J. W. C., Lukas, D. S., Redo, S. F., and Engle, M. A. (1962): Glycogen-storage disease of the myocardium with obstruction to left ventricular outflow. *Circulation*, 25:96–109.

21. Epstein, S. E., Henry, W. L., Clark, C. E., Roberts, W. C., Maron, B. J., Ferrans, V. J., Redwood, D. R., and Morrow, A. G. (1974): Asymmetric septal hypertrophy. NIH Combined Clinical Staff Conference. *Ann. Intern. Med.*, 81:650–680.

22. Eslami, B., Aryanpur, I., Tabaeezadeh, M. J., Alipour, M., Nazarian, I. and Shakibi, J. G. (1979): Midventricular obstruction. *Jpn. Heart J.*, 20:117–126.

23. Falicov, R. E., Resnekov, L., Bharati, S., and Lev, M. (1976): Mid-ventricular obstruction: a variant of obstructive cardiomyopathy. *Am. J. Cardiol.*, 37:432–437.

24. Ferrans, V. J., Buja, L. M., and Jones, M. (1973): Ultrastructure and cytochemistry of glycogen in cardiac diseases. In: *Recent Advances in Studies on Cardiac Structure and Metabolism, Vol. 3, Myocardial Metabolism*, edited by N. S. Dhalla, pp. 97–144. University Park Press, Baltimore.

25. Ferrans, V. J., and Butany, J. W. (1983): Ultrastructural pathology of the heart. In: *Diagnostic Electron Microscopy, Vol. 4*, edited by B. F. Trump and R. T. Jones, pp. 319–473. John Wiley & Sons, New York.

26. Ferrans, V. J., Jones, M., Maron, B. J., and Roberts, W. C. (1975): The nuclear membranes in hypertrophied human cardiac muscle cells. *Am. J. Pathol.*, 78:427–460.

27. Ferrans, V. J., Maron, B. J., Buja, L. M., Ali, N., and Roberts, W. C. (1975a): Intranuclear glycogen deposits in human cardiac muscle cells: ultrastructure and cytochemistry. *J. Mol. Cell. Cardiol.*, 7:373–386.

28. Ferrans, V. J., Morrow, A. G., and Roberts, W. C. (1972): Myocardial ultrastructure in idiopathic hypertrophic subaortic stenosis. A study of operatively excised left ventricular outflow tract muscle in 14 patients. *Circulation*, 45:769–792.

29. Ferrans, V. J., Thiedemann, K.-U., Maron, B. J., Jones, M., and Roberts, W. C. (1976): Spherical microparticles in human myocardium. An ultrastructural study. *Lab. Invest.*, 35:349–368.

30. Goldstein, M. A., Schroeter, J. P., and Sass, R. L. (1979): The Z lattice in canine cardiac muscle. *J. Cell Biol.*, 83:187–204.

31. Goodman, J. R., Warshaw, J. B., and Dallman, P. R. (1970): Cardiac hypertrophy in rats with iron and copper deficiency: quantitative contribution of mitochondrial enlargement. *Pediatr. Res.*, 4:244–256.

32. Grabner, W., and Pfitzer, P. (1974): Number of nuclei in isolated myocardial cells of pigs. *Virchows Arch. [Cell Pathol.]*, 15:279–294.

33. Gutgesell, H. P., Speer, M., and Rosenberg, H. S. (1980): Characterization of the cardiomyopathy in infants of diabetic mothers. *Circulation*, 61:441–450.

34. Hatt, P. Y., Berjal, G., Moravec, J., and Swynghedauw, B. (1970): Heart failure: an electron

microscopic study of the left ventricular papillary muscle in aortic insufficiency in the rabbit. *J. Mol. Cell. Cardiol.* 1:235–247.

35. Hort, W. (1971): Quantitative morphology and structural dynamics of the myocardium. In: *Methods and Achievements in Experimental Pathology*, Vol. 5, edited by E. S. Bajusz and G. Jasmin, pp. 3–21. Karger, Basel.

36. Jones, M., and Ferrans, V. J. (1979): Myocardial ultrastructure in children and adults with congenital heart disease. In: *Congenital Heart Disease in Adults*, edited by W. C. Roberts, pp. 501–530. F. A. Davis Company, Philadelphia.

37. Jones, M., Ferrans, V. J., Morrow, A. G., and Roberts, W. C. (1975): Ultrastructure of crista supraventricularis muscle in patients with congenital heart diseases associated with right ventricular outflow tract obstruction. *Circulation*, 51:39–67.

38. Krayenbuehl, H. P., Schneider, J., Turina, M., and Senning, A. (1982): Myocardial function and structure in aortic valve disease before and after surgery. *Eur. Heart J.*, 3:149–153.

39. Laguens, R. P., and Gómez-Dumm, C. L. A. (1967): Fine structure of myocardial mitochondria in rats after exercise for one-half to two hours. *Circ. Res.*, 21:271–279.

40. Laguens, R. P., Meckert, P. C., and Segal, A. (1972): Effect of acriflavin on the fine structure of the heart muscle cell mitochondria of normal and exercised rats. *J. Mol. Cell. Cardiol.*, 4:185–193.

41. Laks, M. M., Morady, F., Adomian, G. E., and Swan, H. J. C. (1970): Presence of widened and multiple intercalated discs in the hypertrophied canine heart. *Circ. Res.*, 27:391–402.

42. Legato, M. J. (1970): Sarcomerogenesis in human myocardium. *J. Mol. Cell. Cardiol.*, 1:425–437.

43. Linzbach, A. J. (1960): Heart failure from the point of view of quantitative anatomy. *Am. J. Cardiol.*, 5:370–382.

44. Linzbach, A. J. (1976): Hypertrophy, hyperplasia and structural dilatation of the human heart. *Adv. Cardiol.*, 18:1–14.

45. Markwald, R. R. (1973): Distribution and relationship of precursor Z material to organizing myofibrillar bundles in embryonic rat and hamster ventricular myocytes. *J. Mol. Cell. Cardiol.*, 5:341–350.

46. Maron, B. J., Anan, T. J., and Roberts, W. C. (1981): Quantitative analysis of the distribution of cardiac muscle cell disorganization in the left ventricular wall of patients with hypertrophic cardiomyopathy. *Circulation*, 63:882–894.

47. Maron, B. J., Edwards, J. E., Moller, J. H., and Epstein, S. E. (1979): Prevalence and characteristics of disproportionate ventricular septal thickening in infants with congenital heart disease. *Circulation*, 59:126–133.

48. Maron, B. J., and Epstein, S. E. (1980): Hypertrophic cardiomyopathy. Recent observations regarding the specificity of three hallmarks of the disease: asymmetric septal hypertrophy, septal disorganization and systolic anterior motion of the anterior mitral leaflet. *Am. J. Cardiol.*, 45:141–154.

49. Maron, B. J., Epstein, S. E., and Roberts, W. C. (1979a): Hypertrophic cardiomyopathy and transmural myocardial infarction without significant atherosclerosis of the extramural coronary arteries. *Am. J. Cardiol.*, 43:1086–1102.

50. Maron, B. J., and Ferrans, V. J. (1973): Significance of multiple intercalated discs in hypertrophied human myocardium. *Am. J. Pathol.*, 73:81–87.

51. Maron, B. J., and Ferrans, V. J. (1974): The occurrence of α-glycogen in human cardiac muscle cells. *J. Mol. Cell. Cardiol.*, 6:85–90.

52. Maron, B. J., and Ferrans, V. J. (1975): Intramitochondrial glycogen deposits in hypertrophied human myocardium. *J. Mol. Cell. Cardiol.*, 7:697–702.

53. Maron, B. J., Ferrans, V. J., and Roberts, W. C. (1975): Ultrastructural features of degenerated cardiac muscle cells in patients with cardiac hypertrophy. *Am. J. Pathol.*, 79:387–434.

54. Maron, B. J., Gottdiener, J. S., Roberts, W. C., Henry, W. L., Savage, D. D., and Epstein, S. E. (1978): Left ventricular outflow tract obstruction due to systolic anterior motion of the anterior mitral leaflet in patients with concentric left ventricular hypertrophy. *Circulation*, 57:527–533.

55. Maron, B. J., and Roberts, W. C. (1979): Quantitative analysis of cardiac muscle cell disorganization in the ventricular septum of patients with hypertrophic cardiomyopathy. *Circulation*, 59:689–706.

56. Maron, B. J., and Roberts, W. C. (1981): Cardiomyopathies in the first two decades of life. *Cardiovasc. Clin.*, 11:35–78.

57. Meerson, F. Z., Zaletayeva, T. A., Lagutchev, S. S., and Pshennikova, M. G. (1964): Structure and mass of mitochondria in the process of compensatory hyperfunction and hypertrophy of the heart. *Exp. Cell Res.*, 36:568–578.

58. Morganroth, J., Maron, B. J., Henry, W. L., and Epstein, S. E. (1975): Comparative left ventricular dimensions in trained athletes. *Ann. Intern. Med.*, 82:521–524.

59. Morkin, E. (1974): Activation of synthetic processes in cardiac hypertrophy. *Circ. Res.*, 35:37–48.

60. Oberpriller, J. O., Bader, D. M., and Oberpriller, J. C. (1979): The regenerative potential of cardiac muscle in the newt, Notophthalmus viridsecens. In: *Muscle Regeneration*, edited by A. Mauro, pp. 323–333. Raven Press, New York.

61. Oberpriller, J. O., Ferrans, V. J., and Carroll, R. J. (1983): Changes in DNA content, number of nuclei and cellular dimensions of young rat atrial myocytes in response to left coronary artery ligation. *J. Mol. Cell. Cardiol.*, 15:31–42.

62. Oberpriller, J., and Oberpriller, J. C. (1971): Mitosis in adult newt ventricle. *J. Cell Biol.*, 49:560–563.

63. Page, E., and McCallister, L. P. (1973): Quantitative electron microscopic description of heart muscle cells: Application to normal, hypertrophied, and thyroxin-stimulated hearts. *Am. J. Cardiol.*, 31:172–181.

64. Papadimitriou, J. M., Hopkins, B. E., and Taylor, R. R. (1974): Regression of left ventricular dilation and hypertrophy after removal of volume overload. *Circ. Res.*, 35:127–135.

65. Perloff, J. K. (1981): Pathogenesis of hypertrophic cardiomyopathy: hypotheses and speculations. *Am. Heart J.*, 101:219–226.

66. Pfitzer, P., and Capurso, A. (1970): Der DNS-Gehalt der Zellkerne im Herzhor des Menschen. *Virchows Arch. [Cell Pathol.]*, 5:254–267.

67. Richter, G. W., and Kellner, A. (1963): Hypertrophy of the human heart at the level of fine structure. An analysis and two postulates. *J. Cell Biol.*, 18:195–206.

68. Roberts, W. C. (1970): Examining the precordium and the heart. *Chest*, 57:567–571.

69. Roberts, W. C., and Ferrans, V. J. (1975): Pathologic anatomy of the cardiomyopathies. Idiopathic dilated and hypertrophic types, infiltrative types, and endomyocardial disease with and without eosinophilia. *Hum. Pathol.*, 6:287–342.

70. Rumyantsev, P. P. (1974): Ultrastructural reorganization. DNA synthesis and mitotic division of myocytes in atria of rats with left ventricular infarction. *Virchows Arch. [Cell Pathol.]*, 15:357–378.

71. Rumyantsev, P. P. (1977): Interrelations of the proliferation and differentiation processes during cardiac myogenesis and regeneration. *Int. Rev. Cytol.*, 51:187–273.

72. Rumyantsev, P. P., and Kassem, A. M. (1976): Cumulative indices of DNA synthesizing myocytes in different compartments of the working myocardium and conductive system of the rats heart muscle following extensive left ventricular infarction. *Virchows Arch. [Cell Pathol.]*, 20:329–342.

73. Rumyantsev, P. P., and Mirakyan, V. O. (1968): Reactive synthesis of DNA and mitotic division in atrial heart muscle cells following ventricular infarction. *Experientia*, 24:1234–1235.

74. Schwarz, F., Flameng, W., Schaper, J., Langebartels, F., Sesto, M., Hehrlein, F., and Schlepper, M. (1978): Myocardial structure and function in patients with aortic valve disease and their relation to postoperative results. *Am. J. Cardiol.*, 41:661–669.

75. Schwarz, F., Schaper, J., Kittstein, D., Flameng, W., Walter, P., and Schaper, W. (1981): Reduced volume fraction of myofibrils in myocardium of patients with decompensated pressure overload. *Circulation*, 63:1299–1304.

76. Schwarz, F., Schaper, J., Kittstein, D., and Kubler, W. (1981[b]): Quantitative ultrastructural findings of the myocardium in the failing heart. I. Aortic valve insufficiency. *Z. Kardiol.*, 70:729–732.

77. Spotnitz, H. M., Spotnitz, W. D., Cottrell, T. S., Spiro, D., and Sonnenblick, E. H. (1974): Cellular basis for volume related wall thickness changes in the rat left ventricle. *J. Mol. Cell. Cardiol.*, 6:317–331.

78. Streeter, D. D., Jr., Spotnitz, H. M., Patel, D. J., Ross, J., Jr., and Sonnenblick, E. H. (1969): Fiber orientation in the canine left ventricle during diastole and systole. *Circ. Res.*, 24:339–347.

79. Thiedemann, K.-U., and Ferrans, V. J. (1976): Ultrastructure of sarcoplasmic reticulum in atrial myocardium of patients with mitral valvular disease. *Am. J. Pathol.*, 83:1–38.

80. Thiedemann, K.-U., and Ferrans, V. J. (1977): Left atrial ultrastructure in mitral valvular disease. *Am. J. Pathol.*, 89:575–604.
81. Tzagaloff, A., Macino, G., and Sebald, W. (1979): Mitochondrial genes and translation products. *Annu. Rev. Biochem.*, 48:419–441.
82. Wartman, W. B., and Hill, W. T. (1960): Degenerative lesions. In: *Pathology of the Heart*, edited by S. E. Gould pp. 497–554. Charles C. Thomas, Springfield, Ill.
83. Wiener, J., Giacomelli, F., Loud, A. V., Anversa, P. (1979): Morphometry of cardiac hypertrophy induced by experimental renal hypertension. *Am. J. Cardiol.*, 44:919–930.
84. Wollenberger, A., and Schulze, W. (1962): Über das Volumenverhältnis von Mitochondrien zu Myofibrillen im chronisch überlasteten, hypertrophierten Herzen. *Naturwissenchaften*, 49:161–162.
85. Yamaguchi, H., Ishimura, T., Nishiyama, S., Nagasaki, F., Nakanishi, S., Takatsu, F., Nishijo, T., Umeda, T., and Machii, K. (1979): Hypertrophic nonobstructive cardiomyopathy with giant negative T waves (apical hypertrophy): ventriculographic and echocardiographic features in 30 patients. *Am. J. Cardiol.*, 44:401–412.
86. Zak, R. (1974): Development and proliferative capacity of cardiac muscle cells. *Circ. Res.*, 35:17–26.

Growth of the Heart in Health and Disease,
edited by Radovan Zak. Raven Press,
New York © 1984.

Cardiac Hypertrophy with Congenital Heart Disease and Cardiomyopathy

Sanford P. Bishop

Department of Pathology, University of Alabama, Birmingham, Alabama 35294

Normal development of the heart through the embryonic and fetal phases and into the neonatal period involves a complex set of structural developments which takes the developing heart from a small protoplasmic mass of a few cells barely recognizable as muscle tissue to the complex muscular structure that is present in the normally growing and adult animal. The heart changes from a simple tubular structure to a complex chambered organ with several valves and muscular regions. Heart muscle cells undergo a change from a hyperplastic phase of growth in which there is rapid increase in cell number to a hypertrophic phase soon after birth in which the heart muscle cells are no longer able to increase in number but increase only in size. During this complex process of development, there are numerous opportunities for abnormal development to occur which may or may not lead to the production of functional abnormalities at some later period of time during the course of development. Some abnormalities such as the formation of a bicuspid aortic valve rather than the normal tricuspid semilunar valve or the incomplete closure of the foramen ovale may result in no abnormal function until very late in life, if indeed, abnormal function ever develops. At the other extreme are abnormalities leading to functional changes incompatible with life during the fetal or early neonatal period. Such an example would be complete transposition of the aorta and pulmonary artery with normal closure of all other communication between the right and left sides of the heart following birth. Of more clinical interest are those abnormalities of structural development which cause disturbance of the normal flow of blood through the heart and great vessels, resulting in an increased hemodynamic workload on one or more chambers of the heart. Such congenital abnormalities, many of which have been shown to have a genetic basis (88,90,91,97), may lead to the development of cardiac hypertrophy with functional abnormality manifest anytime during fetal development, postnatal growth, or even late in adult life.

Cardiomyopathy is a term applied to abnormal enlargement of the myocardium without an obvious anatomic or functional basis. The diagnosis of cardiomyopathy is made by exclusion of all other known causes of cardiac enlargement. Although a number of cardiomyopathies that occur later in life undoubtedly have toxic, infectious, or metabolic origins that may or may not be recognized, others appear to have a clear familial basis and undoubtedly are associated with specific abnormalities of genetic expression (95,105). The genetic abnormality in these cases results in either morphologic or biochemical changes that affect myocardium function. The common denominator in these cardiomyopathies is cardiac hypertrophy, which may or may not be accompanied by dilation of the heart chambers.

PHYSIOLOGIC HYPERTROPHY

During normal embryonic and fetal growth of the vertebrate heart there is a rapid increase in muscle cell number to reach a finite number of cells characteristic for each species. Heart muscle cells from different species over a wide range in body weight have essentially the same size and structural characteristics at comparable stages of growth (5,40). The difference in heart size in separate species is due to a difference in the total number of cells present in the myocardium. During the early neonatal period, heart muscle cells cease to divide, become binucleated by a process involving one final nuclear mitotic division which is not followed by cellular division, and all further increase in size of the heart is due to increase in the size of individual heart muscle cells (55,56). This normal process of cell growth results in an approximate 30 to 40 times increase in the volume of individual myocardial cells. Normal functional development is occurring during this same time period parallel with structural development of the myocardium (43,54,115). Therefore, normal growth of the heart may be referred to as a form of physiologic hypertrophy.

In the adult individual, changing patterns of physiologic function within normal limits may result in structural alterations of the myocardium, including a moderate degree of hypertrophy of individual muscle fibers; this is referred to as physiologic hypertrophy. An example is exercise training as in a marathon runner or a race horse. In this example there is intermittent increase in workload to the myocardium, as well as other alterations such as increase in vagal tone and adaptations of cellular metabolism to function at altered metabolic levels, which may contribute to changes in cardiac muscle cell size. In the trained athlete, it is well recognized that heart rate under resting conditions is slowed, stroke volume of the myocardium is increased, and there is a modest development of physiologic cardiac hypertrophy. Thyrotoxicosis, on the other hand, is an example with increased metabolic activity; there is an increase in the size of heart muscle cells with associated increase in cardiac function. This may be considered an example of physiologic hypertrophy, since myocardial function is operating at a normal or increased level, and when the stimulus is removed, the heart rapidly returns to normal functional and structural conditions. During physiologic hypertrophy, either in the process of normal growth or in the adult individual, structural alterations are limited to proportional cell and organelle growth, and myocardial function is normal or increased for the particular age of the individual.

PATHOLOGIC HYPERTROPHY

Pathologic hypertrophy is a term that has been applied to the myocardium with depressed myocardial function and certain structural and biochemical abnormalities. It must be recognized that there is no sharp distinction between physiologic hypertrophy on the one hand and pathologic hypertrophy on the other hand. Development of pathologic hypertrophy is a consequence of abnormally increased functional demand which leads to exhaustion of the normal physiologic processes with the gradual development of increased or decreased expressions of various normal functional properties of the myocardium. There will necessarily be a large, poorly defined area between that state which is clearly functionally normal and that which is clearly functionally abnormal. When pathologic hypertrophy has advanced to such a state that severe congestive myocardial failure has occurred, the function of the heart may reach a state in which return to normal with removal of the stimulus is no longer possible. This is then termed irreversible myocardial damage. Exactly where the lines may be drawn between physiologic hypertrophy, pathologic hypertrophy, and irreversible myocardial failure are far from clear. Equally unclear are factors responsible for the progression of cardiac hypertrophy from one phase to the next.

STRUCTURE-FUNCTION RELATIONSHIP OF MYOCARDIAL RESERVE IN CARDIAC HYPERTROPHY

Structural Alterations in Physiologic Hypertrophy

Cardiac hypertrophy, by definition, is an increase in the size of the individual heart muscle cells or cardiac myocytes. Incrementation of nonmuscle components of the heart is variable, depending on the age, cause of hypertrophy, and length of time hypertrophy exists. Several studies in adult animals have shown that with increased load on the heart, there is no mitotic activity in cardiac myocytes, but increased DNA synthesis does occur in nonmuscular components of the myocardium (15,46,81). Logically, one may conclude that even if the capillary-to-fiber ratio does not change in cardiac hypertrophy, as has been shown many times (63,100,103,110,114), if the myocytes increase in length, the length of the capillaries must also increase. Therefore, the number of capillary endothelial cells will increase in number, assuming they do not increase in size. An increase in other nonmuscle components of the myocardium, e.g., fibrocytes, histiocytes, and connective tissue components, may occur as well. It has generally been accepted that hyperplasia of myocytes does not occur in cardiac hypertrophy, at least in currently studied adult animal models. It should be mentioned, however, that very few animal models have resulted in greater than a doubling of the ventricular mass; human hearts and certain spontaneously occurring congenital cardiac conditions in animals do result in an increase in cardiac mass up to three or more times normal. In such very large human hearts, weighing more than 500 g, Linzbach (71) was the first to report, and others (6) have since corroborated, that the morphometric size of heart muscle cells is not commensurate with the increase in heart weight, suggesting that hyperplasia of myocytes has occurred.

Confirmation of these human heart studies awaits development of appropriate animal models to allow use of isolated myocyte measurement techniques, which, to date, have not been applied to human autopsy material.

The question of whether or not adult cardiac myocytes have a latent capacity for hyperplasia remains unanswered. Studies in neonatal animals, however, in contrast to those in adults, have suggested that myocytes may be induced to continue hyperplastic growth beyond the normal period (29,41,84,98). This is discussed in more detail below.

Increase in size of heart muscle cells has generally been documented by measurement of cross-sectional area or diameter of myocytes in tissue sections. Measurements of cell diameter or cross-sectional area in tissue sections is fraught with many technical artifacts such as tissue shrinkage due to dehydrating and embedding agents (up to 50% shrinkage), lack of circular cross section of myocytes, difficulty in ascertaining at the light microscopic level that true cross sections are measured, and difficulty in identifying cell borders in properly fixed tissue without artifactual interstitial cell separation (42). Appreciation of these difficulties may be gained by examination of scanning electron micrographs of individual myocytes prepared by collagenase perfusion of the myocardium (Fig. 1). With increasing size of the myocytes due to normal growth or to cardiac hypertrophy, there is increased irregularity of the cells (Fig. 2), which makes accurate cross-sectional measurements in tissue sections even more difficult (17). Nevertheless, numerous studies have demonstrated that in the presence of increased workload on the heart, and associated increase in heart weight, there is a detectable increase in the cross-sectional area or diameter of heart muscle cells.

Increase in cell length with cardiac hypertrophy has been much more difficult to accurately measure than increase in cross-sectional area. Within tissue sections it is particularly difficult, since the intercalated disc regions are not always located at the ends of the cell, as may be seen from scanning electron micrographs of isolated cells (Figs. 1 and 2). Use of isolated myocyte preparations, however, does allow accurate measurement of cell length, and during normal growth there is a proportionate increase in cell length with increase in cell cross-sectional area (66).

Only a few investigators have reported changes in cell length with cardiac hypertrophy. Laks et al. (67) reported an increase in cell length from 67 ± 2.5 μm (SEM) in normal dog hearts to 105 ± 5 μm in the right ventricle of dogs with pulmonary artery banding. They measured the distance between intercalated discs in 1-μm sections of plastic-embedded sections, which may account for the shorter length they observed in the dog heart than has been reported for the rat heart. Bishop et al. (16) found that 12-week-old spontaneously hypertensive rats (SHR) had left ventricular myocyte lengths of 109 ± 3 μm (SEM) and that normotensive Wistar Kyoto (WKY) cell lengths were 96 ± 4 μm ($p < 0.05$); measurements were done on isolated myocytes (16). Anversa et al. (2) used morphometric techniques to determine that there was a proportionately greater increase in cell length in

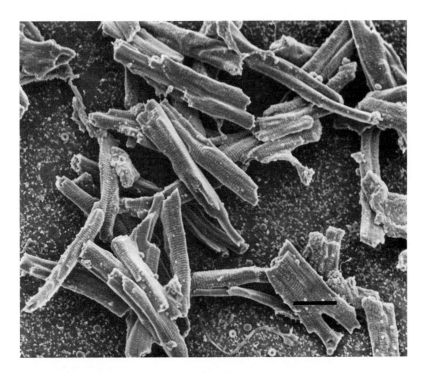

FIG. 1. Scanning electron micrograph of isolated cardiac myocytes from a 12-week-old Wistar Kyoto rat. The individual myocytes are irregular, elongated structures with numerous intercalated disc connection areas not only at the ends of the cells, but also along the edges of the cells. Bar = 20 μm. (Reproduced with permission from Bishop et al., ref. 17.)

outer left ventricular wall myocytes than in inner wall myocytes in rats with renal-vascular-induced cardiac hypertrophy. Studies in our laboratory have also shown a greater increase in cell length in myocytes isolated from the outer left ventricular wall than from the inner wall in aged SHR compared with aged WKY (Table 1). The explanation for the greater increase in cell length in the outer wall than in the inner wall is not clear, but may be related to the greater circumferential increase in the outer versus inner regions with hypertrophy.

Myocardial cell size changes in length and width may be related to the type of work overload placed on the heart. Although there is little experimental evidence to support the concept, it would appear reasonable that myocytes would undergo a relatively greater increase in length than in width in hearts subjected to a volume overload and cardiac dilation, whereas a greater increase in width would occur in hypertrophy due to a pressure overload not accompanied by chamber dilation. In SHR at 2 weeks of age and older we have found a constant length-to-width ratio indicating that there is a proportionate increase in both cell length and width during growth and development of cardiac hypertrophy in this animal model (Table 2). Thyrotoxicosis in the early neonatal rat results in an approximately 25% increase

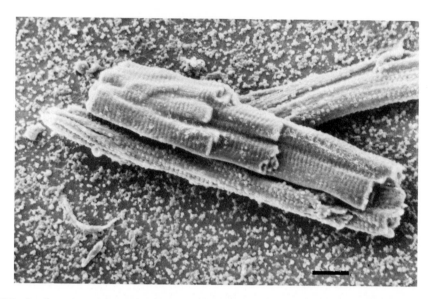

FIG. 2. Scanning electron micrograph of an isolated cardiac myocyte from a 1-year-old SHR. There are numerous irregular areas along the length of the cell as well as at the ends, which are the location of intercalated disc intercellular connections. These cell junction areas are more numerous in the hypertrophied heart than in the normal (compare with Fig. 1). In addition, there are deep longitudinal grooves in the hypertrophied cell due to growth of the cell around adjacent longitudinally oriented capillaries. Bar = 10 μm. (Reproduced with permission from Bishop et al., ref. 17.)

TABLE 1. *Regional isolated myocyte size in 18-month-old rats*

	SHR		WKY	
	Length μm	Volume μm	Length μm	Volume μm
Epicardium mean ± SD	201 ± 7	51,382 ± 7,374	148 ± 6	32,671 ± 4,781
Endocardium mean ± SD	182 ± 6	58,821 ± 11,153	121 ± 8	45,444 ± 7,209
Endocardial/epicardial ratio	0.91	1.14	0.82	1.39

in heart weight with very little increase in heart rate, suggesting an increase in stroke volume in this hypermetabolic model. Cell length, measured in isolated myocytes, was 20% greater after 12 days treatment with thyroxine (T4) from birth than in nontreated littermate controls (41). In this model, at an age when myocytes are normally undergoing rapid size changes, a volume overload results in a disproportionate increase in cell length relative to cell width, thus supporting the concept of differential cell size changes dependent on the nature of the work overload.

Ultrastructural changes in the physiologically hypertrophied myocardium are limited to moderate alterations in the relative proportion of cellular organelles. The increased cellular volume of the myocytes in a heart with stable hypertrophy is

TABLE 2. *Length and width of isolated left ventricular myocytes of SHR and WKY during growth*

	4 Weeks	12 Weeks	12 Months
WKY			
Length (μm)	68 $\pm$ 9	105 $\pm$ 14	122 $\pm$ 9
Width (μm)	12.0 $\pm$ 0.09	18.4 $\pm$ 2.6	21.6 $\pm$ 0.9
L/W ratio	6.01 $\pm$ 0.6	6.02 $\pm$ 0.3	5.90 $\pm$ 0.5
SHR			
Length (μm)	77 $\pm$ 7[a]	117 $\pm$ 8[a]	150 $\pm$ 7[b]
Width (μm)	13.0 $\pm$ 1.0[a]	22.4 $\pm$ 1.6[b]	28.3 $\pm$ 0.9[b]
L/W ratio	6.32 $\pm$ 0.8	5.54 $\pm$ 0.6	5.56 $\pm$ 0.3

[a] $p < 0.05$ compared to WKY.
[b] $p < 0.01$ compared to WKY.

characterized by a normal distribution of all intracellular elements, except for a decrease in nuclear-to-cytoplasmic ratio (Fig. 3). During the early stages of sudden pressure-overload-induced cardiac hypertrophy, mitochondria increase more rapidly than myofibrils (1,78); the mitochondrial to myofibrillar ratio returns to normal when a stable state of hypertrophy is reached (78) or remains normal in models with slowly developing cardiac hypertrophy (125). In thyrotoxicosis-induced cardiac hypertrophy, there is a disproportionate increase in the volume percent of the cell volume occupied by mitochondria (77); this apparently is in response to the increased metabolic requirements of the heart.

Structural Alterations in Pathologic Hypertrophy

When the heart enters a stage of decompensation or pathologic hypertrophy, there are several ultrastructural alterations present. There is a decrease in the volume percent of mitochondria, although the number of mitochondria per unit volume is increased and their size is decreased (11,78). The decreased size of mitochondria may indicate an increased rate of mitochondrial production brought on by the increased workload to the heart. Other ultrastructural changes include activation of the nucleolus with a characteristic ribbon formation of the nucleolar material, increased rough endoplasmic reticulum, and variably increased glycogen content and concentration (18,44). Changes in nuclear membranes consisting of increased folding have been described in human hypertrophied hearts (36). All of these changes are associated with increased protein synthesis.

In the pathologically hypertrophied heart there are characteristic changes in the intercalated disc and the Z-line (11,14,18,35,47,64,68,69,75). These structures are associated with the myofibril—the contractile element of the myocyte. The myofibril itself appears to maintain a normal size and internal structure, except in areas adjacent to intercalated disc or Z-line alterations (14). The intercalated disc shows evidence of increased activity related to assembly of myofilaments into sarcomeres as evidenced by an increase in the longitudinal folding of the disc (Fig. 4). This

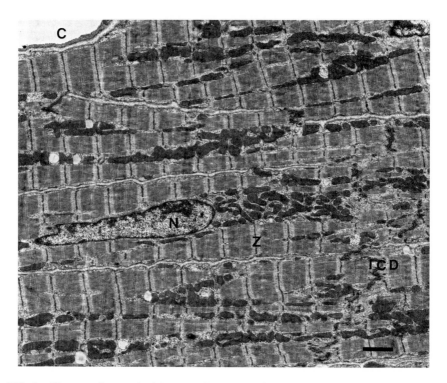

FIG. 3. Electron micrograph of the normally growing left ventricle of a 9-week-old dog. In spite of the rapid rate of growth resulting in rapid increase in myocyte cell volume, normal ultrastructural features are maintained. ICD = intercalated disc; N = nucleus; C = capillary lumen; Z = Z-lines. Bar = 2.0 μm.

increased folding provides increased surface area of the disc, and there is increased amount of dense myofilament attachment area along the disc. Often, poorly organized myofilaments are present, apparently in the process of forming new sarcomeres. The Z-lines also show abnormalities in pathologically hypertrophied hearts (Fig. 5), characterized by expansion of the Z-line material with a periodicity similar to that present in normal Z-line material (11). The electron-dense material in the normal Z-line, the expanded Z-line, and at the myofilament attachment area of the intercalated disc has been identified as α-actinin (23,101). Removal of the dense α-actinin in expanded Z-lines with trypsin or calcium-activated neutral protease reveals thin filaments with the morphologic characteristics of actin, but with an absence or scarcity of thick myosin filaments (126). This suggests that the expanded Z-lines represent incompletely formed sarcomeres that have been temporarily arrested in the process of formation. Whether this explanation is the case, or an alternative explanation is true, remains to be explained. In any event, the expanded Z-lines clearly appear to be a structural marker of pathologically hypertrophied and failing myocardium. They are not found in the normal or physiologically

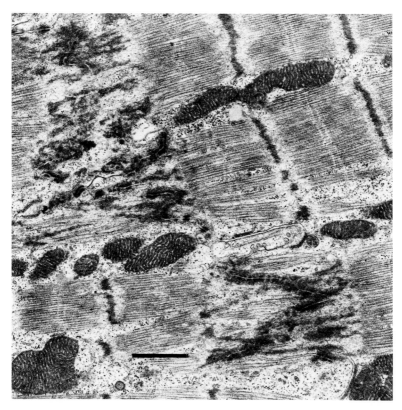

FIG. 4. Electron micrograph of the left ventricular myocardium of an 8-week-old dog with a constricting band placed on the aorta at 5 days of age. Left ventricular weight was more than three times that of a nonbanded littermate. There is marked increase in the folding of the intercalated disc due to increased surface area of the disc region and to increased electron-dense myofilament attachment area material. There are loose myofilaments and poorly organized sarcomeres adjacent to the disc, suggesting formation of new sarcomeres. Bar = 1.0 μm.

hypertrophied myocardium of most animal species. An exception is the occurrence of expanded Z-lines in normal feline myocardium (34). We have found expanded Z-lines in both right and left ventricles of 11 of 18 cats examined, ranging in age from 2 months to 7 years *(unpublished data)*. The explanation for the presence of these dense Z-line structures in the normal cat myocardium is not clear. Similar Z-line structures also occur commonly in the Purkinje fibers of several species of animals (13,24,120).

Metabolic Changes in Cardiac Hypertrophy

The structural changes described in the preceding section are a reflection of the metabolic changes in the hypertrophied heart. Specific metabolic alterations are

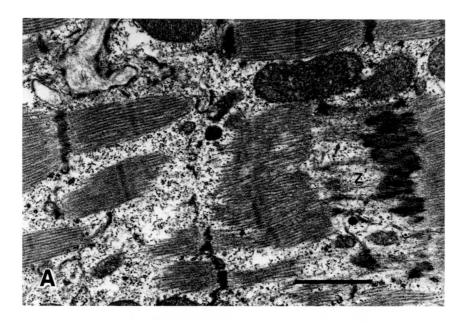

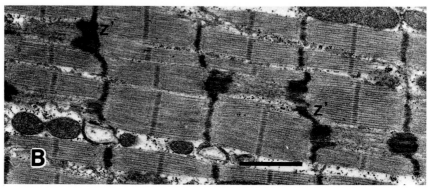

FIG. 5. Electron micrographs of expanded Z-line structures from the hypertrophied failing myocardium of dogs with experimentally produced cardiac hypertrophy. **A:** Right ventricle of a dog with progressive pulmonary artery stenosis. The dense expanded Z-line material (Z') and adjacent loose myofilaments appear to have longitudinally displaced the adjacent sarcomere. Bar = 1.0 μm. **B:** Left ventricle from a dog with progressive constriction of the aortic arch. Dense Z-line expansions (Z') have poorly organized myofilaments between them, suggesting incomplete sarcomere formation. Bar = 1.0 μm.

discussed in detail in other chapters in this volume and need not be discussed here. Suffice it to say that in an increased workload situation, all metabolic functions of the heart are working at an accelerated rate. DNA synthesis in nonmuscular components of the heart is increased in the adult heart subjected to work overload (15,46,81). In the fetal and neonatal heart, there is evidence to suggest that an increased workload will induce additional myocyte DNA synthesis with increased hyperplasia of muscle cells, resulting in an increased number of heart muscle cells in work-overloaded neonatal hearts. We have found an increased number of myocytes with three or four nuclei in neonatal rats exposed to carbon monoxide since birth *(unpublished observations)*. Carbon monoxide (500 ppm) from birth to 30 days of age results in a greater than 50% increase in heart weight compared with control animals maintained in room air (94). This finding, together with prolonged incorporation of tritiated thymidine into cardiomyocyte nuclei in aortic-banded puppies (14) and iron deficiency anemia rats (84), indicates that during the early neonatal period, the heart is able to increase or prolong hyperplastic myocyte activity.

Protein synthesis is obviously increased in the hypertrophying heart beyond that required for normal growth and maintenance of existing proteins. It has also been shown that there is an increased turnover rate of existing protein when the heart is subjected to an increased workload (65,82). Protein synthesis in the failing myocardium has received very little study. It is not known what the limits of protein synthesis are in myocardium. However, it appears reasonable to suggest that in the failing heart, the balance between synthesis required for maintenance and to increase cell size, and breakdown due to normal turnover which may be accelerated with work overload, is altered with the effect that insufficient proteins are produced to maintain normal myocardial contractile function. This would provide a reasonable explanation for the decreased contractile function of the failing myocardium.

Connective Tissue Content of Hypertrophied Myocardium

Increased interstitial connective tissue is found in many forms of cardiac hypertrophy associated with various types of congenital heart disease and cardiomyopathy. Whether the connective tissue is a cause, a consequence, or unrelated to the hypertrophy usually is far from clear, although it is commonly held that hypertrophy directly promotes the deposition of collagenous connective tissue.

In forms of cardiac hypertrophy which represent physiologic hypertrophy, the connective tissue response is absent or mild. In most types of congenital heart diseases, there is minimal connective tissue proliferation. The exception is aortic valvular or subvalvular stenosis, which is characterized by considerable increase in subendocardial connective tissue in dogs (97) and subendocardial ischemia in man (70). Experimentally induced sudden pressure overload, as with pulmonary artery or aortic banding in adult animals, results in multifocal acute necrosis and replacement fibrosis (15). Aortic banding in the rat produces moderate subendocardial fibrosis *(unpublished observations)* but apparently does not prevent the regression of cardiac hypertrophy following removal of the band (26).

Other experimental methods for production of afterload-induced hypertrophy include slowly progressive stenosis of the aorta or pulmonary artery in adult or young-growing animals (14,25,29,44,62,106). Stenosis of the aorta or pulmonary artery in neonatal animals mimics some forms of congenital heart disease in that the constricting band becomes relatively more stenosing as the animal increases in size, thus producing a gradually increasing workload beyond that of normal growth on the heart. Increased hydroxyproline has been reported in the cat with progressive stenosis from weaning (25), but was not found in the rat (62). Fibrosis was not apparent in histologic sections of hypertrophied hearts of dogs with aortic banding from the first week of life *(unpublished observations)*. In SHR and in the car-diomyopathic hamster, there is certainly an increase in connective tissue. However, SHR fibrosis is multifocal to diffuse and predominantly subendocardial (Fig. 6), whereas in the hamster model, fibrosis is multifocal throughout both ventricles (8). Cardiac hypertrophy associated with essential hypertension in man, and in the absence of ischemic heart disease or valve disease, usually is not accompanied by significant increases in hydroxyproline concentration (19,80,87). However, some reports have identified a positive correlation of cardiac hypertrophy and hydroxy-proline (40). In a recent morphometric study of tissue sections, an increase in stainable collagen was found in hypertrophied human hearts which was greatest in those patients with hypertrophy plus myocardial failure (93). In summary, condi-tions associated with very rapid and sudden increase in work overload, and those which result in restriction of blood flow to the myocardium, often have increased connective tissue response. In other nonischemic conditions, cardiac hypertrophy is associated with only a modest or no increase in connective tissue.

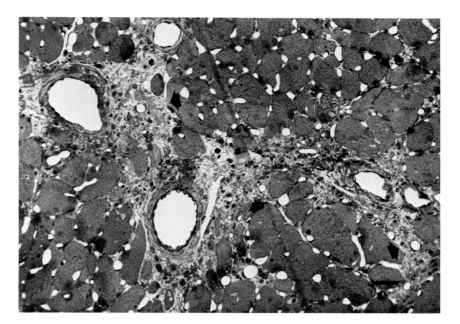

FIG. 6. Photomicrograph of the left ventricular subendocardial region of a 1-year-old SHR. There are multifocal areas of fibrosis *(arrows)* surrounding small arteries and arterioles. Fibrosis was not restricted to perivascular regions. Tissue was perfusion fixed, embedded in epoxy resin, and sectioned at 1 μm. Toluidine blue stain. Bar = 20 μm.

A popular notion for many years has been that the hypertrophied myocardium "outstrips its blood supply," resulting in inadequate oxygen delivery to the cell (especially the innermost portions of a hypertrophied myocyte), inadequate ATP production, and, thus, failure. Many cases have been reported in which the coronary artery size appeared to be inappropriate for the mass of the myocardium. At the cellular level the number of capillaries per myofiber is not increased in most types of cardiac hypertrophy, and maximum diffusion distance is greater in hypertrophied tissue (100,103,110). However, it has recently been proposed (53) that diffusion distance is not a factor, since oxygen is freely and rapidly diffusable through muscle tissue. A more likely candidate for interference with delivery of oxygen to tissues may be the amount of capillary surface area per unit of myocardium available for transport of oxygen from the vessel lumen to the tissue. There has been very little study of this relationship, especially in young individuals with congenital heart disease.

Myocardial Blood Flow

In the presence of a normal coronary vascular system, the myocardium receives an amount of blood proportional to the metabolic requirements of the tissue. Numerous factors, however, including intraluminal and intramural pressure, various humoral substances, and the relative luminal capacity of the coronary vascular system can affect the normal delivery of blood to the myocardium. Whether a measured decrease in myocardial blood flow associated with decreased myocardial function as has been reported in patients with hypertrophy due to aortic stenosis (61) or to hypertrophic or congestive cardiomyopathy (124) is a cause or an effect of that decreased function is unclear. It has been suggested by morphologists for many years that the hypertrophied myocardium may increase in mass beyond the capacity of its vascular system to deliver blood, especially under conditions of increased workload (63,103,110). However, it is also known from classic physiology that a decrease in the contractile function of the heart due to any cause would require less oxygen and, therefore, a decrease in myocardial blood flow (49).

Efforts to determine whether limitations of myocardial blood flow could contribute to the development of myocardial failure with cardiac hypertrophy have concentrated on anatomic and blood flow measurement studies in several experimental animal models. The divergent results appear to be related to the different ages of the animals used and to the duration and severity of cardiac hypertrophy. It appears likely that because of the differing proliferative capacity of myocytes and nonmyocyte components of the heart in immature and adult animals, there are differences in the ability of the vascular system to respond to increased workload. However, the situation is far from clear, since very few studies have been conducted in animal models with stress induced during the fetal or early neonatal period. In the adult, most models produce a relatively mild degree of hypertrophy (usually 30%–80%) compared with the two to four times increase in cardiac mass often found in the human heart.

The early anatomic studies of Wearn (122,123), Shipley (110), Roberts (103), and of others in man and experimental animals demonstrated that with an increase in the fiber cross-sectional area during hypertrophy, there is no increase in number of capillaries, the capillary-to-fiber ratio remaining near 1:1, but intercapillary distance is increased. This observation has led to speculation that a central myofiber core of hypertrophied fibers may be deprived of full oxygenation owing to increased diffusion distance. However, this assumes direct diffusion of oxygen to the tissue and ignores facilitated oxygen transport by myoglobin. More recent studies by Honig and Odoroff (53) have suggested that diffusion distance is unlikely to be a limiting factor in the delivery of oxygen to tissue. A more likely candidate for limitation of oxygen transport is the amount of capillary surface area per unit of tissue. Experimental validation of this hypothesis remains to be obtained.

During development of cardiac hypertrophy in man, there is a proportionate increase in caliber of epicardial coronary vessels (57). This should ensure adequate blood flow to hypertrophied myocardium and argue against theories suggesting that hypertrophied myocardium may outstrip its blood supply. Although the number of capillaries per fiber in cross section does not increase, the capillaries do increase in length as the muscle cells lengthen (3). In adult animals the total vascular capacity is not changed with development of cardiac hypertrophy; however, in young animals there is an increase in the capacity of the terminal vascular bed with hypertrophy (99).

Myocardial blood flow measurements with radioactive tracer microspheres in the hypertrophied hearts of dogs (7,50,83,102) and cats (21) have demonstrated either normal or moderately increased blood flow per gram of tissue. Transmural flow at rest either is normal or shows a slight attenuation of the normal subendocardial to subepicardial flow ratio. However, during maximal vasodilation induced by adenosine, exercise, or other means, there is significant reduction in subendocardial blood flow relative to subepicardial blood flow with a calculated increase in minimal vascular resistance compared with that of normal hearts. This has been interpreted as a failure of vascular capacity to keep pace with the enlarging heart mass, resulting in a reduction in coronary blood flow reserve. Although oxygen supply is adequate under resting conditions, with increased workload, subendocardial ischemia may occur, leading to degenerative and possibly irreversible myocardial changes.

In the fetal or neonatal heart, entirely different results have been obtained. Experimental outflow obstruction of the right or left ventricle in the fetal lamb produces up to a 100% increase in ventricular mass, but no increase in cell cross-sectional area, indicating that myocyte hyperplasia has occurred in this model (38). In lambs with pulmonary artery banding during the first postnatal week, there is continuing myocyte proliferation as well as nonmyocyte proliferation (38) and increased right ventricular myocardial blood flow during rest (4). In these neonatal lambs with enlarged hearts, maximal coronary vasodilation induced by isoproterenol resulted in greater coronary blood flow than in vasodilated control animals. This is in contrast to the reduced coronary vascular reserve reported for adult animals with cardiac hypertrophy (7,83). In another study in dogs with congenital pulmonic valve stenosis, there was no decrease in peak reactive hyperemia debt repayment flow following temporary coronary occlusion (73). There was an attenuation of phasic systolic right coronary flow, which was most pronounced in animals with the highest right ventricular pressure.

In the neonatal rat with nutritional anemia or constriction of the abdominal aorta (66,84) and in the neonatal dog with the aorta banded during the first week of life (14), there was both myocyte and nonmyocyte proliferation. To evaluate the difference between neonatal- and adult-onset myocardial hypertrophy, Dowell (29) induced hypertrophy of similar duration and severity in 21-day-old and 12-week-old rats. Myocardial function indexes remained unaltered in hypertrophied neonatal rat hearts, but there was significant depression of function in the hypertrophied adult animals. These studies support the concept that cardiac hypertrophy induced during fetal or neonatal life, in contrast to the adult, is accompanied by coronary microvascular growth commensurate with increase in myofiber mass. This provides greater coronary blood flow reserve than in adult hearts with comparable degrees of hypertrophy.

CHARACTERIZATION OF HYPERTROPHY IN CONGENITAL HEART DISEASE AND CARDIOMYOPATHY

Enlargement of the heart is a response to a variety of stimuli which stresses the myocardium beyond normal physical limits, but falls short of producing actual cellular necrosis. In many forms of congenital heart disease the cause of the stress appears to be obvious as an alteration in the hemodynamic load on the heart. Thus, an increased left ventricular mass in patients with aortic valve stenosis or right ventricular mass in the presence of pulmonic valve stenosis appears clearly related to increased pressure generated in the corresponding ventricle. Similarly, an enlarged left ventricle associated with a deformed mitral valve or patent ductus arteriosus appears to have a clear relationship to the increased volume that must be pumped by the ventricle. However, in many cases there is enlargement of a chamber without obvious cause, which is then termed cardiomyopathy for lack of a better understanding. There is increasing evidence that many apparently obvious causes of cardiac hypertrophy may, in fact, not be the sole factor, or perhaps even the prime factor, responsible for the development of hypertrophy. For example, how does one explain the increase in right ventricular mass commonly found in patients with a pure left-sided lesion such as aortic stenosis? Or, one could ask if hypertension is a cause, an effect, or unrelated to the cardiac hypertrophy often but not always present in hypertensive patients. The possibility that some humoral factor may be operating must be considered.

In the various nonspecific cardiomyopathies, unknown factors operate to change the structure of the heart. The fact that many cardiomyopathies are familial indicates that some aspect of genetic control has malfunctioned. There are several animal models of genetic cardiomyopathy which provide the opportunity to study these specific abnormalities.

Increased Afterload

Congenital abnormalities of the heart which result in an increase in the resistance to blood flow through all or part of the vascular system cause the ventricle to generate greater pressure to ensure adequate blood flow to meet the body needs. The myocardial wall thickness increases to return the increased wall stress toward normal. Although moderate increase in end-diastolic volume may occur during some stages of the development of such afterload-induced hypertrophy, usually the wall is thickened without increase in chamber diameter; in fact, the lumen may even be compromised. Hypertrophy without ventricular dilation is often referred to as concentric hypertrophy.

The biochemical mechanisms responsible for translating increased luminal pressure and wall stress into increased protein synthesis in myocytes are poorly understood and are discussed in other chapters in this volume. Nevertheless, wall mass does increase until a normalized wall stress is achieved, and a stable state of cardiac hypertrophy is achieved. Whether the increase in muscle mass associated with afterload conditions is due to increased number or size of cells depends on the age of the subject. Abnormalities that cause afterload increases during the fetal period, when cellular hyperplasia is normally occurring, cause increased cell proliferation and increased cell numbers rather than increased size of cells as occurs when afterload occurs after the neonatal period.

Isolated Outflow Tract Obstruction

Obstruction of the left or right ventricular outflow tract in the fetus may produce redistribution of blood flow in addition to increased pressure load on the affected ventricle. Redistribution of blood flow may produce volume load on contralateral chambers in addition to afterload on the obstructed chambers. This may lead to increased muscle cell proliferation in both chambers, depending on the severity of the obstruction. For example, congenital deformity of the pulmonic valve region produces not only right ventricular increased mass, but also increased mass of the left ventricle owing to increased flow across the ostium secundum resulting in volume overload on the left ventricle. Shunting of increased amounts of poorly oxygenated blood from the superior vena cava to the left ventricle rather than normally traversing the right ventricle may produce reduced oxygen supply to the heart and brain, since this blood normally enters the aorta through the ductus arteriosus, distal to the origin of blood vessels to these organs.

Coarctation of the Aorta

Congenital constriction of the aorta may occur either proximal or distal to the ductus arteriosus. In either case, the left ventricle is subjected to increased flow resistance and enlarges. If the coarctation is proximal to the ductus, the right ventricle faces normal systemic resistance. However, if the coarctation is distal to the ductus arteriosus, both ventricles have increased resistance and undergo mass increase.

Following birth and normal closure of the ductus arteriosus, only the left ventricle is faced with increased resistance. With further normal growth the aortic stenosis becomes progressively more severe, requiring increased pressure generation by the left ventricle to force blood through the stenosis. Cellular proliferation persists for a short time in the early neonatal period, followed by increased rate of cellular hypertrophy due to the increased pressure load. The combination of both increased number of cells and increased cell size may result in very large hearts in this and other forms of congenital heart disease.

Increased Systemic or Pulmonary Vascular Resistance

In the fetus, pulmonary vascular resistance is normally high, with blood shunted through the ductus arteriosus. Since both ventricles face approximately equal pressure, left and right ventricular masses are normally approximately equal in the fetus. There are few documented cases of fetal increased systemic vascular resistance. SHR may represent such a case, since increased femoral artery pressures relative to those in normotensive rat strains have been found at birth. This is discussed in more detail below.

Complex Anomalies

Other anomalies such as tetralogy of Fallot, which involve both outflow resistance and abnormal development or failure of normal closure of structures, result in complex effects on the myocardium. Many possible combinations of cardiac enlargement are possible which are beyond the scope of this chapter to discuss.

Preload or Volume Overload

Increased volume of blood may be shunted through one chamber in the fetus owing to flow obstruction in other chambers as described above. Valve abnormalities resulting in insufficiency, such as the cleft anterior mitral valve leaflet in A-V cushion defect, result in left ventricular regurgitant flow and volume overload, even in the fetal period. Others, such as a persistent atrial septal defect, will result in overload only after birth and may not produce signs until late in life, if ever.

The increased blood pumped by the overloaded chamber causes the chamber to dilate at end diastole to accommodate the increased volume. However, most volume overload situations are manifested only after birth owing to failure of closure of a structure normally open in the fetus.

Extracardiac Shunts

Failure of closure of the ductus arteriosus or the persistence of an aortic to pulmonary artery window causes changes only after birth since the ductus is normally patent in the fetus. Patent ductus arteriosus may be associated with two types of flow abnormalities: (a) flow from aorta to pulmonary artery (left to right) occurs when pulmonary vascular resistance drops normally after birth; (b) if pulmonary vascular resistance fails to drop after birth or becomes secondarily increased owing to large volume flow or other factors, flow then is right to left through the ductus. The introduction of poorly oxygenated blood into the distal thoracic aorta often produces cyanotic changes in the caudal portions of the body.

In left-to-right shunt, very large volumes may be pumped by the left ventricle to accommodate the runoff to the pulmonary vascular low-resistance system. Dilation and hypertrophy of the left ventricle may be massive. In right-to-left shunt, the predominant change is right ventricular hypertrophy due to pressure load on the right ventricle equal to or greater than systemic pressure.

Intracardiac Shunts

Failure of closure of developmental structures such as the ostium secundum, ostium primum, or ventricular septum causes abnormal flow between chambers after birth, which is proportional to the size of the defect and the pressure differential across the defect. Ventricular septal defects tend to cause hypertrophy of both ventricles whereas atrial septal defects cause hypertrophy of only the right ventricle.

Reduced Oxygen-Carrying Capacity of Blood

Chronic anemia and carbon monoxide exposure are examples of conditions that result in reduced oxygen-carrying capacity of the blood. Therefore, larger volumes of blood must be delivered to the tissues to supply sufficient oxygen to meet metabolic needs. Cardiac output is greatly increased, partly owing to increased heart rate and partly to increased stroke volume. The ventricular chambers are dilated and there is increased myocardial mass in chronic states.

During the neonatal period, exposure to carbon monoxide or development of iron deficiency anemia produces marked cardiac enlargement resulting from cellular hypertrophy and hyperplasia. Iron deficiency anemia in weanling rats has previously been reported to stimulate myocyte hyperplasia, as demonstrated by tritiated thymidine autoradiography (84). Rats exposed to 200 or 500 ppm carbon monoxide from birth to 30 days of age have increased cell numbers compared with animals reared in air, as determined by cardiac weight and cell volume determined on enzymatically prepared isolated myocytes (*unpublished observation*). Similar conditions producing reduced oxygen-carrying capacity of blood in adult animals result in cardiac hypertrophy and dilation, but there is no hyperplastic response.

Increased Metabolic Activity

Hyperthyroidism is the most commonly studied example of increased metabolic activity which results in cardiac hypertrophy. Increased serum level of T4 or 3,5,3'-triiodothyronine (T3) results in a hypermetabolic rate of all body tissues, requiring increased oxygen delivery to meet these needs. The resulting increased cardiac output causes a volume load on the heart in addition to probable direct actions of

T3 on promotion of protein synthesis in myocardium. The increased energy requirements of heart tissue are reflected by an increase in mitochondrial volume percent composition of hyperthyroid hearts (77). The increased myocyte volume in hyperthyroidism is not accompanied by increased connective tissue, and the muscle mass rapidly returns to normal when T3 is removed (9,121).

Neonatal animals exposed from birth to increased T3 develop significant cardiac hypertrophy, but only a mild increase in heart rate, compared with the relatively large heart rate increase found in adult hyperthyroid rats (41). Isolated myocytes were used to determine cell volume, cell length, and to calculate cell number in normal and hyperthyroid 12-day-old rats given T4 injections from birth. Cell number is increased at 12 days of age and cell volume is increased, indicating that both hypertrophy and hyperplasia occurred with this model. Cell volume was increased principally because of increased cell length, rather than because of increased cross-sectional area. The increased cell length in hypertrophied neonatal myocytes of T4 treated animals, particularly in the absence of proportional heart rate increase, suggests that the neonatal growing myocyte is molded by the hemodynamic load into longer cells to accommodate increased end-diastolic volume. The increased cell number and remodeling of cell shape may have importance in the heart's ability to respond to overload in later life.

Cardiomyopathy

There are numerous specific substances or conditions that are known to have a direct effect on the myocardium. When cardiac hypertrophy with or without dilation is associated with such a substance, the name of the substance is linked with the general term "cardiomyopathy"; e.g., alcoholic, cobalt, adriamycin, viral, or ischemic cardiomyopathy; the specific mechanism of action is usually not understood. When no specific cause for cardiac disease can be identified, the term cardiomyopathy alone is used to designate the condition. That is, the diagnosis is made by exclusion of all other known causes.

Cardiomyopathies of various known or unknown origins are further classified as hypertrophic, dilated or restrictive; the dilated form virtually always has hypertrophy present.

The hypertrophic form of cardiomyopathy may or may not be accompanied by outflow tract obstruction of the left ventricle, the chamber most commonly affected. Specific examples of several cardiomyopathies are discussed in the next section and in other chapters in this volume. The usual outcome of most types of cardiomyopathy is progressive deterioration of myocardial function leading to fatal congestive heart failure.

SELECTED ANIMAL MODELS OF CONGENITAL CARDIAC HYPERTROPHY AND CARDIOMYOPATHY

The purpose of this section is to review specific anatomic features of selected hypertrophic myocardial diseases. Particular attention will be given to naturally occurring and experimental animal models available to study the human disease.

Stenosis of the Pulmonic Outflow Tract Region

Isolated lesions of the pulmonary outflow tract may be valvular, infundibular (subvalvular), or supravalvular in location. Valve lesions are the most common and are due to defective cusp formation with fusion and thickening of the cusps. Infundibular lesions usually are fibrous or muscular rings located in the outflow tract below the valve. Supravalvular lesions may be anywhere from just distal to the valve to the terminal pulmonary artery branches. In all cases, right ventricular hypertrophy is the prominent feature with variable degrees of left ventricular enlargement, depending on the severity of stenosis, whether stenosis was present during the fetal period, and on the presence or absence of other associated anomalies.

Stenotic lesions of the pulmonary outflow tract region occur as congenital lesions in dogs (89,90) and cats (127), but have been more thoroughly studied in the dog (92). Pulmonic valve lesions are most frequent, followed by fibrous thickening of the infundibular outflow tract; supravalvular lesions occur rarely. Planned matings of a family of Beagle dogs at the University of Pennslvania has shown this to be an inherited condition, with valvular and subvalvular forms in varying degrees of severity occurring most frequently in the offspring. In one litter from this colony resulting from mating an affected male with a nonaffected female from a litter with affected siblings, two affected and four normal pups were delivered by Cesarian section. One affected and one normal pup were dead at the time of surgery; the other affected pup lived for a few minutes only and the heart was immediately perfusion fixed with 2% glutaraldehyde. The other three normal pups were perfusion fixed within 12 hr of delivery. Heart and body weights are shown in Table 3. Both affected pups had massive enlargement of the left ventricle, and pup 1 had massive right ventricular enlargement as well. In pup 2, right ventricular free wall weight was normal; there was endocardial fibrosis in the right ventricle of this pup. By electron microscopy, the right and left ventricles of pup 1 had increased folding of the intercalated disc regions and extensive Z-line expansions associated with disrupted sarcomere formation.

Experimental models of pulmonary artery stenosis have been produced by single or repeated banding or implantation of inflatable cuffs in adult and neonatal or weanling animals (12,15,25,67). The degree of stenosis determines whether right ventricular hypertrophy alone develops or if congestive heart failure will also be produced (111). Right ventricular hypertrophy and failure may be produced by single banding in adult cats and rabbits (15,111), but multiple banding or progressive stenosis of inflatable cuffs is required to produce myocardial failure in the dog (12,28). Single-banding models have a serious limitation in that the sudden pressure overload on the ventricle results in multifocal areas of necrosis and replacement fibrosis in the acutely stressed ventricle (15). This results in increased connective tissue content of the ventricle which is an artifact and could produce changes that would obscure the interpretation of functional, biochemical, and structural studies of the hypertrophied ventricle.

TABLE 3. *Heart weights of a litter of beagle dogs including two with pulmonary outflow tract obstruction*

	Body weight (g)	Heart weight (g)	RV free wall weight (g)	LV + septum weight (g)	HW/BW	RV/BW	LV + S/BW	RV/LV+S
Pup 1[a]	240	5.03	2.07	2.50	20.95	8.62	10.41	0.83
Pup 2[b]	220	3.28	0.70	2.24	14.90	3.18	10.18	0.31
Normal (N = 4) mean ± SD	240 ± 16	1.90 ± 0.17	0.72 ± 0.11	0.92 ± 0.10	7.92 ± 0.78	3.00 ± 0.41	3.86 ± 0.59	0.79 ± 0.15

[a] Isolated pulmonic valve stenosis.
[b] Hypoplastic pulmonary artery and RV endocardial fibrosis.
RV = right ventricular free wall; LV + S = left ventricle plus septum.

Banding of the pulmonary artery in neonatal or weanling lambs (4,38), dogs (83), cats (25), and rats (62) produces a gradual increase in right ventricular pressure as the animal increases in size with the fixed stenosis. Greater than 100% increase in right ventricular mass is often produced with this method, but myocardial failure is seldom reported. Since pressure load is present only after intracardiac shunts are closed, left ventricular hypertrophy is absent or mild, in contrast to the massive left ventricular hypertrophy present in naturally occurring congenital pulmonic outflow tract obstruction.

Left Ventricular Outflow Obstruction

In man, congenitally bicuspid aortic valve commonly leads to calcific aortic stenosis in later life, with fixed valve leaflets producing aortic stenosis and insufficiency (104). Other valve malformations occur but are rare. Coarctation of the aorta may occur either proximal or distal to the ductus arteriosus. Subvalvular fibrous ring formation occurs, but is less common than bicuspid aortic valve (30,76). Left ventricular hypertrophy develops in response to the outflow obstruction.

In animals, congenital abnormalities of the aortic valve and coarctation of the aorta are quite rare conditions. Subaortic fibrous ring stenosis, however, is a frequent congenital lesion in dogs (90,97) and also has been reported in cats (127). In the dog, the lesion occurs most frequently in German shepherds, boxers, and Newfoundlands, and has been studied extensively in Newfoundlands, where a definite polygenic genetic basis has been demonstrated (97). The lesion occurs in varying degrees of severity and consists of a well-developed fibrous band that completely encircles the left ventricular outflow tract just below the aortic valve. Left heart failure and sudden death are frequent. There is massive left ventricular hypertrophy with many expanded Z-lines and widened intercalated disc lesions present (107). There is multifocal fibrosis and intimal proliferation of small coronary arteries and arterioles, particularly within the endocardial half of the left ventricle and interventricular septum (Fig. 7) (39).

Experimentally, banding of the aorta at various levels from the arch to the abdominal aorta has been used in many species (7,9,21,26,29,44,82,106). Left ventricular hypertrophy develops as a result of the increased outflow resistance and probable contributions of renal mechanisms, but congestive heart failure is uncommon when bands are placed in adult animals. Banding the aorta of newborn dogs results in progressive aortic stenosis as the animal increases in size, and death due to congestive heart failure develops by 6 to 10 weeks of age (14). The aortic banding models, especially in neonatal animals, provide a useful model for the study of left ventricular hypertrophy similar to that produced by coarctation of the aorta. Study of the hyperplastic versus hypertrophic response of the myocardium in neonatal animals with aortic banding is possible, since the heart muscle cells are still growing by hyperplasia during the first days to weeks after birth, and the pressure load is gradually increasing with normal growth, similar to the situation in congenital

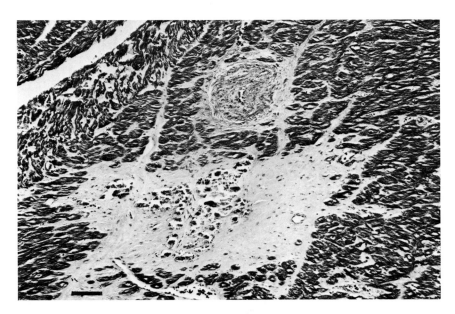

FIG. 7. Photomicrograph of left ventricular myocardium from a 7-month-old dog with congenital subaortic stenosis. There is focal fibrosis with central mineralization and severe intimal smooth-muscle cell proliferation of an adjacent small artery resulting in severe luminal narrowing. These lesions were extensive throughout the inner half of the left ventricular myocardium. H and E stain. Bar = 50 μm.

lesions of man. Spontaneous subaortic stenosis in the dog is a useful model to study the effects of outflow tract obstruction with normal coronary artery perfusion pressure, in contrast to increased coronary perfusion pressure produced by the banding models.

The Spontaneously Hypertensive Rat

The SHR has become one of the most widely used strains of rats to study mechanisms of hypertension in a model not requiring various mechanical, drug, or dietary manipulation. This genetically derived strain was developed in Japan by Okamoto and Aoki (86) by selective sibling matings from an original strain of Wistar rats. The strain was returned to the United States in the 1960s and is readily available from several commercial breeders. Hypertension develops early in this strain with increased systolic pressure compared with normotensive strains, detectable by the tail-cuff method by 4 to 6 weeks of age (109). Cardiac hypertrophy involving both right and left ventricles is present in the neonatal animal (27), indicating an increased pressure load on the heart *in utero*. By several weeks of age, only left ventricular hypertrophy is present, which continues to increase relative to body weight throughout the life-span of the animal (109). Hemodynamic deterioration occurs after 18 months age (96), associated with a marked increase in myocyte cross-sectional area and increased myocardial fibrosis, particularly in the inner half of the myocardial wall. In addition to focal fibrosis, ultrastructural evidence of myocardial failure (pathologic hypertrophy) is found in SHR as widened intercalated discs and Z-line expansion (64).

Hereditary Cardiomyopathy in the Golden Syrian Hamster

A myopathic strain of hamsters (Bio. 1.50) was described by Homberger and associates (51,52) which was derived from inbred lines of *Mesocricetus auratus*. Subsequently, several outbred lines have been developed and are commercially available today (Bio Research Institute, Cambridge, MA). Both cardiac and skeletal muscle are involved with multiple foci of myocytolysis starting at about 30 days of age. In the myocardium, lesions are randomly distributed throughout inner and outer layers of both right and left ventricles. Active lesions are replaced with fibrous connective tissue, and few active lesions are found after 100 days of age. Connective tissue content continues to increase with further healing and there is continuous development of cardiac hypertrophy. Hypertrophy includes both ventricles and eventually leads to ventricular dilation with death due to congestive heart failure in most cases. The specific cause of this cardiomyopathy remains unclear, although there appears to be disturbance of calcium control. Myocardial calcium stores show more than a 10-fold increase during the myocytolytic stage which persists throughout the life-span of the animal (108). Recently, a deficiency of sialyltransferase has been identified in this model (74); the enzyme is required for maintenance of normal basement membrane glycocalyx and control of calcium flux across the plasma membrane. Treatment with calcium antagonistic agents such as verapamil have a potent ameliorating effect on the course of the disease (60).

During the myocytolytic stage, lesions are limited to multifocal areas of myocyte degeneration, necrosis, and replacement with mineralized fibrous connective tissue. In some strains, cardiac hypertrophy may exceed 100% by late in life. In the hypertrophied dilated heart, ultrastructural changes in the intercalated disc and Z-lines as described above are present. These characteristic changes of pathologic hypertrophy make this a good model for study of genetically controlled cardiomyopathy.

Cardiomyopathy of Man, Dog, and Cat

Cardiomyopathies with many similar features occur sporadically in man, dog, and cat. The condition has been most extensively studied in man, but several reports have appeared describing the clinical and pathologic features of cardiomyopathies in animals and comparisons made with the human condition. Cardiomyopathy is usually classified as hypertrophic, either with or without outflow tract obstruction; congestive; or restrictive (105). The hypertrophic type may be symmetrical, in which the left ventricular free wall and septum are uniformly thickened and there is no obstruction to blood flow through the outflow tract. In the obstructive type of hypertrophic cardiomyopathy, the interventricular septum is disproportionately thicker than the free wall by a ratio of 1.3 or greater (33,112). In addition, the anterior leaflet of the mitral valve moves cranially during systole, striking the septum and resulting in fibrous thickening of the endocardium (37). The left ventricular cavity is smaller than normal, there is left atrial dilatation, and there is fibromuscular proliferation with increased medial thickness in small intramuscular coronary arteries. A characteristic feature of hypertrophic cardiomyopathy is myofiber disarray involving the septum, less frequently the left ventricular free wall and right ventricle, and rarely the atria (35). The myofibers are arranged in nonparallel order with adjacent muscle fibers often coursing at sharp angles to each other (Fig. 8). The disarray is even present within individual fibers, with myofibrils within the cell coursing at sharp angles to each other. The obstructive form of cardiomyopathy has been shown to have a familial basis in man (95). In animals no genetic studies have been done, but in cats the hypertrophic cardiomyopathy occurs most commonly in Persian cats (113) and in the dog is more common in German shepherds than in other breeds (72).

The nonobstructive form of cardiomyopathy in man is not characterized by asymmetrical septal hypertrophy, but atrial dilatation and intramyocardial coronary artery lesions are often present (105). These features were also present in dogs (72) and in 50% of cats (117) with hypertrophic cardiomyopathy. In one series of 10 cats with hypertrophic cardiomyopathy (117) none was found to have asymmetrical septal thickening beyond that found in normal cats. However, in another

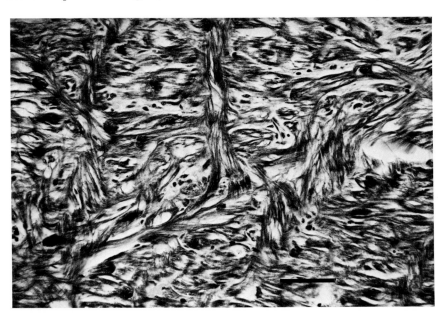

FIG. 8. Left ventricular myocardium from a 12-year-old boy with obstructive hypertrophic cardiomyopathy. Muscle fiber disarray characteristic of this condition is present with fibers coursing at sharp angles to each other. Gomori aldehyde fuchsin trichrome stain. Bar = 50 μm.

series of 27 cats with hypertrophic cardiomyopathy, eight had disproportionate septal thickening with endocardial fibrosis in the outflow tract region at the point of contact with the anterior leaflet of the mitral valve (113). In dogs, both symmetrical and asymmetrical types have been reported (72).

Electron microscopic examination of hypertrophic cardiomyopathy in man (35) and the cat (117) has revealed widening of the intercalated disc due to increased folding and characteristic expansions of Z-line material such as found in pathologic hypertrophy. Hypertrophic cardiomyopathy has not been studied by electron microscopy in the dog. The presence of intercalated disc and Z-line changes in hypertrophic cardiomyopathy lends support to the hypothesis that these changes are indicative of myocardial failure. However, Z-line expansions must be interpreted with caution in the cat, since very similar structures have been reported in the normal cat (34).

The dilated type of cardiomyopathy with congestion occurs in all three species. There is no disproportionate septal thickening, and hypertrophy is often less severe than in the hypertrophic form. All four chambers are often dilated (Fig. 9). There is no muscle fiber disarray, and myofibers often appear thin and wavy. In man there appears to be no genetic association; in the dog the condition is found most commonly in large breeds such as Great Dane, St. Bernard, Doberman, Labrador Retriever, and Irish Setter (72). Ultrastructurally, dense Z-line expansions have been reported in the cat with congestive cardiomyopathy (117), but not in the dog (118).

The restrictive type of cardiomyopathy with endocardial thickening is rare in man and animals. In cats, focal areas of endocardial fibrosis often occur with the congestive type of cardiomyopathy and sometimes may be so extensive as to interfere with normal contraction, thus giving rise to a small subgroup which has been classified as a restrictive type of cardiomyopathy (113). Etiology is unknown.

In summary, the cardiomyopathies of man, dog, and cat have many similarities and provide an intriguing group of conditions with hypertrophy with or without

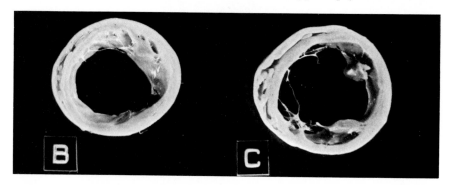

FIG. 9. Cross sections of the ventricles from a cat with congestive cardiomyopathy. There was cardiac hypertrophy with marked dilation of the left ventricle resulting in thinning of the left ventricular wall. Scale = 3.0 cm.

myocardial failure. The hypertrophy appears to be unrelated to either pressure or volume overload, and further investigations into these conditions may provide important clues to the control of myocardial cell enlargement.

Cardiomyopathy of Turkeys

A cardiomyopathy characterized by hypertrophy and dilation occurs sporadically in turkey flocks. By selective breeding, a flock has been developed in which 90% or more of the birds develop congestive failure by about 1 month of age (85). Virus-like particles have been found in the myocardium of affected birds, but a causal relationship has not been shown. There is cardiac hypertrophy with dilation and decreased cardiac output in 34-day-old birds. There is reduced left ventricular shortening fraction, systemic hypotension, and relative subendocardial underperfusion (31,32).

Histologically there is mononuclear cell infiltration associated with focal areas of myocardial necrosis which may be identified even in the embryo (45). Lesions become progressively more severe after hatching. Endocardial fibroelastosis occurs, first in the ventricular outflow tract, then becoming generalized as ventricular dilation develops.

Doxorubicin HCl (Adriamycin) Cardiomyopathy

Numerous compounds are capable of inducing severe and even fatal myocardial damage. Few have claimed more interest or clinical importance than doxorubicin HCl, since this drug has a very broad spectrum of antitumor activity. Clinical usefulness of the drug, however, is limited by a dose-related fatal congestive cardiomyopathy. Extensive clinical monitoring with right ventricular endomyocardial biopsies (10) has led to the development of a grading system useful in evaluating when toxic doses of the drug have been given to an individual. In general, myocardial toxicity appears morphologically when a total body dose of more than 240 mg/m^2 has been given, and the incidence of fatal congestive failure sharply increases when over 500 mg/m^2 is given.

In the human heart, lesions appear first in single cells in the subendomyocardium of the right and left ventricles, later involve clusters of cells, and finally become widely disseminated (22). There is loss of myofibrils and vacuolar formation of sarcoplasmic reticulum; lipid accumulation and dilation of the transverse tubular system also occur. Myocytes become separated from each other and undergo atrophy. The extensive myofibril loss leads to decreased contractile ability of the myocardium with irreversible congestive myocardial failure. Characteristically, lesions of doxorubicin cardiotoxicity progress after the last dose, and congestive failure may develop months later.

In experimental animals, chronic doxorubicin toxicity has been induced in several species including the rabbit (58), dog (116), pig (119), monkey (48), and rat (79), among others. The drug is given intravenously several times weekly over a period of several weeks to months. Similar lesions to those found in man occur in animals, including myofibrillar loss and vacuolization leading to necrosis, fibrosis, and congestive myocardial failure. In rabbits, lesions progress for several weeks after the last dose as in man (59).

The mechanisms of cardiotoxicity of doxorubicin remain unknown. It is known that the drug readily intercalates DNA both *in vitro* and *in vivo*, with blockade of DNA, RNA, and protein synthesis. Other theories have proposed that free radical formation associated with the reduction of doxorubicin to its semiquinone induces damage to myocyte membranes. However, treatment of experimental animals with the antioxidant vitamin E failed to protect against chronic doxorubicin cardiotoxicity (20,116,119). Doxorubicin is taken up into phospholipid membranes and is a strong chelator of divalent cations, both being mechanisms that could contribute to the cardiotoxicity of the drug. These and other possible mechanisms are being actively investigated in several laboratories in an effort to reduce the cardiotoxicity of this powerful antitumor agent.

CONCLUSION

Enlargement of the heart occurs in response to increased hemodynamic load, but other nonhemodynamic factors also appear to play a role. Enlargement of the opposite ventricle to the one facing the load and cardiac enlargement in various cardiomyopathies support the concept of other nonhemodynamic factors participating in the pathogenesis.

Enlargement of the heart appears to be limited to a hypertrophic response of cardiac myocytes if development starts after the early neonatal period. A possible exception is reported hyperplasia in very large human hearts, a thesis that has not been tested in animal models owing to lack of a model with cardiac hypertrophy comparable to that in man. Proliferation of nonmyocyte components of the heart does occur, however.

By way of contrast, in the fetal and neonatal heart, myocyte proliferation is the rule when the heart is exposed to overload. The capacity for myocyte proliferation is retained for several weeks after birth and is a feature of cardiac enlargement, together with hypertrophy, when overload is applied to neonatal animals.

Cardiac hypertrophy in adult animals is associated with reduced coronary blood flow reserve, particularly in the inner myocardial wall regions. This reduced coronary reserve may be influential in the development of myocardial failure. In the fetal and early neonatal animal, however, there appears to be no reduction in coronary blood flow reserve, suggesting that there is proportionate growth of myocytes and the coronary vascular bed during overload induced in this period. Very little is known of coronary blood flow reserves in animal models of cardiomyopathy, but reduced coronary blood flow has been reported in human cardiomyopathy.

During early and functionally compensated stages of cardiac hypertrophy, or physiologic hypertrophy, there are few changes in myocardial ultrastructure. With the gradual progression to a decompensated stage, however, ultrastructural changes in mitochondria, Z-lines, and intercalated discs occur. These changes include decreased mitochondrial volume percent composition of myofibers, deformed and expanded Z-lines suggesting abnormal sarcomere formation, and increased surface area of intercalated discs with increased myofilament attachment areas. These changes are compatible with decreased or altered protein synthesis in the severely hypertrophied myocyte, which may be contributory to development of congestive myocardial failure. The ultrastructural changes provide a morphologic marker for pathologic hypertrophy.

Several naturally occurring and experimental models of cardiac hypertrophy and cardiomyopathy are available for study. Although much information has been obtained characterizing functional, biochemical, and structural features of these conditions, the mechanisms responsible for stimulated growth of the heart await further investigation.

ACKNOWLEDGMENTS

This work was supported in part by a grant from the Alabama Heart Association and by National Heart, Lung, and Blood Institute grants RO1HL 23255, Ischemic Heart Disease SCOR P17HL 17667, and Hypertension SCOR P50HL 25451. The author would like to acknowledge the expert assistance of Irene Lynn in the preparation of this manuscript.

REFERENCES

1. Anversa, P., Loud, A. V., and Vitali-Mazza, L. (1976): Morphometry and autoradiography of early hypertrophic changes in the ventricular myocardium of adult rat. An electron microscopic study. *Lab. Invest.*, 35:475–483.
2. Anversa, P., Loud, A. V., Giacomelli, F., and Wiener, J. (1978): Absolute morphometric study of myocardial hypertrophy in experimental hypertension. II. Ultrastructure of myocytes and interstitium. *Lab. Invest.*, 38:597–609.
3. Arai, S., Machida, A., and Nakamura, T. (1968): Myocardial structure and vascularization of hypertrophied hearts. *Tohoku J. Exp. Med.*, 95:35–54.
4. Archie, J. P., Fixler, D. E., Ullyot, D. J., Buckberg, G. D., and Hoffman, J. I. E. (1974): Regional myocardial blood flow in lambs with concentric right ventricular hypertrophy. *Circ. Res.*, 34:143–154.
5. Ashley, L. M. (1945): A determination of the diameters of ventricular myocardial fibers in man and other mammals. *Am. J. Anat.*, 77:325–363.
6. Astorri, E., Bolognesi, R., Colla, B., Chizzola, A., and Visioli, O. (1977): Left ventricular hypertrophy: a cytometric study on 42 human hearts. *J. Mol. Cell. Cardiol.*, 9:763–775.
7. Bache, R. J., Vrobel, T. R., Ring, W. S., Emery, R. W., and Andersen, R. W. (1981): Regional myocardial blood flow during exercise in dogs with chronic left ventricular hypertrophy. *Circ. Res.*, 48:76–87.
8. Bajusz, E., Homburger, F., Baker, J. R., and Opie, L. H. (1966): The heart muscle in muscular dystrophy with special reference to involvement of the cardiovascular system in the hereditary myopathy of the hamster. *Ann. NY Acad. Sci.*, 138:213–231.
9. Bartosova, D., Chvapil, M., Korecky, B. Poupa, O., Rakusan, K., Turek, Z., and Vizek, M. (1969): The growth of the muscular and collagenous parts of the rat heart in various forms of cardiomegaly. *J. Physiol. (Lond).*, 200:285–295.
10. Billingham, M. E., Mason, J. W., Bristow, M. R., and Daniels, J. R. (1978): Anthracycline cardiomyopathy monitored by morphologic changes. *Cancer Treat. Rep.*, 62:865–872.
11. Bishop, S. P., and Cole, C. R. (1969): Ultrastructural changes in canine myocardium with right ventricular hypertrophy and congestive heart failure. *Lab. Invest.*, 20:219–229.

12. Bishop, S. P., and Cole, C. R. (1969): Production of externally controlled progressive pulmonic stenosis in the dog. *J. Appl. Physiol.*, 26:659–663.
13. Bishop, S. P. (1972): Structural alterations of myocardium induced by chronic work overload. In: *Advances in Experimental Medicine and Biology, Comparative Pathophysiology of Circulatory Disturbances*, edited by C. M. Bloor, pp. 289–314. Plenum Press, New York.
14. Bishop, S. P. (1973): Effect of aortic stenosis on myocardial cell growth, hyperplasia, and ultrastructure in neonatal dogs. In: *Recent Advances in Studies on Cardiac Structure and Metabolism: Myocardial Metabolism*, edited by N. S. Dhalla, 3:637–656. University Park Press, Baltimore.
15. Bishop, S. P., and Melsen, L. R. (1976): Myocardial necrosis, fibrosis and DNA synthesis in experimental cardiac hypertrophy induced by sudden pressure overload. *Circ. Res.*, 39:238–245.
16. Bishop, S. P., Oparil, S., Reynolds, R. H., and Drummond, J. L. (1979): Regional myocyte size in normotensive and spontaneously hypertensive rats. *Hypertension*, 1:378–383.
17. Bishop, S. P., Dillon, D., Naftilan, J., and Reynolds, R. (1980): Surface morphology of isolated cardiac myocytes from hypertrophied hearts of aging spontaneously hypertensive rats. *Scan. Electron Microsc.*, 2:193–199.
18. Bishop, S. P. (1983): Ultrastructure of the myocardium in physiologic and pathologic hypertrophy in experimental animals. In: *Perspectives in Cardiovascular Research, Vol. 7. Myocardial Hypertrophy and Failure*, edited by N. R. Alpert, pp. 127–147. Raven Press, New York.
19. Blumgart, H., Gilligan, D. R., and Schlesinger, M. J. (1940): The degree of myocardial fibrosis in normal and pathological hearts as estimated chemically by the collagen content. *Trans. Assoc. Am. Physicians*, 55:313–315.
20. Breed, J. G. S., Zimmerman, A. N. E., Dormans, J. A. M. A., and Pinedo, H. M. (1980): Failure of the antioxidant vitamin E to protect against adriamycin-induced cardiotoxicity in the rabbit. *Cancer Res.*, 40:2033–2038.
21. Breisch, E. A., Houser, S. R., Carey, R. A., Spann, J. F., and Bove, A. A. (1980): Myocardial blood flow and capillary density in chronic pressure overload of the feline left ventricle. *Cardiovasc. Res.*, 14:469–475.
22. Buja, L. M., Ferrans, V. J., Mayer, R. J., Roberts, W. C., and Henderson, E. S. (1973): Cardiac ultrastructural changes induced by daunorubicin therapy. *Cancer*, 32:771–788.
23. Busch, W. A., Stromer, M. H., Goll, D. E., and Suzuki, A. (1972): Ca^{24+} specific removal of Z-lines from rabbit skeletal muscle. *J. Cell Biol.*, 52:367–381.
24. Challice, C. E. (1969): Microstructure of "specialized" tissues in the mammalian heart. *Ann. NY Acad. Sci.*, 156:14–33.
25. Cooper, G., IV, Tomanek, R. J., Ehrhardt, J. C., and Marcus, M. L. (1981): Chronic progressive pressure overload of the cat right ventricle. *Circ. Res.*, 48:488–497.
26. Cutilletta, A. F., Dowell, R. T., Rudnik, M., Arcilla, R. A., and Zak, R. (1975): Regression of myocardial hypertrophy. I. Experimental model, changes in heart weight, nucleic acids and collagen. *J. Mol. Cell. Cardiol.*, 7:767–781.
27. Cutilletta, A. F., Benjamin, M., Culpepper, W. S., and Oparil, S. (1978): Myocardial hypertrophy and ventricular performance in the absence of hypertension in spontaneously hypertensive rats. *J. Mol. Cell. Cardiol.*, 10:689–703.
28. Davis, J. O., Hyatt, R. E., and Howell, D. S. (1955): Right-sided congestive heart failure in dogs produced by controlled progressive constrictions of the pulmonary artery. *Circ. Res.*, 3:252–258.
29. Dowell, R. T., and McManus, R. E., III (1978): Pressure-induced cardiac enlargement in neonatal and adult rats: left ventricular functional characteristics and evidence of cardiac muscle cell proliferation in the neonate. *Circ. Res.*, 42:303–310.
30. Edwards, J. E. (1965): Pathology of left ventricular outflow tract obstruction. *Circulation*, 31:586–599.
31. Einzig, S., Jankus, E. F., and Moller, J. H. (1972): Round heart disease in turkeys: a hemodynamic study. *Am. J. Vet. Res.*, 33:557–561.
32. Einzig, S., Staley, N. A., Mettler, E., Nicoloff, D. M., and Noren, G. R. (1980): Regional myocardial blood flow and cardiac function in a naturally occurring congestive cardiomyopathy of turkeys. *Cardiovasc. Res.*, 14:396–407.
33. Epstein, S. E., Henry, W. L., Clark, C. E., Roberts, W. C., Maron, B. J., Ferrans, V. J., Redwood, D. R., and Morrow, A. G. (1974): Asymmetric septal hypertrophy. *Ann. Intern. Med.*, 81:650–680.
34. Fawcett, D. W. (1968): The sporadic occurrence in cardiac muscle of anomalous Z-bands exhibiting a periodic structure suggestive of tropomyosin. *J. Cell Biol.*, 36:266–270.

35. Ferrans, V. J., Morrow, A. G., and Roberts, W. C. (1972): Myocardial ultrastructure in idiopathic hypertrophic subaortic stenosis. *Circulation*, 45:769–792.
36. Ferrans, V. J., Jones, M., Maron, B. J., and Roberts, W. C. (1975): The nuclear membranes in hypertrophied human cardiac muscle cells. *Am. J. Pathol.*, 78:427–460.
37. Ferrans, V. J., Muna, W. F. T., Jones, M., and Roberts, W. C. (1978): Ultrastructure of the fibrous ring in patients with discrete subaortic stenosis. *Lab. Invest.*, 39:30–40.
38. Fishman, N. H., Hof, R. B., Rudolph, A. M., and Heymann, M. A. (1978): Models of congenital heart disease in fetal lambs. *Circulation*, 58:354–364.
39. Flickinger, G. L., and Patterson, D. F. (1967): Coronary lesions associated with congenital subaortic stenosis in the dog. *J. Path. Bact.*, 93:133–140.
40. Fuster, V., Danielson, M. A., Broadbent, J. C., Brown, A. L., Jr., and Elveback, L. R. (1977): Quantitation of left ventricular myocardial fiber hypertrophy and interstitial tissue in human hearts with chronically increased volume and pressure overload. *Circulation*, 55:504–508.
41. Gerdes, A. M., Kriseman, J., and Bishop, S. P. (1983): Changes in myocardial cell size and number during the development and reversal of hyperthyroidism in neonatal rats. *Lab. Invest.*, 48:598–602.
42. Gerdes, A. M., Kriseman, J., and Bishop, S. P. (1982): Morphometric study of cardiac muscle: the problem of tissue shrinkage. *Lab. Invest.*, 46:271–274.
43. Gerstenblith, G., Lakatta, E. G., and Weisfeldt, M. L. (1976): Age changes in myocardial function and exercise response. *Prog. Cardiovasc. Dis.*, 19:1–21.
44. Goldstein, M. A., Sordahl, L. A., and Schwartz, A. (1974): Ultrastructural analysis of left ventricular hypertrophy in rabbits. *J. Mol. Cell. Cardiol.*, 6:265–273.
45. Gough, A. W., Pinn, S., Hulland, T. J., Thomson, R. G., and De la Iglesia, F. (1981): Spontaneous cardiomyopathy: histopathologic and ultrastructural alterations of turkey heart tissue. *Am. J. Vet. Res.*, 42:1290–1297.
46. Grove, D., Zak, R., Nair, K. G., and Aschenbrenner, V. (1969): Biochemical correlates of cardiac hypertrophy: IV. Observations on the cellular organization of growth during myocardial hypertrophy in the rat. *Circ. Res.*, 25:473–485.
47. Hatt, P. Y., Berjal, G., Moravec, J., and Swynghedauw, B. (1970): Heart failure: an electron microscopic study of the left ventricular papillary muscle in aortic insufficiency in the rabbit. *J. Mol. Cell. Cardiol.*, 1:235–247.
48. Herman, E., Mhatre, R., Lee, I. P., Vick, J., and Waravdekar, V. S. (1971): A comparison of the cardiovascular actions of daunomycin, adriamycin and N-acetyldaunomycin in hamsters and monkeys. *Pharmacology (Basel)*, 6:230–241.
49. Hoffman, J. I. E., and Buckberg, G. D. (1978): The myocardial supply: demand ratio—a critical review. *Am. J. Cardiol.*, 41:327–332.
50. Holtz, J., vonRestorff, W., Bard, P., and Bassenge, E. (1977): Transmural distribution of myocardial blood flow and of coronary reserve in canine left ventricular hypertrophy. *Basic Res. Cardiol.*, 72:286–292.
51. Homburger, F., Baker, J. R., Nixon, C. W., and Wilgram, G. (1962): New hereditary disease of Syrian hamsters. Primary, generalized polymyopathy and cardiac necrosis. *Arch. Intern. Med.*, 110:660–662.
52. Homburger, F., Baker, J. R., Wilgram, G. F., Caulfield, J. B., and Nixon, C. W. (1966): Hereditary dystrophy-like myopathy: the histopathology of hereditary dystrophy-like myopathy in Syrian hamsters. *Arch. Pathol.*, 81:302–307.
53. Honig, C. R., and Odoroff, C. L. (1981): Calculated dispersion of capillary transit times: significance for oxygen exchange. *Am. J. Physiol.*, 240:H199–H208.
54. Hopkins, S. F., Jr., McCutcheon, E. P., and Wekstein, D. R. (1973): Postnatal changes in rat ventricular function. *Circ. Res.*, 32:685–691.
55. Hort, W. (1953): Quantitative histologische Untersuchungen an wachsenden Herzen. *Virchows Arch.*, 323:223–242.
56. Hort, W. (1966): The normal heart of the fetus and its metamorphosis in the transitional period. In: *Heart and Circulation in the Newborn and Infant*, edited by D. E. Cassels, pp. 210–224. Grune and Stratton, New York.
57. Hutchins, G. M., Bulkley, B. H., Miner, M. M., and Boitnott, J. K. (1977): Correlation of age and heart weight with tortuosity and caliber of normal human coronary arteries. *Am. Heart J.*, 94:196–202.

58. Jaenke, R. S. (1974): An anthracycline antibiotic-induced cardiomyopathy in rabbits. *Lab. Invest.*, 30:292–304.
59. Jaenke, R. S. (1976): Delayed and progressive myocardial lesions after adriamycin administration in the rabbit. *Cancer Res.*, 36:2958–2966.
60. Jasmin, G., and Solymoss, B. (1975): Prevention of hereditary cardiomyopathy in the hamster by verapamil and other agents. *Proc. Soc. Exper. Biol. Med.*, 149:193–198.
61. Johnson, L. L., Sciacca, R. R., Ellis, K., Weiss, M. B., and Cannon, P. J. (1978): Reduced left ventricular myocardial blood flow per unit mass in aortic stenosis. *Circulation*, 57:582–590.
62. Julian, F. J., Morgan, D. L., Moss, R. L., Gonzalez, M., and Dwivedi, P. (1981): Myocyte growth without physiological impairment in gradually induced rat cardiac hypertrophy. *Circ. Res.*, 49:1300–1310.
63. Karsner, H. T., Saphir, O., and Todd, T. W. (1925): The state of the cardiac muscle in hypertrophy and atrophy. *Am. J. Pathol.*, 1:351–372.
64. Kawamura, K., Kashii, C., and Imamura, K. (1976): Ultrastructural changes in hypertrophied myocardium of spontaneously hypertensive rats. *Jpn. Circ. J.*, 40:1119–1145.
65. Koide, T., and Ozeki, K. (1971): Increased amino acid transport in experimentally hypertrophied rat heart. *Jpn. Heart J.*, 12:177–184.
66. Korecky, B., and Rakusan, K. (1978): Normal and hypertrophic growth of the rat heart. Changes in cell dimensions and number. *Am. J. Physiol.*, 234:H123–128.
67. Laks, M. M., Morady, F., and Swan, H. J. C. (1969): Canine right and left ventricular cell and sarcomere lengths after banding the pulmonary artery. *Circ. Res.*, 24:705–710.
68. Laks, M. M., Morady, F., Adomian, G. E., and Swan, H. J. C. (1970): Presence of widened and multiple intercalated discs in the hypertrophied canine heart. *Circ. Res.*, 27:391–402.
69. Legato, M. J. (1970): Sarcomerogenesis in human myocardium. *J. Mol. Cell. Cardiol.*, 1:425–437.
70. Lewis, A. B., Heymann, M. A., Stanger, P., Hoffman, J. I. E., and Rudolph, A. M. (1974): Evaluation of subendocardial ischemia in valvar aortic stenosis in children. *Circulation*, 49:978–984.
71. Linzbach, A. J. (1960): Heart failure from the point of view of quantitative anatomy. *Am. J. Cardiol.*, 5:370–382.
72. Liu, S. K., and Tilley, L. P. (1980): Animal models of primary myocardial diseases. *Yale J. Biol. Med.*, 53:191–211.
73. Lowensohn, H. S., Khouri, E. M., Gregg, D. E., Pyle, R. L., and Patterson, R. E. (1976): Phasic right coronary artery blood flow in conscious dogs with normal and elevated right ventricular pressures. *Circ. Res.*, 39:760–766.
74. Ma, T. S., Baker, J. C., and Bailey, L. E. (1979): Excitation-contraction coupling in normal and myopathic hamster hearts. III: Functional deficiencies in interstitial glycoproteins. *Cardiovasc. Res.*, 13:568–577.
75. Maron, B. J., Ferrans, V. J., and Roberts, W. C. (1975): Ultrastructural features of degenerated cardiac muscle cells in patients with cardiac hypertrophy. *Am. J. Pathol.*, 79:387–434.
76. Maron, B. J., Redwood, D. R., Roberts, W. C., Henry, W. L., Morrow, A. G., and Epstein, S. E. (1976): Tunnel subaortic stenosis: left ventricular outflow tract obstruction produced by fibromuscular tubular narrowing. *Circulation*, 54:404–416.
77. McCallister, L. P., and Page, E. (1973): Effects of thyroxin on ultrastructure of rat myocardial cells: a stereological study. *J. Ultrastruct. Res.*, 42:136–155.
78. Meerson, F. Z., Zaletayeva, T. A., Lagutchev, S. S., and Pshennikova, M. G. (1964): Structure and mass of mitochondria in the process of compensatory hyperfunction and hypertrophy of the heart. *Exp. Cell. Res.*, 36:568–578.
79. Mettler, F. P., Young, D. M., and Ward, J. M. (1977): Adriamycin-induced cardiotoxicity (cardiomyopathy and congestive heart failure) in rats. *Cancer Res.*, 37:2705–2713.
80. Montfort, I., and Perez-Tamayo, R. (1962): The muscle collagen ratio in normal and hypertrophic human hearts. *Lab. Invest.*, 11:463–470.
81. Morkin, E., and Ashford, T. P. (1968): Myocardial DNA synthesis in experimental cardiac hypertrophy. *Am. J. Physiol.*, 215:1409–1413.
82. Morkin, E., Kimata, S., and Skillman, J. J. (1972): Myosin synthesis and degradation during development of cardiac hypertrophy in the rabbit. *Circ. Res.*, 30:690–702.
83. Murray, P. A., and Vatner, S. F. (1981): Reduction of maximal coronary vasodilator capacity in conscious dogs with severe right ventricular hypertrophy. *Circ. Res.*, 48:25–33.

84. Neffgen, J. F., and Korecky, B. (1972): Cellular hyperplasia and hypertrophy in cardiomegalies induced by anemia in young and adult rats. *Circ. Res.*, 30:104–113.

85. Noren, G. R., Staley, N. A., Jankus, E. F., and Stevenson, J. E. (1971): Myocarditis in round heart disease of turkeys. A light and electron microscopic study. *Virchows Arch. (Pathol. Anat.)*, 352:285–295.

86. Okamoto, K., and Aoki, K. (1963): Development of a strain of spontaneously hypertensive rats. *Jpn. Circ. J.*, 27:282–293.

87. Oken, D. E., and Boucek, R. J. (1957): Quantitation of collagen in human myocardium. *Circ. Res.*, 5:357–361.

88. Patterson, D. F., Pyle, R. L., Buchanan, J. W., Trautvetter, E., and Abt, D. A. (1971): Hereditary patent ductus arteriosus and its sequelae in the dog. *Circ. Res.*, 29:1–13.

89. Patterson, D. F. (1971): Canine congenital heart disease: epidemiology and etiological hypotheses. *J. Small Anim. Pract.*, 12:263–287.

90. Patterson, D. F., Pyle, R. L., and Buchanan, J. W. (1972): Hereditary cardiovascular malformations of the dog. In: *Birth Defects: Orig. Art. Ser., Part XV, The Cardiovascular System*, edited by D. Bergsma, 8:160–174. Williams and Wilkins Co., Baltimore.

91. Patterson, D. F., Pyle, R. L., VanMierop, L., Melbin, J., and Olson, M. (1974): Hereditary defects of the conotruncal septum in Keeshond dogs: pathologic and genetic studies. *Am. J. Cardiol.*, 34:187–205.

92. Patterson, D. F. (1976): Congenital defects of the cardiovascular system of dogs: studies in comparative cardiology. *Adv. Vet. Sci. Comp. Med.*, 20:1–37.

93. Pearlman, E. S., Weber, K. T., Janicki, J. S., Pietra, G. G., and Fishman, A. P. (1982): Muscle fiber orientation and connective tissue content in the hypertrophied human heart. *Lab. Invest.*, 46:158–164.

94. Penney, D., Benjamin, M., and Dunham, E. (1974): Effect of carbon monoxide on cardiac weight as compared with altitude effects. *J. Appl. Physiol.*, 37:80–84.

95. Perloff, J. K. (1981): Pathogenesis of hypertrophic cardiomyopathy: hypotheses and speculations. *Am. Heart J.*, 101:219–226.

96. Pfeffer, J., Pfeffer, M., Fletcher, P., and Braunwald, E. (1979): Alterations of cardiac performance in rats with established spontaneous hypertension. *Am. J. Cardiol.*, 44:994–998.

97. Pyle, R. L., Patterson, D. F., and Chacko, S. (1976): The genetics and pathology of discrete subaortic stenosis in the Newfoundland dog. *Am. Heart J.*, 92:324–334.

98. Rakusan, K., and Poupa, O. (1966): Differences in capillary supply of hypertrophic and hyperplastic heart. *Cardiologia*, 49:293–298.

99. Rakusan, K., deRochemont, W. M., Braasch, W., Tschopp, H., and Bing, R. J. (1967): Capacity of the terminal vascular bed during normal growth, in cardiomegaly, and in cardiac atrophy. *Circ. Res.*, 21:209–215.

100. Rakusan, K., Moravec, J., and Hatt, P. Y. (1980): Regional capillary supply in the normal and hypertrophied rat heart. *Microvasc. Res.*, 20:319–326.

101. Reddy, M. K., Etlinger, J. D., Rabinowitz, M., Fischman, D. A., and Zak, R. (1975): Removal of Z-lines and α-actinin from isolated myofibrils by a calcium-activated neutral protease. *J. Biol. Chem.*, 250:4278–4284.

102. Rembert, J. C., Kleinman, L. H., Fedor, J. M., Wechsler, A. S., and Greenfield, J. C. (1978): Myocardial blood flow distribution in concentric left ventricular hypertrophy. *J. Clin. Invest.*, 62:379–386.

103. Roberts, J. T., and Wearn, J. T. (1941): Quantitative changes in the capillary muscle relationship in human hearts during normal growth and hypertrophy. *Am. Heart J.*, 21:617–633.

104. Roberts, W. C. (1970): The congenitally bicuspid aortic valve. A study of 85 autopsy cases. *Am. J. Cardiol.*, 26:72–83.

105. Roberts, W. C., and Ferrans, V. J. (1975): Pathologic anatomy of the cardiomyopathies. Idiopathic dilated and hypertrophic types, infiltrative types and endomyocardial disease with and without eosinophilia. *Hum. Pathol.*, 61:287–342.

106. Rogers, W. A., Bishop, S. P., and Hamlin, R. L. (1971): Experimental production of supravalvular aortic stenosis in the dog. *J. Appl. Physiol.*, 30:917–920.

107. Schaper, J., Thiedemann, K. U., Flameng, W., and Schaper, W. (1974): The ultrastructure of sarcomeres in hypertrophied canine myocardium in spontaneous subaortic stenosis. *Basic Res. Cardiol.*, 69:509–515.

108. Schwartz, A., Sordahl, L. A., Crow, C. A., McCollum, W. B., Harigaya, S., and Bajusz, E.

(1972): Several biochemical characteristics of the cardiomyopathic Syrian hamster. In: *Recent Advances in Studies of Cardiac Structure and Metabolism*, edited by E. Bajusz and G. Rona, 1:235–242. University Park Press, Baltimore.

109. Sen, S., Tarazi, R. C., Khairallah, P. A., and Bumpus, F. M. (1974): Cardiac hypertrophy in spontaneously hypertensive rats. *Circ. Res.*, 35:775–781.
110. Shipley, R. A., Shipley, L. J., and Wearn, J. T. (1937): The capillary supply in normal and hypertrophied hearts of rabbits. *J. Exp. Med.*, 65:29–42.
111. Spann, J. F., Jr., Buccino, R. A., and Sonnenblick, E. H. (1967): Production of right ventricular hypertrophy with and without congestive heart failure in the cat. *Proc. Soc. Exp. Biol. Med.*, 125:522–524.
112. Teare, D. (1958): Asymmetrical hypertrophy of the heart in young adults. *Br. Heart J.*, 20:1–8.
113. Tilley, L. P., Liu, S. K., Gilbertson, S. R., Wagner, B. M., and Lord, P. F. (1977): Primary myocardial disease in the cat: A model for human cardiomyopathy. *Am. J. Pathol.*, 86:493–522.
114. Turek, Z., Grandtner, M., and Kreuzer, F. (1972): Cardiac hypertrophy, capillary and muscle fiber density, muscle fiber diameter, capillary radius and diffusion distance in the myocardium of growing rats adapted to a simulated altitude of 3500 m. *Pfluegers Arch.*, 355:19–28.
115. Urthaler, F., Walker, A. A., Kawamura, K., Hefner, L. L., and James, T. N. (1978): Canine atrial and ventricular muscle mechanics studied as a function of age. *Circ. Res.*, 42:703–713.
116. VanVleet, J. F., Ferrans, V. J., and Weirich, W. E. (1980): Cardiac disease induced by chronic adriamycin administration in dogs and an evaluation of vitamin E and selenium as cardioprotectants. *Am. J. Pathol.*, 99:13–41.
117. VanVleet, J. F., Ferrans, V. J., and Weirich, W. E. (1980): Pathologic alterations in hypertrophic and congestive cardiomyopathy of cats. *Am. J. Vet. Res.*, 41:2037–2048.
118. VanVleet, J. F., Ferrans, V. J., and Weirich, W. E. (1981): Pathologic alterations in congestive cardiomyopathy of dogs. *Am. J. Vet. Res.*, 42:416–424.
119. VanVleet, J. F., Greenwood, L. A., and Rebar, A. H. (1981): Effect of selenium-vitamin E on hematologic alterations of adriamycin toxicosis in young pigs. *Am. J. Vet. Res.*, 42:1153–1159.
120. Viragh, S., and Challice, C. E. (1969): Variations in filamentous and fibrillar organization, and associated sarcolemmal structures, in cells of the normal mammalian heart. *J. Ultrastruct. Res.*, 28:321–334.
121. Edgnen, J., VonKnorring, J., Lindy, S., and Turto, H. (1976): Heart volume and myocardial connective tissues during development and regression of thyroxine-induced cardiac hypertrophy in rats. *Acta Physiol. Scand.*, 97:514–518.
122. Wearn, J. T. (1928): The extent of the capillary bed of the heart. *J. Exp. Med.*, 47:273–292.
123. Wearn, J. T. (1940): Morphological and functional alterations of the coronary circulation. *Harvey Lec.*, 243–270.
124. Weiss, M. B., Ellis, K., Sciacca, R. R., Johnson, L. L., Schmidt, D. H., and Cannon, P. J. (1976): Myocardial blood flow in congestive and hypertrophic cardiomyopathy. *Circulation*, 54:484–494.
125. Winkler, B., Schaper, J., and Thiedemann, K-U. (1977): Hypertrophy due to chronic volume overloading in the dog heart. A morphometric study. *Basic Res. Cardiol.*, 72:222–227.
126. Yamaguchi, M., Robson, R. M., Stromer, M. H., Dahl, D. S., and Oda, T. (1978): Actin filaments form the backbone of nemaline myopathy rods. *Nature*, 271:265–267.
127. Zook, B. C. (1974): Same spontaneous cardiovascular lesions in dogs and cats. Comparative pathology of the heart. *Adv. Cardiol.*, 13:148–168.

Growth of the Heart in Health and Disease,
edited by Radovan Zak. Raven Press,
New York © 1984.

Cardiac Hypertrophy and Hypertension

Suzanne Oparil

Department of Medicine, University of Alabama, Birmingham,
Birmingham, Alabama 35294

Cardiac enlargement was known to be a feature of hypertensive disease long before routine measurement of systemic arterial pressure was possible. Bright described marked left ventricular hypertrophy unassociated with valvular disease or other known organic cause in patients with proteinuria and small contracted kidneys (15). He further observed a correlation between the extent of hypertrophy and the apparent severity of the renal disease:

> It is observable that the hypertrophy of the heart seems, in some degree, to have kept pace with the advance of disease in the kidneys; for in by far the majority of cases, where the muscular power of the heart was increased, the hardness and contraction of the kidney bespoke the probability of a long continuance of the disease . . . The enlarged state of the heart would seem to bespeak some cause of obstruction to the circulation through the system beyond what we discovered, nor will I venture to say what share this might have had in giving rise to the dropsy . . .

In modern times the Framingham Study has underscored the importance of the relationships between blood pressure, particularly systolic pressure, and left ventricular hypertrophy and between left ventricular hypertrophy and congestive heart failure in a hypertensive population (83). In a representative population sample followed for 16 years, the dominant etiologic precursor of congestive heart failure was hypertension, which was present in 75% of cases. Congestive heart failure was six times as common in hypertensive as in normotensive persons. Further, electrocardiographic evidence of left ventricular hypertrophy in the Framingham cohort was strongly associated with both hypertension and coronary disease. Persons with definite electrocardiographic evidence of left ventricular hypertrophy had 10 times the risk of developing congestive heart failure as those with normal electrocardiograms. The authors concluded that the markedly increased risk of congestive heart failure in hypertensive subjects with left ventricular hypertrophy probably reflects the severity and duration of underlying hypertension and the compensatory cardiac hypertrophy with or without the added complication of myocardial ischemia due to associated accelerated coronary atherosclerosis. Whatever the mechanism, left ventricular hypertrophy in the setting of systemic hypertension appears to be an ominous harbinger of congestive heart failure. This finding underscores the importance of the mechanism(s) that underlies the development of left ventricular hypertrophy in the hypertensive subject and determines its reversibility.

Whether the abnormalities of cardiac structure and function that occur in the hypertensive subject are entirely secondary to the increased intracavitary pressure and/or the neurohumoral correlates of the hypertension or whether the heart plays a primary role in the pathogenesis of hypertensive disease remains a matter of conjecture. According to the theory of autoregulation, increased cardiac output is central to the pathogenesis of systemic hypertension (20,57,60a). (Guyton et al., 1971). Systemic resistance vessels respond to an increased cardiac output by constricting in order to reduce tissue blood flow to normal, thus causing blood pressure to rise. This theory, although controversial, is supported by the finding of transient elevations in cardiac output early in the course of several forms of experimentally induced hypertension in animals and of essential hypertension in man (38,52).

The remainder of this chapter is devoted to a discussion of the structure and function of the heart in hypertensive animals and man. Abnormalities in the myocardium and coronary arteries that are found in systemic hypertension is considered secondary to the hypertensive process rather than primary. Emphasis is placed on evidence that factors other than increased intracavitary pressure contribute to myocardial hypertrophy in systemic hypertension, on the role of echocardiography in the evaluation of the heart in hypertensive man, and on recent studies of the regression of myocardial hypertrophy after surgical or medical treatment of hypertension.

ETIOLOGY OF MYOCARDIAL HYPERTROPHY IN SYSTEMIC HYPERTENSION

Mechanical Factors

Normal cardiac muscle grows to compensate for the workload imposed upon the ventricle. The relationship between left ventricular wall tension, intracavitary pressure, and heart size can be expressed by the law of La place. Assuming that the ventricle is a thin-walled sphere, wall tension (T_w) is proportional to pressure (P) and the radius of curvature (r) (47):

$$T_w = Pr/2$$

When a chronically increased pressure load, whether due to systemic hypertension, aortic stenosis, or some other lesion, is imposed on the ventricle, left ventricular wall thickness increases so that the left ventricular peak systolic wall stress remains relatively constant and within normal limits (58,75,154). Pressure overloaded left ventricles tend to develop concentric hypertrophy and an increased ratio of wall thickness to radius of the left ventricular cavity (h/R ratio). To account for these observations, Grossman has hypothesized that when the primary stimulus to hypertrophy is left ventricular pressure overload, the resultant acute increase in peak systolic wall stress leads to parallel replication of sarcomeres, wall thickening, and concentric hypertrophy (58). The wall thickening is just sufficient to return peak systolic stress to normal, thus acting as feedback inhibition.

Neurohumoral Factors

The close correlation between intracavitary pressure and left ventricular wall thickness that is characteristic of the heart in aortic stenosis has not generally been found in systemic hypertension. Whether this is entirely due to moment-to-moment variability in blood pressure and to the difficulty in extrapolating from measurements of peripheral arterial pressure to intraventricular pressure or whether it is due in part to the contribution of factors other than pressure per se to the pathogenesis of myocardial hypertrophy in systemic hypertension is not known. Among the factors that have been implicated in the pathogenesis of myocardial hypertrophy in hypertension are genetic influences, the presence of concomitant processes that have a deleterious influence on the myocardium, such as aging, diabetes mellitus, and cardiomyopathy, increased activity of the renin-angiotensin system, increased circulating catecholamines and/or discharge of the cardiac sympathetic nerves, thyroxine, and growth hormone (19,51).

Evidence for involvement of the renin-angiotensin system in the pathogenesis of myocardial hypertrophy in hypertension is indirect and largely based on cardiac response to treatment with various antihypertensive drugs: agents such as hydralazine or minoxidil, which tend to elevate renin levels, fail to reverse left ventricular hypertrophy despite adequate control of blood pressure, whereas drugs such as alpha-methyldopa, clonidine, and captopril, which lower angiotensin II levels cause left ventricular hypertrophy to regress (162–166,171). The differential effects of these agents on the myocardium may be related to factors other than the renin-angiotensin system, such as hemodynamics, catecholamine release, and direct stimulation of myocyte and connective tissue growth. Attempts to correlate severity of left ventricular hypertrophy with circulating renin levels in patients with essential hypertension have been unsuccessful: blood pressure was found to be a more important determinant of hypertrophy than was renin status (29,79). Further study is needed to define the role of renin and/or angiotensin per se in the pathogenesis of myocardial hypertrophy in hypertension.

Several lines of evidence have implicated catecholamines in the pathogenesis of cardiac hypertrophy (129,176). Exogenous catecholamines were shown to induce myocardial hypertrophy (95,149), and myocardial catecholamine stores and turnover were found to be altered in the hypertrophic heart (45). Further, long-term treatment of normal animals with β-adrenergic receptor antagonists has been shown to reduce myocardial growth (186). Evidence that catecholamines are involved in hypertension-related myocardial hypertrophy is less clear, however, despite the fact that activity of the cardiac sympathetic nerves, as assessed by turnover and synthesis of norepinephrine in the myocardium, is increased in several animal models of hypertension. These include aortic coarctation, renovascular hypertension, desoxycorticosterone acetate (DOCA)-NaCl hypertension, and genetic spontaneous hypertension (129). Further, circulating norepinephrine concentration, a generally accepted clinical index of sympathetic nervous system activity, is elevated in at least a subset of patients with essential hypertension. Pharmacologic agents such as alpha-methyldopa and clonidine, which have a sympatholytic effect on the heart, can prevent or reverse myocardial hypertrophy. These drugs also have effects on systemic hemodynamics, myocardial contractility, and the renin-angiotensin system, which complicate the interpretation of these data. In contrast, systemic vasodilators such as hydralazine or minoxidil, which cause reflexly mediated myocardial stimulation, fail to reverse or even exacerbate myocardial hypertrophy despite adequate control of blood pressure. Further, administration of β-adrenergic receptor blocking agents does not prevent or cause reversal of myocardial hypertrophy in hypertensive rats even when blood pressure is lowered significantly (133,188).

Studies of the effects of sympathetic denervation of the heart on the development of myocardial hypertrophy have yielded conflicting results. Chemical sympathectomy with 6-hydroxydopamine (6-OHDA) has been shown not to prevent the development of cardiac hypertrophy in the DOCA-NaCl hypertensive rat, a model in which increased sympathetic activity has been demonstrated (19). Further, neonatal immunosympathectomy with nerve-growth factor antiserum does not prevent cardiac hypertrophy in the spontaneously hypertensive rat (SHR) of the Okamoto strain despite prevention of the hypertension and extensive depletion of myocardial norepinephrine stores (27). In contrast, chemical sympathectomy with guanethidine was shown in one study to prevent exercise-induced cardiac hypertrophy in the normotensive rat (128). As in the case of the renin-angiotensin system, further study is needed to assess the role of neural influences and catecholamines in mediating myocardial hypertrophy associated with systemic hypertension.

THE HEART IN ANIMAL MODELS OF SYSTEMIC HYPERTENSION

Morphology

It is well recognized that heart muscle cells undergo a dramatic increase in size in the course of myocardial hypertrophy induced by systemic hypertension. Since myocytes lose their ability to divide early in the neonatal period, the pressure-induced increase in heart size is accomplished by myocyte hypertrophy rather than hyperplasia. In contrast, nonmuscle cells of the heart undergo hyperplastic change in response to pressure-induced cardiac hypertrophy. The hypertrophic myocytes seen in chronic pressure overloading of the left ventricle generally manifest a significant increase in the volume fraction of myofibrils and a decrease in that of mitochondria, resulting in a decrease in the mitochondria/myofibril ratio (115). Examination of the ultrastructure of the myocardium in the maturing SHR has revealed the development of marked hypertrophy of left ventricular myocytes in association with the establishment of sustained hypertension (86). In these myocytes the myofibrils were significantly increased in mass in association with altered intercalated discs, extended subsarcolemmal dense mats, and unorganized filamentous structures in the periphery of preexisting myofibrils (Fig. 1). Focal interstitial fibroses occurred in the myocardium, and tunnel capillaries appeared in some hypertrophied myocytes. There were also marked changes in the intercalated discs associated with numerous immature sarcomeres and frequent abnormal Z-band expansions. In animals with established hypertension, intracellular volume ratios of myofibrils and T-tubular system were significantly increased, whereas mitochondrial volume was markedly decreased, resulting in a significant increase in the myofibril/mitochondria volume ratio.

Mitochondria in hypertrophic cells, although reduced in number, appeared to be normal in structure. This suggests that the decrease in mitochondrial mass is related to a developmental defect rather than to secondary degeneration. Thus there appears to be independent control of mitochondrial and myofibrillar mass in hypertrophying myocytes. This formulation is consistent with the observation of Page and Oparil (130) that prevention of hypertension in the SHR with neonatal administration of nerve-growth factor antiserum does not alter the development of myocardial hypertrophy but does prevent the fall in cellular concentration of mitochondria characteristic of sham-treated (hypertensive) control animals. Myofibrillar concentrations were identical in nerve-growth factor antiserum treated and sham-treated animals. The data are insufficient to permit us to determine whether immunosympathectomy affects mitochondrial concentration via its effect on arterial blood pressure or via some other, unidentified mechanism. The findings do suggest, however, that the decreased mitochondrial concentration found in myocardial cells of untreated SHR need not be causally related to the cardiac dysfunction observed in these animals.

In SHR with stable, established hypertension of many months' duration, malalignment of the contractile apparatus has been observed. In such cases a proportion of myofibrils are found to be obliquely oriented with respect to the long axis of the myocyte and terminate on the free lateral sarcolemma rather than the intracalated disc. This disadvantageous geometric arrangement of the contractile material could impair the contractile performance of the hypertrophied myocyte.

Similar ultrastructural alterations were reported in Wistar Kyoto rats (WKY) in which two-kidney Goldblatt hypertension was induced (187). Substantial (34%–54%) increments in left ventricular weight and myocyte size, enlargements of the T-tubular system, and increases in the ratio of myofibril volume-to-total cell volume appeared within the first 4 weeks of renal artery clipping in two-kidney one-clip Goldblatt hypertensive Wistar rats (190). Mitochondrial volume decreased, while mitochondrial structure remained normal during this early stage of hypertrophy. Myofibrillar malalignment also appeared early in the course of hypertrophy in this model. At 8 weeks following placement of the renal artery clip, left ventricular weight was greater than at 4 weeks and myofibrillar volume, although significantly higher than in control hearts from normotensive animals, was less than at 4 weeks. Mitochondrial volume and the ratio of mitochondria to myofibrils were also lower

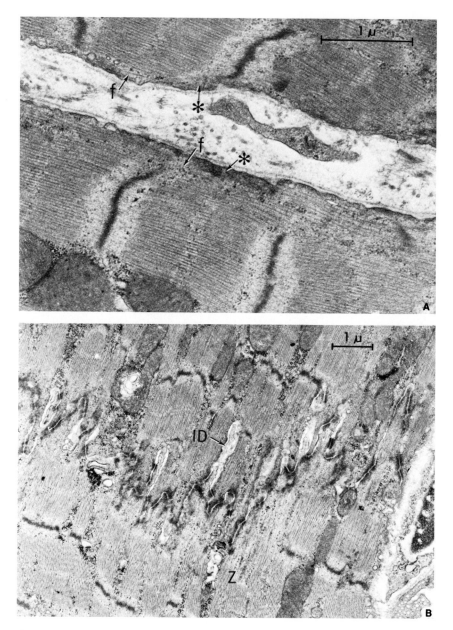

FIG. 1. Hypertrophied cardiocytes in 15-week-old SHR.   **A:** Subsarcolemmal dense mats (*) are larger than in control hearts and are in close contact association with fine filamentous structures (f). Scale, 1 μ. Final magnification ×36,900.   **B:** Intercalated disc (ID) exhibits irregular and marked convolutions. In the vicinity of intercalated discs, Z bands (Z) are often indistinct, fragmented, and dislocated so that the sarcomeres cannot be identified as completely formed structural units. Scale, 1 μ. Final magnification ×16,200. (Reprinted by permission of *Jpn. Circ. J.* and K. Kawamura, ref. 86.)

than at 4 weeks. Further, distortion in the intercalated discs and myofibrillar malalignment became more prominent, although sarcomere length did not appear to change. At 24 weeks, all of these changes became more marked: left ventricular weight continued to increase and myofibrillar volume continued to increase and mitochondrial volume to decrease, so that the ratio of mitochondria to myofibrils decreased further. Mitochondrial degeneration appeared: the matrix of the mitochondria became lighter, and the cristae were decreased in number and showed transversal links to each other. Lipid droplets appeared in myocytes, signifying cell degeneration. Some hearts showed evidence of connective tissue proliferation at this stage. The functional properties of these hypertrophied hearts were examined in the same series of animals (190). These are discussed later in the chapter.

The similarity in myocardial ultrastructure at comparable levels of blood pressure in these genetic and acquired models of hypertension suggests that the morphological abnormalities observed are secondary to the hypertension rather than the primary result of independent genetic or neurohumoral influences. It should be noted that hypertension develops gradually over a period of approximately 4 weeks in both of these models. In contrast, there are major differences in myocyte ultrastructure, biochemistry, and capillary density between SHR and WKY in which hypertension is induced abruptly by constricting the abdominal aorta (105). This finding indicates that aortic constriction models should not be used interchangeably with hypertensive models in studies of myocardial hypertrophy.

Traditional methods of estimating myocyte size from tissue sections are limited by the difficulty of obtaining measurements of cell length from fixed tissue. The development of the isolated heart muscle cell preparation has provided the opportunity to measure cell length accurately and, when combined with width measurements, to calculate cell volume. Bishop and associates (13) have used this preparation to determine the size of myocytes from the right ventricle and from inner and outer halves of the left ventricle of SHR and of control normotensive WKY and Fischer-344 rats. They found (Fig. 2) that calculated left ventricular cell volume in SHR was greater than in age- and weight-matched WKY or Fischer-344 rats. Cell size

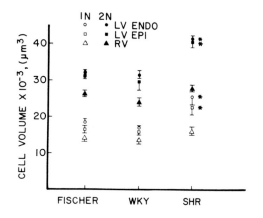

FIG. 2. Calculated cell volume for double nucleated (2N; *solid symbols*) and single nucleated (1N; *open symbols*) isolated myocytes from three strains of rats. Each symbol represents the mean ± SEM of six animals. There was no difference between inner and outer halves of left ventricle within each strain. Asterisk = significant difference (*p*<0.05) from normotensive strains; LV Endo = left ventricular free-wall inner half; LV Epi = left ventricular free-wall outer half; RV = right ventricle. (Reprinted by permission of the American Heart Association, Inc. and S. Bishop, *Hypertension*, ref. 13.)

measurements of isolated myocytes from endocardial and epicardial regions were not significantly different within any of the three strains. Left ventricular cells from the hypertrophied hearts of SHR were larger than from the normotensive control strains. Right ventricular cells were smaller than left ventricular cells but were not different in size among the three strains, which is consistent with the absence of right ventricular hypertrophy in the adult SHR (24).

The issue of whether there are regional differences in the size of heart muscle cells is potentially an important one, as such differences could have an influence on the susceptibility of different regions of myocardium to degenerative changes, leading to decreased functional performance or cell death. The predilection of the inner half of the left ventricular wall to ischemic cell death in severe coronary artery disease and in conditions associated with severe left ventricular pressure overload such as aortic stenosis is well known. Whether the size of individual myocytes plays a role in the development of mechanical dysfunction or ischemic cell death is unknown, but it has been suggested that greater cell diameter and therefore longer diffusion distances from the capillaries would increase the probability of ischemic cell damage. Investigators using traditional histologic techniques have reported slightly larger mean cross-sectional areas for subendocardial versus subepicardial cells from the hearts of normotensive WKY. Following induction of renal hypertension in these animals, the cross-sectional area of subepicardial cells increased at a faster rate than that of subendocardial cells, so that with the development of hypertrophy, cells in the two left ventricular regions became nearly equal in cross-sectional area (5,104). Calculated cell length increased more in the subepicardium than in the subendocardium, however, resulting in a greater increase in calculated cell volume for subepicardial cells. The apparent inconsistencies in these studies point up the need for further investigation to determine whether regional differences in cell size are present in severely hypertrophied hearts with myocardial dysfunction.

The development of ultrastructural changes in left atrial myocytes from hearts of Wistar rats with DOCA/NaCl hypertension was recently shown to precede the development of five structural changes in ventricular myocytes from the same hearts (1). Following 6 weeks of sustained but modest (mean systolic blood pressure for the group $= 144$ mm Hg) arterial hypertension, marked ultrastructural abnormalities were found in the left atrial contractile cells of treated animals. These included sarcoplasmic accumulation of dense particles associated with thick (presumably myosin) filaments, isolated helical arrangements of dense particles, irregular nuclei, and enlarged mitochondria (Fig. 3). The size and arrangement of the dense particles suggest ribosomes or polyribosomes. Their association with myofilaments and their helical arrangement may represent morphological evidence of active myosin synthesis *in situ* by polyribosomes. At the same time left ventricular myocytes appeared to be less affected by the pressure overload, manifesting only slight mitochondrial enlargement without evidence of mitochondrial degeneration or increased myofibrillar volume. This study documents an early response of left atrial cells to pressure overload: atrial cells appear to be carrying out increased myofibrillar synthesis at

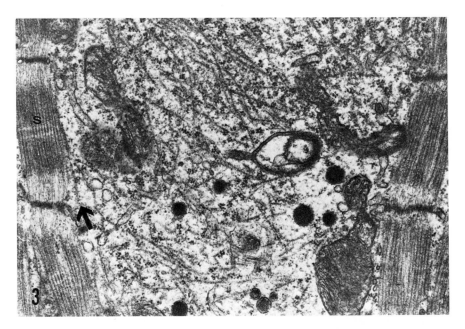

FIG. 3. Longitudinal section of central portion of atrial myocyte from 6-week-treated hypertensive rat. Unorganized thick filaments associated with groups of ribosomes (polyribosomes) occupy most of the sarcoplasmic core. A thick filament partially assembled in a sarcomere (S) is also coated by ribosomes *(arrow).* ×28,800. (Reprinted by permission of the American Heart Association, Inc. and J. N. da Costa, *Hypertension,* ref. 1.)

a stage when the left ventricle presents changes of hyperfunction (mitochondrial enlargement) only. These findings are consistent with the clinical observation that electrocardiographic alterations of the atrial complex appear in hypotensive patients prior to definite clinical evidence of left ventricular involvement (31,33,53), and with the recording of increased left atrial pressure and decreased left atrial distensibility in hypertensive rats (125,145). Further examination of the ultrastructure of the atrium in various stages of experimental hypertension are needed to fully elucidate its role in the pathogenesis of hypertension-induced heart disease. Hearts from rats with streptozotocin-induced diabetes and one-kidney Goldblatt hypertension have been shown to develop focal myocytolysis and dense interstitial fibrosis, a finding similar to that shown in hearts from hypertensive diabetic patients (39,40). Deposition of periodic acid-Schiff (PAS)-positive material in the fibrotic regions and intramyocardial small vessel disease were observed, as described in hypertensive diabetic man. None of these abnormalities was seen in normotensive nondiabetic, normotensive diabetic, or hypertensive nondiabetic control rats. Thus, the combination of diabetes and hypertension in the rat appears to produce significant myocardial damage of a kind similar to that seen in diabetic cardiomyopathy in man. Use of the hypertensive diabetic rat model may allow more precise assessment of the role of hypertension in the pathogenesis of human diabetic cardiomyopathy.

Biochemistry

The biochemical alterations observed in the hypertrophied myocardium of the hypertensive animal are qualitatively similar to those described in hearts subjected to pressure overload induced by aortic or pulmonary artery constriction. Most published studies of the biochemistry and molecular biology of pressure-induced hypertrophy have been carried out using the latter models. As pointed out by Rabinowitz and Zak (136), the characteristics of pressure-overload-induced cardiac growth may differ, depending on a number of experimental variables, including the severity and duration of the overload, the rapidity with which it is imposed, the species and age of the animal, and the underlying condition of the myocardium. Because the pressure overload associated with systemic hypertension is of gradual onset, the associated myocardial changes are usually less extensive than in ligation models, where pressure is suddenly elevated, leading to ischemic damage and fibrotic repair.

The biochemistry and molecular biology of pressure overload-induced cardiac hypertrophy have been well reviewed (41,136,137,159,191,195) and are discussed in detail in this volume. Accordingly, the biochemical aspects of hypertension-induced myocardial hypertrophy will be considered here only insofar as they appear to be distinct from other forms of pressure-induced hypertrophy and as they relate in an important way to myocardial performance in hypertensive subjects or play a primary or secondary role in the pathogenesis of hypertensive disease.

Increased RNA polymerase has been demonstrated in nuclei from isolated cardiac myocytes of SHR with established hypertension (97), as well as in nuclei from both isolated cardiac myocytes and nonmuscle cells during the development of acute pressure-overload hypertrophy induced by constricting the ascending aorta of the rat (25). In the SHR both template-engaged and free RNA polymerases were increased compared with WKY controls. The ratio of RNA polymerases I/II was lower in SHR for both functional pools of the enzyme. Increased numbers of enzyme molecules were present in nuclei from SHR without appreciable change in the rate of polyribonucleotide-chain elongation. Enhanced myocardial RNA synthesis in SHR with established cardiac hypertrophy was associated with increased numbers of RNA polymerase molecules, perhaps reflecting altered chromatin structure with resultant increased polymerase binding and/or chain initiation.

In the rat subjected to aortic binding, total RNA polymerase activity in both muscle and nonmuscle cells began to increase at 48 hr after aortic constriction and reached maximal levels at 72 hr. By 72 hr after aortic constriction, RNA polymerases II and III were increased twofold in both muscle and nonmuscle nuclei; RNA polymerase I activity showed a fivefold increase in muscle nuclei but was unchanged in nonmuscle nuclei. The data demonstrate enhancement of the activity and/or amount of RNA polymerases in cardiac muscle and nonmuscle cells during the development of acute pressure overload hypertrophy. The 24- to 48-hr delay in onset of the increase in RNA polymerase activity following imposition of pressure overload is remarkable, since increased myocardial RNA synthesis has been demonstrated within a few hours of aortic constriction. This finding suggests that the immediate stimulation of RNA synthesis following aortic constriction may be regulated by processes other than changes in the activity or amount of RNA polymerase, such as a change in chromatin template activity. Further study is needed to delineate the molecular events that initiate and sustain increased protein synthesis in the pressure-overloaded heart.

Myocardial hypertrophy occurring after sustained augmentation in afterload or preload of any etiology is usually characterized by increments in RNA and DNA content per unit cardiac mass (136). The change in RNA reflects a change in muscle cell mass, whereas the change in DNA in the adult heart usually is associated with hyperplasia of nonmuscle cells. In the SHR, the most commonly used animal model of systemic hypertension, left ventricular RNA and DNA, expressed as milligram per gram left ventricular wet weight, have been shown to be significantly elevated compared with normotensive WKY controls (25). The increments in RNA and DNA were found in association with elevated left ventricular to body weight ratios in SHR from age 1 day to 24 weeks (Fig. 4). Myocardial hypertrophy in association with increased myocardial RNA and DNA were found in animals 1 day to 8 weeks of age, which had not yet developed hypertension, and in immunosympathectomized animals, which never developed hypertension.

The dissociation between myocardial hypertrophy and hypertension in this model was interpreted by Cutilletta et al. as evidence that myocardial hypertrophy may be a manifestation of an underlying genetic abnormality of the heart which could play a role in the pathogenesis of the hypertensive syndrome (27) (Fig. 5). According to this hypothesis, a primary myocardial abnormality in an animal genetically predisposed to hypertension results in myocardial dysfunction and hypertrophy. This is followed by a compensatory increase in sympathetic activity to maintain cardiac output; myocardial function returns toward, but not completely to, normal. Because of increased sympathetic activity, vasoconstriction occurs and results in increased peripheral vascular resistance and elevated systemic pressure. Other genetically determined factors, such as increased reactivity of the arteriolar musculature or increased levels of circulating catecholamines, may also play a role. Because of high peripheral vascular resistance and continued hypertension, cardiac output is further diminished and left ventricular hypertrophy increases. In the above scheme, if increased sympathetic activity is prevented by immunosympathectomy or some other maneuver, myocardial hypertrophy will still develop. Even though pressure remains normal, ventricular function and cardiac output are still compromised.

Direct evidence for a biochemical defect in myocytes of SHR comes from studies in which Ca^{2+} uptake and binding and Ca^{2+}-ATPase activity of microsomal preparations from hearts of SHR and control WKY were compared (65,99). Ca^{2+} uptake and binding were depressed, whereas Ca^{2+}-ATPase activity was significantly elevated in SHR compared with WKY, suggesting uncoupling of the ATPase from Ca^{2+} transport. These differences were apparent in 10-week-old animals and increased progressively to 22 weeks of age. Cyclic AMP-dependent phosphorylation

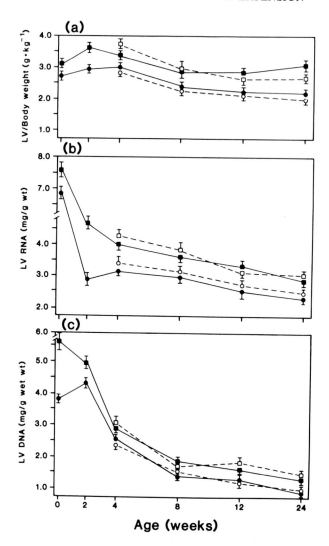

FIG. 4. Age-related changes in **(a)** left ventricular to body weight ratios (mg/g), **(b)** left ventricular RNA (mg/g wet weight), and **(c)** left ventricular DNA (mg/g wet weight of sham (●——●) and NGFAS (○---○)-treated WKY rats and sham (■——■)- and NGFAS (□---□)-treated SH rats at 1 day and 2, 4, 8, 12, and 24 weeks of age. Means ± SEM; $n = 8$ for each group and age. At any given age all three parameters were significantly greater in SHR than WKY ($p < 0.01$ or better by the unpaired Student's t-test). (Reproduced with modification by permission of Academic Press, London, and A. F. Cutilleta, ref. 24.)

of sarcoplasmic reticulum was significantly decreased in SHR and was correlated with Ca^{2+} uptake. Limas and Cohn (99) postulated that differences in endogenous cyclic AMP-dependent protein kinase activity may partly explain the decreased Ca^{2+} transport in SHR, though the molecular basis of the altered Ca^{2+} transport

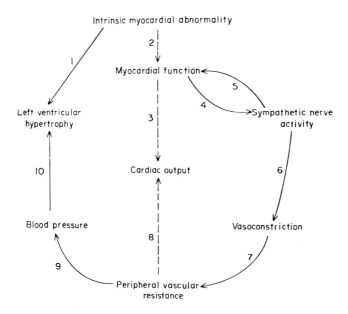

FIG. 5. Diagram of a possible mechanism for the development of hypertension and myocardial hypertrophy in the SH rat. *Solid arrows* indicate an increase; *dashed arrows* indicate a decrease. A genetically transmitted primary myocardial abnormality results in left ventricular hypertrophy (1) and myocardial dysfunction (2). Because of diminished ventricular performance, cardiac output is decreased (3) and sympathetic nerve activity is increased (4) as a compensatory mechanism (5). Enhanced sympathetic activity, however, also results in vasoconstriction of the systemic arterioles (6) which in turn leads to an increase in peripheral vascular resistance (7). As peripheral vascular resistance rises, cardiac output is further compromised (8) and hypertension develops (9). An increase in afterload as a result of hypertension further stimulates the development of left ventricular hypertrophy (10). (Reprinted with permission from Academic Press, London. A. F. Cutilletta, ref. 24).

was not fully elucidated by the study. These biochemical defects could explain the depressed myocardial contractile performance, impaired isometric relaxation, and blunted response to exogenous catecholamines that have been reported in hearts from SHR.

Reduced concentrations of α- and β-adrenergic receptors, cyclic AMP and cyclic GMP and depressed cyclic GMP-dependent protein kinase and specific actomyosin activities have been reported in the hypertrophied hearts of hypertensive rats and rabbits (SHR, DOCA-NaCl, coarctation, and one-kidney Goldblatt models) (14,18, 92,93,98,113,194). Further, altered proportions of myosin isozymes have recently been demonstrated in pressure-overload-induced and thyroxine-induced hypertrophy and have been related to altered cardiac performance in these models (101,103). Pressure overloading of the rat heart has been shown to induce the preferential synthesis of a cardiac myosin isoenzyme which has specific immunologic and electrophoretic properties and diminished ATPase activity. Since the contractile activity of the heart is controlled, at least in part, by the rate of hydrolysis of ATP by its myosin isoenzyme, this adaptive change could account for the reduced shortening speed (V_{max}) of cardiac muscle that has undergone pressure-overload-induced hypertrophy. In contrast, administration of thyroid hormone increases cardiac performance and V_{max} and induces the synthesis of a cardiac myosin isoenzyme of higher ATPase activity. These alterations are tissue-specific, so do not appear to be secondary to the desensitizing effects of increased circulating catecholamines or other humoral mediators. The reduced concentrations of cardiac adrenergic receptors have been ascribed to the specific enhancement in cardiac sympathetic drive characteristic of the hypertensive animal (194) and to myocyte hypertrophy (14). Affinities of α- and β-adrenergic receptors in the hearts of hypertensive animals remained unchanged in most reported studies. These findings, coupled with the observation that hearts from hypertensive animals show reduced isoproterenol-induced stimulation of adenylate cyclase activity (3,193) and the previously described demonstration of impaired cyclic AMP-dependent Ca^{2+} transport in membrane fractions from hypertensive hearts, provide a biochemical basis for the blunted inotropic and chromotropic response to adrenergic stimulation seen in hypertensive animals.

Increased collagen deposition occurs as a consequence of proliferation of connective tissue cells in hearts with pressure-overload hypertrophy. Collagen content of the heart is usually assessed by measuring myocardial hydroxyproline concentration. Hydroxyproline determination alone provides an inadequate quantitative assessment of total myocardial collagen content because the heart contains other hydroxyproline-containing proteins such as elastin, as well as several molecular species of collagen which vary in hydroxyproline content (117). Nevertheless, useful qualitative and comparative data are derived from hydroxyproline measurements. Hydroxyproline concentration has been shown to be increased in left ventricles, particularly in endomyocardial areas of SHR and of two-kidney Goldblatt hypertensive rats (27,111,112,114). The increased hydroxyproline levels characteristic of SHR appeared even when hypertension was prevented by neonatal immunosympathectomy with nerve-growth factor antiserum, indicating that, in this model at least, collagen deposition is not secondary to hypertension-induced myocardial damage (27).

Patterns of collagen deposition have been shown to differ in various models of pressure-overload hypertrophy. In one study, in which the experimental animals were sacrificed at age 16 weeks, myocardial hydroxyproline concentration was increased in WKY with hypertension induced by constriction of the abdominal aorta but not in age- and sex-matched SHR despite the fact that blood pressure levels were comparable in both groups (106). Further, the difference was apparent in both stressed (left) and unstressed (right) ventricles. These findings indicate that in the SHR the myocardial connective tissue response to pressure overload lags behind myocyte hypertrophy and that growth of connective tissue is less vigorous than that seen in the aortic constriction model. Whether these differences can be related to the rapidity of development of the pressure-overload stimulus or to genetic factors is unclear. These findings do, however, suggest that the factors governing myocardial connective tissue proliferation may be independent of those governing muscle fiber hypertrophy. Whether increased collagen deposition in pressure-overload-induced hypertrophy is a fundamental part of adaptive myocardial growth or a reparative response to myocyte death is unknown. Further study is needed to fully elucidate the nature of the process. Whatever its mechanisms of development, the functional significance of increased collagen deposition in hearts with pressure-induced hypertrophy is to cause an increase in passive stiffness of the myocardium.

Increased activities of a variety of enzymes involved in cardiac metabolism have been described in SHR (173). These include glucose-6-phosphate, dehydrogenase, lactate dehydrogenase, isocitrate dehydrogenase, succinate dehydrogenase, β-hydroxybutyrate dehydrogenase, and monoamine oxidase. The most striking finding was a dramatic increase in β-hydroxybutyrate dehydrogenase from age 5 to 11 weeks, the stage of developing hypertension in SHR. Control Wistar rats did not develop these increments in enzyme activity. Tanijiri interpreted these data and similar results from studies performed in other hypertensive rat models as consistent with the interpretation that there may be impaired oxidative metabolism and increased anerobic glycolysis in hypertrophic hearts from animals with systemic hypertension. The appearance of these abnormalities during the developmental stage of the hypertension suggests that they may play a role in the pathogenesis of the syndrome.

Conversely, there is no evidence that activities and distribution of the lysosomal enzymes cathepsin D, acid phosphatase, and β-acetylglucosaminidase are altered during the development of cardiac hypertrophy induced by systemic hypertension (192). This suggests that lysosomal activity does not play an important role in controlling the net changes in protein balance that characterize this form of pressure-overload-induced hypertrophy. Further study in other hypertensive models is needed to document alterations in activity of various myocardial enzymes in the hypertrophic heart and to determine whether these are primary or secondary to the elevation in blood pressure.

Electrophysiology

Left ventricular hypertrophy resulting from the chronic pressure overload of systemic hypertension is associated with characteristic electrophysiological alterations (6,60). These include marked prolongation of the action potential and a lesser prolongation of the time-course of repolarization to the resting membrane potential without accompanying changes in the transmembrane resting potential or in the amplitude, overshoot, or maximum upstroke velocity of the action potential. In the two-kidney one-clip Goldblatt model, prolongation of the action potential was shown to increase progressively with time postrenal artery clipping and to be directly proportional to the extent of hypertrophy. Depression of the fast inward Na^+ current with tetrodotoxin or augmentation of extracellular potassium concentration did not alter the duration of the action potential. In contrast, varying extracellular Ca^{2+} concentration at a time when the fast Na^+ channels were blocked or reducing extracellular sodium concentration altered the duration of the action potential. These findings suggest that membrane sensitivity to these ions is altered in hypertrophied myocardium and that prolongation of the action potential in this model may be explained by slowed inactivation of a Ca^{2+}-inactivated inward current. This could be accomplished by partial inhibition of the Na^+-Ca^{2+} exchange system or by development of a new slow channel capable of carrying Na^+ and regulated by Ca^{2+}. Prolongation of the action potential could contribute to the increase in time to peak force, augmentation of isometric force, and slowed relaxation seen in this model of pressure-induced myocardial hypertrophy. This would tend to preserve the contractile strength of the hypertrophied myocardium in the face of the biochemical lesions of the contractile apparatus which have been described previously (60,78).

Similar alterations in electrical and mechanical properties have been described in hypertrophied papillary muscles from hearts of DOCA-NaCl hypertensive rats, SHR, and aorta-constricted rats (67,67a,68) and in isolated Langendorf-perfused ventricles from adult SHR (67a). When compared with papillary muscles from normotensive WKY rat hearts, hypertrophied papillary muscles were found to have longer action potentials, longer contraction times, and longer electrical and mechanical refractory periods. When subjected to paired-pulse or high-frequency, short-duration stimulation, hypertrophied preparations developed larger aftercontractions and larger transient depolarizations than did nonhypertrophied preparations. Hyperexcitable periods of SHR ventricles were significantly longer than those of control WKY ventricles. Propranolol treatment did not eliminate these differences, suggesting that endogenous catecholamines were not responsible for them. Evidence from studies of nonhypertrophied muscle preparations suggests that transient depolarizations are associated with a slow inward Na^+ current and an oscillatory release of Ca^{2+} from intracellular stores. The observation of altered Ca^{2+} handling by the sarcoplasmic reticulum could provide a biochemical basis for the development of aftercontractions and transient depolarization in hypertrophied cardiac muscle (99).

Recent evidence suggests that the action potential prolongation that occurs in the hearts of rats with two-kidney, one-clip Goldblatt hypertension is not uniform throughout the myocardium (88). The entire course of repolarization appears to be prolonged in endocardial and papillary muscle fibers, but only the latter half of repolarization is prolonged in epicardial fibers. Further, endocardial action potentials, particularly those that occur in hypertrophied muscle, have a distinctive steep relation between duration and drive rate which may be due to a difference in the rate dependence of a membrane conductance(s), a relatively greater accumulation of extracellular K^+, and/or altered activity of the Na^+-K^+ pump. The similarity in the profile of spatial voltage decrement and the values for effective input resistance observed in hypertensive and control hearts in this study suggest that alterations in electrotonic coupling between cells probably do not account for the prolonged action potentials observed in hypertrophied myocardium.

Electrophysiological alterations that could predispose to the development of arrhythmias have been described in the hypertrophied hearts of rats with two-kidney, one-clip Goldblatt hypertension (7). Afterpotentials can be induced selectively in hypertrophied myocardium from rats with this form of hypertension. Three kinds of afterpotentials have been recorded by standard microelectrode techniques: early afterdepolarizations, delayed afterdepolarizations, and early afterhyperpolarizations. The first two could give rise to triggered spontaneous activity. The coupling interval from the upstroke of the last driven action potential to the peak of the delayed afterdepolarization decreased when the stimulation frequency or number of preceding driven beats increased. Hypertrophied fibers treated with high Ca^{2+} that gave rise to triggered activity showed a characteristic relationship between delayed afterpotential magnitude and drive cycle length. In hypertrophied muscles treated with tetraethylammonium, triggered activity developed from an early afterdepolarization but terminated with delayed afterdepolarization. The relationship of the previously described structural and biochemical abnormalities of the hypertrophied myocardium to the occurrence of afterpotentials and triggered activity is uncertain, although alterations in the distribution, binding, uptake, and free concentration of ions such as Ca^{2+} might well foster these events (7). Further studies of the Ca^{2+} release and uptake system and of sarcolemmal Na^+-K^+-ATPase will be required to establish whether biochemical alterations may contribute to the generation of afterpotentials in this model of cardiac hypertrophy. Sustained rhythmic activity that depends on afterpotentials for its initiation has been demonstrated in the two-kidney, one-clip Goldblatt hypertensive model of myocardial hypertrophy as well as in atrial fibers from diseased human hearts (108). This finding suggests that afterpotentials and triggered activity could predispose hypertrophied hearts to arrhythmias (7). Further study is needed to determine whether arrhythmias are more frequent in hypertension-induced myocardial hypertrophy.

Cardiac Function

Cardiac hypertrophy alters the entire excitation-contraction sequence of cardiac muscle performance. Meerson (116) observed that when hemodynamic overload is imposed on the left ventricle for prolonged periods, the mechanical functions of the heart improve initially to handle the increased load, but in later stages of hypertrophy, the performance of the stressed ventricle gradually deteriorates. The nonstressed right ventricle develops concomitant augmentation and then deterioration in function following imposition of a pressure overload on the left ventricle. The mechanisms that lead to increased myocardial protein synthesis and therefore to increased myocardial performance in the early phase of pressure-overload-induced hypertrophy have been discussed in this volume and in several reviews (41,136,137,159,191,195). According to Meerson (116), the factors leading to diminution in maximum attainable force and contraction rate of cardiac muscle include disturbances in ion transport and muscle relaxation, decreased coronary reserve, diminished capacity of energy supply mechanisms, reduced myofibrillar ATPase activity, and disturbances in adrenergic regulation of the heart (Fig. 6). The time required for these factors to produce a significant diminution in cardiac performance and, thereby, congestive failure may be measured in years. Compensatory mechanisms that tend to delay the development of heart failure include the increase in myocardial mass, which compensates for the defect in contractile function of the hypertrophied myocardium, and peripheral mechanisms that tend to decrease the metabolic demands of tissues and increase the efficiency of delivery of oxygen and nutrients by an impaired circulation.

Left ventricular performance has been shown to be enhanced in two-kidney, one-clip Goldblatt hypertensive rats at 4 and 8 weeks after clipping (89,90). Developed stress and maximum rate of stress development were increased, probably as a result of increased density of contractile proteins, in these hearts, which developed a 40% increase in left ventricular weight following induction of hypertension. The improvement in myocardial performance was reflected in alterations in isovolumic systolic and diastolic pressure-volume relations, stress development during after-loaded and isovolumic contractions, and the force-velocity relation. Diastolic and systolic pressure-volume relations of the isovolumetrically beating left ventricles of Goldblatt hypertensive rats at 4 and 8 weeks postclipping are shown in Fig. 7. At 4 weeks the diastolic minimum curves of the hypertrophied ventricles were shifted to greater volumes. The maximum developed pressure increased and moved to the range of greater volumes. Neither the maximum nor the minimum curves changed significantly between the fourth and eighth week, indicating that hypertrophy became functionally significant soon after development of the hypertension and remained stable for a considerable period thereafter. The work capacity of the whole ventricle, as estimated by the distance between the diastolic and systolic pressure-volume curves, was increased in these hypertensive rats. At any given end-diastolic wall stress, the elastic modulus of the hypertrophied ventricle was slightly increased, whereas the sarcomere length remained unchanged. In addition, the rate of development of pressure was increased in the hypertrophied ventricle: the maximum dP/dt was increased for a given end-diastolic pressure. Ejection fraction and maximum flow and acceleration of ejected blood were not influenced by hypertrophy: at any given end-diastolic volume the hypertrophied ventricles of hypertensive rats ejected the same stroke volume as normotensive controls. In contrast, the maximum shortening velocity (V_{max}) was decreased in this model of myocardial hypertrophy, suggesting that the contractile state of a single contractile unit is diminished. This is consistent with the observations of decreased Ca^{2+}-ATPase activity of myosin in the hearts of Goldblatt hypertensive rats (114) and SHR (99) and of impaired Ca^{2+} uptake and binding in microsomal preparations from hearts of SHR (65,99). The decrease in V_{max} is compensated by an increase in P_o, resulting in enhancement of contractile performance of the whole left ventricle. These observations are consistent with data obtained from other models of pressure-induced myocardial hypertrophy (2,85,155,170).

Later in the course of two-kidney one-clip Goldblatt hypertension (8,16,190), impairment in left ventricular performance appeared. Maximum developed tension

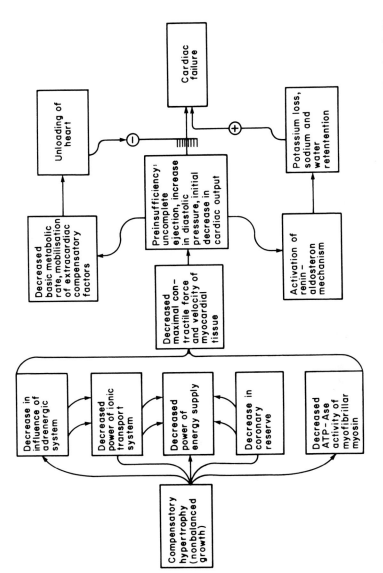

FIG. 6. Diagram of the mechanism of development of congestive failure in the hypertrophied heart. (Reprinted with permission from German Association of Cardiovascular Research and F.Z. Meerson, ref. 116.)

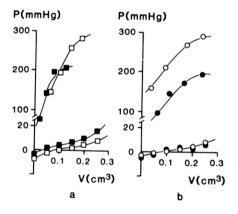

FIG. 7. Isovolumic systolic and diastolic pressure-volume relations of the left ventricle of rats 4 weeks (a) and 8 weeks (b) after narrowing one renal artery. ■ control 4 weeks; ● control 8 weeks; ▲ control 14 weeks; □ Goldblatt 4 weeks; ○ Goldblatt 8 weeks. (Reprinted with permission from German Association of Cardiovascular Research and G. Kissling, ref. 89.)

and V_{max} were depressed, particularly in hearts with fibrosis and coronary artery damage. The resting tension curve of hypertrophied muscle became progressively steeper and the constants of parallel elasticity progressively higher with duration of the hypertension, reflecting increased myocardial stiffness that was presumed to be secondary to increased collagen deposition. Rats with chronic renal hypertension have normal resting cardiac outputs and left ventricular diastolic pressures but diminished cardiac reserve (8). When cardiac function is evaluated by measuring left ventricular end-diastolic pressure, stroke volume, and cardiac output during rapid alterations in venous return, analysis of the relationship between stroke volume and left ventricular end-diastolic pressure reveals a significant decrease in ventricular performance in the hypertrophied heart. Alterations in stroke volume and cardiac output are unassociated with significant changes in work performed at matched end-diastolic pressures. Taken together, these data suggest that the impairment in cardiac function in chronic renal hypertension is related to diminished myocardial contractility and/or reduced left ventricular compliance.

To determine whether the enhanced performance of the hypertrophied ventricle is due entirely to the increase in muscle mass or to an enhanced contractile state of the hypertrophied muscle, it is necessary to determine the force generated per unit of cross-sectional area (89). To approximate this, the mechanical performance of isolated trabecular muscle strips or papillary muscles of the left ventricle of one- and two-kidney Goldblatt hypertensive rats and rats subjected to banding of the ascending aorta was examined (16,80). Muscle was obtained from two-kidney Goldblatt rats at intervals between 4 and 30 weeks after clipping, from one-kidney Goldblatt rats at 4 and 8 weeks, and from aortic banded rats at 4 and 6 weeks. Length-tension and force-velocity relations were established on the basis of afterloaded contractions and quick-release experiments. Myocardial distensibility was reduced in all Goldblatt rats tested. Increased muscle stiffness appeared earlier in the course of hypertrophy than did increased myocardial connective tissue content, as reflected in increased hydroxyproline concentration. This suggests that the increased resting tension may have an active tonic component, possibly resulting from residual activation of the contractile system in diastole (70) or from hypertrophy of inner membranes. In contrast, myocardial distensibility was not altered in the early phases of hypertrophy associated with aortic banding, genetic hypertension (10-week-old SHR), or swimming training, suggesting that decreased myocardial distensibility is not an inherent property of the hypertrophy process (77). Maximum shortening velocity of the unloaded myocardium ("apparent V_{max}") was found to be significantly reduced at all stages of investigation and in all forms of pressure-induced hypertrophy. Isometric tension development, on the other hand, was enhanced in the early stages of Goldblatt hypertension and was not decreased in rats with aortic stenosis. Shortening velocity and developed tension showed a decrease in later stages of hypertrophy, most impressively in preparations with high connective tissue content. Force-velocity curves in muscles from hypertensive animals demonstrated a significant depression in velocity of shortening at all relative loads that progressed with the duration of hypertension. Thus the development of myocardial hypertrophy appears to confer the ability to maintain ventricular performance by preserving force development even while speed of shortening delays (16). These findings are in excellent agreement with those obtained using intact hearts from each of these experimental models of hypertension (90).

The finding of enhanced myocardial performance early in the course of hypertension-induced left ventricular hypertrophy is consistent with the observation that cardiac output is elevated early in the course of several forms of experimentally induced and spontaneously occurring hypertension in animals (20,107,131). The concept of total body autoregulation has been used to explain the adaptation of resistance vessels to such increases in cardiac output. According to the theory of autoregulation, systemic resistance vessels respond to an increased cardiac output and intravascular volume by constricting in order to reduce blood flow to normal, thus causing blood pressure to rise (20). Animals with long-standing established hypertension usually have a normal or somewhat decreased cardiac output and increased peripheral and renal vascular resistance. The fall in cardiac output, which occurs during the natural history of systemic hypertension, may be related to myocardial changes as well. Studies have shown a decline in left ventricular performance with increased duration of hypertension in several animal models (8,16, 24,132,134,190). This may be related in part to impairment of the contractile properties of the ventricle and in part to reduced diastolic compliance, which shifts the Frank-Starling relationship to the right (62). To compensate for this shift in the pressure-volume relationship the heart must either climb upwards on the Frank-Starling curve by increasing the diastolic filling pressure of the left ventricle and/ or shift to a steeper Frank-Starling curve by operating in a higher inotropic state (125). Left atrial pressure measured in the unanesthetized SHR at 4 to 5 months of age was found elevated to levels more than twice those found in normotensive control rats (125). Mechanisms that may contribute to the elevated left atrial pressure in hypertension include redistribution of blood flow to the cardiopulmonary region and increased stiffness of the pulmonary veins and/or left atrium secondary to increased sympathetic discharge or pressure-induced hypertrophy. Decreased dynamic distensibility of left atrial walls in mature SHR has recently been demonstrated (147). Whatever its mechanism, enhanced left atrial pressure in SHR with established hypertension represents a real rise in diastolic filling pressure of the left ventricle and rightward shift of the Frank-Starling curve. Without this compensation the stroke volume of the hypertrophied SHR heart would be drastically reduced. The critical dependence of cardiac performance on left ventricular filling in the hypertrophied heart, along with the effects of anesthesia, may explain the apparently inconsistent values for cardiac output and ventricular performance obtained in various studies of animal models of hypertension (168).

Coronary Arteries

Pressure-induced left ventricular hypertrophy increases the susceptibility of the heart to ischemic damage. This results from a combination of increased myocardial workload, myocardial mass, and myocyte size in the face of decreased intramyocardial capillary density (138). These abnormalities, in turn, cause increased diffusion distances from nutrient capillaries to myocytes, decreased coronary reserve (120,144), and redistribution of coronary blood flow with relative endocardial hypoperfusion. Hypertension-related damage to intramyocardial vessels (126) and accelerated intracoronary atherosclerosis also increase the likelihood of ischemic damage to the heart. Further, intrinsic electrophysiological abnormalities that may predispose to arrhythmias have been described in hypertrophied myocardial cells (6). Although these changes are of the greatest practical significance in man, where they predispose to myocardial infarction, congestive heart failure, and sudden death, animal studies of the effects on the coronary circulation of left ventricular hypertrophy secondary to experimentally induced or genetic hypertension are useful in elucidating the pathogenesis of the human disease.

Mortality from acute occlusion of the left circumflex coronary artery has been shown to be significantly greater in dogs with left ventricular hypertrophy secondary to one-kidney Goldblatt hypertension than in normotensive control animals (91). The perfusion fields of the occluded vessel as defined by postmortem coronary angiography were similar in the two groups, indicating that the increased mortality rate in hypertensive animals cannot be explained by increased size of the occluded vascular bed. Decreased coronary reserve and/or electrophysiologic abnormalities that predispose to the development of fatal arrhythmias could explain the increased incidence of sudden cardiac death after coronary occlusion in animals with hypertension-induced left ventricular hypertrophy. Hypertrophied cardiac muscle cells manifest a prolongation of action potential duration. Since myocardial ischemia shortens the action potential after coronary occlusion, the dispersion of action potential durations in normal and ischemic tissue would tend to be greater in hypertrophied than in normal ventricles, thus introducing a second mechanism by which arrhythmias could be generated.

To examine the hypothesis that decreased coronary vascular capacity and capillary density contribute to the increased mortality rate associated with acute coronary occlusion in this model, further experiments were carried out in which myocardial blood flow was measured before and at intervals after coronary artery occlusion, and the extent of infarction was quantified histologically in selected myocardial segments (121). Coronary occlusion reduced flows to a similar extent, and over a 48-hr period, collateral flow increased to a similar extent in both normotensive and hypertensive animals. In addition, the amount of necrosis associated with a given degree of ischemia was similar in the two groups. Although the extent of the left ventricle that became ischemic was greater in the hypertensive dogs, chronic hypertension and left ventricular hypertrophy did not limit the recruitment of collateral blood flow or increase the amount of necrosis associated with a given degree of ischemia. These data tend to support the concept that coronary occlusion does not have greater adverse effects in pressure-hypertrophied ventricles than in the normal heart. Other evidence from the same study shows that coronary occlusion does produce the following undesirable effects in the hypertrophied heart: (a) The resistance of coronary collateral vessels was higher in hypertrophied ventricles than in controls. Thus if coronary occlusion resulted in a major decrease in arterial pressure, which is often the case clinically, flow to the ischemic region could be severely compromised. (b) Blood flow to the subendocardium in the hypertrophied ventricles was more severely affected after the onset of ischemia. (c) The ischemic region was larger in the ventricles of hypertensive dogs; both the proportion of the left ventricle affected and the mass of ischemic tissue were greater. Further study is needed to determine the mechanisms which predispose to sudden death following coronary occlusion in the pressure-hypertrophied left ventricle. These may be of major importance in the prevention and treatment of myocardial infarction in the hypertensive patient.

The effect of systemic hypertension per se on extent of myocardial ischemic injury following acute coronary occlusion was examined in a dog model in which phenylephrine was infused to elevate blood pressure (71). Alterations in systemic arterial pressure were shown to influence the extent of ischemic injury by altering both oxygen supply and demand, and the magnitude of the effect was related directly to the level of blood pressure. Small increases in systemic arterial pressure (diastolic pressure 95–115 mm Hg) did not alter blood flow to the ischemic myocardium and reduced ischemic injury, as reflected by a smaller rise of intramural carbon dioxide tension during coronary artery occlusion. Moderate increases in systemic arterial pressure (diastolic pressure 116–140 mm Hg) augmented blood flow to the ischemic myocardium but exerted no consistent effect on ischemia. A drastic rise in systemic arterial pressure (diastolic pressure >140 mm Hg) worsened ischemic injury, presumably by increasing the oxygen demand of the tissue, even though blood flow to the ischemic tissue was greatly augmented. These observations may bear on the clinical issue of blood pressure control in hypertensive patients with acute myocardial infarction.

Hypertension produced by renal artery constriction (135) or aortic coarctation (73) accelerated the development of atherosclerotic narrowing of the coronary arteries in monkeys fed an atherogenic diet compared with normotensive monkeys fed the same diet. In monkeys with coarctation of the aorta fed an atherogenic diet, ECG evidence of ischemic heart disease and sudden cardiac death occurred more frequently than in normotensive animals fed the same diet. Postmortem examination of hearts from monkeys with hypertension and hypercholesterolemia showed evidence of both hypertensive and atherosclerotic disease, whereas monkeys with hypertension or hypercholesterolemia alone had either hypertensive or atherosclerotic heart disease but not both. Hypertensive heart disease was characterized by hypertrophy of the left ventricle and by focal myocardial degeneration and fibrosis and focal thickening and narrowing of the small coronary arteries, particularly the sinus node artery and the atrioventricular node artery. Transmural myocardial infarction was found in monkeys with patent coronary arteries, suggesting a possible role for coronary artery spasm in ischemic heart disease associated with hypertension. Taken together, these data suggest that accelerated coronary atherosclerosis is one of the mechanisms that predisposes to myocardial infarction in the hypertrophied heart of the hypertensive patient.

Data from dogs with myocardial hypertrophy secondary to one-kidney Goldblatt hypertension or aortic coarctation hypertension indicate that the endocardium may not be adequately perfused in situations requiring high flow (9,74,120,127,144). This deficiency is not apparent in the resting state, since both blood flow per unit mass of myocardium and regional distribution of coronary flow are normal in resting hypertrophied hearts of hypertensive animals (120). In contrast, the endocardial/epicardial flow ratio is reduced even at rest in hearts in which left ventricular hypertrophy is secondary to aortic banding (144). The difference in myocardial blood flow distribution between these two models of hypertrophy may relate to a combination of higher diastolic pressure in the hypertensive hearts, which results in an increased diastolic perfusion pressure, and differences in degree of hypertrophy. In both models the endocardial/epicardial flow ratio is decreased in situations in which flow is increased, such as during exercise, pacing, maximal vasodilation produced by intravenous infusion of adenosine or carbochrome, or ischemia-induced vasodilatation. The mechanism of the relative decrease in endocardial perfusion in high flow states is uncertain, but may relate to reduced capillary density in the subendocardium of the hypertrophied heart and/or to impingement on arteries that supply the endocardium by the stiff and thickened left ventricle (134).

Thus, in situations requiring high flow to meet heart metabolic requirements, e.g., exercise, the endocardial layer of the markedly hypertrophied left ventricle may not receive adequate flow and could become truly ischemic. This is consistent with the frequent clinical observation of subendocardial underperfusion and angina pectoris in patients with left ventricular hypertrophy secondary to systemic hypertension or valvular aortic stenosis and without obstructive lesions in the coronary arteries. Additional evidence suggesting that the hypertrophied ventricle may be at increased risk of ischemic injury is the observation that during maximal coronary vasodilatation, the coronary vascular resistance of the left ventricle is the same in normal hearts, hypertrophied hearts of animals with one-kidney Goldblatt hypertension, and hypertrophied hearts of animals in which hypertension has been cured by unclipping the renal artery and resection of the stenotic segment (121). Further, elevated coronary vascular resistance has been demonstrated both at rest and following maximal coronary vasodilatation due to adenosine or carbochrome in all regions of the left ventricle and in the right ventricle of coarcted dogs (127). Assuming that minimal coronary vascular resistance measured during maximal vasodilatation is a valid index of the functional cross-sectional area of the coronary bed, these findings suggest that the cross-sectional area of the coronary vascular bed either remains unchanged or decreases with hypertrophy. Failure of the cross-sectional area of the coronary bed to increase as hypertrophy develops appears to be due to an anatomical or architectural alteration of the relationship between the coronary bed and cardiac muscle rather than to a functional alteration caused by hypertension alone.

Effects of Antihypertensive Treatment

Regression of experimentally induced myocardial hypertrophy has been demonstrated in a number of models following removal of the stimulus. Hall et al. (61) showed that cardiac hypertrophy produced by a constricting ligature on one renal artery or by the subcutaneous implantation of a desoxycorticosterone (DOC) pellet regressed after the ligated kidney or the DOC pellet was removed. More recently Beznak et al. (11) produced myocardial hypertrophy in the rat by four methods: hypertension secondary to DOC/NaCl treatment, hyperthyroidism, aortic coarctation, and nutritional anemia. In all cases hypertrophy regressed when the provoking stimulus was removed. In the DOC/NaCl hypertensive model, cardiac enlargement was impressive: the increase in weight of the whole heart was 38% in 2 weeks, 58% in 4 weeks, 64% in 6 weeks, and 78% in 9 weeks. Following removal of the DOC pellet and replacement of NaCl with tap water, blood pressure rapidly returned to normal, and cardiac hypertrophy regressed from 38% to 4% in 2 weeks, from 58% to 7% in 4 weeks, and from 64% to 11% in 6 weeks (Fig. 8). Comparable results were obtained following removal of the aortic band in animals with aortic coarctation hypertension. In neither case did heart size return completely to normal,

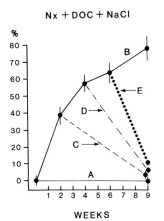

FIG. 8. Percentage change in the weight of the heart during cardiac hypertrophy and its regression. Ordinate: percentage change in heart weight. Abscissa: experimental period in weeks. (A) Normal control; (B) unilateral nephrectomy + DOC pellet implantation + salt-loading starting at week 0; (C) same as B but with removal of the stimuli after 2 weeks; (D) same as B but with removal of the stimuli after 4 weeks; (E) same as B but with removal of the stimuli after 6 weeks. The vertical lines indicate ± one standard error. (Reprinted with permission from *The Canadian Journal of Physiology and Pharmacology*, the National Research Council of Canada, and M. Beznak, ref. 11.)

however. Possible explanations for incompleteness of regression of myocardial hypertrophy include failure to remove the DOC pellet or to open the constricting aortic ring completely, scarring of the hypertrophied myocardium with connective tissue, and/or the development of structural lesions of the systemic resistance vessels which cause fixed elevation of peripheral resistance and persistent hypertension.

The biochemical consequences of mechanical removal of pressure overload have been examined in the aortic constriction model (26,137) and the two-kidney, one-clip Goldblatt hypertension model (166) in the rat. In the aortic constriction model, stable left ventricular hypertrophy developed within 1 week of constricting the ascending aorta to approximately 30% of its original cross-sectional area. Removal of the constricting band either 10 days (early debanding) or 38 days (late debanding) later completely relieved the obstruction to left ventricular outflow. After early debanding, left ventricular mass decreased from 35% to 11% above control values in 3 days and remained at control levels for the rest of the study period. Left ventricular RNA of the debanded animals fell from 37% to 19% above the control group 3 days after surgery and remained at control levels for the rest of the study period. Left ventricular DNA of the debanded group remained elevated for as long as 28 days postdebanding, however. Similarly, left ventricular hydroxyproline levels of the debanded group remained substantially elevated above those of controls. Following late debanding, left ventricular mass and RNA fell less rapidly than after early debanding, although both eventually decreased to control values. In contrast, left ventricular DNA and hydroxyproline content did not decline, remaining 25% and 118% above control values, respectively, at 28 days postdebanding. The data show that while left ventricular mass and RNA content decrease after relief of a pressure overload, left ventricular DNA and hydroxyproline content do not. DNA and hydroxyproline content per gram of tissue actually increased in debanded animals because of the fall in left ventricular mass.

Results obtained following removal of the clipped kidney in two-kidney, one-clip Goldblatt rats following 6 weeks of hypertension were compatible with those seen following late debanding. There were significant reductions in arterial pressure (but not to normotensive levels) and left ventricular weight, no change in ventricular RNA or DNA concentration, and increases in ventricular hydroxyproline concentration (166). Plasma renin activity fell, and ventricular catecholamine concentration increased following nephrectomy. It is not known why connective tissue does not regress as readily as cardiac muscle, but explanations that have been put forward include the fact that the increase in connective tissue is mainly due to cellular hyperplasia, whereas the changes in muscle cells are chiefly those of hypertrophy. Also, collagen fibers, once formed and extruded into the interstitial space, may not be as accessible to destruction as are intracellular components. This problem merits further investigation, as does the question of whether increased myocardial collagen impairs cardiac performance by interfering with diastolic compliance.

Prevention or reversal of left ventricular hypertrophy has been reported in association with lowering of blood pressure in SHR following treatment with alpha-methyldopa (163,167,179,180). Alpha-methyldopa administered for a 10-week period to SHR with stable hypertension lowered blood pressure to normal range and reduced left ventricular weight to a value intermediate between that found in sham-treated SHR and control normotensive WKY (163,167). Results were similar when the development of hypertension was prevented by administering alpha-methyldopa to young SHR. Alpha-methyldopa also reduced ventricular weight in normotensive WKY rats without altering blood pressure. Reversal of cardiac hypertrophy in SHR was associated with an increase in DNA concentration toward normal without an accompanying change in DNA content, reflecting reversal of hypertrophy. RNA concentration was reduced, reflecting a decrease in cellular protein synthesis. Hydroxyproline concentration was increased without an accompanying change in hydroxyproline content. Similar alterations in RNA and hydroxyproline were induced in the myocardium of normotensive WKY by alpha-methyldopa, but DNA concentration was reduced rather than increased as in SHR. Persistence of the hypertrophy-related abnormalities in myocardial DNA and hydroxyproline in the face of regression of left ventricular hypertrophy in SHR provides additional evidence that connective tissue does not regress as readily as cardiac muscle following removal of the stimulus for hypertrophy.

Administration of alpha-methyldopa to SHR from 4 to 16 weeks of age has been shown to prevent or modify the ultrastructural abnormalities previously reported in this model (181). Interestingly, alpha-methyldopa produced these changes even when administered in doses too small to lower blood pressure. Heart weights of treated animals were in the high normal range; myocytes in the epicardial region of treated animals were similar in size to those of normotensive animals whereas those in the subendocardial region were only slightly hypertrophic. The volume ratio of mitochondria to myofibrils in myocytes of treated animals was restored to normal. Conversely, the enhanced folding of the intercalated disc which is observed in the untreated SHR was accentuated in alpha-methyldopa-treated animals. These findings support the hypothesis that cardiac hypertrophy in the SHR is not due to elevated blood pressure alone. They further suggest that the effectiveness of alpha-methyldopa in reducing heart size is not entirely related to its antihypertensive action, but may be mediated by central adrenergic mechanisms or a direct effect on the myocyte.

Recent evidence indicates that structural abnormalities characteristic of myocardial hypertrophy in SHR may be influenced by the aging process, the duration of hypertension and/or hypertrophy, and the magnitude of the hypertrophy and severity of the hypertension (182). The decrement in mitochondria/myofibrillar volume ratio that is seen in hypertension-induced hypertrophy has been shown to progress with increased duration of the hypertension. Further, myocardial hypertrophy in SHR becomes stabilized over time and thus is relatively refractory to reversal following antihypertensive treatment of older animals. To examine this stabilization effect, Tomanek (180) administered alpha-methyldopa to SHR and normotensive control WKY rats between the ages of 1 and 12 months, a period that encompassed the developmental and early-established phases of hypertension. A second group of SHR and WKY rats received alpha-methyldopa beginning at age 12 months for a total of 3 months. The antihypertensive effects of alpha-methyldopa were identical in both groups of SHR. In contrast, left ventricular weight and cell size were significantly reduced following early long-term treatment SHR, but remained unchanged following delayed treatment. Despite the effectiveness of early long-term treatment in modifying left ventricular mass, the relative volumes of mitochondria, myofibrils, and other cellular components were not altered. Delayed treatment, on the other hand, caused a twofold increase in relative sarcoplasmic volume and a decrease in myofibrillar volume in both SHR and WKY. These findings indicate that shifts in relative volumes of intracellular components following alpha-methyldopa treatment are independent of cell size and blood pressure and suggest that the effects of alpha-methyldopa on the cardiac myocyte are dependent on aging and/or factors associated with the development or stabilization of hypertrophy. The efficacy of alpha-methyldopa in reversing hypertrophy is markedly attenuated once stabilized myocardial growth is attained (180). Whether these observations are pertinent to the treatment of hypertension in man is a matter of conjecture.

Further evidence for a dissociation between the blood pressure lowering actions of antihypertensive drugs and their effects on cardiac hypertrophy comes from studies in which a vasodilator (hydralazine or minoxidil) was administered to SHR in doses sufficient to lower blood pressure into the normal range (164,167,175,180). Left ventricular weight was unchanged following hydralazine administration and actually increased following administration of minoxidil despite adequate blood pressure control. In addition, characteristic alterations in myocardial RNA, DNA, and hydroxyproline content and concentration that accompany regression of myocardial hypertrophy were not seen in these hearts. Both hydralazine and minoxidil stimulate renin release and activate the sympathetic nervous system via reflex mechanisms, and either or both of these effects could stimulate myocardial hypertrophy. Additional factors to be taken into account are the positive inotropic effects of the vasodilators and possible direct trophic effects of the drugs on the myocardium. Further study is needed to elucidate the mechanism by which cardiac hypertrophy is preserved in the face of adequate blood pressure control by hydralazine and minoxidil. The demonstration by Limas and Spier (100) of improvement in Ca^{2+} transport by cardiac sarcoplasmic reticulum of mature SHR following treatment with effective antihypertensive doses of alpha-methyldopa but not hydralazine may be a clue to such a mechanism.

In contrast, the angiotensin-converting enzyme inhibitor captopril, which acts as a vasodilator, is effective in preventing myocardial hypertrophy when administered to young SHR and in reversing hypertrophy in mature SHR and two-kidney, one-clip Goldblatt hypertensive rats (165,166). In these studies blood pressure fell, left ventricular weight decreased, and alterations in myocardial RNA and DNA appropriate to regression of myocardial hypertrophy appeared in captopril-treated rats. In addition, captopril therapy was associated with a reduction in myocardial hydroxyproline content, a result observed after surgical cure of renovascular hypertension but not associated with alpha-methyldopa treatment. The mechanism(s) by which captopril effects reversal of cardiac hypertrophy is unknown but may include prevention of angiotensin II formation, failure to activate sympathetic nervous system responses to a fall in blood pressure, production of vasodilator prostaglandins, preservation of circulating bradykinin, and/or a direct effect on the heart and blood vessels.

Most studies have shown that chronic administration of β-adrenergic receptor blocking agents does not prevent or cause reversal of myocardial hypertrophy in hypertensive rats even when blood pressure is lowered significantly (133,180,188). In contrast, Fernandes et al. (44) and Richer et al. (146) reported that propranolol and atenolol attenuated the development of myocardial hypertrophy in rats with renal hypertension and in SHR, respectively. In the former case, propranolol did not ameliorate the hypertension; in the latter, atenolol did cause an attenuation in the severity of genetic hypertension. The mechanisms by which β-adrenergic blocking agents can influence the development and reversal of hypertension-induced myocardial hypertrophy are incompletely understood but may involve decreases in cardiac workload and inotropic activity, blockade of catecholamine effects on the heart, or inhibition of neurally mediated renin release. It is uncertain why these effects are evident in only a minority of experimental studies.

The effects of reversing pressure-overload hypertrophy on cardiac pumping ability have been evaluated in a cat model of right ventricular hypertrophy following debanding of the pulmonary artery (21), in adult SHR following alpha-methyldopa treatment (171), and in a single cat papillary muscle following pressure unloading secondary to transection of the chordae tendinae (22). Functional abnormalities of the hypertrophied right ventricular myocardium were fully reversed with restoration of normal myocardial loading conditions (21). Treatment of SHR with alpha-methyldopa was associated with reversal of cardiac hypertrophy and improvement in ventricular function, which was, in part, related to the observed reduction in arterial pressure (171). In this study left ventricular pumping ability was determined by maximum levels of stroke volume and cardiac output reached during rapid intravenous volume loading with blood. Therapy increased heart rate and cardiac output and decreased peripheral resistance. During volume-loading, the levels of stroke volume and cardiac output at matched left ventricular end-diastolic pressures were significantly higher in treated than in untreated SHR. To evaluate the role of blood pressure in the improved peak pumping ability observed in treated rats, a phenylephrine infusion was used to equalize pressures while repeating cardiac function studies. In normotensive WKY and untreated SHR, left ventricular pump function was not greatly affected. A pronounced depression in peak stroke volume and peak cardiac output was observed only in treated SHR. The mechanism of the ventricular decompensation that follows an acute rise in pressure in treated SHR is unknown, but the response raises questions about the state of pump performance and/or contractile properties of the myocardium after reversal of cardiac hypertrophy with alpha-methyldopa.

Methyldopa can affect myocardial contractility either directly or as a result of decreasing the adrenergic drive to the heart. Further, the structural abnormalities associated with reduced pump performance in SHR may not be corrected by treatment with methyldopa. Myocardial hydroxyproline concentration increases significantly during reversal of cardiac hypertrophy induced by methyldopa treatment (163). An increase in fibrous tissue during development of cardiac hypertrophy was considered by Averill et al. (8) to account for the reduced ventricular performance in experimental renal hypertension. On this basis, it is possible that the smaller and presumably more fibrous heart of treated SHR is unable to cope with acute stresses that call for an increase in ventricular tension to overcome an increase in impedance to left ventricular ejection. Alterations in cardiac collagen might also decrease myocardial compliance. It is therefore possible that ventricular compliance remained depressed following treatment with methyldopa. Direct determinations of pressure-volume curves in treated animals are needed to determine the influence of increased hydroxyproline concentration in hearts with reversed hypertrophy. These studies may have clinical relevance in predicting myocardial responses to antihypertensive therapy.

It has been shown that under some circumstances reduction of myocardial loading may lead to degeneration of myocardial ultrastructure, depression of isotonic and isometric contractile function, and a negative shift of force-velocity and active length-tension relationships (22). Whether such changes could occur with reduction of systemic arterial pressure into the normal range in a previously hypertensive animal or patient remains to be determined.

THE HEART IN HYPERTENSIVE MAN

Morphology

Gross Anatomy

Systemic hypertension in man is related to increased mass of the whole heart and particularly of the left ventricle. Reiner and associates (142,143) examined postmortem hearts from a series of 292 adult patients (160 men and 132 women), of whom 60 (29 men and 31 women) had systemic hypertension (blood pressure >170/90 mm Hg recorded at the time of final admission to the hospital) without significant coronary artery disease, previous myocardial infarction, macroscopic myocardial fibrosis, valvular heart disease, or disproportionate right ventricular hypertrophy. All of the component muscle weights, including left ventricular free wall, right ventricular free wall, and interventricular septum and atria, were greater in hearts from hypertensive patients than in those from normotensive controls. The difference between hypertensive and normotensive hearts was most pronounced for the left ventricular free wall and interventricular septum. The normal left ventricle of the adult male was found to weigh 203 g or less; of the adult female, 141 g or less (142a). The upper limit of normal heart weight in men was set at 400 g; in women, at 300 g. The thickness of the left ventricular free wall and the interventricular septum tended to be greater in hypertensive hearts than in normotensive ones and greater in males than in females. However, thickness measurements of the left ventricle showed more overlap between hypertensive and normotensive hearts than did left ventricular weight and appeared to be of limited usefulness in the diagnosis of left ventricular hypertrophy. The degree of left ventricular hypertrophy was significantly correlated with systolic blood pressure in both sexes; a similar relationship was not apparent for diastolic blood pressure or pulse pressure. For any given level of blood pressure elevation, left ventricular hypertrophy was greater in men than in women and in younger patients than in older ones. Anatomic standards of left ventricular size such as these provide the basis for standardization of cineangiographic and echocardiographic methods of assessing left ventricular hypertrophy.

Microscopic Anatomy

Quantitative morphometric studies of the heart in patients with hypertensive heart disease have been limited by the difficulties inherent in examining autopsy material. Fuster and associates (54) performed a quantitative analysis of left ventricular myocardial fiber cross-sectional area and interstitial tissue volume in 22 hearts from patients with chronic systemic hypertension and mild left ventricular failure (NYHA Class II-III) who did not have significant coronary artery disease and who died from causes other than cardiac failure. Hearts from hypertensive subjects showed a significant increase in myocardial fiber diameter (7.1 ± 0.8 μm vs control 5.8 ± 0.5 μm, $p<0.001$). Myocardial cell dimensions were similar in basal and apical regions and subendocardial and subepicardial areas of the left ventricle. The proportion of interstitial tissue was 31.5%, unchanged from the value in normal hearts. Thus hearts from patients with systemic hypertension have evidence of myocyte hypertrophy similar to that seen in animal models of experimentally induced or genetic hypertension (see earlier part of chapter).

The combination of systemic hypertension and diabetes mellitus produces myocardial abnormalities rarely found in patients with either disorder alone (40). These abnormalities, which occur in the absence of significant coronary lesions, include focal myocytolysis and dense interstitial fibrosis with deposition of PAS-positive, diastase-resistant material in the fibrotic regions. It is uncertain if the myocytolysis and interstitial scarring are related to disease of small intramyocardial blood vessels. On the basis of these observations, it has been suggested that the cardiomyopathy associated with diabetes mellitus is a specific entity that may be secondary to the combined effects of diabetes and hypertension on the myocardium. Similar observations in rats with streptozotocin-induced diabetes and one-kidney Goldblatt hypertension (39) add strength to this interpretation. Use of the hypertensive diabetic rat model may allow more precise assessment of the role of hypertension in the pathogenesis of diabetic cardiomyopathy in man.

Echocardiography in the Evaluation of Left Ventricular Hypertrophy and Function

Measurements of left ventricular wall thickness and cavity dimensions using the M-mode echocardiogram have been used to calculate ventricular mass in normal and hypertrophic hearts (10,30,185). These estimates of left ventricular mass have been validated against biplane angiography and against left ventricular weights obtained at autopsy (30,87,138). Figure 9 is a diagrammatic representation of the method for obtaining left ventricular dimensions recommended by the American Society of Echocardiography (42,153). Posterior left ventricular wall thickness (PWT) and septal wall thickness (SWT) can be measured during any phase of the cardiac cycle. Diastolic measurements are taken at the peak of the R wave of the electrocardiogram; systolic measurements, at the peak downward motion of the interventricular septum. Wall thickness measurements should be taken from leading edge to leading edge of the septal and endocardial echoes (42,153). The diastolic left ventricular internal dimension (LVID$_d$) is taken between the left side of the interventricular septum and the posterior left ventricular endocardium at end-diastole (Fig. 10). The systolic left ventricular internal dimension (LVID$_s$) is taken at the peak downward motion of the interventricular septum (Fig. 10). There is controversy in the literature as to precisely how these measurements should be made (23,30,42,153). For instance, whether the thickness of endocardial echoes should be included in measurements of septal and posterior wall thickness is a point of debate among investigators (30,42). Whatever conventions are adopted, it is important to standardize measurements within any given laboratory in order to obtain a reproducible assessment of left ventricular wall thickness and cavity dimensions.

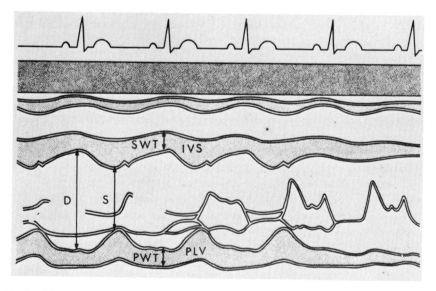

FIG. 9. Diagram of the M-mode echocardiogram demonstrating the left ventricular measurements as recommended by the American Society of Echocardiography. D = left ventricular diastolic dimension; S = left ventricular systolic dimension; SWT = septal wall thickness; IVS = interventricular septum; PWT = posterior left ventricular wall thickness; PLV = posterior left ventricular wall. (Reprinted by permission of Lea and Febiger, and H. Feigenbaum, *Echocardiography*, 3rd edition, 1981.)

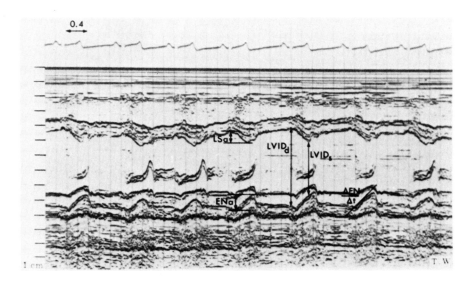

FIG. 10. Left ventricular M-mode echocardiogram showing some of the measurements that can be obtained from such an examination. This recording also demonstrates some cyclical variations that may occur with respiration. LS_a = amplitude of motion of left septal echo; EN_a = amplitude of motion of posterior left ventricular endocardial echo; $LVID_d$ = diastolic left ventricular internal dimension; $LVID_s$ = systolic left ventricular internal dimension; $\Delta EN/\Delta t$ = rate of rise of posterior left ventricular endocardial echo. (Reprinted by permission of Lea and Febiger, and H. Feigenbaum, *Echocardiography*, 3rd edition, 1981.)

Once measurements of left ventricular wall thickness and cavity dimensions have been obtained, it is possible to calculate ventricular mass. The theory behind such a calculation is to estimate the volume of the epicardial surface of the ventricle and to subtract the volume of the ventricular cavity. The difference represents the volume of the left ventricular wall. A number of formulas, all of which involve assumptions about geometric uniformity of the left ventricle, have been used to estimate total left ventricular volume and end-diastolic intraventricular volume (30,140,178). The weaknesses of this technique lie in the imprecision of echocardiographic determinations of volume and in inaccuracies introduced with assumptions about a uniform ventricular configuration. Despite their defects, estimates of left ventricular mass based on M-mode echocardiographic measurements are strongly correlated with anatomic left ventricular mass ($r = 0.86$ to $r = 0.96$, depending on the method of estimating volume and mean myocardial thickness) (30) and with angiographic estimates of left ventricular mass ($r = 0.83$, ref. 122, to $r = 0.88$) (185). It has been shown that the echocardiographic estimation of left ventricular mass is a more sensitive indicator of left ventricular hypertrophy than left ventricular posterior wall or interventricular septal thickness (110).

In a recent study, anatomic, echocardiographic, and electrocardiographic findings of left ventricular hypertrophy were compared in 34 subjects who had been studied shortly before death (141). Echocardiographic estimates of left ventricular mass correlated well with postmortem left ventricular weight even when myocardial infarction was present or the left ventricle was dilated ($r = 0.96$). The M-mode echocardiogram diagnosed left ventricular hypertrophy accurately. Sensitivity of the diagnosis was 93%:

$$\frac{\text{True positives correctly diagnosed}}{\text{Total true positives}} \times 100$$

Specificity was 95%:

$$\frac{\text{True negatives correctly diagnosed}}{\text{Total true negatives}} \times 100$$

In contrast, ECG criteria for left ventricular hypertrophy were insensitive (Romhilt-Estes point score 50% and Sokolow-Lyon voltage criteria 21% for both sets of criteria) but specific (95%). In the same study, echocardiographic and electrocardiographic diagnoses of left ventricular hypertrophy were compared in an unselected clinical series of 100 patients, 20 of whom had hypertensive heart disease. Results were similar: established electrocardiographic criteria were insensitive but specific indices of left ventricular hypertrophy. The investigators found that correction of voltage for distance from the left ventricle did not substantially improve results. Further, they were unable to devise new electrocardiographic criteria to improve diagnostic accuracy. Data from this study predicted that when the prevalence of left ventricular hypertrophy in a population is less than 10%, conventional electrocardiographic criteria will identify more false positives than true positives. Comparison of electrocardiographic and cineangiographic criteria of left ventricular hypertrophy in a series of 93 patients, 47 of whom had left ventricular hypertrophy on the electrocardiogram, yielded similar results (4). Wall thickening sufficient to result in increased left ventricular mass was not reflected in left ventricular hypertrophy on the electrocardiogram unless the left ventricle was also dilated. These data indicate that a critical geometric relationship resulting from a combination of increased wall thickness and chamber dilatation is necessary for left ventricular hypertrophy to appear on the electrocardiogram. Thus it appears unwise to use electrocardiographic estimates in the assessment of left ventricular hypertrophy, even for screening or epidemiologic purposes.

In order to determine normal echocardiographic values for cardiac dimensions and functional parameters in older subjects, Gardin et al. (55) studied 136 adults (78 men and 58 women, 20 to 97 years of age) without evidence of cardiovascular disease. When the oldest group (>70 years) was compared with the youngest group (21–30 years), significant ($p < 0.01$) increases in aortic root (22%) and left atrial (16%) dimensions, interventricular septal (20%) and left ventricular free-wall (18%) thickness, and estimated left ventricular mass (15%) were noted. In addition, a significant (<0.01) decrease in mean mitral E-F slope (43%) and slight decreases in mean left ventricular systolic and diastolic internal dimensions (5% and 6%, respectively; $p<0.05$) were noted. Left ventricular ejection fraction and percentage fractional shortening were found to be independent of age. These data were used to derive regression equations that are related to both age and body surface area which can be used to calculate mean normal values and 95% prediction intervals for echocardiographic measurements in adults.

Recently the reliability of two-dimensional echocardiographic quantitation of left ventricular mass has been assessed in man *in vivo* (182a) and in canine and human hearts *in vitro* (142,189). The correlation between estimates of left ventricular volume made by two-dimensional echocardiography and those made by angiography has been excellent ($r = 0.89$–0.97) (66,182a), as has the correlation between estimates of left ventricular mass made by two-dimensional echocardiography and actual left ventricular weight ($r = 0.93$) (142). The latter of the diagnosis was 93%: correlation was obtained using two-dimensional echo short-axis area-length estimates of left ventricular mass corrected for the specific image area properties of the echo instrument used. Short-axis imaging techniques have the advantage of permitting sharper definition of endocardial and epicardial borders than do other views in the same subject because the echo beam has a relatively favorable angle of incidence throughout much of the short-axis image. Use of a short-axis image at the papillary muscle level at approximately the midpoint in left ventricular length in combination with apical left ventricular length has given accurate estimates of left ventricular mass and volume in both symmetric and asymmetric ventricles (142). The two-dimensional echo is superior to the M-mode echo for estimating volumes of irregularly shaped ventricles because mean myocardial thickness can be better estimated by two-dimensional techniques and because the formula for estimating the left ventricular length/diameter ratio from the M-mode echo is inaccurate when applied to irregularly shaped ventricles. Nevertheless, two-dimensional echocardiography tends to underestimate left ventricular volume and therefore to overestimate ventricular mass (17,46,160). This error can be minimized by using equations that relate echocardiographic measurements to angiographic volumes (Tortoledo et al., 1983). In summary, two-dimensional echocardiography is the method of choice in the noninvasive diagnosis of left ventricular hypertrophy and estimation of left ventricular mass, particularly in irregularly shaped ventricles and hearts in which there is segmented impairment of left ventricular wall motion.

Echocardiography is useful in the assessment of left ventricular function in patients with normal or hypertrophic ventricles (42,109) (Tortoledo et al., 1983). Excellent correlations ($r = 0.87$–0.96) have been reported between total left ventricular ejection fraction determined (50). These methods can be applied to the problem of assessing ventricular performance in patients with myocardial hypertrophy.

M-mode echocardiography has been used to examine the effects of acute (72) and chronic (36,84,156,161,183) alterations in systemic arterial pressure on left ventricular performance in man. Augmentation of systemic arterial pressure by means of a phenylephrine infusion in a group of normal human subjects resulted in significant decreases in both by two-dimensional echocardiography and by cineangiography (Tortoledo et al., 1983). Left ventricular ejection fraction is calculated using left ventricular (LV) volumes:

$$\frac{\text{LV diastolic volume } - \text{ LV systolic volume}}{\text{LV diastolic volume}}$$

An additional means of assessing left ventricular function involves determination of circumferential shortening (42,48). In such calculations the left ventricle is represented as a series of circles, and the rate of circumferential shortening is used to describe ventricular contractions. If the left ventricular internal diameter obtained from the M-mode echocardiogram is assumed to be a diameter of the circle, it is possible to calculate circumferential shortening:

$$\frac{\text{LVIDd } - \text{ LVIDs}}{\text{LVIDd}}$$

By obtaining a measurement of ejection time (ET), it is then possible to calculate a mean rate of circumferential shortening (VC$_f$).

$$\text{Mean VC}_f = \frac{\text{LVIDd } - \text{ LVIDs}}{\text{LVIDd}}$$

Fractional shortening of the left ventricle is similar to circumferential shortening except that no assumptions are made about volumes or circumferences. Instead, one merely calculates the percent shortening of the left ventricular dimension: Percent fractional shortening of the left ventricle =

$$\frac{\text{LVIDd } - \text{ LVIDs}}{\text{LVIDd}} \times 100$$

Another echocardiographic measurement commonly used in the assessment of left ventricular performance is wall motion (42). The total amplitude or excursion of the septal echo or of the posterior ventricular endocardial echo (ENa) can be measured. Mean velocity is calculated by dividing the amplitude by the ejection time:

$$\text{Mean velocity } = \frac{\text{ENa}}{\text{ET}}$$

The measurement is then normalized by dividing it by the diastolic dimension:

$$\text{Normalized velocity } = \frac{\text{ENa}}{\text{LVIDd } \times \text{ ET}}$$

Sophisticated assessments of rates of wall motion, changes in wall motion, absolute cavity dimension, and rates of change in cavity dimensions and wall thickening can be obtained through the use of computers and a sonic or light pen to trace left ventricular echoes (50), normalized and nonnormalized VC_f, and posterior wall velocity (72). End-diastolic diameter increased and ejection fraction decreased significantly when blood pressure was elevated. These observations are consistent with the results of animal studies in which there was a reduction in the extent and velocity of myocardial shortening as resistance to ejection was increased. These data also indicate that when echocardiographic measurements are used to assess left ventricular performance, the level of systemic arterial pressure at which studies are carried out must be taken into consideration.

Karliner and associates (84) used M-mode echocardiographic assessment of left ventricular performance to study the adaptation of the left ventricle to chronic pressure overload. They studied 18 patients with left ventricular hypertrophy secondary to systemic arterial hypertension who lacked clinical evidence of ischemic heart disease or congestive failure. All had increased posterior wall and/or interventricular septal thickness. Ejection phase indexes of left ventricular performance, including mean VC_f, fractional percent of shortening, normalized posterior wall velocity, and ejection fraction, were within the normal range in the resting state. Wall stress in the hypertensive patients was identical to that obtained in a group of normal subjects. Thus the hypertrophic response to a chronic increase in afterload in the form of elevated systemic arterial pressure did not cause depression of the basal inotropic state of the left ventricle. Karliner and associates (84) postulated that resting left ventricular performance was normal in their patients because values for wall stress remained within the normal range. Similarly, Toshima and associates (183) reported a normal echocardiographic ejection fraction in 11 patients with concentric left ventricular hypertrophy caused by systemic arterial hypertension.

Echocardiographic techniques have been used to study left ventricular relaxation and filling in various forms of left ventricular hypertrophy (64). In this study echocardiograms in 24 patients with hypertrophic obstructive cardiomyopathy and 24 patients with chronic left ventricular pressure overload (due to aortic stenosis in 6 and to severe arterial hypertension in 18) were analyzed by computer and compared with those of normal subjects. The relaxation time index (minimal left ventricular dimension to mitral valve opening) was 13 ± 15 msec in normal subjects and was prolonged in patients with cardiomyopathy (93 ± 37 msec) and pressure overload (66 ± 31 msec). During the interval from minimal left ventricular dimension to mitral valve opening, both groups with hypertrophy had a marked increase in left ventricular dimension, which was significantly greater than in normal subjects. This was probably a result of an abnormal change in left ventricular shape during isovolumic relaxation.

The rapid filling phase and the increase in dimension during this period were significantly reduced in both hypertrophic obstructive cardiomyopathy and chronic pressure overload. In patients with pressure overload the reduced increase in left ventricular dimension during the rapid diastolic filling period was compensated for by a greater dimensional increase due to atrial contraction, resulting in a normal end-diastolic dimension. These data indicate that significant prolongation of isovolumic relaxation, often associated with an abnormal diastolic filling pattern, is seen in various forms of left ventricular hypertrophy in man.

Echocardiography in Adults with Established Hypertension

Use of invasive techniques for assessment of cardiac dimensions and function in hypertensive patients has been limited by ethical considerations. Echocardiography has proved to be a broadly applicable noninvasive method for examination of the heart in clinical hypertension. The method provides sufficiently accurate measurements of left ventricular wall thickness and wall motion to permit useful assessment of heart size and function in the clinical setting. Echocardiography reveals alterations in left ventricular structure and/or function in adult hypertensive patients who lack both electrocardiographic and roentgenographic evidence of left ventricular hypertrophy and the symptoms of left ventricular failure (35,156,161). Thus echocardiography is the most sensitive and specific noninvasive technique currently available for the detection of cardiac abnormalities in hypertensive subjects. There is evidence that serial echocardiograms may be useful in following hypertensive patients in order to monitor the response of the heart to antihypertensive treatment (28,36,49,76,161,169).

Echocardiographic abnormalities have been common in all reported studies in hypertensive patients, whether treated or not, but the nature of the abnormalities reported has varied from study to study. As a part of the Atlanta Hypertension Detection and Follow-up Program, Schlant et al. (161) obtained standard M-mode echocardiograms on 94 asymptomatic patients with untreated and uncomplicated essential hypertension (diastolic blood pressure >90 mm Hg). Patients with a history of past or current antihypertensive treatment, coronary artery disease, alcohol abuse, diabetes mellitus, congestive heart failure, or renal insufficiency were excluded because it was felt that these conditions might have independent effects on left ventricular anatomy and/or function. Most of the patients were black. Results of the study are summarized in Tables 1 and 2. In hypertensive subjects there was evidence of left ventricular hypertrophy directly proportional in extent to the severity of the hypertension. The thickness of the posterior wall of the left ventricle was increased significantly at both end-diastole and end-systole in hypertensive patients compared with normotensive controls. The thickness of the interventricular septum was also increased in patients with severe hypertension, but no patient met standard echocardiographic criteria for either asymmetric septal hypertrophy or idiopathic subaortic stenosis. The calculated left ventricular mass index was increased in all three hypertensive groups, indicating that left ventricular hypertrophy was present even in mild hypertensives. Left ventricular internal diameter was not significantly increased at end-diastole or end-systole, and left atrial internal diameter was not altered, indicating that the left ventricle was not dilated and the left atrium was not enlarged in hypertensive patients. Table 2 summarizes mean values for six indices of left ventricular performance in hypertensive patients and normotensive controls. Significant decreases in calculated left

TABLE 1. *Echocardiographic determinations of left ventricular anatomy*

| | Normal | Diastolic hypertension | | |
		Mild (90–104 mm Hg)	Moderate (105–115 mm Hg)	Severe (116–155 mm Hg)
Posterior wall thickness (mm)				
End-diastole	9.6 ± 1.4	10.9 ± 1.8[a]	11.0 ± 0.9[a]	11.9 ± 2.1[a]
End-systole	15.7 ± 2.0	17.2 ± 2.0[a]	17.3 ± 1.9[a]	17.9 ± 2.7[a]
Interventricular septal thickness at end-diastole (mm)	10.4 ± 1.1	11.0 ± 1.9	11.4 ± 1.6	14.0 ± 2.0[a]
Internal diameter (mm)				
End-diastole	48.6 ± 4.3	46.6 ± 6.9	48.0 ± 5.6	50.6 ± 10.4
End-systole	31.5 ± 4.5	31.8 ± 6.3	33.1 ± 5.0	37.2 ± 11.8[a]
Mass index at end-diastole (g/m²)	105.4 ± 19.5	130 ± 40.0[a]	147.5 ± 35.8[a]	172.3 ± 54.3[a]
Volume index at end-diastole (ml/m²)	62.2 ± 14.5	64.0 ± 24.2	69.6 ± 23.3	81.9 ± 48.9
Left atrial internal diameter at end-systole (mm)	34.1 ± 4.4	30.8 ± 5.7	30.1 ± 5.7	35.6 ± 5.6

[a]Least significant difference multiple range test indicates that these patients differ from the normal group at the 0.05 level.
Reprinted with permission from *Cardiovascular Medicine* and R. C. Schlant (161).

TABLE 2. *Echocardiographic determinations of left ventricular function*

		Diastolic hypertension		
	Normal	Mild (90–104 mm Hg)	Moderate (105–115 mm Hg)	Severe (116–155 mm Hg)
Decrease in internal diameter	0.357 ± 0.053	0.32 ± 0.064[a]	0.312 ± 0.048[a]	0.273 ± 0.075
Ejection fraction	0.72 ± 0.07	0.68 ± 0.09[a]	0.67 ± 0.07[a]	0.61 ± 0.13[a]
Velocity of circumferential shortening (circ/sec)	1.29 ± 0.22	1.24 ± 0.25	1.16 ± 0.16	1.04 ± 0.26
Posterior wall excursion (mm)	11.4 ± 1.3	11.1 ± 1.4	10.7 ± 2.6	10.5 ± 1.9
Posterior wall velocity (mm/sec)	51.6 ± 12.1	49.3 ± 10.8	43.4 ± 14.6	46.0 ± 12.2
Posterior wall thickening (%)	65.7 ± 19.9	60.1 ± 19.7	58.6 ± 17.3	51.9 ± 22.6

[a]Least significant difference multiple range test indicates that these patients differ from the normal group at the 0.05 level.
Reproduced with permission from *Cardiovascular Medicine* and R. C. Schlant (161).

ventricular ejection fraction and in the fractional decrease in left ventricular internal diameter from end-diastole to end-systole were found in all three hypertensive groups compared with normotensive controls. The other indices of left ventricular performance were not significantly altered in hypertensive subjects.

Resting diastolic blood pressure was weakly but positively correlated with left ventricular mass index ($r = 0.239$, $p < 0.05$) but not with the thickness of the posterior wall of the left ventricle ($r = 0.082$) or of the interventricular septum ($r = 0.212$). Interestingly, there was a significant negative correlation between left ventricular mass index and decrease in ventricular performance as assessed by the decrease in left ventricular internal diameter at end-diastole. These findings suggest that the magnitude of left ventricular enlargement in hypertensive patients is directly, although not precisely, related to the severity of hypertension and that in hypertensive patients the performance of the hypertrophying ventricle is impaired prior to the onset of congestive failure. Whether echocardiographic indices of left ventricular dysfunction are predictive of congestive heart failure in a given patient is unknown. Longitudinal studies of hypertensive patients with and without adequate antihypertensive treatment will be needed to answer this question.

There were weak positive correlations between left ventricular mass index and electrocardiographic evidence of left ventricular hypertrophy ($r = 0.26$, $p < 0.05$) and baseline diastolic blood pressure ($r = 0.34$, $p < 0.01$). There were also statistically significant positive correlations between the echocardiographic measurement of left ventricular internal diameter at end-diastole and the heart volume index calculated from chest films ($r = 0.406$, $p < 0.001$) and between the echocardiographic left ventricular mass index and the radiologic heart volume index ($r = 0.498$, $p < 0.001$). Schlant et al. (149) pointed out that in individual hypertensive patients, however, echocardiography appeared to be more sensitive than the electrocardiogram or chest film in detecting left ventricular abnormalities.

Dunn et al. (37) obtained similar results in a study of 31 patients with sustained hypertension (blood pressure $>140/90$ mm Hg) and 14 normotensive control subjects. Patients with a history of angina pectoris, or evidence of previous myocardial infarction, atrial fibrillation, or congestive heart failure, or who were more than 55 years of age were excluded from the study because of possible independent effects of these conditions on left ventricular anatomy and/or function. Patients were classified into three groups on the basis of the electrocardiogram and chest film: group I—normal electrocardiogram and chest film; group II—evidence of left atrial abnormality on electrocardiogram and normal chest film; and group III— evidence of left ventricular hypertrophy on chest film and/or electrocardiogram. Mean arterial pressure was greater in group II than I and in group III than II (Fig. 11). Septal and posterior wall thicknesses and the left ventricular mass index were significantly increased in groups II and III but not in group I, indicating that increased left ventricular mass was present in some patients (group II) who lacked electrocardiographic and roentgenographic evidence of left ventricular hypertrophy. This was interpreted as confirming the earlier finding of Frolich and associates (53) that left atrial abnormalities are sensitive indices of early cardiac pathology

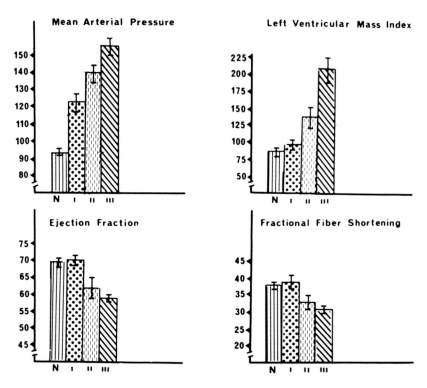

FIG. 11.   Mean arterial pressure (mm Hg), left ventricular mass index (g/m²) and two derived indexes of left ventricular performance [ejection fraction (%) and fractional fiber shortening (%)] are shown. (All *bars* represent mean ± 1 SEM.) The progressive rise in mean arterial pressure and left ventricular mass index is associated with a decrease in ejection fraction and fractional fiber shortening. N = normal subjects; I-III = patient groups I to III. (Reprinted with permission from the American College of Cardiology, and F. G. Dunn, *Am. J. Cardiol*, ref. 37.)

in hypertension. Left ventricular mass was greatest in those patients with the most severe hypertension. Cardiac index, ejection fraction, and fractional fiber shortening were reduced in groups II and III, indicating that left ventricular function was abnormal in those patients with the most severe hypertension and the greatest left ventricular mass. Further, these indices of left ventricular function tended to become progressively more abnormal as the left ventricular mass index increased (Fig. 11). There was no evidence of disproportionate septal hypertrophy, and no patient had systolic anterior motion of the mitral valve after administration of amyl nitrate. Systolic and diastolic dimensions were within normal limits in all groups, a finding compatible with the absence of overt cardiac failure.

Savage et al. (156) studied a larger group of 234 asymptomatic patients with mild-to-moderate systemic hypertension and 124 normotensive control subjects. Exclusion criteria were similar to those employed by Dunn et al. (37). Of the 234 hypertensive patients, 134 were receiving antihypertensive therapy at the time of study and 100 had had therapy discontinued for at least 3 weeks prior to study.

Most of the patients were white and none had evidence of a secondary cause of hypertension. Echocardiographic measurements were adjusted for the effects of age and body surface using a series of regression equations that were derived in the investigators' laboratory (55). Age-related changes in echocardiographic measurements in hypertensive patients were qualitatively and quantitatively similar to those seen in normotensive subjects. Ventricular septal thickness, free-wall thickness, left atrial dimension, and aortic root dimension were found to increase and mitral E-F slope to decrease with advancing age. The authors concluded that the magnitude of these changes is so large that the effects of both age and body surface area should be accounted for in any attempt to assess the effects of hypertension on echocardiographic measurements.

The prevalence of echocardiographic abnormalities in the 234 hypertensive patients is summarized in Table 3. The echocardiogram identified an increase in estimated left ventricular mass in more than 50% of hypertensive patients studied; chest film and electrocardiogram, in less than 10%. This study further supports the concept that the echocardiogram is more sensitive than the standard 12-lead electrocardiogram or the chest film for detecting cardiac abnormalities in hypertensive subjects. The frequencies of echocardiographic abnormalities in patients who remained on therapy, including the subgroup on propranolol, were not significantly different from those in patients who had had antihypertensive therapy withdrawn, so the data were pooled. As in the reports of Schlant et al. (161) and

TABLE 3. *Prevalence of echocardiographic abnormalities in 234 hypertensive subjects*

Electrocardiographic measurement	Patients[a] (%)
Ventricular septal thickness	50
Left ventricular free-wall thickness	61
Disproportionate septal thickening[b]	4
Left ventricular mass	51
Left ventricular transverse dimension at end-diastole	5
Left ventricular transverse dimension at end-systole	12
Left atrial dimension	5
Aortic root dimension	7
Ejection fraction	15
Percent fractional shortening	13
Mitral valve E-F slope[c]	6

[a]Echocardiographic values were considered abnormal if they were above (or below for ejection fraction, percent fractional shortening, and mitral valve E-F slope) the 95% prediction interval derived from normotensive subjects.

[b]Disproportionate septal thickening ratio of ventricular septal thickness to free-wall thickness 1.3.

[c]The number of subjects who had mitral valve E-F slope measured was 227.

Reproduced with permission of the American Heart Association, Incorporated and D. D. Savage, *Circulation*, ref. 156.

Dunn et al. (37), mean ventricular septal thickness, left ventricular free-wall thickness, and calculated left ventricular mass were significantly greater in hypertensive patients than in normotensive subjects. The infrequency (5%) of left atrial enlargement in this series contrasts with the findings of Dunn and associates (37). Savage explained this difference by pointing out that the hypertensive patients in the Dunn study were older than the normotensive subjects and that Dunn and associates had not corrected their findings for the effects of age and body surface area. Thus, the larger left atrial dimensions recorded by Dunn might represent the effects of aging rather than hypertension. Savage then concluded that left atrial enlargement does not appear to be an early indicator of cardiac involvement in hypertensive disease. Further study is needed to resolve this controversy.

Assessments of left ventricular function in this study, which did not include patients with severe hypertension, are consistent with those of Schlant and Dunn. Ejection fraction was reduced in 15% of the hypertensive subjects, and left ventricular diastolic function as estimated by the mitral valve E-F slope was lower in the hypertensive population than in the normotensive controls.

There were statistically significant positive correlations between diastolic pressure and ventricular septal thickness ($r = 0.346$, $p < 0.001$), left ventricular free-wall thickness ($r = 0.468$, $p < 0.001$) and left ventricular mass ($r = 0.319$, $p < 0.001$). Left atrial dimension was weakly correlated ($r = 0.208$, $p < 0.05$) with mean arterial pressure. These correlations were stronger than those reported by Schlant et al. (161) for the relationship between diastolic pressure and left ventricular wall thickness. This difference may be attributed to the larger number of patients or to the greater number of blood pressure determinations in the Savage study, or to some difference in patient populations, such as racial predominance or the presence or absence of antecedent antihypertensive treatment.

Nine (4% of the series) hypertensive patients had ventricular septal thickening that was disproportionate to the left ventricular free-wall thickness (septal-free wall ratio 1.3), but none of these had systolic anterior motion of the anterior leaflet of the mitral valve. According to Doi et al. (32), the echocardiographic diagnosis of hypertrophic cardiomyopathy versus hypertensive heart disease requires the presence of either systolic anterior movement of the mitral valve or midsystolic closure of the aortic valve, both of which are commonly found in hypertrophic cardiomyopathy but not in hypertensive heart disease. The conventional echocardiographic features of left ventricular hypertrophy and function do not permit distinction between these two disease entities. Toshima et al. (183) found a 30% prevalence of disproportionate septal hypertrophy in a series of unselected hypertensive patients. Their patients had more severe hypertension than those reported by the three other groups. In addition, eight of Toshima's 40 patients complained of chest pain and 15 of the 40 had had dizziness and/or syncope. Eight of these patients were in the New York Heart Association functional class III or IV. The presence of symptomatic heart disease in the Toshima study makes it impossible to attribute the disproportionate septal hypertrophy to hypertension alone. Nevertheless, the demonstration of asymmetric septal hypertrophy in hypertensive hearts raises the question of whether this cardiac abnormality is etiologically related to the hypertension or whether it represents an independent genetically mediated event.

There have been several reports of the coexistence of hypertrophic subaortic stenosis or asymmetrical septal hypertrophy and systemic hypertension (63,118,158a). Safar et al. (152) found increases in interventricular septal thickness without a corresponding increase in thickness of the left ventricular posterior wall in adults with borderline hypertension. Safar suggested that this finding may relate to increased sympathetic activity. The question of an etiologic relationship between systemic hypertension and subaortic stenosis has been raised but convincing evidence for such a relationship has not been adduced. Further study, including morphologic examination of autopsy material and echocardiographic examination of the relatives of hypertensive patients who also have disproportionate septal thickening, will be needed to determine whether this abnormality represents genetically transmitted hypertrophic cardiomyopathy or an atypical response to hypertension.

Whether the severity of left ventricular hypertrophy in hypertensive patients correlates with the severity and duration of the hypertension is a matter of controversy. Ross and associates (150) reported a series of 47 asymptomatic hypertensive patients in whom left ventricular wall thickness correlated with duration of known hypertension, initial diastolic pressure, and the presence of hypertensive retinopathy. Increased left atrial diameter was observed only in the presence of long-standing disease. In contrast, Cohen and associates (19) found in a series of 73 patients evaluated with M-mode and two-dimensional echocardiography that the development of left ventricular hypertrophy was not influenced by duration of severity of hypertension or age, body surface area or race of the patients. The presence of increased left ventricular mass was, however, associated with a greater incidence of target organ damage. The apparent inconsistency between these studies may relate to the antihypertensive treatment that was administered to the study subjects: all but two of Cohen's patients were receiving antihypertensive treatment at the time of study and most were adequately controlled. Patients who were receiving two or more antihypertensive drugs tended to have normal left ventricular mass. The treatment status and level of blood pressure control attained in Ross's patients were not specified.

Impaired left (102,174) and right (43,59) ventricular performance and left atrial emptying (34) were demonstrated in patients with systemic hypertension. Takahashi and colleagues used echocardiography and simultaneous recording of brachial artery pressure to assess left ventricular performance in 22 patients with long-standing systemic hypertension and left ventricular hypertrophy. Meridional wall stress (WSt) was used to express force per unit cross-sectional area. The WSt-diameter relation obtained during dynamic responses to acute pressure reduction by nitroprusside infusion was compared with the same relation obtained in 10 normal subjects over a range of matched systolic pressure induced by methoxamine administration. In 15 patients in whom end-diastolic wall thickness increased to 1.1 cm (range 1.0–1.2 cm), the linear WSt-diameter relation at end-systole did not differ from the control group, indicating a normal inotropic state. In the 7 patients with an end-diastolic wall thickness of 1.3 cm or more, the end-systolic WSt-diameter relation was clearly shifted to the right and had a less steep slope, indicating that in advanced left ventricular hypertrophy induced by pressure overload, myocardial contractility may be depressed.

Logan et al. (102) studied by M-mode echocardiography a group of 24 untreated patients with mild hypertension at baseline and after 1 year to assess the cardiac response to the increased pressure load over time. The patients had no clinical evidence of heart disease and normal electrocardiograms and chest X-rays at baseline. At entry, hypertensive patients had a significantly smaller left ventricular internal diameter in diastole and systole and a significantly larger left atrium than normotensive subjects matched for age, sex, and level of activity. There were no significant differences between groups in thickness of the left ventricular posterior wall or in interventricular septum in systole or diastole or in fractional fiber shortening. One year later, hypertensive subjects had developed an increase in the systolic dimension of the left ventricle and a decrease in percent fractional fiber shortening. These findings suggest that in the early stages of hypertension, before left ventricular hypertrophy can be detected by echocardiography, there is a reduction in left ventricular compliance, with subsequent gradual deterioration in contractile function. Dreslinski and associates (34) confirmed this interpretation in a study in which the atrial-emptying index [the first one-third (rapid phase) of left atrial emptying divided by the total left atrial emptying as quantitated from the posterior aortic wall echocardiogram] was used to assess diastolic filling of the left ventricle. Left atrial-emptying index was moderately decreased in hypertensive patients who lacked evidence of cardiac involvement and markedly decreased in hypertensive patients with echocardiographic evidence of left ventricular hypertrophy. These data suggest that rapid filling of the left ventricle is reduced early in hypertension, even before systolic echocardiographic abnormalities are detectable. The atrial-emptying index therefore appears to be an early indicator of abnormalities of left ventricular diastolic compliance in uncomplicated hypertension.

Ferlinz (43) documented increased right-sided pressures and volumes and impaired right ventricular performance (depressed right ventricular ejection fraction) in patients with uncomplicated asymptomatic essential hypertension using invasive techniques. Guazzi and associates (59) observed a similar pattern of right ventricular function in a combined echocardiographic and hemodynamic study. These findings indicate that systemic hypertension has an adverse effect on both ventricles and that both represent a single functional unit. To evaluate the mechanisms responsible for this phenomenon, simultaneous right and left ventricular pressure-volume relationships must be examined.

Echocardiography in Adults with Labile or Early Established Hypertension

In keeping with hemodynamic evidence for increased cardiac output and a "hyperdynamic circulation" in patients with labile or early established essential hypertension (39,52), echocardiographic studies have demonstrated increased left ventricular performance, increased cardiac work, and myocardial hypertrophy in these groups (33,35,96). As hypertension progresses, left ventricular performance diminishes and myocardial hypertrophy increases.

Echocardiography in Children and Adolescents with Borderline or Developing Hypertension

In order to detect pathologic changes in cardiac structure and function in children, it is important to document the effects of normal growth and development on echocardiographic measurements of chamber size, thickness, and function and to establish the reliability of such measurements. To this end, Henry et al. (69) obtained echocardiographic measurements of left ventricular and left atrial dimensions and assessments of left ventricular function in 105 normal subjects ranging from 1 day to 23 years of age. Each parameter was found to follow a linear regression on one of three functions (linear, square root, or cube root) of the body surface area. Schieken et al. (158) reported on the reproducibility achieved both within and between observers in measuring left heart dimensions of school-aged children with standard echocardiographic techniques. The within observer intraclass correlation coefficient for interventricular septum, diastolic dimension, systolic dimension, left ventricular posterior wall, left atrium and aorta averaged 0.94. The coefficient of variation averaged 3.6% (range 2%–7.5%). The least reproducible dimension was left ventricular posterior wall. Day-to-day variability within a single subject was small for all measurements. The standard deviation of error for all variables was no more than 0.3 mm. The authors concluded that standardized echocardiographic measurement techniques can provide the degree of precision necessary to begin studies of groups of hypertensive children.

Echocardiographic studies of children and adolescents with increased blood pressure have generally yielded results similar to those in hypertensive adults: indices of left ventricular wall mass, when corrected for body size, tend to be greater in those children and adolescents who have higher blood pressures (94,124, 157,196). Schieken et al. (1982) measured left ventricular dimensions and derived estimates of cardiac output in 264 randomly selected school children whose systolic blood pressure levels were in the lowest, middle, or highest quintile of the distribution for their age and sex. Most of the children in the study were white and the sexes were equally represented. Children with blood pressures in the upper quintiles were taller, heavier, and more obese than the remaining children. Even after correction for height, weight, and triceps skinfold thickness, thickness of the interventricular septum, left atrial size, and left ventricular wall mass were significantly greater in children with the highest blood pressures. There was no evidence in those children of disproportionate septal hypertrophy or left ventricular dysfunction as assessed by systolic time intervals and echocardiographically derived estimates of stroke volume and cardiac output. Cardiac output among children in the upper quintiles of blood pressure was variable, so that some had increased cardiac output and others elevated peripheral resistance as the basis for their blood pressure elevations. The authors emphasized that longitudinal studies are needed to determine whether the children in the upper quintiles of blood pressure will go on to develop fixed hypertension and progressive left ventricular hypertrophy secondary to increased peripheral vascular resistance.

Zahka et al. (196) found similar evidence of increased left ventricular mass unassociated with impairment of left ventricular function in 61 adolescents with systolic or diastolic blood pressures above the 90th percentile for age and sex compared with 49 normotensive adolescents. Blood pressure elevations were modest (mean blood pressure $\pm$ SEM = 141 $\pm$ 21/94 $\pm$ 20 mm Hg) in the hypertensive group. Most of the subjects studied were black, and none had received antihypertensive therapy or had a prior history of heart disease. There was an increased incidence of obesity in the hypertensive subjects: 40% were above the 95th percentile for weight. Accordingly, a separate set of comparisons was carried out with an obese subset of the normotensive control group. Mean posterior wall thickness was 23% greater and mean ventricular septal thickness 20% greater in hypertensive subjects than in normotensive controls. There was little evidence of disproportionate septal hypertrophy, as the ratio of ventricular septal to posterior wall thickness was greater than 1.3 in only one hypertensive subject. Calculated indices of left ventricular mass indicated that the left ventricle was 45% heavier in hypertensive patients than in normotensive subjects, even when obesity was taken into account. In contrast, abnormalities in left ventricular function were not found in the hypertensive group. The authors commented that it was impossible to determine from these whether ventricular function is preserved in adolescent hypertensives or whether there are minor abnormalities in ventricular function which are not detected by the echocardiogram.

Laird and Fixler (94) examined chest roentgenograms, electrocardiograms, and echocardiograms of 50 adolescents with elevated blood pressure (systolic or diastolic pressure above the 95th percentile on three separate occasions over a 5-month period) and 50 matched normotensive control subjects in an effort to assess the prevalence of left ventricular hypertrophy in adolescents with persistently elevated blood pressures. No subject in either group demonstrated cardiomegaly on X-ray. Similar numbers of both hypertensive (7 of 50) and control subjects (8 of 50) had electrocardiographic evidence of left ventricular hypertrophy. None of the hypertensives and 5 of 8 control subjects were athletes. No subject in either group demonstrated left atrial hypertrophy on electrocardiogram. The echocardiograms showed that the mean left ventricular wall thickness (LVWT) in the hypertensive adolescents was 7.8 mm $\pm$ 0.1 (SE), compared with 6.5 $\pm$ 0.1 in the control subjects ($p<0.001$). When the measurements were indexed to body surface area, the difference remained highly significant. Indexed left ventricular mass (LVM)/body surface area (BSA) was also significantly greater ($p<0.001$) in the hypertensive (84.2 g/sq m $\pm$ 2.1) than in the control subjects (72.0 $\pm$ 2.1). Among hypertensive adolescents, 9 of 50 had LVWT/BSA and 8 of 50 had LVM/BSA above the 95th percentile. In contrast, only 1 of 50 normotensive control subjects had elevated

LVWT/BSA values and 2 of 50 had elevated LVM/BSA values. This study demonstrates that hypertensive adolescents have an increased prevalence of left ventricular hypertrophy and that echocardiography is the most useful noninvasive method to detect these changes. It is unclear whether the small changes in myocardial mass noted in this study represent target organ damage. The authors emphasized that while it is important to document these changes and follow the patients longitudinally, left ventricular hypertrophy per se should not be considered an indication for specific pharmacologic treatment of mild hypertension in adolescents.

The findings of Goldring et al. (54) in a study of 114 hypertensive (systolic and/or diastolic pressures 1.65 SD above the mean at initial screening) high-school students, most of whom were white, contrast with those of the other groups. They found no significant differences between hypertensive and normotensive boys in interventricular septal and posterior wall thicknesses or in left atrial and aortic root diameter. The ventricular septum was actually thicker and the aortic diameter greater in normotensive than in hypertensive girls. Echocardiographic indices of left ventricular function were significantly higher in the hypertensive males than in normotensive controls, suggesting that the hypertensive subjects were in a hyperdynamic circulatory state. Further study is needed to reconcile these apparently inconsistent results and to more clearly delineate the morphologic and functional characteristics of early myocardial involvement in the hypertensive syndrome in man.

Coronary Arteries

According to the Framingham Study, the incidence of sudden cardiac death after acute myocardial infarction is markedly increased in patients with systemic hypertension and electrocardiographic evidence of left ventricular hypertrophy (81,82). The pathogenesis of sudden death in such patients is incompletely understood, but potential explanations include increased size of the occluded coronary vascular bed secondary to extensive atherosclerotic coronary artery disease, decreased coronary reserve secondary to left ventricular hypertrophy, intrinsic electrophysiologic abnormalities in hypertrophied cardiac muscle, and alterations in autonomic tone related to hypertension (91). Pathologic studies of human coronary arteries have shown that atherosclerotic lesions are more extensive and more severe in hypertensive than in normotensive subjects (148). Extensive coronary atherosclerosis secondary to hypertension may increase the size of the vascular bed involved and, secondarily, increase infarct size and the incidence of ventricular dysrhythmia and sudden cardiac death after myocardial infarction.

Strauer (172) presented data on coronary blood flow and ventricular function in 158 patients with essential hypertension. Sixty-seven percent of patients who underwent coronary angiography had significant (>75%) stenoses in at least one coronary artery. Angina pectoris was common, occurring in 100% of hypertensives with coronary artery disease and in 62% of those without detectable lesions. Half of the patients had experienced prior myocardial infarction. Left ventricular coronary blood flow increased by a mean 16% compared with normal subjects, whereas coronary vascular resistance was increased by 38%. The relative increase in coronary vascular resistance persisted when maximal coronary vasodilatation was induced by infusion of adenosine or dipyridamole, consistent with the findings of animal studies (see preceding pages). The increase in total left ventricular blood flow found in hypertensive subjects was presumably related to the greater left ventricular mass, as other investigators have reported normal or decreased left ventricular blood flow in the hypertensive heart when normalized for heart weight (12,123,151,184).

Nichols and associates (123) reported that resting left ventricular myocardial blood flow was reduced in hypertensive patients with left ventricular hypertrophy compared with both normotensive subjects and hypertensive patients without left ventricular hypertrophy. Coronary vascular resistance was elevated at rest in hypertensive patients with left ventricular hypertrophy but decreased significantly during atrial pacing, indicating a functional rather than a structural basis. Nichols and associates developed a multivariate regression equation to relate myocardial blood flow (MBF) to heart rate (HR), mean velocity of circumferential fiber shortening (MV_{cf}) and peak left ventricular wall stress:

$$MBF = 22.2\ MV_{cf} + 10.6\ \text{stress} + 0.38\ HR - 48.2\ (r = 0.89, p < 0.01)$$

When myocardial blood flow was adjusted for differences in wall stress among patients using the regression equation, there was no significant difference in myocardial blood flow between hypertensive patients with and without left ventricular hypertrophy. These data indicate that resting left ventricular myocardial blood flow is normal in hypertensive patients without left ventricular hypertrophy and reduced in controlled hypertensive patients with left ventricular hypertrophy as a consequence of reduced wall stress. The apparent discrepancy between these results and those of Strauer (172) may be related to arterial pressure at the time of study: All antihypertensive medications were discontinued at least 8 to 10 days prior to study in Strauer's patients, so they probably had higher levels of arterial pressure and systolic wall stress. Nichols' patients were not subjected to cardiac catheterization until their arterial pressures were reduced by bedrest and/or antihypertensive treatment, and some received antihypertensive agents until the day of catheterization.

Coronary vascular reserve of the left ventricle determined by the response to intravenous injection of dipyridamole was reduced to 72% of normal in compensated hypertensives without coronary artery disease and to 42% of normal in compensated hypertensives with coronary artery disease (172). Coronary vascular reserve was inversely related to peak systolic wall stress but unrelated to end-diastolic pressure, end-diastolic volume, or degree of hypertrophy (mass-volume ratio). Left ventricular oxygen consumption was increased in hypertensive subjects in positive linear relation to left ventricular mass and peak systolic wall stress. Strauer concluded that both impairment of coronary regulatory capacity and increase in myocardial oxygen demand may contribute to the pathogenesis of angina in patients with essential hypertension who have normal coronary angiograms.

The effects on coronary hemodynamics and myocardial oxygen consumption of acute β-adrenergic receptor blockade with atenolol and acute afterload reduction with intravenous hydralazine were examined as part of the same study (172). Eleven patients with essential hypertension and left ventricular hypertrophy, seven of whom also had angina pectoris and three of whom had high-grade coronary artery stenosis, were studied. Atenolol administration was associated with a 14.5% reduction in left ventricular coronary blood flow, a 12.7% increase in coronary vascular resistance, and a 13.6% reduction in left ventricular oxygen consumption. Coronary perfusion pressure and arterial-venous oxygen difference were not altered. The fall in myocardial oxygen consumption was interpreted as a consequence of decreases in heart rate, systolic pressure, and indices of left ventricular function, e.g., cardiac index, cardiac work, and dp/dt. The decrease in coronary blood flow and increase in coronary vascular resistance that occurred during β-adrenergic blockade were interpreted as consequences of the decrease in myocardial oxygen demand. In contrast, afterload reduction with intravenous hydralazine was associated with large increases (41%) in coronary blood flow and decreases (36%) in coronary vascular resistance. The arterial-venous oxygen difference was markedly reduced, and myocardial oxygen consumption remained unchanged. The constancy of myocardial oxygen consumption in the face of increases in stroke volume index, external cardiac work, heart rate, and dp/dt_{max} reflects the fall in myocardial oxygen demand induced by reductions in systolic wall stress. These findings point up the therapeutic value of hydralazine as an afterload-reducing agent in hypertensive heart disease: it enhances left ventricular function without increasing myocardial oxygen consumption.

Effects of Treatment on Left Ventricular Dimensions and Performance in Hypertension

Evidence (28,36,49,76,161,169) is accumulating that patients with systemic hypertension may show regression of left ventricular hypertrophy and/or improvement in left ventricular function after successful antihypertensive treatment. Schlant and associates performed M-mode echocardiographic examinations of 31 patients with essential hypertension prior to and 12 to 24 months following initiation of antihypertensive therapy (161). Their results are summarized in Table 4. They found that regression of left ventricular hypertrophy and improvement in left ventricular function were most likely to occur in those patients whose blood pressures decreased significantly. The effects of specific antihypertensive regimens on left ventricular structure and function were not discussed.

More recently the effects of various classes of antihypertensive agents on echocardiographic indices of left ventricular mass and function were assessed in a series of 60 patients with essential hypertension (28). Patients were studied at an interval of 40 ± 5 months. In 36 patients whose blood pressure did not respond to treatment, left ventricular mass index rose significantly while percent systolic shortening of the LVID fell slightly but not significantly. In 24 patients whose mean blood

TABLE 4. *Changes in left ventricular anatomy and function in 31 patients after therapy for hypertension*

	Baseline (mean ± SD)	12–24 months (mean ± SD)	Significance of paired t-test
Diastolic blood pressure (mm Hg)	101.5 ± 10.5	87.3 ± 9.4	<0.01
Left ventricular anatomy posterior wall thickness (mm) end-diastole	10.8 ± 1.0	10.1 ± 1.0	<0.05
End-systole	17.2 ± 1.8	16.0 ± 2.0	<0.01
Interventricular septal thickness at end-diastole (mm)	11.8 ± 1.7	10.7 ± 1.5	<0.01
Internal diameter (mm) end-diastole	47.8 ± 8.5	45.9 ± 7.3	NS
End-systole	33.4 ± 9.1	30.7 ± 6.4	NS
Mass index at end-diastole (g/m²)	135.7 ± 41.4	114.3 ± 27.9	<0.05
Volume index at end-diastole (ml)	65.6 ± 33.3	57.4 ± 24.2	NS
Left atrial internal diameter (mm)	32.8 ± 6.7	32.2 ± 4.0	NS
Left ventricular function decrease in internal diameter	0.311 ± 0.068	0.347 ± 0.053	<0.05
Ejection fraction	0.66 ± 0.12	0.72 ± 0.07	<0.05
Velocity of circumferential shortening (circ/sec)	1.22 ± 0.26	1.38 ± 0.23	<0.05
Posterior wall excursion (mm)	10.73 ± 2.1	10.9 ± 1.7	NS
Posterior wall velocity (mm/sec)	48.6 ± 12.6	48.8 ± 9.4	NS

Reprinted with permission from *Cardiovascular Medicine* and R. C. Schlant (161).

pressure fell by 6 to 42 mmHg, left ventricular mass index fell slightly but not significantly while percent systolic shortening of the LVID increased significantly. A subgroup of 10 patients treated with sympatholytic drugs alone or in combination with captopril had a significant reduction in left ventricular mass index. In contrast, there was no significant change in either left ventricular mass index or percent systolic shortening of the LVID in 12 patients treated with diuretics alone or in 14 patients treated with a combination of diuretics and sympatholytic drugs despite comparable reductions in blood pressure. Thus, blood pressure reduction by sympatholytic agents but not by diuretics or combinations of diuretics and sympatholytic agents appears to reduce left ventricular mass in patients with essential hypertension. These data give evidence that patients in whom antihypertensive therapy is ineffective show progression of left ventricular hypertrophy and progressive impairment of left ventricular performance.

Administration of the cardioselective β-blocker atenolol for a period of 8 weeks to patients with uncomplicated essential hypertension has been shown to alter echocardiographic indices of left ventricular mass and function (76). During this period mean blood pressure decreased from 197/119 to 160/98 mmHg. Septal thickness, left ventricular mass index, mean circumferential wall stress, end-diastolic diameter, and urinary epinephrine did not change. Posterior wall thickness and the ratio of left ventricular wall thickness to radius decreased significantly during the treatment period. The change in left ventricular mass index was significantly ($r = 0.42$) related to the change in mean circumferential wall stress, weakly related to the changes in systolic blood pressure ($r = 0.32$) and urinary epinephrine ($r = 0.22$), and not related to the change in diastolic blood pressure ($r = 0.03$). Thus atenolol in adequate antihypertensive doses can produce a rapid decrease in left ventricular mass. Some of the changes may have been related to a decrease in end-diastolic dimensions, as the ratio of left ventricular wall thickness to radius did not change. These data suggest that regression of myocardial hypertrophy following β-blockade with atenolol is more dependent on the reduction in wall stress than on the hypotensive effect or the decrease in adrenergic activity.

A recent study in patients with essential hypertension and myocardial hypertrophy confirmed the finding from animal studies that alpha-methyldopa causes regression of hypertrophy by a mechanism independent of its antihypertensive effect (45). Ten patients with essential hypertension and left ventricular hypertrophy were treated with small doses (500–750 mg/day) of alpha-methyldopa added to long-term diuretic therapy. Blood pressure was not significantly altered by the added treatment. Nevertheless, sequential M-mode echocardiography showed a significant reduction in left ventricular mass in four treated patients, and three of these reductions in left ventricular mass appeared as early as 12 weeks after institution of treatment. Neither the left ventricular mass-to-volume ratio nor fractional shortening was significantly altered by the reduction in left ventricular mass. There was no apparent relationship between changes in blood pressure and alterations in left ventricular mass. Whether alpha-methyldopa mediates regression of myocardial hypertrophy via its sympatholytic effect, as has been suggested (175), remains to be determined.

Dunn and associates (36,169) confirmed the observation that control of blood pressure with antihypertensive drugs is associated with regression of left ventricular hypertrophy and improvement in left ventricular function in patients with essential hypertension. They studied 22 patients with uncomplicated essential hypertension prior to initiation of treatment and after 9 months of blood pressure control. Nine patients had normal baseline echocardiograms; 13 had echocardiographic evidence of left ventricular hypertrophy (posterior wall thickness ≥ 1.2 cm and septal thickness ≥ 1.3 cm). Therapeutic regimens included stepped care (diuretic-β-blocker vasodilator or a diuretic plus alpha-methyldopa). Most patients received multiple drugs. A reduction of at least 15 mmHg in systolic and/or diastolic pressure was achieved in all patients. The group with left ventricular hypertrophy showed a fall in mean blood pressure from 200/129 to 154/98 mm Hg accompanied by significant reductions in mean posterior wall thickness, septal thickness, and left ventricular mass and significant increases in fractional fiber shortening and stroke volume. Sonotani et al. (169) obtained similar results in 34 patients who were treated for periods of 1 to 2 years with a variety of antihypertensive agents, including trichlormethiazide, β-adrenergic blocking agents, alpha-methyldopa, clonidine, and guanethidine, usually as multiple drug therapy. The magnitude of regression of hypertrophy was unrelated to pretreatment blood pressure, the fall in blood pressure induced by treatment, or duration of follow-up. The factors that determine which hypertensive patients will develop regression of left ventricular hypertrophy while on antihypertensive therapy have therefore not been elucidated by these or any other clinical study. Data from animal experiments (see earlier pages) may bear on this point, but it is not clear that they can be extrapolated to man. Further clinical studies are needed to determine the effects of adequate blood pressure control and of specific antihypertensive agents on the structure and function of the hypertrophic left ventricle in hypertensive man. Moyer and associates (119) cautioned that in any such study the acute effects of antihypertensive agents on ventricular structure and function must be taken into account, as these drugs can alter the configuration and performance of the left ventricle directly via an acute reduction in afterload without regression of hypertrophy.

REFERENCES

1. Aguas, A. P., Abecasis, P., Mariano, V., and Nogueria da Costa, J. (1981): Myofilament-polyribosome association in muscle cells of rat left atrium after short-term hypertension. *Hypertension*, 3:725–729.
2. Alpert, N. R., Hamrell, B. B., and Halpern, N. (1974): Mechanical and biochemical correlates of cardiac hypertrophy. *Circ. Res.*, 34/35[Suppl. II]:71–81.
3. Amer, M. S., Doba, N., and Reis, D. J. (1975): Changes in cyclic nucleotide metabolism in aorta and heart of neurogenically hypertensive rats: possible trigger mechanism of hypertension. *Proc. Natl. Acad. Sci. USA*, 72:2135–2139.
4. Antman, E. M., Green, L. H., and Grossman, W. (1979): Physiologic determinants of the electrocardiographic diagnosis of left ventricular hypertrophy. *Circulation*, 60:386–396.
5. Anversa, P., Loud, A. V., Giacomelli, F., and Wiener, J. (1978): Absolute morphometric study of myocardial hypertrophy in experimental hypertension. II. Ultrastructure of myocytes and interstitium. *Lab. Invest.*, 38:597–609.
6. Aronson, R. S. (1980): Characteristics of action potentials of hypertrophied myocardium from rats with renal hypertension. *Circ. Res.*, 47:443–454.
7. Aronson, R. S. (1981): Afterpotentials and triggered activity in hypertrophied myocardium from rats with renal hypertension. *Circ. Res.*, 48:720–727.
8. Averill, D. B., Farrario, C. M., Tarazi, R. C., Sen, S., and Bajbus, R., (1976): Cardiac performance in rats with renal hypertension. *Circ. Res.*, 38:280–288.
9. Bache, R. J., Vrobel, T. R., Arentzen, C. E., and Ring, W. S. (1981): Effect of maximal coronary vasodilation on transmural myocardial perfusion during tachycardia in dogs with left ventrical hypertrophy. *Circ. Res.*, 49:742–750.
10. Bennett, D. H., and Evans, D. W. (1974): Correlation of left ventricular mass determined by echocardiography with vectorcardiographic and electrocardiographic voltage messages. *Br. Heart J.*, 36:981–987.
11. Beznak, M., Korecky, B., and Thomas, G. (1969): Regression of cardiac hypertrophies of various origin. *Can. J. Physiol. Pharmacol.*, 47:572–586.
12. Bing, R. J., Hammond, M. M., Handelsman, J. C., Powers, S. R., Spencer, F. C., Eckenhoff, J. E., Goodale, W. T., Hafkenschiel, J. H., and Kety, S. S. (1949): The measurement of coronary blood flow, oxygen consumption and efficiency of the left ventricle in man. *Am. Heart J.*, 38:1–24.
13. Bishop, S. P., Oparil, S., Reynolds, M. D., and Drummond, J. L. (1979): Regional myocyte size in normotensive and spontaneously hypertensive rats. *Hypertension*, 1:378–383.
14. Bobik, A., and Korner, P. (1981): Cardiac beta adrenoceptors and adenylate cyclase in normotensive and renal hypertensive rabbits during changes in autonomic activity. *Clin. Exp. Hypertens.*, 3:257–280.
15. Bright, R. (1846): Tabular view of the morbid appearances in 100 cases connected with albuminous urine. With observations. *Guy's Hosp. Rep.*, 1:380–400.
16. Capasso, J. M., Strobeck, J. E., and Sonnenblick, E. H. (1981): Myocardial mechanical alterations during gradual onset long-term hypertension in rats. *Am. J. Physiol.*, 241:H435–H441.
17. Carr, K. W., Engler, R. L., Forsythe, J. R., Johnson, A. D., and Gosnick, B. (1979): Measurement

of left ventricular ejection fraction by mechanical cross-sectional echocardiography. *Circulation*, 59:1196–1201.

18. Cervoni, P., Herzlinger, H., Lai, F. M., and Tanikella, T. (1981): A comparison of cardiac reactivity and β-adrenoceptor number and affinity between aorta-coarcted hypertensive and normotensive rats. *Br. J. Pharmacol.*, 74:517–523.

19. Cohen, A., Hagan, A. D., Watkins, J., Mitas, J., Schvartzman, M., Mazzoleni, A., Cohen, I. M., Warren, S. E., and Vieweg, W. V. R. (1981): Clinical correlates in hypertensive patients with left ventricular hypertrophy diagnosed with echocardiography. *Am. J. Cardiol.*, 47:335–341.

20. Coleman, T. G., Granger, H. J., and Guyton, A. C. (1971): Whole-body circulatory autoregulation and hypertension. *Circ. Res.*, 29[Suppl. II]:76–87.

21. Cooper, G., IV, Satava, R. M., Harrison, C. E., and Coleman, H. N., III (1974): Normal myocardial function and energetics after reversing pressure-overload hypertrophy. *Am. J. Physiol.*, 226:1158–1165.

22. Cooper, G., IV, and Tomanek, R. J. (1982): Load regulation of the structure, composition and function of mammalian myocardium. *Circ. Res.*, 50:788–798.

23. Crawford, M. H., Grant, D., O'Rourke, R. E., Starling, M. R., and Groves, B. M. (1980): Accuracy and reproducibility of new M-mode echocardiographic recommendations for measuring left ventricular dimensions. *Circulation*, 61:137–143.

24. Cutilletta, A. F., Benjamin, M., Culpepper, W. S., and Oparil, S. (1978a): Myocardial hypertrophy and ventricular performance in the absence of hypertension in spontaneously hypertensive rats. *J. Mol. Cell Cardiol.*, 10:689–703.

25. Cutilletta, A., Rudnick, M., and Zak, R. (1978b): Muscle and non-muscle cell RNA polymerase activity during the development of myocardial hypertrophy. *J. Mol. Cell Cardiol.*, 10:677–687.

26. Cutilletta, A. F., Dowell, R. T., Rudnik, M., Arcilla, R. A., and Zak, R. (1975): Regression of myocardial hypertrophy. I. Experimental model, changes in heart weight, nucleic acids and collagen. *J. Mol. Cell Cardiol.*, 7:767–781.

27. Cutilletta, A. F., Erinoff, L., Heller, A., Low, J., and Oparil, S. (1977): Development of left ventricular hypertrophy in young spontaneously hypertensive rats after peripheral sympathectomy. *Circ. Res.*, 40:428–434.

28. Devereux, R. B., Savage, D. D., Sachs, I., and Laragh, J. H. (1980): Effect of blood pressure control and antihypertensive medication on left ventricular hypertrophy and function in hypertension. *Circulation*, 62(Suppl. III):III–36.

29. Devereux, R. B., Savage, D. D., Drayer, J. I. M., and Laragh, J. H. (1982): Left ventricular hypertrophy and function in high, normal and low-renin forms of essential hypertension. *Hypertension*, 4:524–531.

30. Devereux, R. B., and Reichek, N. (1977): Echocardiographic determination of left ventricular mass in man. *Circulation*, 55:613–618.

31. DiBianco, R. R., Gottdiener, J. S., Flecher, R. D., and Pipberger, H. V. (1979): Left atrial overload: a hemodynamic, echocardiographic, electrocardiographic, and vectorcardiographic study. *Am. Heart J.*, 98:478–489.

32. Doi, Y. L., Deanfield, J. E., McKenna, W. J., Dargie, H. J., Oakley, C. M., and Goodwin, J. F. (1980): Echocardiographic differentiation of hypertensive heart disease and hypertrophic cardiomyopathy. *Br. Heart J.*, 44:395–400.

33. Dreslinski, G. R., Messerli, F. H., Dunn, F. G., Suarez, D. H., and Frohlich, E. D. (1981a): Patterns of left ventricular adaptation in borderline and mild essential hypertension. Echocardiographic findings. *Chest*, 80:592–595.

34. Dreslinski, G. R., Frohlich, E. D., Dunn, F. G., Messerli, F. H., Suarez, D. H., and Reisin, E. (1981b): Echocardiographic diastolic ventricular abnormality in hypertensive heart disease: atrial emptying index. *Am. J. Cardiol.*, 47:1087–1090.

35. Dreslinski, G. R., Messerli, F. H., Dunn, F. G., and Frohlich, E. D. (1982): Early hypertension and cardiac work. *Am. J. Cardiol.*, 50:149–151.

36. Dunn, F. G., Bastian, B., Lawrie, T. D. V., and Lorimer, A. R. (1980): Effect of blood pressure control on left ventricular hypertrophy in patients with essential hypertension. *Clin. Sci.*, 59:441s–443s.

37. Dunn, F. G., Chandraratna, P., deCarvalho, H. G. R., Basta, L. L., and Frohlich, E. D. (1977): Pathophysiologic assessment of hypertensive heart disease with echocardiography. *Am. J. Cardiol.*, 39:789–795.

38. Eich, R. H., Cuddy, R. P., Smulyna, H., and Lyons, R. G. (1966): Hemodynamics in labile hypertension. *Circulation*, 34:299–307.
39. Factor, S. M., Bhan, R., Minase, T., Wolinsky, H., and Sonnenblick, E. H. (1981): Hypertensive-diabetic cardiomyopathy in the rat. *Am. J. Pathol.*, 102:219–228.
40. Factor, S. M., Minase, T., and Sonnenblick, E. H. (1980): Clinical and morphologic features of human hypertensive-diabetic cardiomyopathy. *Am. Heart J.*, 99:446–458.
41. Fanburg, B. L. (1970): Experimental cardiac hypertrophy. *N. Engl. J. Med.*, 282:723–732.
42. Feigenbamm, H. (1981): *Echocardiography*, 3d Ed. Lea and Febiger, Philadelphia.
43. Ferlinz, J. (1980): Right ventricular performance in essential hypertension. *Circulation*, 61:156–162.
44. Fernandes, M., Onesti, G., Fiorentini, R., Kim, K. E., and Swartz, C. (1976): Effect of chronic administration of propranolol on the blood pressure and heart weight in experimental renal hypertension. *Life Sci.*, 18:967–970.
45. Fischer, J. E., Horst, W. D., and Kopin, I. J. (1965): Norepinephrine metabolism in hypertrophied rat hearts. *Nature*, 207:951–953.
46. Folland, E. D., Parisi, A. F., Moynihan, B. S., Jones, D. R., Feldman, C. L., and Tow, D. E. (1979): Assessment of left ventricular ejection fraction and volumes by real-time, two-dimensional echocardiography. *Circulation*, 60:760–766.
47. Ford, L. E. (1976): Heart size. *Circ. Res.*, 39:297–303.
48. Fortuin, N. J., Hood, W. P., and Craige, E. (1972): Evaluation of left ventricular function by echocardiography. *Circulation*, 46:26–35.
49. Fouad, F. M., Nakashima, Y., Tarazi, R. C., and Salcedo, E. E. (1982): Reversal of left ventricular hypertrophy in hypertensive patients treated with methyldopa. *Am. J. Cardiol.*, 49:795–801.
50. Friedman, M. J., Sahn, D. J., Burris, H. A., Allen, H. D., and Goldberg, S. J. (1979): Computerized echocardiographic analysis to detect abnormal systolic and diastolic left ventricular function in children with aortic stenosis. *Am. J. Cardiol.*, 44:478–486.
51. Frohlich, E. D., and Tarazi, R. C. (1979): Is arterial pressure the sole factor responsible for hypertensive cardiac hypertrophy? *Am. J. Cardiol.*, 44:959–963.
52. Frohlich, E. D., Tarazi, R. C., and Dustan, H. P. (1969): Reexamination of the hemodynamics of hypertension. *Am. J. Med. Sci.*, 257:9–23.
53. Frohlich, E. D., Tarazi, R. C., and Dustan, H. P. (1971): Clinical-physiological correlations in the development of hypertensive heart disease. *Circulation*, 44:446–455.
54. Fuster, V., Danielson, M. A., Robb, R. A., Broadbent, J. C., Brown, A. L., Jr., and Elveback, L. R. (1977): Quantitation of left ventricular myocardial fiber hypertrophy and interstitial tissue in human hearts with chronically increased volume and pressure overload. *Circulation*, 55:504–508.
55. Gardin, J. M., Henry, W. L., Savage, D. D., Ware, J. H., Burn, C., and Borer, J. S. (1979): Echocardiographic measurements in normal subjects: evaluation of an adult population without clinically apparent heart disease. *J. Clin. Ultrasound*, 7:439–447.
56. Goldring, D., Hernandez, A., Choi, S., Lee, J. Y., Londe, S., Lindgren, F., and Burton, R. M. (1979): Blood pressure in a high school population. II. Clinical profile of the juvenile hypertensive. *J. Pediatr.*, 95:298–304.
57. Granger, H. J., and Guyton, A. C. (1969): Autoregulation of the total systemic circulation following destruction of the central nervous system in the dog. *Circ. Res.*, 25:379–388.
58. Grossman, W., Jones, D., and McLaurin, L. P. (1975): Wall stress and patterns of hypertrophy in the human left ventricle. *J. Clin. Invest.*, 56:56–64.
59. Guazzi, M., Fiorentini, C., Olivari, M. T., and Polese, A. (1979): Cardiac load and function in hypertension. Ultrasonic and hemodynamic study. *Am. J. Cardiol.*, 44:1007–1012.
60. Gulch, R. W., Baumann, R., and Jacob, R. (1979): Analysis of myocardial action potential in left ventricular hypertrophy of Goldblatt rats. *Basic Res. Cardiol.*, 74:69–82.
60a. Guyton, R. W., Granger, H. J., and Coleman, T. G. (1971): Autoregulation of the total systemic circulation and its relation to control of cardiac output and arterial pressure. *Circ. Res.*, 28:93.
61. Hall, O., Hall, C. E., and Ogden, E. (1953): Cardiac hypertrophy in experimental hypertension and its regression following reestablishment of normal blood pressure. *Am. J. Physiol.*, 174:175–178.
62. Hallback, M., Isaksson, O., and Noresson, E. (1975): Consequences of myocardial structural adaptation on left ventricular compliance and the Frank-Starling relationship in spontaneously hypertensive rats. *Acta Physiol. Scand.*, 94:259–270.

63. Hamby, R. I., Roberts, G. S., and Meron, J. M. (1971): Hypertension and hypertrophic subaortic stenosis. *Am. J. Med.*, 51:474–481.
64. Hanrath, P., Mathey, D. G., Siegert, R., and Bleifeld, W. (1980): Left ventricular relaxation and filling pattern in different forms of left ventricular hypertrophy: an echocardiographic study. *Am. J. Cardiol.*, 45:15–22.
65. Heilmann, C., Lindl, T., Muller, W., and Pette, D. (1980): Characterization of cardiac microsomes from spontaneously hypertonic rats. *Basic Res. Cardiol.*, 75:92–96.
66. Helak, J. W., and Reichek, N. (1981): Quantitation of human left ventricular mass and volume by two-dimensional echocardiography in vitro anatomic validation. *Circulation*, 63:1398–1407.
67. Heller, L. J. (1979): Augmented aftercontractions in papillary muscles from rats with cardiac hypertrophy. *Am. J. Physiol.*, 237:H649–H654.
67a. Heller, L. J. (1981): Isovolumetric properties of ventricles of spontaneously hypertensive rats. *Am. J. Physiol.*, 240:H927–H933.
68. Heller, L. J., and Stauffer, E. K. (1981): Membrane potentials and contractile events of hypertrophied rat cardiac muscle (41036). *Proc. Soc. Exp. Biol. Med.*, 166:141–147.
69. Henry, W. L., Ware, J., Gardin, J. M., Hepner, S. I., McKay, J., and Weiner, M. (1978): Echocardiographic measurements in normal subjects. Growth-related changes that occur between infancy and early adulthood. *Circulation*, 57:278–285.
70. Hill, D. K. (1968): Tension due to interaction between the sliding filaments in resting striated muscle. *J. Physiol. (Lond.)*, 199:637–684.
71. Hillis, L. D., Izquierdo, C., Davis, C., Brotherton, S., Eberhart, R., Roan, P. G., and Willerson, J. T. (1981): Effect of various degrees of systemic arterial hypertension on acute canine myocardial ischemia. *Am. J. Physiol.*, 240:H855–H861.
72. Hirschleifer, J., Crawford, M., O'Rourke, R. A., and Karliner, J. S. (1975): Influence of acute alterations in heart rate and systemic pressure on echocardiographic measures of left ventricular performance in normal human subjects. *Circulation*, 52:835–841.
73. Hollander, W., Prusty, S., Kirkpatrick, B., Paddock, J., and Nagraj, S. (1977): Role of hypertension in ischemic heart disease and cerebral vascular disease in the cynomolgus monkey with coarctation of the aorta. *Circ. Res.*, 40[Suppl. I]:I-70–83.
74. Holtz, J., Restoriff, W. V., Bard, P., and Bassenge, E. (1977): Transmural distribution of myocardial blood flow and of coronary reserve in canine left ventricular hypertrophy. *Basic Res. Cardiol.*, 72:286–292.
75. Hood, W. P., Rackley, C. E., and Rolett, E. L. (1968): Wall stress in the normal and hypertrophied human left ventricle. *Am. J. Cardiol.*, 22:550–558.
76. Ibrahim, M. M., Madkour, M. A., and Mossallam, R. (1981): Effect of beta blockade therapy on hypertensive cardiac hypertrophy. *Am. J. Cardiol.*, 47:469.
77. Jacob, R., Brenner, B., Ebrecht, G., Holubarsch, Ch., and Medugorac, I. (1980): Elastic and contractile properties of the myocardium in experimental cardiac hypertrophy of the rat. Methodological and pathophysiological considerations. *Basic Res. Cardiol.*, 75:253–261.
78. Jacob, R., Ebrecht, G., Kammereit, A., Medugorac, I., and Wendt-Gallitelli, M. F. (1977): Myocardial function in different models of cardiac hypertrophy. An attempt at correlating mechanical, biochemical and morphological parameters. *Basic Res. Cardiol.*, 72:160–167.
79. Jorgensen, H., and Sundsfjord, J. A. (1974): The relation of plasma renin activity to left ventricular hypertrophy and retinopathy in patients with arterial hypertension. *Acta Med. Scand.*, 196:307–313.
80. Kammereit, A., and Jacob, R. (1979): Alterations in rat myocardial mechanics under Goldblatt hypertension and experimental aortic stenosis. *Basic Res. Cardiol.*, 74:389–405.
81. Kannell, W. B. (1974): Role of blood pressure in cardiovascular morbidity and mortality. *Prog. Cardiovasc. Dis.*, 17:5–24.
82. Kannel, W. B., Gordon, T., and Offutt, D. (1969): Left ventricular hypertrophy by electrocardiogram. Prevalence, incidence and mortality in the Framingham Study. *Ann. Intern. Med.*, 71:89–101.
83. Kannel, W. B., Castelli, W. P., McNamara, P. M., McKee, P. A., and Feinleib, M. (1972): Role of blood pressure in the development of congestive heart failure. The Framingham Study. *N. Engl. J. Med.*, 287:781–787.
84. Karliner, J. S., Williams, D., Gorwit, J., Crawford, M. H., and O'Rourke, R. A. (1977): Left ventricular performance in patients with left ventricular hypertrophy caused by systemic arterial hypertension. *Br. Heart J.*, 39:1239–1245.

85. Kaufmann, R. L., Homburger, H., and Wirth, H. (1971): Disorder in excitation-contraction coupling of cardiac muscle from cats with experimentally produced right ventricular hypertrophy. *Circ. Res.*, 28:356–357.

86. Kawamura, K., Kashii, C., and Imamura, K. (1976): Ultrastructural changes in hypertrophied myocardium on spontaneously hypertensive rats. *Jpn. Circ. J.*, 40:1119–1145.

87. Kennedy, J. W., Reichenbach, D. D., Baxley, W. A., and Dodge, H. T. (1967): Left ventricular mass: A comparison of angiocardiographic measurements with autopsy weight. *Am. J. Cardiol.*, 19:221–223.

88. Keung, E. C. H., and Aronson, R. S. (1981): Non-uniform electrophysiological properties and electronic interaction in hypertrophied rat myocardium. *Circ. Res.*, 49:150–158.

89. Kissling, G., and Wendt-Gallitelli, M. F. (1977): Dynamics of the hypertrophied left ventricle in the rat. Effects of physical training and chronic pressure load. *Basic Res. Cardiol.*, 72:178–183.

90. Kissling, G., Gassenmaier, T., Wendt-Gallitelli, M. F., and Jacob, R. (1977): Pressure-volume relations, elastic modulus, and contractile behaviour of the hypertrophied left ventricle of rats with Goldblatt II hypertension. *Pflügers Arch.*, 369:213–221.

91. Koyanagi, S., Eastham, C., and Marcus, M. L. (1982): Effects of chronic hypertension and left ventricular hypertrophy on the incidence of sudden cardiac death after coronary artery occlusion in conscious dogs. *Circulation*, 65:1192–1197.

92. Kuchii, M., Fukuda, K., Hano, T., Ohtani, H., Mohara, O., Nishio, I., and Masuyama, Y. (1981): Changes in cardiac beta-adrenoceptor concentrations in spontaneously hypertensive and experimental renal hypertensive rats. *Jpn. Circ. J.*, 45:1104–1110.

93. Kuo, J. F., Davis, C. W., and Tse, J. (1976): Depressed cardiac cyclic GMP-dependent protein kinase in spontaneously hypertensive rats and its further depression by guanethidine. *Nature*, 261:335–336.

94. Laird, W. P., and Fixler, D. E. (1981): Left ventricular hypertrophy in adolescents with elevated blood pressure: assessment by chest roentgenography, electrocardiography and echocardiography. *Pediatrics*, 67:255–259.

95. Laks, D. M., Morady, F., and Swan, J. J. C. (1973): Myocardial hypertrophy produced by chronic infusion of subhypertensive doses of norepinephrine in the dog. *Chest*, 64:75–78.

96. Lehner, J. P., Safar, M. E., Dimitriu, V. M., Simon, A. Ch., Carrez, J. P., and Plainfosse, M. T. (1979): Systolic time intervals and echocardiographic findings in borderline hypertension. *Eur. J. Cardiol.*, 9:319–331.

97. Limas, C. J. (1980): Ribonucleic acid synthesis in the myocardium of spontaneously hypertensive rats: quantification of transcribing ribonucleic acid polymerases. *Biochem. J.*, 188:67–73.

98. Limas, C., and Limas, C. J. (1978): Reduced number of β-adrenergic receptors in the myocardium of spontaneously hypertensive rats. *Biochem. Biophys. Res. Commun.*, 83:710–714.

99. Limas, C. J., and Cohn, J. N. (1977): Defective calcium transport by cardiac sarcoplasmic reticulum in spontaneously hypertensive rats. *Circ. Res.*, [Suppl. I] 40:62–69.

100. Limas, C. J., and Spier, S. S. (1980): Effect of antihypertensive therapy on calcium transport by cardiac sarcoplasmic reticulum of SHRs. *Cardiovasc. Res.*, 14:692–699.

101. Litten, R. Z., Martin, B. J., Low, R. B., and Alpert, N. R. (1982): Altered myosin isozyme patterns from pressure-overloaded and thyrotoxic hypertrophied rabbit hearts. *Circ. Res.*, 50:856–864.

102. Logan, A. G., Gilbert, B. W., Haynes, R. B., Milne, B. J., and Flanagan, P. T. (1981): Early effects of mild hypertension on the heart. A longitudinal study. *Hypertension*, 3[Suppl.II]:II-187–II-190.

103. Lompre, A-M., Schwartz, K., d'Albis, A., Lacombe, G., Van Thiem, N., and Swynghedauw, B. (1979): Myosin isoenzyme redistribution in chronic heart overload. *Nature*, 282:105–107.

104. Loud, A. V., Anversa, P., Giacomelli, F., and Wiener, J. (1978): Absolute morphometric study of myocardial hypertrophy in experimental hypertension. I. Determination of myocyte size. *Lab. Invest.*, 38:586–596.

105. Lund, D. D., and Tomanek, R. J. (1978): Myocardial morphology in spontaneously hypertensive and aortic-constricted rats. *Am. J. Anat.*, 152:141–152.

106. Lund, D. D., Twietmeyer, T. A., Schmid, P. G., and Tomanek, R. J. (1979): Independent changes in cardiac muscle fibres and connective tissue in rats with spontaneous hypertension, aortic constriction and hypoxia. *Cardiovasc. Res.*, 13:39–44.

107. Lundin, S. A., and Hallback-Nordlander, M. (1980): Background of hyperkinetic circulatory state in young spontaneously hypertensive rats. *Cardiovasc. Res.*, 14:561–567.

108. Mary-Rabine, L., Hordoff, A. J., Danilo, P., Jr., Malm, J. R., and Rosen, M. R. (1980): Mechanisms for impulse initiation in isolated human atrial fibers. *Circ. Res.*, 47:267–277.
109. McDonald, I. G., Feigenbaum, H., and Chang, S. (1972): Analysis of left ventricular wall motion by reflected ultrasound. Application to assessment of myocardial function. *Circulation*, 45:14–25.
110. McFarland, T. M., Alam, M., Goldstein, S., Pickard, S. D., and Stein, P. D. (1978): Echocardiographic diagnosis of left ventricular hypertrophy. *Circulation*, 57:1140–1144.
111. Medugorac, I. (1980a): Collagen content in different areas of normal and hypertrophied rat myocardium. *Cardiovasc. Res.*, 14:551–554.
112. Medugorac, I. (1980b): Myocardial collagen in different forms of heart hypertrophy in the rat. *Res. Exp. Med.*, 177:201–211.
113. Medugorac, I. (1977): Characteristics of the hypertrophied left ventricular myocardium in Goldblatt rats. *Basic Res. Cardiol.*, 72:261–267.
114. Medugorac, I., and Jacob, R. (1976): Concentration and adenosinphosphatase activity of left ventricular actomyosin in Goldblatt rats during the compensatory stage of hypertrophy. *Hoppe-Seylers Z. Physiol. Chem.*, 357:1495–1503.
115. Meerson, F. Z. (1969): The myocardium in hyperfunction and heart failure. *Circ. Res.*, 25[Suppl. II]:1–163.
116. Meerson, F. Z. (1976): Insufficiency of hypertrophied heart. *Basic Res. Cardiol.*, 71:343–354.
117. Miller, E. J. (1976): Biochemical characteristics and biological significance of the genetically distinct collagens. *Mol. Cell. Biochem.*, 130:165–192.
118. Moreyra, E., Knibbe, P., and Brest, A. N. (1970): Hypertension and muscular subaortic stenosis. *Chest*, 57:87–90.
119. Moyer, J. P., Pittman, A. W., Belasco, R. N., and Woods, J. W. (1979): Echocardiographic assessment of the effect of an antihypertensive regimen on left ventricular performance. *Am. J. Cardiol.*, 43:594–599.
120. Mueller, T. M., Marcus, M. L., Kerber, R. E., Young, J. A., Barnes, R. W., and Abboud, F. M. (1978): Effect of renal hypertension and left ventricular hypertrophy on the coronary circulation in dogs. *Circ. Res.*, 42:543–549.
121. Mueller, T. M., Tomanek, R. J., Kerber, R. E., and Marcus, M. L. (1980): Myocardial infarction in dogs with chronic hypertension and left ventricular hypertrophy. *Am. J. Physiol.*, 239(*Heart Circ. Physiol.* 8):H731–H735.
122. Murray, J. A., Johnston, W., and Reid, J. M. (1972): Echocardiographic determination of left ventricular dimensions, volumes and performance. *Am. J. Cardiol.*, 30:252–257.
123. Nichols, A. B., Sciacca, R. R., Weiss, M. B., Blood, D. K., Brennan, D. L., and Cannon, P. J. (1980): Effect of left ventricular hypertrophy on myocardial blood flow and ventricular performance in systemic hypertension. *Circulation*, 62:329–340.
124. Nishio, T., Mori, C., Saito, M., Soeda, T., Abek, T., and Nakao, Y. (1978): Left ventricular hypertrophy in early hypertensive children: its importance as a risk factor for hypertension. *Shimane J. Med. Sci.*, 2:63–68.
125. Noresson, E., Ricksten, S-E., and Thoren, P. (1979): Left atrial pressure in normotensive and spontaneously hypertensive rats. *Acta Physiol. Scand.*, 107:9–12.
126. Ohtaka, M. (1980): Vectorcardiographical and pathological approach to the relationship between cardiac hypertrophy and coronary arteriosclerosis in spontaneously hypertensive rats (SHR). *Jpn. Circ. J.*, 44:283–293.
127. O'Keefe, D. D., Hoffman, J. I. E., Cheitlin, R., O'Neill, M. J., Allard, J. R., and Shapkin, E. (1978): Coronary blood flow in experimental canine left ventricular hypertrophy. *Circ. Res.*, 43:43–51.
128. Ostman-Smith, I. (1976): Prevention of exercise-induced cardiac hypertrophy in rats by chemical sympathectomy (guanethidine treatment). *Neuroscience*, 1:497–507.
129. Ostman-Smith, I. (1981): Cardiac sympathetic nerves as the final common pathway in the induction of adaptive cardiac hypertrophy. *Clin. Sci.*, 61:265–727.
130. Page, E., and Oparil, S. (1978): Effect of peripheral sympathectomy on left ventricular ultrastructure in young spontaneously hypertensive rats. *J. Mol. Cell. Cardiol.*, 10:301–305.
131. Pfeffer, M. A., and Frohlich, E. D. (1973): Hemodynamic and myocardial function in young and old normotensive and spontaneously hypertensive rats. *Circ. Res.*, 32/33[Suppl. I]:28–35.
132. Pfeffer, M. A., Pfeffer, J. M., and Frohlich, E. D. (1976): Pumping ability of the hypertrophying left ventricle of the spontaneously hypertensive rat. *Circ. Res.*, 38:423–429.

133. Pfeffer, M. A., Pfeffer, J. M., Weiss, A. K., and Frohlich, E. D. (1977): Development of SHR hypertension and cardiac hypertrophy during prolonged beta blockade. *Am. J. Physiol.*, 232(6):H639–H644.

134. Pfeffer, J. M., Pfeffer, M. A., Fishbein, M. C., and Frohlich, E. D. (1979): Cardiac function and morphology with aging in the spontaneously hypertensive rat. *Am. J. Physiol.*, 237(4):H461–H468.

135. Pick, R., Johnson, P. J., and Glick, G. (1974): Deleterious effects of hypertension on the development of aortic and coronary atherosclerosis in stumptail macaques (Macaca speciosa) on an atherogenic diet. *Circ. Res.*, 35:472–482.

136. Rabinowitz, M., and Zak, R. (1972): Biochemical and cellular changes in cardiac hypertrophy. *Annu. Rev. Med.*, 23:245–261.

137. Rabinowitz, M. (1974): Overview on pathogenesis of cardiac hypertrophy. *Circ. Res.*, 34/35[Suppl. II]:II-3–II-11.

138. Rackley, C. E., Dodge, H. T., Cable, Y. D., and Hay, R. E. (1964): A method for determining left ventricular mass in man. *Circulation*, 29:666–671.

139. Rakusan, K. (1971): Quantitative morphology of capillaries of the heart. Number of capillaries in animal and human hearts under normal and pathological conditions. *Methods Achiev. Exp. Pathol.*, 5:272–286.

140. Ratshin, R. A., Rackley, C. E., and Russell, R. O. (1974): Quantitative echocardiography: accuracy of ventricular volume analysis by area-length, linear regression and quadratic regression formulae. *Am. J. Cardiol.*, 35:165.

141. Reichek, N., and Devereux, R. B. (1981): Left ventricular hypertrophy: relationship of anatomic, echocardiographic and electrocardiographic findings. *Circulation*, 63:1391–1398.

142. Reichek, N., Helak, J., Plappert, T., Sutton, M. St. J., and Weber, K. T. (1983): Anatomic validation of left ventricular mass estimates from clinical two-dimensional echocardiography: initial results. *Circulation*, 67:348–352.

142a. Reiner, L., Mazzoleni, A., Rodriguez, F. L., and Freudenthal, R. R. (1959): The weight of the human heart. I. "Normal" cases. *AMA Arch. Path.*, 68:58–73.

143. Reiner, L., Mazzoleni, A., Rodriguez, F. L., and Freudenthal, R. R. (1961): The weight of the human heart. II. Hypertensive cases. *Arch. Path.*, 71:74–95.

144. Rembert, J. C., Kleinman, L. H., Fedor, J. M., Wechsler, A. S., and Greenfield, J. C., Jr. (1978): Myocardial blood flow distribution in concentric left ventricular hypertrophy. *J. Clin. Invest.*, 62:379–386.

145. Ricksten, S. E., Yao, T., Ljung, B., and Thoren, P. (1980): Distensibility of left atrium in normotensive and spontaneously hypertensive rats. *Acta Physiol. Scand.*, 110:413–418.

146. Richer, C., Boissier, J-R, and Ciudicelli, J-F. (1978): Chronic atenolol treatment and hypertension development in spontaneously hypertensive rats. *Eur. J. Pharmacol.*, 47:393–400.

147. Ricksten, S-E, Yao, T., Ljung, B., and Thoren, P. (1980): Distensibility of left atrium in normotensive and spontaneously hypertensive rats. *Acta Physiol. Scand.*, 110:413–418.

148. Robertson, W. B., and Strong, J. P. (1968): Atherosclerosis in persons with hypertension and diabetes mellitus. *Lab. Invest.*, 18:538–551.

149. Rona, G., Chappel, C. I., Balazs, T., and Gaudry, R. (1959): An infarct-like myocardial lesion and other toxic manifestations produced by isoproterenol in the rat. *Arch. Pathol.*, 67:443–455.

150. Ross, A. M., Pisarczyk, M. J., and Calabresi, M. (1978): Echocardiographic and clinical correlations in systemic hyper-tension *J. Clin. Ultrasound*, 6:95–99.

151. Rowe, G. G., Afonso, S., Lugo, J. E., Castillo, C. A., Boake, W. C., and Crumpton, C. W. (1965): Coronary blood flow and myocardial oxidative metabolism at rest and during exercise in subjects with severe aortic valve disease. *Circulation*, 32:251–257.

152. Safar, M. E., Weiss, Y. A., Levenson, J. A., London, G. M., and Milliez, P. L. (1979): Hemodynamic study of 85 patients with borderline hypertension. *Am. J. Cardiol.*, 31:315–318.

153. Sahn, D. J., De Maria, A., Kisslo, J., and Weyman, A. (1978): Recommendations regarding quantitation in M-mode echocardiography: results of a survey of echocardiographic measurements. *Circulation*, 58:1072–1083.

154. Sandler, H., and Dodge, H. T. (1963): Left ventricular tension and stress in man. *Circ. Res.*, 13:91–104.

155. Sasayama, S., Franklin, D., and Ross, J., Jr. (1977): Hyperfunction with normal inotropic state of the hypertrophied left ventricle. *Am. J. Physiol.*, 232(4):H418–H425.

156. Savage, D. D., Drayer, J. I. M., Henry, W. L., Mathews, E. D., Ware, J. H., Gardin, J. M., Cohen,

E. R., Epstein, S. E., and Laragh, J. H. (1979): Echocardiographic assessment of cardiac anatomy and function in hypertensive subjects. *Circulation*, 59:623–632.

157. Schieken, R. M., Clarke, W. R., Lauer, R. M., and Rainbolt, M. J. (1981): Left ventricular hypertrophy in children with blood pressures in the upper quintile of the distribution: the Muscatine study. *Hypertension*, 3:669–675.

158. Schieken, R. M., Clarke, W. R., Mahoney, L. T., and Lauer, R. M. (1979): Measurement criteria for group electrocardiographic studies. *Am. J. Epidemiol.*, 110:504–514.

158a. Schieken, R. M., Clarke, W. R., Prineas, R., Klein, V., Lauer, R. M. (1982): Electrocardiographic measures of left ventricular hypertrophy in children across the distribution of blood pressure: The muscatine study. *Circulation*, 66:428–432.

159. Schreiber, S. S., Evans, C. D., Oratz, M., and Rothschild, M. A. (1981): Protein synthesis and degradation in cardiac stress. *Circ. Res.*, 48:601–611.

160. Schiller, N. B., Acquatella, H., Ports, T. A., Drew, D., Goerke, J., Ringertz, H., Silverman, N. H., Brundage, B., Botvinick, E. H., Boswell, R., Carlsson, E., and Parmley, W. W. (1979): Left ventricular volume from paired biplane two-dimensional echocardiography. *Circulation*, 60:547–555.

161. Schlant, R. C., Felner, J. M., Heynsfield, S. B., Gilbert, C. A., Shulman, N. B., Tuttle, E. P., and Blumenstein, B. A. (1977): Echocardiographic studies of left ventricular anatomy and function in essential hypertension. *Cardiovasc. Med.*, 2:477–491.

162. Sen, S., Tarazi, R. C., and Bumpus, F. M. (1974): Cardiac hypertrophy in spontaneously hypertensive rats. *Circ. Res.*, 35:775–781.

163. Sen, S., Tarazi, R. C., and Bumpus, F. M. (1976): Biochemical changes associated with development and reversal of cardiac hypertrophy in spontaneously hypertensive rats. *Cardiovasc. Res.*, 10:254–261.

164. Sen, S., Tarazi, R. C., and Bumpus, F. M. (1977): Cardiac hypertrophy and antihypertensive therapy. *Cardiovasc. Res.*, 11:427–433.

165. Sen, S., Tarazi, R. C., and Bumpus F. M. (1980): Effect of converting enzyme inhibitor (SQ 14,225) on myocardial hypertrophy in spontaneously hypertensive rats. *Hypertension*, 2:169–176.

166. Sen, S., Tarazi, R. C., and Bumpus, F. M. (1981): Reversal of cardiac hypertrophy in renal hypertensive rats: medical vs. surgical therapy. *Am. J. Physiol.*, 240 *(Heart Circ. Physiol. 9)*:H408–H412.

167. Sen, S., Tarazi, R. C., Khairallah, P. A., and Bumpus, F. M. (1974): Cardiac hypertrophy in spontaneously hypertensive rats. *Circ. Res.*, 35:755–781.

168. Smith, T. L., and Hutchens, P. M. (1980): Anesthetic effects on hemodynamics of spontaneously hypertensive and Wistar-Kyoto rats. *Am. J. Physiol.*, 238:H539–H544.

169. Sonotani, N., Kubo, S., Nishioka, A., and Takatsu, T. (1981): Electrocardiographic and echocardiographic changes after one to two years' treatment of hypertension. Analyses of voltages (Sv1 + RV5), wall thickness, cavity, mass and hemodynamics of the left ventricle. *Jpn. Heart J.*, 22:325–333.

170. Spann, J. F., Jr., Covell, J. W., Eckberg, D. L., Sonnenblick, E. H., Ross, J., Jr., and Braunwald, E. (1972): Contractile performance of the hypertrophied and chronically failing cat ventricle. *Am. J. Physiol.*, 223:1150–1157.

171. Spech, M. M., Ferrario, C. M., and Tarazi, R. C. (1980): Cardiac pumping ability following reversal of hypertrophy and hypertension in spontaneously hypertensive rats. *Hypertension*, 2:75–82.

172. Strauer, B. E. (1980): *Hypertensive Heart Disease.* Springer-Verlag, New York.

173. Tanijiri, H. (1975): Cardiac hypertrophy in spontaneously hypertensive rats. *Jpn. Heart J.*, 16:174–188.

174. Takahashi, M., Sasayam, S., Kawai, C., and Kotoura, H. (1980): Contractile performance of the hypertrophied ventricle in patients with systemic hypertension. *Circulation*, 62:116–126.

175. Tarazi, R. C. (1979): Reversal of cardiac hypertrophy: possibility and clinical implications. In: *Left Ventricular Hypertrophy in Hypertension: Royal Society of Medicine International Congress and Symposium Series No. 9*, edited by J. I. S. Robertson, and A. D. S. Caldwell, pp. 55–66. Royal Society of Medicine (London), Academic Press, London, New York.

176. Tarazi, R. C., and Sen, S. (1979): Catecholamines and cardiac hypertrophy. In: *Catecholamines and the Heart: Royal Society of Medicine International Congress and Symposium Series No. 8*, edited by K. Mezy and A. D. S. Caldwell, pp. 47-57, World Society of Medicine, London, Academic Press, Inc., London, and Grune and Stratton, New York.

177. Deleted in proof.
178. ten Cate, F. J., Kloster, F. E., van Dorp, W. G., Meester, G. T., and Roelandt, J. (1974): Dimensions and volumes of left atrium and ventricle determined by single-beam echocardiography. *Br. Heart J.*, 36:737–746.
179. Tomanek, R. J. (1979): The role of prevention or relief of pressure overload on the myocardial cell of the spontaneously hypertensive rat. A morphometric and sterologic study. *Lab. Invest.*, 40:83–91.
180. Tomanek, R. J. (1982): Selective effects of α-methyldopa on myocardial cell components independent of cell size in normotensive and genetically hypertensive rats. *Hypertension*, 4:499–506.
181. Tomanek, R. J., Davis, J. W., and Anderson, S. C. (1979): The effects of alpha-methyldopa on cardiac hypertrophy in spontaneously hypertensive rats: ultrastructural, stereological and morphometric analysis. *Cardiovasc. Res.*, 13:173–182.
182. Tomanek, R. J., and Hovanec, J. M. (1981): The effects of long-term pressure overload and aging on the myocardium. *J. Mol. Cell. Cardiol.*, 13:471–489.
182a. Tortoledo, F. A., Quinones, M. A., Fernandez, G. C., Waggoner, A. D., and Winters, W. L. (1983): Quantification of left ventricular volumes by two-dimensional echocardiography: A simplified and accurate approach. *Circulation*, 67:579–584.
183. Toshima, H., Koga, Y., Yoshioka, H., Akiyoshi, T., and Kimura, N. (1975): Echocardiographic classification of hypertensive heart disease: a correlation study with clinical features. *Jpn. Heart J.*, 16:377–393.
184. Trenouth, R. S., Phelps, N. C., and Neill, W. A. (1975): Determinants of left ventricular hypertrophy and oxygen supply in chronic aortic valve disease. *Circulation*, 53:644–650.
185. Troy, B. L., Pombo, J., and Rackley, C. E. (1972): Measurement of left ventricular wall thickness and mass by echocardiography. *Circulation*, 45:602–611.
186. Vaughan-Williams, E. M., Raine, A. E. G., Cabrera, A. A., and Whyte, J. M. (1975): The effects of prolonged β-adrenoreceptor blockade on heart weight and cardiac intracellular potentials in rabbits. *Cardiovasc. Res.*, 9:579–592.
187. Weiner, J., Giacomelli, F., Loud, A. V., and Anversa, P. (1979): Morphometry of cardiac hypertrophy induced by experimental renal hypertension. *Am. J. Cardiol.*, 22:909–929.
188. Weiss, L., and Lundgren, Y. (1978): Left ventricular hypertrophy and its reversibility in young spontaneously hypertensive rats. *Cardiovasc. Res.*, 12:635–638.
189. Weiss, L., Eaton, L. W., Kallman, C. H., and Maughan, W. L. (1983): Accuracy of volume determination by two-dimensional echocardiography: defining requirements under controlled conditions in the ejecting canine left ventricle. *Circulation*, 67:889–895.
190. Wendt-Gallitelli, M. F., Ebrecht, G., and Jacob, R. (1979): Morphological alterations and their functional interpretation in the hypertrophied myocardium of Goldblatt hypertensive rats. *J. Mol. Cell Cardiol.*, 11:275–287.
191. Wilkman-Coffelt, J., Parmley, W. W., and Mason, D. T. (1979): The cardiac hypertrophy process. Analyses of factors determining pathological vs. physiological development. *Circ. Res.*, 45:697–707.
192. Wildenthal, K., and Mueller, E. A. (1977): Lysosomal enzymes in the development and regression of myocardial hypertrophy induced by systemic hypertension. *J. Mol. Cell Cardiol.*, 9:121–130.
193. Woodcock, E. A., Funder, J. W., and Johnston, C. I. (1979): Decreased cardiac β-adrenergic receptors in deoxycorticosterone-salt and renal hypertensive rats. *Circ. Res.*, 45:560–565.
194. Woodcock, E. A., and Johnston, C. I. (1980): Changes in tissue alpha- and beta-adrenergic receptors in renal hypertension in the rat. *Hypertension*, 2:156–161.
195. Zak, R., and Rabinowitz, M. (1979): Molecular aspects of cardiac hypertrophy. *Annu. Rev. Physiol.*, 41:539–552.
196. Zahka, K. G., Neill, C. A. Kidd, L., Cutilletta, M. A., and Cutilletta, A. F. (1981): Cardiac involvement in pediatric hypertension: Electrocardiographic determination of myocardial hypertrophy. *Hypertension*, 3:664–668.

Growth of the Heart in Health and Disease,
edited by Radovan Zak. Raven Press,
New York © 1984.

Carbon Monoxide Induced Cardiac Hypertrophy

David G. Penney

Department of Physiology, Wayne State University School of Medicine, Detroit, Michigan 48201

Carbon monoxide (CO) is an odorless, tasteless, colorless gas of about the same density as air. It is a product of incomplete combustion of carbonaceous fuels. However, the oceans are a major worldwide source of natural background levels of CO. It is also produced in the human body by the catabolism of hemoglobin.

Aristotle was the first to mention the lethal effect of coal fumes, although humans have been exposed to the gas since prehistory. The Roman philosopher Seneca reportedly committed suicide by shutting himself in a bath heated with coal. In 1902, Emile Zola, the French novelist, was killed by CO leaking from a faulty flue.

CO levels in urban areas have generally declined during the last 60 years. For example, the CO in auto exhaust, a major contributor, has fallen from 7% in 1930 to 3.8% in the 1960s to 0.5% presently. However, cigarette smoke, a major personal source, is 4% CO, and smokers show COHb saturations as high as 10% to 13%.

John Scott Haldane in the late 19th and early 20th centuries carried out heroic studies of the acute physiologic effects of CO. Using dangerously high CO levels and himself as a test subject, Haldane showed that its primary effect was exerted in binding to blood hemoglobin. First, the oxygen-carrying capacity of the blood is depressed as CO with its far higher binding affinity is taken up and oxygen displaced. Second, the oxygen association/dissociation curve of the hemoglobin not binding CO is shifted to the left, forcing tissue and venous P_{O_2} lower in order to release oxygen. Third, the shape of the curve changes from sigmoidal to a rectangular hyperbola in the presence of CO. Although arterial P_{O_2} is not normally altered in mild CO poisoning, it is with certain attendant pathological conditions.

CO EXPOSURE

J. Argyll Campbell working with mice in 1933 (2) was the first to report that chronic CO exposure induces cardiac enlargement. Our studies over the last 12 years have explored this phenomenon at different stages of myocardial development and over a range of CO concentrations. Throughout this chapter the term "cardiomegaly" will be used to refer to abnormal enlargement of the whole heart and any gross subdivisions thereof, whereas the terms hypertrophy and hyperplasia are reserved for changes occurring at the cellular level.

The CO model of cardiomegaly presents a number of characteristics which confer advantages over other experimental models in that (a) it does not require surgery, (b) the intensity of the stressor is variable and is easy to monitor, (c) it is initiated by hypotensive volume overloading, (d) the process may be started and stopped at will, (e) it is applicable to very small animals, e.g., fetuses, neonates, (f) the variability of effects is small, and (g) the method is convenient and inexpensive.

CO exposure of the laboratory rat was carried out in large, inflated polyethylene bags, each enclosing 1 to 3 plastic cages, as seen in Fig. 1 (6). Each cage accomodates two adults, one dam with pups, up to 15 preweanlings, or 6 to 12 weanlings, depending on age. With six bags in use and two cages per bag, 24 adults can be exposed simultaneously. Pure CO from a commercial high-pressure cylinder is mixed with room air from a carbon vane compressor, and the gas mixture is continuously pumped through the bags. CO flow rate is monitored by a floating ball flow meter and air flow rate by an electromagnetic turbine flow meter. CO concentration of the air-CO mixture is monitored by an infrared gas analyzer. Both CO concentration and air flow rate are continuously recorded by a pen recorder. A signal from the CO analyzer in turn serves to control the flow of pure CO gas mixing with the air, maintaining CO concentration constant $\pm 3\%$ of the set point. Air-CO flow rate is adjusted to 25 liters/min/bag to keep waste gases generated by the animals, urine and fecal matter, at a low level. Waste gases are carried away through a fume hood. Control animals are kept in the same room, and CO concentration there is monitored by a second electrochemical CO analyzer.

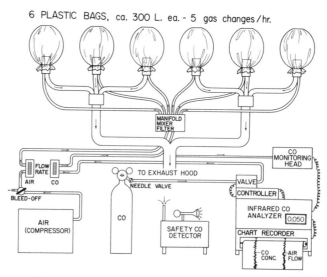

FIG. 1. Apparatus used for CO exposure. Each bag holds two or three plastic rodent cages (R.T. = room temperature 22–25°C, L./D. = 24-hr light-dark cycle).

The CO concentration never exceeds 5 ppm. The rats are allowed Purina rodent chow and water *ad libitum*. As the compressor operates within a baffle and is muffled, noise level in the treatment room is no higher than that present in the average research laboratory. Relative humidity is not controlled.

CHANGES IN BLOOD AND HEART DURING CHRONIC INHALATION

Adult

Exposure of adult and juvenile rats to 500 ppm CO resulted in mortality rates of less than 5% over 6 weeks. As CO concentration rose above that level, mortality rate mounts. At least a 6-week period of exposure was used in most experiments, since by then the major changes involving the blood and heart reached a plateau.

Exposure of adults to 500 ppm CO resulted in nearly the steady state concentration of COHb (40%) within 1 hr, because rats take up CO at a rate about 10-fold that of humans. Hemoglobin concentration, hematocrit and erythrocyte count began to rise within 3 days, reaching levels 65% above normal over a period of 6 weeks (10,11). With fully developed polycythemia, that fraction of the hemoglobin not binding CO (60%) returned to near pre-exposure levels, although blood viscosity was now above normal and binding affinity has increased.

Reticulocyte count rose sixfold within 10 days and then settled back to a 3% basal level during established polycythemia (10). Paralleling this change was a similar increase in mean corpuscular volume and hemoglobin, whereas mean corpuscular hemoglobin concentration was somewhat depressed. Oxygen tension at half-saturation (P_{50}) fell from 37 torr in normal rats to 27.5 torr in rats treated for 3 to 9 weeks (15). The left-shifted curve and polycythemic condition are presumably responsible for the enhanced survivability during acute hypobaric testing. Lowered 2,3-diphosphoglycerate may contribute to the decline in P_{50}, as it tends to decrease over this period. Although platelet count declined during CO exposure, this probably resulted from dilution as the expanding red cell mass contributed to an expanded blood volume. There was no change in white cell count.

Even somewhat faster than blood changes, fresh heart weight increased, reaching a value 40% above equal body weight controls within 2 weeks (Fig. 2) (11). This state of cardiomegaly was maintained as long as CO treatment continued. The increase in heart mass occurred in both ventricles and the atria although to a somewhat greater extent on a percent basis in the right ventricle (RV) than in the left ventricle plus interventricular septum (LV + S) (9). Over a somewhat more rapid time-course, myocardial lactate dehydrogenase (LDH) isozyme composition in percent of the M subunit (skeletal muscle type) increased and plateaued 10% to 12% higher than normal (11).

The cardiomegaly produced by 500 ppm CO was absolute, not simply relative, as heart weight was greater than same-age controls. Increased heart mass cannot be ascribed to myocardial edema, as neither percent water content nor percent dry weight changed during compensatory growth. Since protein content increased apace

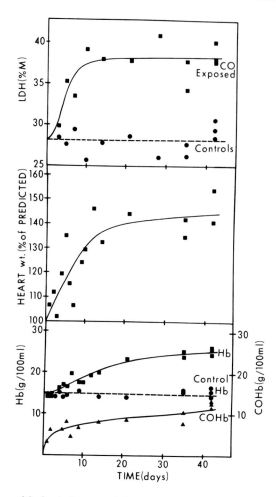

FIG. 2. Time-course of changes in blood, heart weight, and lactate dehydrogenase isozymes in adult male rats exposed to 500 ppm CO.

with fresh heart weight, the cardiomegaly represented additional cardiac constituents.

Lower CO concentrations produced lesser degrees of cardiomegaly: 100 to 200 ppm CO, in our hands, being the threshold for detectable effects in adult rats (5). However, significant polycythemia was demonstrated in these studies at 100 ppm. Through the use of a larger number of animals, heart and hematologic effects would probably have been observed at still lower CO concentrations.

That CO is a stressor there is little doubt. However, rate of body weight gain was not depressed in adult rats following long-term 500 ppm CO inhalation as it was, for example, with high-altitude exposure. Two groups of littermate male rats were made up such that mean group body weights were identical. They then inhaled 500 ppm CO continuously for 47 days during which time body weight and food and water consumption were monitored on a daily or semi-daily basis. All three parameters fell below normal during the first 5 days, as seen in Fig. 3. Afterward,

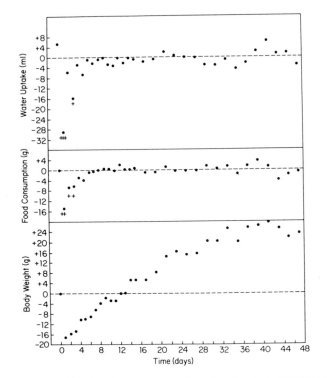

FIG. 3. Body weight and food and water consumption of male rats exposed to 500 ppm CO (difference from controls).

TABLE 1. *Food consumption (Purina Rodent Chow) of male rats exposed to 500 ppm CO for 47 days and their littermate controls*

Group	Consumption per rat (g)		
	Days 0–5	Days 6–47	Total
CO (7)	111.6 ± 6.9	1,156.9 ± 67.6	1,268.5 ± 73.9
Air (6)	147.5 ± 5.5	1,189.2 ± 28.8	1,336.7 ± 32.5
Probability	<0.01	>0.05	>0.05

Note: Values are means ± SE. Number of animals used in each group is given in parentheses.

food and water consumption were at control values (Table 1). Body weight, however, increased faster than in the controls, such that by the time of sacrifice, body weight of CO-exposed rats was 28.5 g greater than that of controls (Table 2). We also observed during food restriction experiments that to maintain constant body weight in CO-exposed and control rats, the former require less food. How might this be explained? Several studies show that whole body metabolic rate is depressed

TABLE 2. *Body weight, hematocrit, heart weight, and heart dimensions of male rats exposed to 500 ppm CO for 47 days and their littermate controls*

Group	BW (g)	Hct (%)	HW (mg)	HW/BW (mg/g)	Apex to valve distance (mm)	LV diam. (mm)	Wall thickness (mm)		
							LV	S	RV
CO (6)	534.7 ± 8.3	67.59 ± 0.32	1,757 ± 70	3.30 ± 0.10	16.66 ± 0.19	12.43 ± 0.30	3.62 ± 0.09	3.07 ± 0.11	1.29 ± 0.03
Air (6)	506.2 ± 8.4	48.44 ± 0.40	1,335 ± 56	2.63 ± 0.08	15.65 ± 0.22	11.17 ± 0.14	3.49 ± 0.25	3.06 ± 0.23	1.25 ± 0.09
Probability	<0.05	<0.001	<0.001	<0.001	<0.01	<0.01	>0.05	>0.05	>0.05

Note: Values are means ± SE. Number of animals in each group is given in parentheses.

by CO poisoning. Thus, continuation of normal food consumption after an initial period of anorexia (Table 1) results in a greater than normal rate of body weight gain in the CO-exposed animals, because less food is utilized for movement and body heat and more is added to body mass.

Compensatory heart growth may be concentric (i.e., increased wall thickness), eccentric (i.e., increased lumen volume), or some intergrade between these extremes. Morphologic measurements on K^+ relaxed hearts, frozen and then sectioned, demonstrated that CO-induced cardiomegaly is primarily of the eccentric variety. In rats inhaling CO, hematocrit rose from 48.4% to 67.6% and heart weight to body weight ratio increased from 2.63 to 3.30, as seen in Table 2. Apex to valve distance and left ventricle diameter of these larger hearts were increased, whereas left ventricle, septal, and right ventricle wall thickness were not. Estimates of left ventricle end-diastolic lumen volume based on a simplified geometric shape suggest an increase of approximately 33%. The morphologic alterations observed in the CO-enlarged heart dovetail with the hemodynamic data (discussed below) and are reminiscent of endurance exercise, where heart changes represent a functional-anatomical adaptation necessary to maintain greater stroke volume and cardiac output. An essential difference from exercise, however, as discussed below, is the hypotension produced by carboxyhemoglobinemia.

Previous studies have established an approximate inverse relationship between muscle contractility and taurine concentration. This being the case, cardiac taurine was assayed in left ventricle, septum, and right ventricle at 0, 2, 9, and 22 days after initial exposure of 62- to 64-day-old male rats to 500 ppm CO. Although heart weight and heart weight to body weight ratio progressively increased (not shown) with the period of carboxyhemoglobinemia, as indicated earlier, there was, in general, no change in taurine concentration, as seen in Table 3. This suggests

TABLE 3. *Myocardial taurine concentration (μmoles per g wet wt) of male rats 62–64 days of age (controls) exposed to 500 ppm CO for 2, 9, and 22 days and their littermate controls*

Days in CO	LV	S	RV
2 (3)	29.37 ± 0.41	31.13 ± 0.73	28.63 ± 2.60
0 (3)	29.40 ± 2.91	31.23 ± 1.04	32.37 ± 1.25
Probability	>0.05	>0.05	>0.05
9 (4)	22.95 ± 0.69	23.10 ± 0.31	21.95 ± 0.61
0 (4)	24.53 ± 0.40	26.87 ± 1.14	26.58 ± 0.15
Probability	>0.05	<0.05	<0.001
22 (5)	29.08 ± 0.82	30.96 ± 1.48	28.86 ± 1.32
0 (4)	30.35 ± 0.55	32.38 ± 1.65	31.40 ± 0.78
Probability	>0.05	>0.05	>0.05

Note: Values are means ± SE. Number of animals used in each group is given in parentheses.
Courtesy of Charles Parker of Wayne State University.

that the CO-enlarged heart, at least as produced by this CO concentration, was not in hyperfunction or in failure.

Neonate

Our studies with rats of various ages exposed to 500 ppm CO showed that cardiomegaly was much more dramatic in the young than in the old (13). For example, in those exposed initially at 1 day of age for 35 days, heart weight rose to 70% above that predicted for rats of equal body weight. In those initially exposed at 265 days of age, heart weight was only 25% above the predicted value. There may be two reasons for the exaggerated cardiomegalic response in CO treated neonates: (a) accentuation of postnatal anemia (16), and (b) greater stimulation of myocyte hyperplasia. Presumably, since rats older than 3 to 4 weeks retain the potential for myocyte hypertrophy alone, the heart weight response to stress is smaller. Even those exposed to CO at 21 days of age for 35 days showed only a 35% increase in heart weight (13), highlighting the special effect a stressor exerts when applied immediately after birth.

In recent studies with neonates inhaling 500 ppm CO (7), LV + S weight at first increased more rapidly than RV, becoming 50% above predicted values within 1 week. By 14 days of age, however, RV enlargement was greater, being 100% above the predicted value, while LV + S was 77% above that predicted. As CO treatment continued, relative cardiomegaly declined somewhat, as polycythemia developed following weaning and the change to solid food. Thus, for some reason not yet clear, there is a proportionally greater increase in RV than in LV + S. This is more exaggerated than in adult CO-induced cardiomegaly.

Myocardial LDH M subunit composition was also elevated in neonates exposed to CO, but to an even greater extent than in adults. As in adults, however, total LDH enzyme activity was unchanged. This is due in part to a retardation, produced by CO hypoxia, of the normal decline in M subunit composition which comes about as the metabolism of the heart becomes increasingly aerobic after birth.

Cytochrome c was measured in order to address the question whether CO-induced cardiomegaly produces mitochondrial alterations (17). In adults exposed to CO from 38 to 45 days, myocardial cytochrome c content increased directly with heart mass in both RV and LV + S (Fig. 4). However, in 5-day-old rats exposed to CO over a period of 48 to 55 days, cytochrome c concentration declined significantly. Although content increased, it did not keep pace with increasing heart weight. Two additional experiments with large numbers of 5-day-old rats exposed for 25 and 47 days, respectively, again showed depressed cytochrome c concentrations in LV, S, and RV. No changes were noted in atria. This suggests that mitochondrial mass is depressed by 500 ppm CO exposure in neonates, but not in adults. It is unknown, however, whether this comes about as a result of changes in mitochondrial number and/or size or in content of individual mitochondria, and whether this alters functional oxidative capacity. The CO-induced alterations in cytochrome c and LDH are probably related to lowered tissue P_{O_2}, since proliferation of mitochondria and

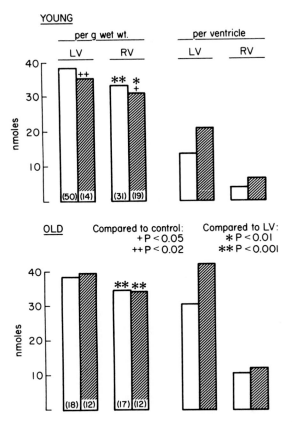

FIG. 4. Effect of 500 ppm CO exposure in 5-day-old rats exposed for 48–55 days and in adult rats exposed for 38–45 days on myocardial cytochrome *c* concentration and content.

synthesis of mitochondrial enzymes and synthesis of the M and H subunits of LDH are strongly influenced by it. These changes once again illustrate the more plastic nature of the developing heart and the differential effects relative to the adult which stress produces.

Pulmonary structure and function were examined in young rats that inhaled 500 ppm CO from birth until 33 days of age (3). Wet lung weight and the lung displaced volume were not changed. Lung alveolar macrophages obtained by bronchoalveolar lavage did not change with respect to number, viability, maximal diameter, surface area, or acid phosphatase activity. The phagocytic ability of the cells, however, was enhanced in CO-exposed rat pups and was correlated with an increased percentage of spread forms of alveolar macrophages adhering to glass coverslips. The surface features of the cells were also somewhat modified. The number and percentage of granular leukocytes were increased in lavages following chronic CO exposure. Although carboxyhemoglobinemia strongly affected the neonatal cardio-vascular system, the effects on the lung appeared relatively small.

Fetus

Exposure of pregnant female rats to 200 ppm CO for the final 18 days of gestation resulted in cardiomegaly of the newborn (6,8). At birth, heart weight was 20% larger and body weight 14% smaller than that of controls. More recent studies showed that both fresh and dry weights of the two ventricles were significantly larger than that of controls at 4, 3, 2, and 1 days before birth and at birth (8). Fetal cardiomegaly was not a result of myocardial edema. Again, the body weights of the treated fetuses and newborn were less than that of controls. In addition, placental weight was significantly greater than controls and litter size marginally smaller. At birth, the erythrocyte indexes mean corpuscular hemoglobin (MCH) and mean corpuscular volume (MCV), suggest a population of cells less mature than normal for that developmental stage. As in older animals inhaling CO, LDH M subunit composition was elevated, although total LDH enzyme activity was not altered. Cardiac myoglobin content and concentration were both increased, while cytochrome *c* was unchanged. Total heart DNA content was marginally elevated, while hydroxyproline was not. Recent studies (F. J. Clubb, Jr., Dallas, Texas, *unpublished data*) showed increased myocardial cell numbers at birth following CO exposure. This probably accounts for the increased DNA and indicates that CO stimulates muscle cell hyperplasia *in utero*.

Exposure of fetuses to 157 and 166 ppm CO over the same period (16 days) produced somewhat smaller, although clearly discernible degrees of cardiomegaly, depressed birth weight, increased placental weight, and alterations in hematology.

REGRESSION OF CHRONIC CO EFFECTS

Adult

Upon termination of 500 ppm CO inhalation in adult rats, COHb saturation returned to normal within 3 to 5 hours. Within 5 to 10 days the established polycythemia began to decline noticeably (10). Hemoglobin concentration, hematocrit and erythrocyte count returned to normal within 30 to 35 days. Reticulocyte count fell transiently from 3% to 0.2% within 5 days post CO exposure. Platelet count rose again to the normal value with the change in red cells. We did not see any lasting hematologic effects of chronic CO inhalation.

Heart weight began to decline within a few days on return to room air. The regression process was essentially completed within 30 to 36 days (19). This was the case whether heart mass was expressed as a ratio-to-body weight or as a difference from the predicted value for a normal animal of identical body weight.

When male rats were exposed to 500 ppm CO that was then gradually raised to 1,100 ppm over 6 weeks, greater cardiomegaly was induced: heart weight was 50% above predicted (19). Regression occurred with the same time-course as at the lower CO concentration, but did not proceed to completion. Heart mass remained 10% to 12% higher than in normal rats for as long as 47 days. This suggests the induction of an irreversible myocardial lesion in rats with extreme cardiac enlargement, which does not occur in more modest cardiomegaly.

This was supported by biochemical data (19). LDH percent M subunit composition, which was elevated at 500 ppm CO in LV, S, and RV, regressed bimodally after termination of CO exposure, reaching normal levels within 15 to 20 days. In the rats with more massive cardiomegaly, M subunit composition failed to wholly regress.

Neonate

In neonates with extreme cardiomegaly induced by 500 ppm CO, regression did not proceed to completion, at least within the time frame of our studies (6,7). The weight ratio of the two ventricles to body weight remained significantly elevated 36, 75, and 185 days after termination of CO inhalation. As an average, the LV + S and RV remained elevated approximately 5% and 15%, respectively, above normal animals over this time period. We termed this phenomenon "persistent cardiomegaly." The excess mass in the RV at 75 and 185 days post CO exposure were the same, suggesting permanence for the life of the animal. Thus, the substantial increase in weight ratio of RV to LV + S established early in neonatal cardiomegaly also persisted. In addition, the depressed rate of body weight gain of males, but not females, persisted for as long as 9 months. Thus CO-exposed males exhibited lower mean body weight for many months postexposure, whereas females did not.

This finding of persistent cardiomegaly may be important from the standpoint of human cardiovascular birth defects (e.g., atrial septal defects, A-V fistulas) when significant cardiomegaly is involved. Does normalization of heart mass depend on whether surgical correction is performed early or later in life? In the CO rat model at least, persistent cardiomegaly is probably favored by (a) cardiomegalic induction immediately after birth, (b) cardiomegaly of large magnitude, and (c) prolongation of cardiomegaly. It is not necessarily assumed, however, that persistent cardiomegaly is deleterious. It could conceivably be neutral or even beneficial with respect to myocardial function, health, and life-span. More than once it has been suggested that "super hearts" might result from cardiovascular conditioning at an early age.

In support of the suggestion made earlier that muscle cell hyperplasia contributes to cardiomegaly in stressed neonates, myocardial DNA was measured in 5-day old rat pups continuously inhaling CO. DNA content increased sharply over equal-age controls within 5 days (16). Content reached a plateau after 20 to 25 days of exposure in both groups, but the level of the treated group was above that of the controls. Similar studies with newborn pups exposed to 500 ppm CO for 32 days (7) showed that DNA content of RV increased an average of 18.8% over age-matched controls when compared with 14, 21, 32, 65, and 105 days of age. In LV + S a similar comparison showed that content was elevated 6.7%. These findings make several points: (a) that CO-cardiomegaly in neonates is accompanied by increased DNA synthesis, (b) that the extra DNA formed does not disappear upon stress removal, and (c) that the extent of the increase in DNA content relative to controls, in RV and LV + S, is remarkably similar to the observed heart mass excess (see above).

Is it possible that the increased DNA resulted from nonmuscle cell proliferation? In order to test this possibility, hydroxyproline content was measured, a commonly used index of collagen. Hydroxyproline content was no greater in treated hearts than in controls at any of the five measurement points (7). In fact, hydroxyproline concentration was considerably depressed during CO exposure, suggesting it was "diluted out" by the more rapid growth of other cardiac components. Rate of hydroxyproline synthesis, and presumably connective tissue, was simply unaffected by this form of cardiomegaly. Thus, fibroblast DNA could not be responsible for the increased total heart DNA observed. Based on the data of others, endothelial cell numbers do not change significantly and the incidence of polyploidy is very low in the rat.

Recently, myocardial cells were isolated from neonates that had inhaled 500 ppm CO (F. J. Clubb, Jr., Dallas, Texas, *unpublished data*). LV + S cell volume of controls increased steadily from 1,461 μm^3 at birth to 32,225 μm^3 at 200 days of age. The percentage of cells in LV + S and RV containing two nuclei was depressed at 6 days of age, indicating that CO exposure delays the final round of nuclear division, which normally results in the heart containing 90% binucleated myocardial cells. Binucleated cells in LV + S of the CO rats were longer than that of the controls at 15 and 28 days of age, but LV + S and RV cell volumes of CO rats were smaller at 15 days of age. The ratio of LV + S volume to body weight, however, was greater than that of controls at 6, 15, and 28 days of age, demonstrating cell hypertrophy. By 15 days of age CO rats had more total myocardial cells than the controls, demonstrating hyperplasia. Similar experiments involving 200 ppm CO exposure also showed increases in cell numbers, although of smaller magnitude, suggesting a dose-response relationship of CO-stimulated myocardial cell hyperplasia. We believe that the early delay of binucleation in CO rats permits some fraction of myocardial cells to continue on through cytokinesis after completing karyokinesis, producing an additional generation. This is the mechanism by which hyperplasia proceeds and by which additional cells are generated under stress.

Following 32 days of CO inhalation, these rats were removed to room air. At 200 days of age there were 9.5% more cells in LV + S; however, this increase just missed statistical significance. Cell length and binucleated cell volume in these rats were less than that of the controls. Apparently hearts showing persistent cardiomegaly contain more, but smaller, myocardial cells. Thus it appears likely that muscle cell numbers (a) increase abnormally during development of neonatal cardiomegaly, (b) contribute to the extreme response at that age, and (c) remain abnormally elevated in persistent cardiomegaly.

Both cytochrome *c* concentration and LDH isozyme composition, grossly altered in the CO-exposed neonate, return to normal following termination of treatment.

Fetus

Fetal cardiomegaly induced by CO exposure disappears within 1 to 3 months postexposure (6). There is some evidence (F. J. Clubb, Jr., Dallas, Texas, *unpublished data*), however, that RV myocardial cell number remains elevated and cell volume depressed long after CO exposure is discontinued.

EFFECTS OF CO ON CARDIOVASCULAR FUNCTION

Acute Hemodynamic Changes

Heart rate and systolic arterial blood pressure have been measured in conscious male rats during acute exposure to 500 ppm CO (4). This was done noninvasively by the tail-cuff method while the animals were in restraint and being warmed to assure tail-artery blood flow. Heart rate rose 20% and blood pressure fell 30% in the first half hour when COHb saturation reached 23%. After 2 hr when a 38% COHb level was attained, heart rate rose 37% and blood pressure fell 27% below that of rats breathing room air. These changes remained for the duration of the 24-hr exposure period, then normalized within 2 hr of return to room air.

In order to examine the effect of CO on a broader spectrum of functional parameters, studies have been executed with an open-chest animal preparation (14). Rats were anesthetized with chloralose-urethan, an agent eliciting little sympathetic action on the cardiovascular system, an unfortunate effect of sodium pentobarbital. The animals were ventilated through a tracheostomy with either air or an air-CO mixture. A catheter was inserted into the left iliac artery to monitor arterial pressure. After midline thoracotomy, an electromagnetic flow probe was placed around the ascending aorta. Finally, a stainless steel hypodermic needle directly attached to a micro pressure transducer was inserted through the chest and heart walls into the left ventricular cavity. Using this procedure a number of indexes of muscle and pump function were assessed.

As in the conscious rat, heart rate rose and mean arterial blood pressure fell during initial CO inhalation (4). In fact, sizable changes in these two parameters occurred at COHb saturation as low as 7%. For example, total peripheral resistance fell by 46%. Cardiac output and stroke volume increased gradually as COHb saturation approached 40%. There were no significant changes in either stroke work or LV $+ dP/dt$. For the remainder of the 48-hr-exposure period the changes in these parameters moderated somewhat, but remained different from animals breathing room air.

We believe that as arterial hemoglobin-oxygen saturation falls during CO uptake, profound arteriolar vasodilation is produced. The major effect probably takes place via local tissue control of blood flow, although there may be a CNS component. The fall in venous Po_2 with increasing COHb saturation reflects increased tissue hypoxia, which is probably responsible for release of enzymes such as LDH and creatine phosphokinase into the plasma at such times (12). This in turn produces hypotension, which reflexly elevates heart rate and secondarily enhances inotropic state of the myocardium through increased sympathetic drive. In addition, the falling arterial blood pressure provides lower afterload, which, in turn, permits elevated stroke volume (hence cardiac output) at no greater level of stroke work. Thus, CO inhalation produces a hypotensive volume loading of the heart.

Chronic Hemodynamic Changes

In rats inhaling CO for several weeks, studied in an open-chest preparation, cardiac output was elevated an average of 53% over the first week, largely because of enhanced stroke volume (14). Both declined somewhat thereafter. Total systemic resistance, extremely depressed in the first week, rose afterward, but remained below that of normal rats. After 5 to 6 weeks, cardiac output, stroke volume, and peak aortic flow were still somewhat higher than normal. Since total peripheral resistance was now only slightly subnormal, stroke work was marginally elevated. Of course, both polycythemia and cardiomegaly were well established by this time. Heart rate and arterial blood pressure measured with the cuff in conscious rats at this time were significantly elevated and depressed, respectively (Table 4).

We believe that the initial stimulus to CO-induced cardiac enlargement is enhanced cardiac output mainly via increased stroke volume and to a lesser extent heart rate. Although it is vexing that stroke work remains normal, it is possible that increased wall tension is required as a result of changes in mean ejection pressure and end-diastolic volume interacting through LaPlace's equation. Since we have data on neither end-diastolic nor end-systolic volumes, this possibility cannot be evaluated at present. Although it is possible that CO exerts a direct cardiomegalic effect on the heart, no supporting data exist.

Beyond 1 week, polycythemia develops, re-establishing oxygen-carrying capacity. However, since CO increases the oxygen affinity of hemoglobin, tissue oxygen

TABLE 4. *Conscious heart rate and systolic blood pressure of male rats exposed to 500 ppm CO for 27–42 days, as determined by the tail-cuff method and their controls*

Group	HR[a] (beats/min)	BP[b] (mm Hg)
CO (13)	392.8 ±6.8	90.0 ±4.0
Air (12)	356.3 ±4.7	104.9 ±4.7
Probability	<0.001	<0.05

Note: Values are means ± SE. Number of animals used in each group is given in parentheses.
[a]Measurements were made on all animals in each group on six different days.
[b]Measurements were made on all animals in each group on five different days.

delivery remains impaired. Cardiac output then slowly wanes mainly via decreases in stroke volume. Meanwhile peripheral resistance and blood pressure rise as blood viscosity climbs. With well-established polycythemia after several weeks, it appears that both elevated blood viscosity and modestly increased cardiac output, requiring enhanced stroke work, act to maintain cardiomegaly. The sequence of these changes are seen in Fig. 5. Thus, myocardial volume loading produced by CO is of major importance both prior to, during development of, and in the stable state of cardiomegaly, with some decrement in magnitude as increasing blood viscosity comes to assume a greater role.

Figure 5 also shows the effect of cardiomegaly and polycythemia in the absence of CO. This was done by withdrawing rats from the exposure chambers 1 day prior to hemodynamic measurements. Resistance was elevated 52% and blood pressure 40%, presumably because of high viscosity in the absence of peripheral vasodilation. Cardiac output returned to the normal level. Stroke volume on the other hand was depressed, probably as a result of increased afterload. Mild tachycardia takes up

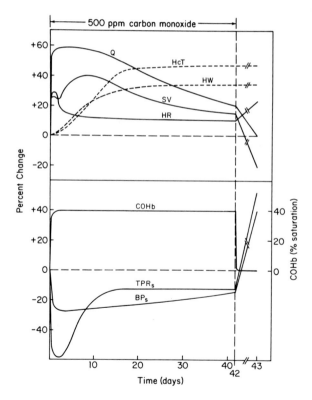

FIG. 5. Time-course of the hemodynamic and hematologic changes that may underlie development and maintenance of cardiomegaly during CO exposure. Q = cardiac output; SV = stroke volume; HR = heart rate; HW = heart weight; Hct = hematocrit; COHb = carboxyhemoglobin saturation; TPR$_s$ = total systemic peripheral resistance; BP$_s$ = systolic arterial blood pressure.

the slack to assure normal output. This illustrates the importance of vasodilation during carboxyhemoglobinemia, maintaining heart work at a far lower level than would otherwise be the case.

Contrasting CO hypoxia and hypoxic hypoxia, very different hemodynamic mechanisms are responsible for development of cardiomegaly. In the latter, increase in heart mass in adult animals is unilateral, occurring only in the RV and that part of the S which contributes to its function (9). This comes about as pulmonary vascular resistance increases, elevating pulmonary arterial pressure and RV afterload. On the other hand, CO hypoxia, as we have seen, produces profound systemic arterial hypotension and increased volume loading, which in turn results in biventricular (and atrial) enlargement. Rats inhaling CO showed no evidence of pulmonary hypertension. Measurements of RV diastolic and systolic pressures showed them to be normal. Thus they are very different hypoxic stressors—one volume, the other pressure—and produce quite different forms of cardiomegaly.

Hypoxic Myocardial Adaptation?

Does chronic exposure to hypoxia induce changes in the myocardium which provide it with greater acute tolerance to depressed arterial hemoglobin saturation and venous P_{O_2}? Over the last two decades more than a score of studies, mainly using RV strips from animals acclimated to simulated high altitude, report "enhanced anoxia tolerance" and recovery of function when returned to oxygen as compared with normals (e.g., ref. 5). Using the RV preparation obtained from rats chronically exposed to CO, we reported a similar phenomenon (1). A number of tissue-level changes have been suggested as contributing factors, including (a) increased efficiency of oxidative metabolism, (b) increased myoglobin content, (c) increased anaerobic (glycolytic) capacity, (d) increased storage of intracellular carbohydrates (glycogen), and (e) necessity of adequate thyroid hormone titer. These studies, however, failed to account for the effect of differences in muscle dimensions produced by cardiomegaly on muscle performance. In addition, all of them used the same test resting force for both treated and control muscles. Since hypoxic hypoxia produces increases in RV mass and wall thickness, this leads to varying rest muscle tension and, hence, performance.

In order to examine this question, the enlarged left ventricular anterior papillary muscle from male rats chronically exposed to 500 ppm CO for 38 to 50 days was used (18).

After decapitation and thoracotomy, the heart was excised from the rat. With the LV slit open, the anterior papillary muscle was removed. The chordae tendinae were held by a miniature spring-loaded clip fashioned from piano wire. The opposite end was held by a similar clip connected to a force-displacement transducer. Length and, consequently, preload changes were imparted to the muscle through a micrometer adjustment. The papillary muscle was positioned in the center of a water-jacketed chamber containing oxygenated Tyrode's solution at 22°C. Following a 2- to 3-hr-equilibration period at 1.0-g preload, contractions were initiated at 15/min by square wave pulses 25% over threshold voltage. Through use of two external reservoirs containing Tyrode's solution, one in equilibrium with 95% O_2 - 5% CO_2 and the other in equilibrium with 95% N_2 - 5% CO_2, changeover from an aerobic to an anaerobic medium was effected in 30 sec.

In the first experiment, groups of CO-treated rats of similar body weight were used. As seen in Table 5, body weights were not different at the time of muscle testing. Hemoglobin concentration, heart weight, heart weight to body weight ratio, and weight of the LV + S were, however, elevated in the CO-exposed group. Papillary muscle weight and cross-sectional area were much greater than that of the control group. The latter was computed by dividing muscle weight by the product of muscle length and specific gravity, assuming the muscle to be a perfect cylinder.

Papillary muscles were tested at a resting force of 3.0 *g*, a preload that was found to lie on the ascending limb of the length-tension curve for most of the muscle preparations in the size range we were using. Although initial aerobic-developed tension was less in the treated group, the time taken for tension to decline to 50% of this value in anoxia was nearly twice as long as in the controls, suggesting that enhanced anoxia tolerance was present in the former group.

To examine the possibility that this difference in apparent anoxia tolerance was due to differences in papillary muscle dimensions, a second experiment was carried out in which rats of smaller body weight were exposed to CO. Although final body weight was 125 g less than controls, the CO-treated rats were polycythemic, and

TABLE 5. *Body weight, blood, heart weight, papillary muscle dimensions, and contractile performance of male rats exposed to 500 ppm CO for 38–50 days, and their controls of similar body weight*

	CO (9)	Air (6)	Probability
BW (g)	442.7 ± 13.8	429.5 ± 21.5	>0.5
Hb (g/100 ml)	22.63 ± 0.42 (8)	15.10 ± 0.35 (5)	<0.001
HW (mg)	1,303.6 ± 55.9	1,017.4 ± 58.9	<0.01
HW/BW (mg/g)	2.95	2.37	<0.01
LV + S wt (mg)	934.7 ± 39.5	746.4 ± 39.9	<0.01
PM wt (mg)	10.52 ± 0.61	5.66 ± 0.51	<0.001
X-sect area (mm²)	2.09 ± 0.14	1.37 ± 0.07	<0.01
DT_i[a] (g/mm²)	0.82 ± 0.10	1.15 ± 0.08	<0.05
1/2 DT_A[b] (min)	9.07 ± 1.28	4.66 ± 1.32	<0.05

Note: Values are means ± SE. Number of animals used in each group is given in parentheses.

[a]Initial preanoxic-developed tension.

[b]Time in anoxia for developed tension to reach half of preanoxic developed tension.

Abbreviations used: BW = body weight, Hb = hemoglobin concentration, HW = heart weight, LV + S = left ventricle plus interventricular septum, PM = papillary muscle, DT_i = preanoxic developed tension, 1/2 DT_A = time to one-half of preanoxic developed tension.

the elevated heart weight to body weight ratio indicates cardiomegaly was present (Table 6). However, the heart weights, weights of the LV + S and papillary muscles, and papillary muscle cross-sectional areas were not different in the two groups. Testing the muscles in the same manner as in the first experiment produced no differences in either aerobic tension or anoxia tolerance.

A third experiment was performed in order to examine the relationship of anoxia tolerance to preload and muscle length. Groups of treated and control rats were established having similar body weight, hemoglobin concentration, heart weight, heart weight to body weight ratio, LV + S weight, papillary muscle weight and similar cross-sectional area to those used in the first experiment. These muscles were tested at lengths giving maximal developed tension (L_{max}), lengths 15% below L_{max}, and lengths 10% and 20% above L_{max}. L_{max} was determined for each individual muscle by varying resting force. No muscle was tested at more than one of the four muscle lengths.

A plot of time to reach 50% of preanoxic-developed tension versus muscle length-tension positioning is seen in Fig. 6. No significant differences between treated and control muscles were seen at any of the four increments of L_{max} used. This is so, even though the muscles of the treated rats were considerably larger than those of the controls. Furthermore, the increasing values for time to reach 50% of preanoxic-developed tension with shorter muscle lengths indicate that anoxia tolerance is a function of muscle length. Separate regression lines were drawn for control and treated muscles (not shown). This enabled an analysis of covariance to be performed. It indicated no significant difference ($p > 0.05$) between the two lines. A t-test performed on the slopes, as well as the y-intercepts, gave similar results. In addition, there was no correlation between time to 50% of preanoxic-developed tension and cross-sectional area when control and treated muscles were

TABLE 6. *Body weight, blood, heart weight, papillary muscle dimensions, and contractile performance of male rats exposed to 500 ppm CO for 38–50 days, and their controls of similar papillary muscle weight*

	CO (12)	Air (14)	Probability
BW (g)	324.3 ± 9.5	451.3 ± 13.9	<0.001
Hb (g/100 ml)	23.39 ± 0.53 (4)	15.59 ± 0.27 (9)	<0.001
HW (mg)	1,099.6 ± 31.3	1,192.6 ± 44.2	>0.05
HW/BW (mg/g)	3.39	2.64	<0.05
LV + S (mg)	771.8 ± 21.4	829.6 ± 24.3	>0.05
PM (mg)	8.76 ± 0.74	8.99 ± 0.71	>0.5
X-sect area (mm²)	1.73 ± 0.15	1.77 ± 0.14	>0.5
DT_i (g/mm²)	1.03 ± 0.12	1.11 ± 0.11	>0.5
1/2 DT_A (min)	7.77 ± 1.07	6.92 ± 0.91	>0.5

Note: Values are means ± SE. Number of animals used in each group is given in parentheses.
Abbreviations same as in Table 5.

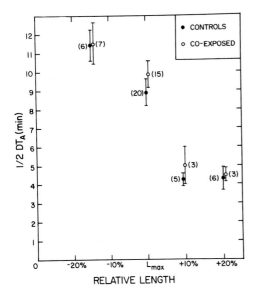

FIG. 6. Relationship between the time required for developed tension to reach one-half preanoxic developed tension and papillary muscle length-tension positioning for muscles from hearts of 500 ppm CO-exposed and control rats. Values in parentheses are numbers of animals used. *Vertical bars* represent SE.

tested at the four muscle lengths along their respective length-tension curves. The data points for the CO-exposed and control muscles were completely interspersed. Again, however, muscles above L_{max} showed a lower anoxia tolerance than muscles at or below L_{max}.

Let us review the results of these experiments and their probable meaning. In the first experiment, aerobic tension development by the treated muscles was less than that of the controls. This resulted from a smaller preload on the former since rest force acted over a larger cross section. Because the ascending limb of the length-tension curve for papillary muscle and cardiac muscle is, in general, steep, small differences in position away from L_{max} result in large differences in developed tension. Thus, larger muscles would have a lower metabolic rate than smaller muscles contracting at the same rate. The slower rate of depletion of tissue oxygen, glycogen, creatine phosphate, and ATP permitted contraction to continue longer in the larger muscles removed from enlarged hearts.

Could diffusional differences between larger and smaller muscles play a role in anoxia tolerance? McGrath et al. (5) reasoned that an increased diffusion path works against enhanced anoxia tolerance in preparations by limiting oxygen uptake. However, oxygen loss to the anoxic medium assumes critical importance during testing, not uptake. Moreover, loss occurs more slowly in a muscle of larger cross-sectional area than in a smaller one. Our data relating anoxia tolerance and cross-sectional area suggest, however, that diffusion is not a significant factor in modifying anoxia tolerance when comparisons are made to muscles operating at the same position on their respective length-tension curves. Thus, we find no evidence that chronic exposure to CO hypoxia results in an adaptation whereby myocardial tissue becomes more tolerant of acute anoxia.

Long-Standing Changes

The phenomenon of persistent cardiomegaly was described earlier in this chapter. Do changes in cardiovascular function induced by CO also persist? Studies were undertaken to determine if so and to what degree.

Again, newborn rat pups inhaled 500 ppm CO for several weeks, after which they were returned to room air. Subsequently, hematology, cardiac morphology, and hemodynamics were examined in the females at 92 and 171 days of age and in the males at 103 and 180 days of age. For the sake of brevity, one group, representative of the data obtained on the other three, is presented in Table 7. At 70 days post CO exposure (103 days of age), body weight was the same as controls and hematocrit was not significantly different. The weight ratio of the two ventricles (2V) to body weight remained elevated, and the weights of the LV + S, RV, and 2V were significantly above those predicted for rats of equal body weight. Predictions based on body weight were made using multiple regression equations derived from data on 289 normal rats in the body weight range, 20 to 500 g (19). The ratio of RV to LV + S weight was also elevated in those previously exposed to CO. The findings on the 92-day-old female rats were similar, with the exception that hematocrit of the treated group remained slightly, but significantly higher. In the 171-day-old female and 180-day-old male rats the same pattern was displayed, although the degree of cardiomegaly that persisted was somewhat smaller.

Using the open-chest preparation previously outlined, the hemodynamic parameters seen in Table 8 were examined. There were no statistically significant differences between previously treated male rats at 103 days of age and age-matched controls, with the exception of the first derivation of LV pressure rise, which was higher in the CO group. Since body weights of the two groups were not different, it was not necessary to index the values on that basis. However, because the LV + S weight of the CO group was absolutely greater than that of the controls, indexing was done on that basis. This permits comparison of pump function and muscle performance of equivalent quantities of heart muscle (lower panel). Again there were no differences between the treated and control groups and the earlier difference in $+dP/dt$ disappeared.

Examination of the heart rates of the anesthetized animals, however, revealed consistently higher values in the previously CO-exposed group (Table 9). Generally, the difference from controls was greater at 92 and 103 days of age than at 171 and 180 days of age. It was displayed equally by males and females. In all the treated groups but one, including the 103-day-old males, stroke volume was marginally lower than that of the respective control group. Because cardiac outputs were nearly identical in all cases when comparing matched treated and control groups, heart rate therefore was elevated. The enhanced $+dP/dt$ (and $-dP/dt$, not shown) we observed is a usual complement of a shortened cardiac cycle.

With one exception, there were no significant differences in aortic systolic blood pressures between treated and control rats (Table 9). Two treated groups displayed a tendency toward lower values and two a tendency toward higher values. A long-

TABLE 7. Body weight, heart weight, and blood data for male rats 103 days of age, exposed to 500 ppm CO for 33 days after birth

Group	BW (g)	$2V^a$/BW (mg/g)	RV/LV+S (mg/mg)	% above predicted			Hematocrit (%)
				LV + S	RV	2V	
CO (22)	493.8 ± 7.5	2.69 ± 0.04	0.3144 ± 0.0054	9.11 ± 1.53	28.39 ± 2.74	13.18 ± 1.61	55.42 ± 0.79
Air (22)	494.8 ± 6.6	2.46 ± 0.03	0.2910 ± 0.0041	1.81 ± 1.20	10.98 ± 2.08	3.75 ± 1.29	53.60 ± 0.76
Probability	>0.05	<0.001	<0.01	<0.01	<0.001	<0.001	>0.05

Note: Values are means ± SE. Number of animals used in each group is given in parentheses.
^{a}2V = RV + LV+S.

TABLE 8. *Hemodynamic data for male rats 103 days of age, exposed to 500 ppm CO for 33 days after birth*

Group	Q̇	Q̇p	SV	SW	+dP/dt	dF/dt	Vp_D	TPR_s	LV+S
CO (22)	38.1 ± 3.9	234.0 ± 13.2	89.8 ± 9.8	7,858 ± 973	4,965 ± 555	23,180 ± 1,559	1.46 ± 0.11	0.98 ± 0.12	1,087.6 ± 39.3
Air (22)	38.0 ± 3.3	212.0 ± 16.3	107.2 ± 9.7	7,612 ± 853	3,595 ± 247	19,674 ± 1,653	1.61 ± 0.12	0.80 ± 0.07	941.2 ± 13.5
Probability	>0.05	>0.05	>0.05	>0.05	<0.05	>0.05	>0.05	>0.05	<0.01
				per g LV+S					
CO (22)	35.0	215.2	82.6	7,225	4,565	21,313			
Air (22)	40.4	225.2	113.9	8,088	3,820	20,903			
Probability	>0.05	>0.05	>0.05	>0.05	>0.05	>0.5			

Note: Values are means ± SE. Number of animals used in each group is given in parentheses.

Abbreviations: Q̇ = cardiac output (ml/min), Q̇p = peak aortic flow (ml/min), SV = stroke volume (μl), SW = stroke work (dyne · cm), +dP/dt = first derivative of left ventricle pressure increase (mm Hg/sec), dF/dt = first derivative of aortic flow (ml/min/sec), Vp_D = end-diastolic left ventricle pressure (mm Hg), TPR_s = total systemic vascular resistance (PRU/kg), LV+S (mg).

TABLE 9. *Heart rate and aortic systolic blood pressure of female and male rats exposed to 500 ppm CO for 33 days after birth and sacrificed later*

Females	92 days of age		171 days of age		Males	103 days of age		180 days of age	
	HR[a]	Ao$_s$[b]	HR	Ao$_s$		HR[a]	Ao$_s$[b]	HR	Ao$_s$
CO	413.8 ± 7.5 (12)	72.3 ± 5.6	389.2 ± 12.2 (19)	83.9 ± 5.7	CO	428.4 ± 10.9 (22)	91.2 ± 4.7	410.3 ± 12.9 (11)	88.8 ± 7.2
Air	378.9 ± 7.5 (12)	81.0 ± 6.1	360.8 ± 7.9 (21)	78.3 ± 5.7	Air	372.9 ± 8.9 (22)	78.1 ± 3.7	368.1 ± 15.7 (13)	98.0 ± 7.8
Probability	<0.01	>0.05	<0.05	>0.05	Probability	<0.001	<0.05	<0.05	>0.05

Note: Values are means ± SE. Number of animals used in each group is given in parentheses.
[a] Beats/min.
[b] mm Hg.

standing effect of CO, therefore, is not hypertension. However, our data suggest that chronic elicitation of elevated heart rate leads, in some degree, to persistence long after CO inhalation is discontinued. This apparently acts to offset chronically depressed stroke volume. The reason for the depression of stroke volume is not clear, as neither LV end-diastolic pressure nor peripheral resistance was abnormal.

It was also desirable to examine heart function under conditions of acutely increased workloading. Following completion of the measurements discussed above, which were made under isovolemic conditions, blood volume was increased first by 10% and then by an additional 10% by infusion of saline. This served to increase venous return, left atrial and LV end-diastolic pressures, and presumably LV end-diastolic volume. With the initial 10% increment, cardiac output, peak aortic flow, stroke volume, $+dP/dt$, and dF/dt increased by 35% to 75%. Stroke work increased by 85% to 160%. A further 10% increase in blood volume resulted in much smaller increases in these parameters. However, examination of the data (not shown) for all four age groups, two male and two female, failed to reveal any significant differences between treated and control hearts. Apparently, CO-induced neonatal cardiomegaly does not compromise the potential of the adult myocardium to respond to acute volume workloading, at least as judged by the parameters examined.

SUMMARY AND CONCLUSIONS

Although the studies described were all carried out on the laboratory rat, the findings probably apply, in general, to humans. The initial cardiovascular effect of CO inhalation is a decline in the oxygen-carrying capacity of the blood and increased affinity. This is quickly compensated, in large measure, by increased tissue blood flow at reduced arterial pressure. Within days the rate of erythrocyte formation increases, inducing polycythemia, and reestablishing oxygen carrying capacity. At the same time, the myocardium is undergoing exaggerated growth. Although volume overloading of the heart appears to later moderate in the presence of greater red cell mass, both factors contribute to maintaining cardiomegaly during chronic CO exposure. Although the thresholds for the blood and cardiac changes were observed to be 100 and 200 ppm CO, respectively, there is no reason to believe that these effects and others do not occur to some degree at much lower concentrations. In fact, since CO has been with us so long (in our evolution), might it not provide unseen benefits?

A number of studies suggest that intrinsic changes occur in the myocardium of animals chronically exposed to environmental hypoxia which provide it with enhanced acute anoxia or hypoxia tolerance. Our results fail to confirm this in hearts of rats treated with CO and reveal the sources of error in earlier studies.

The younger the age at which cardiomegaly is induced by CO, the greater the response. This process is particularly extreme in neonates and is accompanied by alterations in the LDH isozyme pattern and depression of cytochrome c concentration. Possibly of greater importance, this excess heart weight tends to persist into adulthood, long after termination of CO inhalation, i.e., persistent cardiomegaly.

We find that myocardial cell hyperplasia occurs in neonatal cardiomegaly and that the greater cellularity for the most part persists. Evidence suggests that connective tissue does not proliferate.

Exposure of the rat fetus to 200 ppm CO results in mild cardiomegaly, which, however, disappears within a few months after birth. It is accompanied at birth by depressed body weight, enlarged placenta, immature hematology, and enhanced heart LDH M subunit composition and myoglobin concentration.

Functionally the heart with persistent cardiomegaly is abnormal in several respects. Tachycardia, a response to CO, like persistent cardiomegaly, is present as long as 5 months post CO exposure. Although unproven, the mechanism may hinge on subnormal stroke volume, the elevated heart rate reflexly assuring normal cardiac output. Our studies suggest, as have few others, that chronic CO inhalation is capable of producing lasting changes in both cardiac morphology and function. These changes become especially prominent when cardiomegaly occurs in the plastic and vulnerable neonatal heart.

ACKNOWLEDGMENTS

I wish to acknowledge the technical assistance and kind suggestions of the following individuals who contributed to this work: Wayne Kanten, Michael Baylerian, Audrey Stryker, Bernd Barthel, James Thill, Christopher Fanning, Sunita Yedavally, and Kevin Francisco at Wayne State University; and Lawrence Bugaisky and Bud Rasmussen at the University of Illinois, Chicago.

REFERENCES

1. Bugaisky, L., and Penney, D. (1976): Chronic carbon monoxide poisoning: effects on performance of the isolated right ventricle. *J. Appl. Physiol.*, 40:324–328.
2. Campbell, J. (1933): Hypertrophy of the heart in acclimatization to chronic carbon monoxide poisoning. *J. Physiol. (Lond.)*, 77:8P.
3. Chen, S., Weller, M., and Penney, D. (1982): A study of free lung cells from young rats chronically exposed to carbon monoxide from birth. *Scan. Electron Microsc.*, II:859–867.
4. Kanten, W., Penney, D., Francisco, K., and Thill, J. (1983): Hemodynamic responses to acute carboxyhemoglobinemia in the rat. *Am. J. Physiol.*, 244:H320–H327.
5. McGrath, J., Bullard, R., and Komives, G. (1969): Functional adaptation in cardiac and skeletal muscle after exposure to simulated high altitude. *Fed. Proc.*, 28:1307–1311.
6. Penney, D., Baylerian, M., and Fanning, K. (1980): Temporary and lasting cardiac effects of pre- and postnatal exposure to carbon monoxide. *Toxicol. Appl. Pharmacol.*, 53:271–278.
7. Penney, D., Baylerian, M., Thill, J., Fanning, C., and Yedavally, S. (1982): Postnatal carbon monoxide exposure: immediate and lasting effects in the rat. *Am. J. Physiol.*, 243:H328–H339.
8. Penney, D., Baylerian, M., Thill, J., Yedavally, S., and Fanning, C. (1983): Cardiac response of the fetal rat to carbon monoxide exposure. *Am. J. Physiol.*, 244:H289–H297.
9. Penney, D., Benjamin, M., and Dunham, E. (1974): Effect of carbon monoxide on cardiac weight as compared with altitude effects. *J. Appl. Physiol.*, 37:80–84.
10. Penney, D., and Bishop, P. (1978): Hematologic changes in the rat during and after exposure to carbon monoxide. *J. Environ. Pathol. Toxicol.*, 2:407–415.
11. Penney, D., Dunham, E., and Benjamin, M. (1974): Chronic carbon monoxide exposure: time course of hemoglobin, heart weight and lactate dehydrogenase changes. *Toxicol. Appl. Pharmacol.*, 28:493–497.
12. Penney, D., and Maziarka, T. (1976): Effect of acute carbon monoxide poisoning on serum lactate dehydrogenase and creatine phosphokinase. *J. Toxicol. Environ. Health*, 1:1017–1021.

13. Penney, D., Sakai, J., and Cook, K. (1974): Heart growth: interacting effects of carbon monoxide and age. *Growth*, 38:321–328.
14. Penney, D., Sodt, P., and Cutilletta, A. (1979): Cardiodynamic changes during prolonged carbon monoxide exposure in the rat. *Toxicol. Appl. Pharmacol.*, 50:213–218.
15. Penney, D., and Thomas, M. (1975): Hematological alterations and response to acute hypobaric stress. *J. Appl. Physiol.*, 39:1034–1037.
16. Penney, D., and Weeks, T. (1979): Age dependence of cardiac growth in the normal and carbon monoxide-exposed rat. *Dev. Biol.*, 71:153–162.
17. Penney, D., Zak, R., and Aschenbrenner, V. (1983): Carbon monoxide inhalation: effect on heart cytochrome c in the neonatal and adult rat. *J. Toxicol. Environ. Health.*, 20:1–20.
18. Slonek, R. (1979): The effect of carbon monoxide exposure on the anoxia tolerance or rat myocardium. Master of Science degree thesis, University of Illinois at Chicago Circle.
19. Styka, P., and Penney, D. (1978): Regression of carbon monoxide-induced cardiomegaly. *Am. J. Physiol.*, 235:H516–H522.

Growth of the Heart in Health and Disease,
edited by Radovan Zak. Raven Press,
New York © 1984.

Hypertrophic Adaptation of the Heart to Stress: A Myothermal Analysis

Norman R. Alpert and Louis A. Mulieri

Department of Physiology and Biophysics, University of Vermont, College of Medicine, Burlington, Vermont 05405

In the transformation from the basal state to that of maximum activity, such as occurs in exercise, the peripheral metabolic demands of the mammalian organism may increase by more than an order of magnitude. To meet this acute increase in metabolic demand there is a virtually instantaneous increase in cardiac output. The altered contractile performance of the heart is mediated by changes in sarcomere length (18,38), autonomic balance (34), and heart rate (13). In contrast, when the increased demands on the heart are chronic, such as in hypertensive heart disease, aortic stenosis, arteriovenous fistula, or thyrotoxicosis, the heart responds by augmenting its mass. Without the increase in mass, the heart would soon fail. The increase in mass, and thus the adaptation, is not a simple addition of identical units. Cellular and subcellular reorganization of the myocytes occurs. Both the change in mass and the reorganization contribute to meeting the chronic increase in demand. In this process the contractile and noncontractile components are reshaped in a manner that produces distinct changes in the (a) characteristics and quantity of the subcellular constituents, (b) mechanical performance, and (c) thermomechanical economy. The precise nature of these changes is a function of the stress applied to the heart. We have chosen to examine two types of hypertrophy, pressure overload and thyrotoxic, whose characteristics (mechanical V_{max}, curvature of the force velocity relation, myosin ATPase, thermomechanical economy) represent opposite ends of the spectrum which encompasses most types of hypertrophy. Although the similarities between these models and the relevant clinical entities are striking, it is unwarranted to consider them identical.

PREPARATION OF ENLARGED HEARTS

Pressure-overload hypertrophy was produced in male albino rabbits weighing about 2.0 kg by twisting a spiral monel metal spring around the pulmonary artery to induce a 66% constriction of the right ventricular outflow tract (5,24). The animals are used approximately 5 weeks after the surgery. Thyrotoxic hypertrophy was produced in 2.0-kg rabbits by 14 daily intramuscular injections of 0.2 mg/kg

L-thyroxine (10). If body weight fell below 80% of the starting weight, the daily injections were omitted (not more than two) until the 80% level was reached.

NATURE AND EXTENT OF CARDIAC ENLARGEMENT

The right ventricular weight/body weight ratio (g/kg) for control (C), pressure overload (P), and thyrotoxic (T) rabbits was 0.46 ± 0.02, 0.88 ± 0.05 ($p<0.001$), and 0.70 ± 0.02 ($p<0.001$), respectively (28). This ratio may be somewhat misleading because the body weight in the P preparations is somewhat larger than in the T preparations, with both being smaller than that in control animals (C) (P, 1.94 ± 0.06 kg; T, 1.87 ± 0.06 kg; C, 2.56 ± 0.09 kg). The absolute weights of the right ventricles were 1.17 ± 0.05 g, 1.70 ± 0.13 g, and 1.31 ± 0.05 g for the C, P, and T hearts, respectively (28).

Effects of Hyperplasia and Hypertrophy

The heart may enlarge by hyperplasia (increase in number of myocytes), hypertrophy (increase in the size of myocytes), or both (Fig. 1). Heart muscle cells have the capacity to increase in number during the embryonic and neonatal phase of development (23,33) and perhaps after the heart has reached a critical size (500 g in the human) (27). When hyperplastic growth occurs after the critical size is reached, the increase in the number of cells apparently occurs from longitudinal splitting of the enlarged hypertrophic cells. The myocytes increase in both length and width and contribute to the dimensional reorganization of the whole heart (9). The connective tissue also enlarges. Here, in contrast to the myocytes, the main response to the stress involves hyperplasia (15). A collagenous network connects myocytes and surrounds them. In the hypertrophied heart, the collagen content is higher and the struts thicker and longer. Connective tissue hyperplasia does not occur in hearts enlarged secondary to thyrotoxicosis (12,26).

Concentric and Eccentric Hypertrophy

The growth of the myocyte obligates a certain rearrangement of the heart. In response to pressure overload, the heart enlarges in a concentric fashion, with the

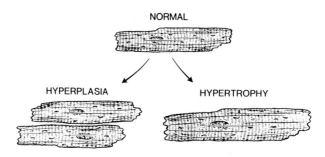

FIG. 1. Myocardial enlargement by hyperplasia or hypertrophy.

walls getting thicker while the lumen size remains within normal limits. In response to volume overload or thyrotoxicosis there is also an increase in the wall mass. However, under these conditions the wall thickness may not increase very much whereas the chamber size increases substantially. Dynamic measurement of intraluminal systolic and diastolic pressure (Table 1) can be used to make calculations of wall stress using the LaPlace relationship:

$$T = P \cdot \frac{R_1 R_2}{R_1 + R_2} \tag{1}$$

where T is the wall tension and R_1 and R_2 are the greater and lesser radii of the heart curvature. Wall stress (S) is then approximated as follows:

$$S = T/h \tag{2}$$

where T is tension per unit circumference and h is wall thickness. Under these circumstances, the heart grows in a manner that tends to normalize active wall stress despite the changes found in systolic intraluminal pressure (Table 1) (20). Diastolic wall stress is normal in the pressure overload but may be increased in the volume-overload preparation. It is very difficult to evaluate the contractile function in the intact heart because of the interdependence of contractile performance and peripheral cardiovascular load as well as the confounding contribution of the complex geometry. For this reason the analysis of hypertrophic myocardial adaption, which follows, is based on (a) measurements of morphological and biochemical changes of the subcellular components resulting from the development of hypertrophy; and (b) mechanical and myothermal measurements on isolated papillary muscles from the hypertrophied hearts.

COMPOSITION AND CHEMISTRY OF MYOCYTES
FROM THE ENLARGED HEART

In pressure-overload hypertrophy the volume of the myocardial cell occupied by the myofibril, sarcoplasmic reticulum, and T-tubular system increases out of proportion to the other components of the myocyte (32). The percent volume occupied by the mitochondria is thus reduced, and there have been reports that the size of

TABLE 1. *Right ventricular intraluminal pressure (mm Hg)* [a]

Preparation	Diastolic	Systolic
Control	1.2	17
Pressure overload	2.2	38
Thyrotoxic	1.2	31

[a]Data from ref. 28.

the individual mitochondrion is also somewhat reduced (25). Thyroxine-stimulated growth (30) or volume overload resulting from aortic insufficiency (22) produces myocytes in which mitochondria occupy a significantly greater percent volume than normal. The individual mitochondria are enlarged and exhibit a complex internal structure with a lacy-appearing inner membrane resulting from expansion of the intracrystal spaces. This increase in percent volume is at the expense of the other intracellular components.

There has been a controversy about the effects of cardiac enlargement on contractile protein ATPase activity. It is clear that the controversy resulted from the unanticipated sensitivity of the adaptive process to the fine details of the applied stress as well as the variability found in the control preparations. Pressure-overload hypertrophy can result in increases, decreases, or no change in myosin ATPase activity (35). In thyrotoxic hypertrophy there is agreement about the increase in myosin ATPase activity (10,11,16,19,41). In the standard enlarged heart preparations used in the studies described below, the calcium-activated myosin ATPase was 0.32 ± 0.01, 0.22 ± 0.02 ($p < 0.001$), and 0.86 ± 0.03 ($p < 0.001$) μmoles Pi/mg min for the C, P, and T hearts, respectively (28). The change in ATPase activity seen in the hypertrophied hearts is believed to result from alterations in the percent composition of the myosin isoenzymes in the myocytes. Distinct differences of the densitometer scans of polyacrylamide pyrophosphate gels from the two types of hypertrophy are clearly discernable (Fig. 2). Analysis of the area under the V_1 (high ATPase myosin), V_3 (low ATPase myosin), and the V_2 (intermediate) peaks gives values for V_1 of 12%, 0%, and 90% of the total for the C, P, and T hearts, respectively (8). There is a linear relationship between percent V_1 and calcium-activated myosin ATPase activity (Fig. 3).

MECHANICAL PERFORMANCE OF ISOLATED PAPILLARY MUSCLES FROM ENLARGED HEARTS

Papillary muscles isolated from the right ventricle of pressure-overload hypertrophy hearts exhibit a depressed maximum velocity of unloaded shortening (1,24,29) and an increase in the curvature of the force velocity relationship (7,24) (Fig. 4). There was an increase in time to peak isometric tension, a slight (20%) but not significant decrease in peak isometric tension, and a decrease in the maximum rate of tension development (1,24) (Fig. 4). Conversely, in thyrotoxic hypertrophy there is an increase in maximum velocity of unloaded shortening and a decrease in the curvature of the force velocity relationship (2,7,21,37,39,40) (Fig. 4). There is a decrease in time to peak isometric tension, a decrease (28%) in peak isometric

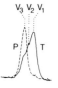

V_3 V_2 V_1

P   T

FIG. 2. Densitometer scan of pyrophosphate gels of myosin from pressure overload (P) and thyrotoxic (T) hypertrophied right ventricles. (Redrawn from Litten et al., ref. 9, with permission.)

force, and an increase in the maximum rate of force development (2,7,21,37,39,40) (Fig. 4.) In the pressure-overload hearts there is a decrease in the passive compliance whereas in the thyrotoxic preparations there is no change in compliance. These changes in mechanical performance, involving the contractile and excitation contraction coupling systems, are a reflection of the morphologic and chemical differences present in these preparations.

MYOTHERMAL ANALYSIS OF MYOCARDIAL HYPERTROPHIC ADAPTATION

General Considerations

The total energy liberated by a muscle is made up of heat and work:

$$E = H + W \tag{3}$$

where E is the total energy liberated in any given period of time, and W is the work done during that period of time. In the case of heart papillary muscle, if the contractions are isometric, and thus no external work is done, all the energy is liberated as heat. Under these circumstances, the heat output is an index of all of the subcellular energy-consuming and energy-releasing reactions. If the time-course and quantity of heat can be measured accurately, then the heat measurements in conjunction with the isometric mechanical studies can be used as a window to the

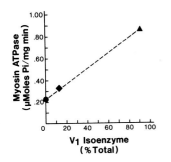

FIG. 3. The relationship between V_1 isoenzyme content and myosin ATPase (9).

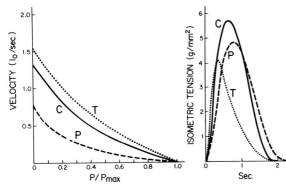

FIG. 4. The mechanical performance of isolated papillary muscles from control, (C), pressure overload (P), and thyrotoxic (T) hypertrophied hearts. The force velocity relationship is presented in the **left panel** and the isometric myogram recorded at l_o is presented in the **right panel**. The *dotted* force velocity curve is unpublished data from Maughan, Mulieri, and Alpert.

intracellular molecular events occurring during activity. The total heat, T, during isometric contractions is made up of two separable entities:

$$T = B + T_A \qquad (4)$$

where B is the resting or basal heat and T_A is the total activity-related heat. The resting heat is a reflection of all the heat-producing and heat-absorbing reactions associated with maintenance of cellular integrity. These include maintenance of ionic and chemical gradients as well as the synthesis and degradation of organelles and enzymes. The total activity-related heat is made up of all the heat liberated as a result of muscle contraction, i.e., the initial heat, I, and the recovery heat, R:

$$T_A = I + R \qquad (5)$$

The initial heat, I, is liberated during contraction and relaxation (Fig. 5, left panel). It consists of the heat liberated or absorbed as a result of all the biophysical and biochemical events involved in the release of free calcium and its final sequestration by the sarcoplasmic reticulum as well as all the heat liberated and absorbed when myosin cross bridges interact with actin and ATP to produce isometric force:

$$I = TIH + TDH \qquad (6)$$

TIH is the tension-independent heat, i.e., all the heat associated with calcium cycling, and *TDH* is the tension-dependent heat, i.e., all the heat associated with cross-bridge cycling. Initial heat can be partitioned into its two components by incubating the papillary muscle in 2.5 times hyperosmotic mannitol Krebs solution. In this incubation medium, stimulation of the muscle produces no force although

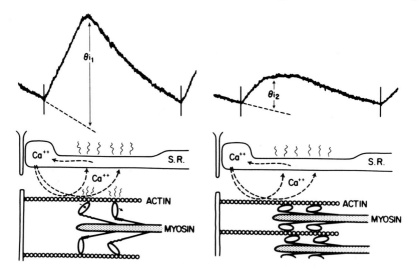

FIG. 5. A diagram of the temperature change **(above)** and the molecular events **(below)** associated with contraction and relaxation in normal Krebs **(left panel)** and 2.5 × mannitol Krebs **(right panel)**. (Reprinted from Alpert and Mulieri, ref. 4, with permission.)

a triggerable heat is present (Fig. 5, right panel). Since cross-bridge cycling and thus contraction is eliminated under these conditions, the remaining triggerable heat is the result of heat-consuming and heat-producing reactions associated with calcium cycling. This heat output is the tension-independent heat, *TIH*. Subtracting the *TIH* from *I* gives the tension-dependent heat:

$$TDH = I - TIH \tag{7}$$

Recovery heat, *R*, is a reflection of all the processes involved in restoring the muscle to the initial steady state conditions prevailing immediately before the stimulus was applied. For the most part, this involves the resynthesis of ATP from ADP.

The Heat-Measuring System

To carry out the precise myothermal measurements described above on isolated right ventricular papillary muscles weighing 1 to 2 mg, low thermal capacity, rapid response time heat-measuring equipment is required. Vacuum-deposited, Hill-type planar thermopiles meet this requirement. The thermopile was fabricated by vacuum deposition of bismuth and antimony through a chemically milled mask onto a thin mica sheet which was then covered with a second mica sheet to provide electrical insulation (31). The papillary muscle is mounted on the central portion of the thermopile (exposed measuring junctions) and fastened to the stationary hook below and the glass rod extension from the force transducer above (Fig. 6, left). The reference junctions are under the brass jaws of the frame. The muscle is held flat against the thermopile by a tether which counteracts the irregular shape of the tendinous end of the muscle (see legend Fig. 6 for details). The entire frame (Fig. 7 left) is placed inside the incubating chamber (Fig. 7 right), and the whole assembly is then lowered into a 70-liter constant-temperature water bath (see legend Fig. 7 for details). The muscle is stimulated at 0.2 Hz for the 2-hr-equilibration period,

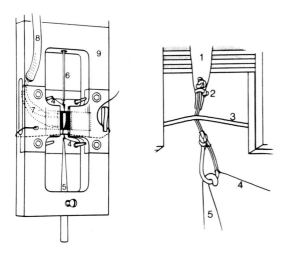

FIG. 6. Thermopile and mounting frame. **1.** Muscle located in the center of the thermopile resting on the measuring junctions. **2.** Knot used to tie connecting loop to the muscle and to place stimulating electrode in contact with the end of the muscle. **3.** Tether to ensure close contact of the muscle with the thermopile surface. **4.** Stimulating electrode wire leading to electrode post. **5.** Glass rod to anchor lower end of the muscle. **6.** Upper glass rod connecting muscle to the force transducer. **7.** Leads from the thermopile. **8.** Conduit for thermopile leads. **9.** Thermopile frame.

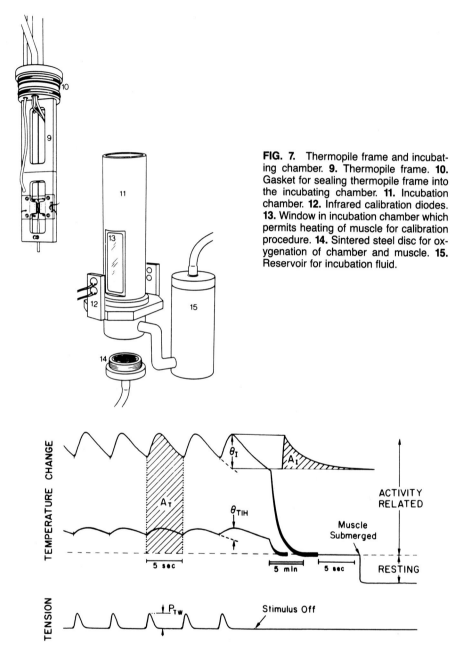

FIG. 7. Thermopile frame and incubating chamber. **9.** Thermopile frame. **10.** Gasket for sealing thermopile frame into the incubating chamber. **11.** Incubation chamber. **12.** Infrared calibration diodes. **13.** Window in incubation chamber which permits heating of muscle for calibration procedure. **14.** Sintered steel disc for oxygenation of chamber and muscle. **15.** Reservoir for incubation fluid.

FIG. 8. A record of force **(below)** and temperature change **(above)**. The topmost oscillating line is the temperature change which occurs during repetitive stimulation of the isometrically contracting papillary muscle. The middle oscillating line is the triggerable temperature change which occurs when the papillary muscle is stimulated repetitively in 2.5 × mannitol Krebs solution. A complete discussion of the methods used to measure the various heats is found in the text.

and the length adjusted in small increments (0.05–0.10 mm) until l_o is reached. The thermopile is calibrated and the thermal capacity of the muscle and system determined as previously described (31).

Analysis of the Heat Records

The thermopile system measures the temperature changes in the papillary muscle during and following activity. When a steady state is reached in the repetitively stimulated muscle there is an oscillating temperature change (Fig. 8, upper trace). The observed temperature change is a function of the time-course and quantity of the heat liberated by the muscle, the thermal capacity of the muscle and system, and the heat-loss characteristics of the muscle and system. The initial heat, which is associated with contraction and relaxation, is obtained by measuring the temperature change, θ_I. This value is obtained by translating the cool-off curve following the last stimulus to the falling portion of the previous heat record (see dashed line, upper record, Fig. 8) and then dropping a vertical line from the peak temperature to the dashed curve. The temperature, θ_I, is then multiplied by the thermal capacity of the muscle and the heat loss conductance to give the initial heat, I (5). The total activity-related heat, T_A, is proportional to the hatched area, A_T, and consists of the initial heat, I, and the recovery heat, R. An area proportional to the initial heat can be obtained by multiplying the temperature change associated with the initial heat, θ_I, by the cool-off time constant. This gives the hatched area, A_I. The recovery/initial heat ratio can then be defined as follows:

$$R/I = (A_T - A_I)/A_I \tag{8}$$

The *TIH* is measured from the oscillating temperature change observed when tension is eliminated by incubation in 2.5 times hyperosmotic manitol Krebs solution (Fig. 8, middle trace). The temperature change associated with the *TIH* is obtained by extrapolating the cool-off curve after the stimulus is turned off so that it forms an extension of the previous falling temperature curve (dashed line). A vertical line is then drawn from the peak of the oscillating temperature curve to the extrapolated falling temperature curve. This temperature, θ_{TIH}, is then multiplied by the heat capacity of the muscle and the heat loss conductance to give the tension-independent heat, *TIH*. Tension-dependent heat *(TDH)* is obtained by subtracting *TIH* from I. Resting heat, B, is obtained by stopping the stimulus and allowing the muscle to cool to its resting temperature (Fig. 8, top record, heavy solid line, 5-min cooling period). The muscle is then fully submerged in normal Krebs solution. The change in temperature is then multiplied by the previously determined heat loss conductance. The success of this method depends on being able to perform the same immersion with no muscle on the thermopile with no more than a 0.1 m°C transient excursion in the temperature base line. The lowest trace (Fig. 8) is a record of the isometric tension. The record of tension obtained while stimulating the muscle in hyperosmotic manitol is not presented. It would be a straight line (less than 5% original twitch tension) superimposed on the base line of the force record.

Mechanical and Thermal Measurements

Papillary muscles from normal hearts exhibited an unloaded shortening velocity of 1.34 muscle lengths per second. This was reduced to 68% of normal in the P preparations and increased to 140% of normal in the T hearts (Table 2) (6,7,36). The peak isometric force developed by the normal muscle was 5.69 g/mm². In the P and T preparations this force was 84% (not significant) and 72% of the control value, respectively (Table 2). Time to peak tension (*TPT*) was 631 msec in the control muscles. This increased to 123% of normal in the P muscles and decreased to 54% of normal in the T hearts (Table 2). The tension time integral was 6.12 gsec/mm² in the control papillary muscles. This value was reduced to 92% (not significant) and 78% of normal in the P and T hearts, respectively (Table 2). The resting heat production for the C and P preparations was 25 and 16 mcal/g min, respectively. The total activity-related heat production, T_A, for the control papillary muscles is 4.15 mcal/g·min (3,5,7,36). This value is reduced to 61% and 69% of normal in the P and T preparations, respectively (Table 3). Initial heat, I, is 1.69 mcal/g in the control muscles. It is reduced to 61% of normal in the P hearts and is unchanged in the T muscles (Table 3). The recovery to initial heat ratio is 1.46 in the control muscles. This value is unchanged in the P and reduced to 54% of normal in the T preparations, respectively (Table 3). It is important to note that the method used for measuring recovery metabolism (14) includes any activity-related changes in the base-line levels. The tension-dependent heat, *TDH*, is 1.29 mcal/g. This is reduced to 65% of normal in the P and is unchanged in the T muscles (Table 4) (3,7). The tension-independent heat is 0.40 mcal/g in the normal

TABLE 2. *Mechanical characteristics of papillary muscle*[a]

Preparation	V_{max}(l_o/sec)	P_{TW}(g/mm²)	*TPT* (msec)	$\int P_{TW}dt$ (gsec/mm²)
C	1.34	5.69	631	6.12
P	0.92	4.81	776	5.64
T	1.88	4.15	339	4.83

[a]Data from refs. 6, 7, and 36.

TABLE 3. *Total activity-related heat, initial heat, and recovery/initial heat ratios*[a]

Preparation	T_A(mcal/g)	I(mcal/g)	R/I
C	4.15	1.69	1.46
P	2.52	1.04	1.42
T	2.88	1.61	0.79

[a]Data from refs. 3, 5, 7, and 36.

TABLE 4. *Tension-dependent and tension-independent heat production[a]*

Preparation	TDH(mcal/g)	TIH(mcal/g)
C	1.29	0.40
P	0.84	0.20
T	1.29	0.32

[a]Data taken from refs. 3 and 7.

muscles. This is reduced to 50% and 80% of normal in the P and T preparations, respectively.

Analysis of Mechanical and Thermal Data in Terms of Molecular Mechanisms

It is clear from the mechanical performance of the isolated papillary muscle that the intracellular morphological and biochemical changes in the hypertrophied myocytes have had an effect. The decrease in V_{max} for the P muscles and the increase for the T preparations is, at least in part, a reflection of the altered ratios of the myosin isoenzymes. To some extent it may also be a reflection of the kinetics of calcium cycling. An index of this is the increase in time to peak tension *(TPT)* seen in the P hearts in contrast to the decrease present in the T preparations (Table 2). The decrease in peak tension (P_{TW}) observed in the P hearts (36) is small and not always significant (7). Since there is an increase in the relative myofibrillar mass, decreases in isometric force may result from a decrease in the amount of calcium cycled and an alteration in the rate at which it is cycled (see *TIH*, Table 4). The decrease in isometric force seen in the T preparations may result from the combination of a decrease in relative myofibrillar mass along with an alteration in the kinetics and quantity of the calcium cycled. A measure of the economy of contraction can be obtained by dividing the twitch tension time integral (Table 2) by the total activity-related heat (T_A) (Table 3). The economy of isometric contraction for the C, P, and T hearts is 1.47, 2.23, and 1.67 g cm sec/μcal, respectively. Thus, both the P and T preparations contract more economically than the C hearts. This result is somewhat misleading and provides little insight into the molecular events involved in the contractions, because the T_A is made up of both the initial heat and the recovery heat. For the C and P preparations the *R/I* ratio is essentially the same (Table 3). For the T hearts the *R/I* ratio is 0.79, indicating that the recovery processes are substantially more economical (Table 3). In order to separate the contractile from the recovery processes one needs to relate initial heat or tension-dependent heat to the mechanical performance. The economy of force development (using initial heat) for the C, P, and T hearts is 3.62, 5.42, and 3.00 g cm sec/μcal, respectively. The initial heat consists of the tension-dependent and tension-independent heats. Focusing on the cross-bridge performance requires that the economy be calculated using the TDH. Under those circumstances, the economy of contraction for the C, P, and T papillary muscles is 4.74, 6.7, and 3.74 g cm sec/μcal, respectively. It is clear that there are substantial differences in the economy of contraction of the three preparations directly related to contractile mechanisms with the P preparations being more economical and the T less economical than the C hearts. The biochemical analyses indicated that the P hearts contained myosin with a lower ATPase activity than normal whereas the T hearts had myosin with a higher ATPase activity than normal. The differences in the ATPase activity were closely correlated with the percent V_1 isoenzyme present (Fig. 3). There is also a good correlation between V_1 isoenzyme content or actin-activated myosin ATPase and the tension-dependent heat per unit tension (Fig. 9). This correlation suggests that an understanding of the change in economy observed in the hypertrophy preparations might be gained by relating the myosin enzyme kinetics to tension-dependent heat production. Force and work are produced in muscle when the globular cross-bridge head (in a nonrefractory state) makes contact with the an actin monomer located in the thin filament and rotates from the 90° to the 45° position. A simple scheme of this cycle (17) is presented in Fig. 10. Myosin exists in two states, a dissociated nonforce-producing state (steps above the dotted line in Fig. 10) and an associated, force-producing state (steps below the dotted line in Fig. 10.) Step 3 is a rate-limiting step in the dissociated state which probably determines the overall cycling rate. Step 5 is the point in the cycle where the head rotation extends the compliant link and produces force or shortening. Although each cycle of any particular bridge produces only a miniscule amount of force, the summing of the force-developing rotation of millions of these bridges, randomly occuring, produces the observed force and/or shortening. The force developed can be analyzed in terms of the average strength of the cross-bridge, the duration of the "on" time and of the cycling rate. For the purpose of this anyalysis the strength of the cross bridge is considered to be unity for all the preparations and is indicated by the height of the square wave pulse (bottom Fig. 10.). The relative cycling rate

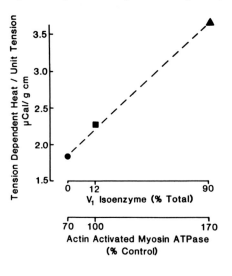

FIG. 9. Relationship of V_1 isoenzyme content or actin-activated myosin ATPase activity to tension-dependent heat per unit tension (8).

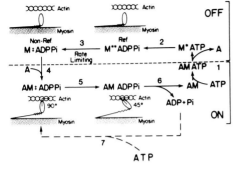

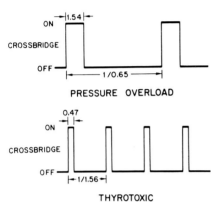

FIG. 10. A kinetic scheme of actin-myosin interaction **(top)** and a representation of the average cross-bridge cycle during contraction and relaxation in terms of cycling rate and "on-time" (see text for details) (30). (Redrawn from Eisenberg and Hill, ref. 17, with permission.)

(f) can be obtained from the tension-dependent heat, TDH, and the twitch time, TT, and is defined in equations 9 and 10:

$$f_P/f_C = (TDH_P/TT_P)/(TDH_C/TT_C) \tag{9}$$

$$f_T/f_C = (TDH_T/TT_T)/(TDH_C/TT_C) \tag{10}$$

The average cycling rate relative to normal for the P and T preparations is indicated by the frequency of appearance of the rectangular pulses (bottom, Fig. 10). The average "on-time", τ, relative to normal muscle is obtained by dividing the tension time integral by the tension-dependent heat:

$$\tau_P/\tau_C = (\textstyle\int Pdt_P/TDH_P) / (\textstyle\int Pdt_C/TDH_C) \tag{11}$$

$$\tau_T/\tau_C = (\textstyle\int Pdt_T/TDH_T) / (\textstyle\int Pdt_C/TDH_C) \tag{12}$$

The relative "on-time" for the P and T preparations is defined in equations 11 and 12 and is indicated in Fig. 10 by the width of the square wave pulses. Thus the economy of force development is increased in the P preparations by increasing the "on-time" and decreasing the cycling rate. Conversely, in the T preparations the economy of force development is reduced by increasing the cycling rate and decreasing the cross-bridge "on-time." Calcium cycling is also involved in the changes observed in isometric force development and in the overall economy of contraction. The quantity of calcium cycled in a complete contraction-relaxation cycle can be calculated from the *TIH* (Table 4) if it is assumed that two calcium ions are transported for every ATP molecule hydrolyzed and that the molar enthalpy of ATP hydrolysis is 11 kcal/mole. Under these circumstances the C, P, and T preparations cycle 0.072, 0.036, and 0.058 μmoles of calcium per gram of papillary muscle per beat. Furthermore, the calcium is removed in 54% of the normal time in the T hearts and 128% of the normal time in the T muscles.

MYOCARDIAL HYPERTROPHY AS AN ADAPTIVE RESPONSE TO STRESS

Long-term demands made on the heart may involve two distinct types of stress. In pressure overload (banding of the pulmonary artery, pulmonary hypertension, systemic hypertension, coarctation of the aorta) there is a requirement for an increase in intraventricular pressure to ensure an adequate circulation to the peripheral tissues. In volume overload (thyrotoxicosis, arteriovenous fistula, valvular insufficiency) the volume pumped by the ventricle must be increased in order to meet the peripheral circulatory demands. Thus, very different demands are made on the heart for the two types of stress. The increase in myocardial mass is compensatory for both types of stress. The success of the compensation is illustrated by the finding of unchanged wall stress during contraction in both types of hypertrophy (20). The concentric hypertrophy in the P hearts, with no change in lumen size and an increase in wall thickness (27), permits the development of high intraluminal pressures with no increase in demands on the individual contractile units (muscle fibers). The contraction, however, is slower and more prolonged. The subcellular alterations that contribute to the P adaptation consist of an increase in relative myofibrillar mass, an increase in V_3 (low ATPase) relative to V_1 (high ATPase) myosin isoenzyme content, and a decrease in the rate and amount of calcium cycled. The increase in relative myofibrillar mass allows for more force to be developed per unit cross-sectional area than would have been possible with a normal myofibrillar mass. The isoenzyme shift permits a more economical development of force as a result of the decrease in the cross-bridge cycling rate and the increase in the duration of the "on-time" during the power stroke of the cross-bridge. The change in the amount and rate of calcium cycled further increases the economy and, for a given amount of calcium released, leaves free calcium available for a longer period of time. Although these hearts can meet the need for an increase in intraluminal pressure more economically (adaptive), they contract more slowly and may have difficulty in meeting an unanticipated demand for an increase in the rate of contraction. In the volume-overloaded heart, the increase in size facilitates the pumping of a larger volume of blood per unit time. This is accomplished while maintaining normal active wall stress (20). At the subcellular and molecular levels, the major changes involve increasing the relative volume of the mitochondria, functional changes in the mitochondria, an increase in the relative amounts of the V_1 (high ATPase) isoenzyme of myosin, and an increase in the rate of calcium cycling. The change from the slow (V_3) to the fast (V_1) myosin type permits a higher velocity of shortening and thus an increase in the cardiac output. This is accomplished at the molecular level by increasing the cross-bridge cycling rate and decreasing the duration of the "on-time." As a result, the economy of force development is decreased and compensated for by a change in the economy of the recovery processes, as indicated by the reduction in the R/I ratio to 0.79 in the T hearts. The overall process thus remains acceptably economical. The increase in the velocity and rate is also facilitated by the increase in the rate of calcium cycling.

Thus the increase in heart mass in response to long-term stress is adaptive. The adaptation involves macroscopic reorganization of the entire heart as well as subcellular reorganization of the organelles and enzymes. The exact profile of the total reorganization is determined by the type, intensity, and duration of the specific stress to which the heart is subjected and produces functional changes specifically designed to meet the stress.

ACKNOWLEDGMENT

This work was supported in part by USPHS Grant 28001-01.

REFERENCES

1. Alpert, N. R., and Mulieri, L. A. (1977): The partitioning of altered mechanics in hypertrophied heart muscle between the sarcoplasmic reticulum and the contractile apparatus by means of myothermal measurements. *Basic Res. Cardiol.*, 72:153–159.
2. Alpert, N. R., Litten, R. Z., and Mulieri, L. A. (1978): Myothermal *vs* enzymatic changes in thyrotoxic cardiac hypertrophy. *Physiologist*, 21:2.
3. Alpert, N. R., Mulieri, L. A., Litten, R. Z., Goulette, R., and Schine, L. (1979): Myothermal and enzymatic analysis of a new cardiac preparation titratable between failing and non-failing hypertrophy. *Circ. Res.*, 60:II-224.
4. Alpert, N. R., and Mulieri, L. A. (1981): The utilization of energy by the myocardium hypertrophied secondary to pressure overload. In: *The Heart in Hypertension*, edited by B. E. Strauer, pp. 153–163. Springer Verlag, Berlin Heidelberg, New York.
5. Alpert, N. R., and Mulieri, L. A. (1982): Increased myothermal economy of isometric force generation in compensated cardiac hypertrophy induced by pulmonary artery constriction in the rabbit. A characterization of heat liberation in normal and hypertrophied right ventricular papillary muscles. *Circ. Res.*, 50:491–500.
6. Alpert, N. R., and Mulieri, L. A. (1982): Heat mechanics and myosin ATPase in normal and hypertrophied heart muscle. *Fed. Proc.*, 41:192–198.
7. Alpert, N. R., and Mulieri, L. A. (1982): Myocardial adaptation to stress from the viewpoint of evolution and development. In: *Basic Biology of Muscles: A Comparative Approach*, edited by B. M. Twarog, R. J. C. Levine and M. M. Dewey, pp. 173–187. Raven Press, New York.
8. Alpert, N. R., Mulieri, L. A., and Litten, R. Z. (1983): Isoenzyme contribution to economy of contraction and relaxation in normal and hypertrophied hearts. In: *Cardiac Adaptation to Hemodynamic Overload, Training and Stress*, edited by R. Jacob, R. W. Gulch, and G. Kissing, pp. 147–157. Darmstadt, Germany.
9. Anversa, P., Loud, A. V., Giacomelli, F., and Wiener, J. (1978): Absolute morphometric study of myocardial hypertrophy in experimental hypertension. *Lab. Invest.*, 38:597–609.
10. Banerjee, S. K., Flink, I. L., and Morkin, E. (1976): Enzymatic properties of native and N-ethylmaleidmide-modified cardiac myosin from normal and thyrotoxic rabbits. *Circ. Res.*, 39:319–326.

11. Banerjee, S. K., and Morkin, E. (1977): Actin-activated adenosine triphosphatase activity of native and N-ethylmaleimide-modified cardiac myosin from normal and thyrotoxic rabbits. *Circ. Res.*, 41:630–634.

12. Bartosova, D., Chvapil, M., Korecky, B., Poupa, O., Rakusan, K., Turek, Z., and Vizek, M. (1969): The growth of the muscular and collagenous parts of the rat heart in various forms of cardiomegaly. *J. Physiol.*, 200:285–295.

13. Bowditch, H. P. (1871): Uber die Eigenthumlich keiten der Reizbarkeit Welche die Muskel Fasern des Herzens Zeigen. *Ber. Verhande. Sachs Akad. Wiss.*, 23:652–689.

14. Bugnard, L. (1934): The relation between total and initial heat in single muscle twitches. *J. Physiol.*, 82:509–519.

15. Caulfield, J. B., and Borg, T. K. (1979): The collagen network of the heart. *Lab Invest.*, 40:364–372.

16. Conway, G., Heazlitt, R. A., Fowler, N. O., Gabel, M., and Green, S. (1976): The effect of hyperthyroidism on the sarcoplasmic reticulum and myosin ATPase of dog hearts. *J. Mol. Cell Cardiol.*, 8:39–51.

17. Eisenberg, E., and Hill, T. L. (1978): A crossbridge model of muscle contraction. *Prog. Biophys. Mol. Biol.*, 33:55–82.

18. Frank, O. (1895): Zur Dynamik des Herzmuskels. *Z. Biol.*, 32:370–447.

19. Goodkind, M. J., Gambach, G. E., Thyrum, P. T., and Luchi, R. J. (1974): Effect of thyroxine on ventricular myocardiac contractility and ATPase activity in guinea pigs. *Am. J. Physiol.*, 226:66–72.

20. Grossman, W., Corabello, B. A., Gunther, S., and Fifer, M. A. (1983): Ventricular Wall Stress and the Development of Cardiac Hypertrophy and Failure. In: *Myocardial Hypertrophy and Failure*, edited by N. R. Alpert, Raven Press, New York.

21. Gunning, J. F., Harrison, Jr., C. E., and Coleman, H. N. III (1974): Myocardial contractility and energetics following treatment with d-thyroxine. *Am. J. Physiol.*, 226:1166–1171.

22. Hatt, P. Y., Berjal, G., Moravek, J., and Swynghedaw, B. (1970): Heart failure: An electron microscopic study of left ventricular papillary muscle in aortic insufficiency in the rabbit. *J. Moll. Cell. Cardiol.*, 1:221–234.

23. Hatt, P. Y., Rakusan, K., Gastineau, P., and LaPlace, M. (1979): Morphometry and Structure of Heart hypertrophy Induced by Chronic Volume overload. (Aorta-caval fistula in the rat). *J. Cell. Mol. Cardiol.*, 11:989–998.

24. Hamrell, B. B., and Alpert, N. R. (1977): The mechanical characteristics of hypertrophied rabbit cardiac muscle in the absence of congestive heart failure: the contractile and series elastic elements. *Circ. Res.*, 40:20–25.

25. Legato, M. J., Mulieri, L. A., and Alpert, N. R. (1983): Parallels Between Normal Growth and Compensatory Hypertrophy in the Rabbit. In: *Myocardial Hypertrophy and Failure*, edited by N. R. Alpert, Raven Press, New York.

26. Limas, C. J., and Chan-Stier, C. (1978): Myocardial chromatin activation in experimental hyperthyroidism in rats. Role of nuclear and non-histone proteins. *Circ. Res.*, 42:311–316.

27. Linzbach, A. J. (1960): Heart failure from the point of view of quantitative anatomy. *Am. J. Cardiol.*, 5:370–382.

28. Litten, R. Z., Martin, B. J., Low, R. B., and Alpert, N. R. (1982): Altered myosin isoenzyme patterns from pressure overload and thyrotoxic hypertrophied hearts. *Circ. Res.*, 50:856–864.

29. Maughan, D., Low, E., Litten, R., Brayden, J., and Alpert, N. (1977): Calcium activated muscle from hypertrophied rabbit hearts. *Circ. Res.*, 44:279–287.

30. McCallister, L. P., and Page, E. (1973): Effects of thyroxine on ultrastructure of rat myocardial cells. A stereological study. *J. Ultrastruct. Res.*, 42:136–155.

31. Mulieri, L. A., Luhr, R., Trefry, J., and Alpert, N. R. (1977): Metal film thermopiles for use with rabbit right ventricular papillary muscles. *Am. J. Physiol.*, 233:146–156.

32. Page, E., and McCallister, L. P. (1973): Quantitative electron microscopic description of heart cells. *Am. J. Cardiol.*, 31:172–180.

33. Rakusan, K., Korecky, B., and Mezl, V. (1983): Cardiac hypertrophy and/or hyperplasia. In: *Myocardial Hypertrophy and Failure*, edited N. R. Alpert, Raven Press, New York.

34. Sarnoff, S. J., and Mitchell, J. H. (1962): The control of function of the heart. In: *Handbook of Physiology*, Section 2. *Circulation*, Vol. 1., edited by W. F. Hamilton and P. Dow, pp. 489–532. Am. Physiological Soc., Washington, D. C.

35. Scheuer, J., and Bhan, A. K. (1979): Cardiac contractile proteins. Adenosine triphosphatase activity and physiological function. *Circ. Res.*, 45:1–12.
36. Schine, L. (1982): The mechanical performance of the pressure overloaded, thyrotoxic and double treated hypertrophied hearts. Masters Thesis. University of Vermont.
37. Skelton, C. L., and Sonnenblick, E. H. (1974): Heterogeneity of contractile function in cardiac hypertrophy. *Circ. Res.*, 34[Suppl. II]:83–96.
38. Starling, E. H. (1918): The Linacre lecture on the law of the heart, given at Cambridge, 1914. Longmans, Green and Co., London.
39. Strauer, B. E., and Scherpe, A. (1975): *Myocardial Mechanics and Oxygen Consumption in Experimental Hyperthyroidism in Recent Advances in Studies on Cardiac Structure and Metabolism. Vol. 8: The Cardiac Sarcoplasm*, edited by Paul-Emile Roy and Peter Harris, pp. 495–502.
40. Strauer, B. E., and Scherpe, A. (1975): Experimental hyperthyroidism. I. Hemodynamics and contractility in situ. *Basic Res. Cardiol.*, 70:115–129.
41. Yazaki, Y., and Raben, M. S. (1975): Effect of thyroid state on enzymatic characteristics of cardiac myosin. A difference in behavior of rat and rabbit cardiac myosin. *Circ. Res.*, 36:208–215.

Growth of the Heart in Health and Disease,
edited by Radovan Zak. Raven Press,
New York © 1984.

Response of the Heart to Exercise Training

Thomas F. Schaible and James Scheuer

*Department of Medicine and Physiology, Albert Einstein College of Medicine, Montefiore
Hospital and Medical Center, Bronx, New York 10467*

Increasingly more attention has been focused on the effects of exercise training on the cardiovascular system. Much of this interest derives from the notion that prolonged physical conditioning may lead to a lower incidence of death from cardiovascular diseases. In fact, exercise is now considered to lower the risk factors for heart disease (54,120). In addition, the cardiac hypertrophy commonly observed in well-trained athletes has intrigued medical scientists because it represents a form of hypertrophy associated with normal or enhanced cardiac function. This "physiological" hypertrophy contrasts with the hypertrophy associated with chronic hemodynamic overloads, or "pathological" hypertrophy, which is generally associated with impaired cardiac function (188). Thus, the mechanisms that allow normal or improved function to occur coinciding with cardiac enlargement in exercise training are of particular interest.

The major physiological consequence of vigorous exercise is an increase in oxygen demand by the working muscles. "Physically trained" describes that state which permits the organism to achieve greater levels of work performance, which is always reflected by the ability to consume greater amounts of oxygen. The trained state involves a complex interplay of adaptations in the skeletal muscle fibers, the nervous system, and the circulatory system. It is not the purpose of this chapter to review all of the systems involved in the response to exercise training, but rather to focus on cardiac adaptations invoked by exercise training. Several recent reviews have covered the cardiovascular and skeletal muscle adaptations to exercise. The reader is referred to those reviews by Clauson (32), Holloszy (80), Rowell (143), and Scheuer and Tipton (157).

This chapter begins with a brief review of the cardiovascular changes that occur during dynamic exercise. Our intention is to characterize those demands placed on the heart during sustained exercise. The changes in morphology and performance of the left ventricle in response to exercise training is discussed, first in human studies and then in animal studies. Differences between cardiac adaptations to dynamic and isometric exercise are discussed. Possible mechanisms that may contribute to cardiac functional alterations are reviewed with regard to the effects of exercise training on the coronary vasculature, subcellular organelles, and cardiac biochemistry. Factors that may modulate the cardiac responses to training are discussed and, finally, the effects of training on cardiac responses to pathological stress are covered.

CARDIOVASCULAR RESPONSES TO DYNAMIC EXERCISE

It is important to have a fundamental knowledge of the hemodynamic changes that occur during exercise, particularly with regard to the load placed on the left ventricle. This is important in characterizing the potential stimulus for cardiac enlargement induced by exercise. In this section we will consider the hemodynamics associated with dynamic exercise (often referred to as isotonic exercise). Dynamic exercise in this discussion denotes the rhythmic contraction and shortening of large muscle groups as would occur in running, swimming, or bicycling. During dynamic exercise large increases in cardiac output and heart rate are observed, yet mean arterial pressure changes vary little (9). Normally, systolic pressure increases with the intensity of the workload (132), but diastolic pressure remains unchanged (9,26). Changes in systolic pressure closely mimic those in cardiac output (1,132). Invariably, during dynamic exercise systemic resistance decreases. The extent to which heart rate and systolic arterial pressure increase during dynamic exercise may depend on the muscle groups being used. For example, performance of arm work elicits a greater pressure, lower cardiac output, and greater resistance when compared with performance of leg work at the same oxygen consumption (143). It is also important to define whether dynamic exercise is performed in the upright or supine position. Cardiac output at a given oxygen uptake is 1 to 2 liters/min higher in the supine position at the same heart rate (9) primarily because of an increase in venous return (32).

Most recent investigations utilizing echocardiographic or radionuclide techniques have shown that stroke volume increases during dynamic exercise (40,132,177,186). However, the mechanisms underlying this increase remain controversial, that is, end-systolic volume may decrease and/or end-diastolic volume may increase (Frank-Starling mechanism). Most studies have shown that associated with an increased stroke volume is a smaller end-systolic volume during exercise (40,132,137,186), results that are consistent with an enhanced contractile state. Supporting this conclusion is evidence of increased rate of systolic pressure development (dP/dt) (177) and rate of dimensional shortening during exercise (186). The response of end-diastolic volume to exercise is not so clear but is very important, since it is difficult to substantiate a true volume overload in the absence of an increased end-diastolic volume. Recent studies have reported increases (132,137,186), no change (40,169), or even a decrease (163) in end-diastolic volume during exercise. Stein et al. (169) reported no change in echocardiographic end-diastolic diameter during supine exercise, but a marked increase during recovery. Few studies have measured end-diastolic volume at maximal exercise loads. Studies in dogs have shown that end-diastolic volume increases only at maximal workloads (83,184). Recently, Weiss et al. (186) and Poliner et al. (132) studying normal volunteers showed that end-diastolic dimension and volume increase with the intensity of the workload.

These results in humans and animals suggest that alterations in end-diastolic volume are dependent on the intensity of the exercise stress. Thus, exercise intensity would appear to be an important factor in determining the volume load associated with exercise. This point will become important in considering the prevalence and degree of cardiac hypertrophy in physically trained humans.

CARDIAC MORPHOLOGICAL AND FUNCTIONAL ADAPTATIONS TO ENDURANCE TRAINING

Cross-Sectional Studies in Athletes

The largest body of data in humans to determine the chronic effects of training on left ventricular size and function has come from cross-sectional studies comparing well-trained champion athletes to sedentary volunteers. These studies have normally employed athletes of a relatively young age (18–30 years of age) comprising a variety of athletic disciplines. This section deals with reports that have studied athletes involved in endurance sports, i.e., sports in which dynamic exercise is performed predominantly.

That endurance-trained athletes have enlarged hearts has been known for sometime (13). Indeed, evidence of cardiac enlargement in athletes either by percussion or chest X-ray along with certain phonocardiographic and electrocardiographic changes led to the concept of the "athlete's heart syndrome," the phrase being suggestive of organic heart disease. In an examination of 25 professional basketball players, Roeske et al. (141) found that all but one had a third heart sound, and 14 had a fourth heart sound. Electrocardiograms from athletes may occasionally simulate those of acute pericarditis or myocardial infarction, but in one study examining athletes with ECG abnormalities suggestive of myocardial infarction, angiographic evidence excluded the presence of coronary artery disease (39). Since athletes manifesting the "athlete's heart syndrome" demonstrate normal basal ventricular function (141) and normal responses to stress tests (135), this condition, rather than reflecting a pathological state, should be regarded as a normal variant (141).

In early studies radiographic measurements were used to demonstrate larger heart volumes in athletes. However, chest X-rays can not distinguish between cardiac dilatation and hypertrophy (increased wall thickness at similar or greater end-diastolic volumes). But over the past decade, the use of echocardiography has overcome this problem, since this method allows measurement of wall thickness and chamber diameter, and by making certain assumptions, left ventricular mass can be calculated. In addition, measurements can be made continuously throughout the cardiac cycle so that end-diastole and end-systole can be precisely defined, a feature lacking in radiographic methods.

Table 1 shows data from several selected recent studies which have used echocardiography to measure cardiac dimension and mass in well-trained endurance athletes. The data are presented in terms of millimeter and percent differences at end-diastole for values obtained in athletes and compared with sedentary controls.

TABLE 1. *Left ventricular size and dimension at end-diastole in cross-sectional studies of athletes*

Study	Athletes	Sex	LVD (mm)	PWT (mm)	SWT (mm)	LVEDV (ml)	LV mass (g)
Roeske et al., 1975 (141)	Basketball players	M	+3.8 (+8%)[a]	+1.3 (+13%)[a]	+0.9 (+7%)	+31 (+25%)[a]	—
Parker et al., 1978 (121)	Long distance runners	M	+5.0 (+10%)[a]	+2.0 (+22%)[a]	+1.0 (+10%)[a]	+48 (+34%)[a]	+86 (+49%)[a]
Zeldis et al., 1978 (201)	Field hockey players	F	+5.0 (+12%)[a]	+0.4 (+4%)	−0.4 (−5%)	+31 (+40%)[a]	+50 (+39%)[a]
Ikaheimo et al., 1979 (84)	Long distance runners	M	+4.5 (+9%)[a]	+3.4 (+40%)[a]	+3.5 (+41%)[a]	+25 (+37%)[a]	+118 (+80%)[a]
Heath et al., 1981 (74)	Long distance runners	M	+6.0 (+14%)[a]	+1.5 (+19%)[a]	+2.0 (+22%)[a]	+22 (+49%)[a,b]	+50 (+67%)[a,b]

Note: Values represent mean absolute and percentage (parentheses) differences from controls.
LVD = left ventricular internal diameter; PWT = posterior wall thickness; LVEDV = left ventricular volume; LV mass = left ventricular mass; SWT = septal wall thickness.
[a]$p < 0.05$ vs controls.
[b]Normalized for body surface area.

By and large, the data demonstrate that the athlete's heart is characterized by an increased end-diastolic volume, i.e., an increase in end-diastolic internal diameter, and an increase in wall thickness. Generally, thickening of the posterior wall and the septal wall occur in tandem, suggesting that cardiac enlargement is basically symmetrical. This is supported by the finding that the septal/posterior wall thickness ratio is usually less than 1.3 in endurance athletes, which excludes the likelihood of asymmetric septal hypertrophy (77). Echocardiographic studies in athletes have not analyzed dimensional alterations with respect to the ratio of wall thickness to internal radius. However, inspection of the data in Table 1 would suggest that this ratio does not change in athletes. Thus, the hypertrophy observed in endurance-trained athletes would appear to represent an eccentric hypertrophy (63), i.e., hypertrophy associated with chamber enlargement. In human studies this type of hypertrophy has been associated with chronic volume overloads (66,82). It has been postulated that the volume overload, leading to increased end-diastolic stress, serves as a stimulus for series replication of sarcomeres, resulting in chamber enlargement (66).

Although Table 1 presents data only for the left ventricle, several cross-sectional studies have also reported increases in right ventricular internal diameter in athletes (60,141,183,202). Little more is known about right ventricular morphological responses to endurance training, and it deserves more in-depth investigation.

In most reports body weight, body surface area, and lean body mass tend to be lower in endurance athletes than in controls, and these differences are generally not taken into account in judging the degree of hypertrophy in the athletes. In this regard the study by Longhurst et al. (96) is important since these workers compared their data in long-distance runners to data in a control group that had greater body weight and body surface area and to a control group that had similar values as the runners. In comparing left ventricular mass, they found a 60% increase in mass in the runners compared with the light controls as opposed to only a 29% increase in the runners compared with the heavier controls.

The changes in left ventricular dimension and mass in response to physical training and detraining can occur quite rapidly. Eshani et al. (52) studied a group of college swimmers that had been inactive for 2 to 7 months before starting their training for competition. As early as 1 week after the start of training, significant increases in left ventricular internal diameter and wall thickness were observed and remained stable at the 1-week level thereon for 9 weeks. Reciprocal changes occurred on detraining and were observed as early as the fourth day of inactivity.

Whether the hypertrophy in athletes is due solely to the intense training they undergo, to preexisting hypertrophy before they undergo training, or to an enhanced cardiac growth response to training has not been established. The last two possibilities would imply a genetic predisposition for a cardiac morphological adaptation in athletes. It has been shown that former athletes, long after they have ceased training, continue to have enlarged hearts (81,134), suggesting that athletes may have inherently large hearts, although the failure to regress does not prove a predisposition. To overcome these interpretive problems, longitudinal studies of the effects of training in nonathletes have been performed, which is the subject of the next section.

Longitudinal Studies in Humans

Longitudinal studies in previously sedentary populations offer several advantages over cross-sectional studies in assessing the cardiac adaptations to chronic exercise training. First, the findings from longitudinal studies bear more meaningful extrapolations to the general population, since randomly selected subjects are used and it may be assumed that a genetic predisposition for a training effect is not present. This assumption cannot be made when athletes are compared cross-sectionally. Second, longitudinal studies provide a more cogent experimental design in that data obtained at the conclusion of training may be compared with data obtained in the same subject prior to training. Therefore, the subject serves as his own control, eliminating variation within experimental groups as a major source of error in comparing sedentary and trained groups. Unfortunately, the number of studies employing a longitudinal design is limited, especially in comparison to the larger number of cross-sectional studies performed in athletes.

Table 2 shows a summary of results from longitudinal studies. Generally, the training regimens required that the subjects trained at least three times a week for periods varying between 30 min to 2 hr a day. The mode of exercise in these studies involved running, either freely or on a treadmill, or bicycle ergometry, and most of the subjects were under 40 years of age. The intensity of the exercise was normally adjusted so that it required 70% to 80% of the maximal oxygen consumption (VO_2 max) or age-predicted maximal heart rate. Periods of regular exercise resulted in the ability to achieve higher rates of maximal oxygen consumption and a resting bradycardia in all of the studies, indicating that a trained state had been achieved.

Table 2 also shows percentage changes from pretraining values for various measurements of cardiac size and dimensions at rest. By comparing the changes in Table 2 to those obtained for athletes in Table 1, one can see that cardiac dimensional adaptations are more profound in athletic populations. In reviewing the data from longitudinal studies, the most notable feature is the ambivalent evidence for cardiac enlargement after training. The study by DeMaria et al. (43) demonstrated the only unequivocal evidence of hypertrophy by virtue of increases in left ventricular diameter, posterior wall thickness, and calculated left ventricular mass. However, these results are in contrast to those from studies using similar intensities of exercise where there was no evidence of cardiac hypertrophy (2,130,194), even though the exercise program elicited a similar if not greater increase in VO_2 max as in the DeMaria study. Indeed, some studies (2,130) have shown trends of a decrease in wall thickness at similar or greater internal diameters, suggesting the possibility of cardiac dilatation following training. ECG evidence of left ventricular hypertrophy (increase in R-wave voltage in leads V_5 and V_6) in longitudinal studies has not always coincided with echocardiographic evidence (146) and vice versa (130). This

TABLE 2. Summary of data from longitudinal studies for left ventricular size and dimension

Study	Subjects (age, yr)	Training program	VO$_{2\,max}$	Heart volume (X-ray)	Diastolic wall thickness (echo)	Diastolic internal diameter (echo)	LV Mass (echo)
Frick et al. 1963 (55)	14 Men (19–26)	Basic training for 2 months	+12%[a]	+8%[a]	—	—	—
Saltin et al., 1968 (146)	5 Men: 3 Sedentary (19–21), 2 Active	Running, ergometer 2 hr/day, 5 days/wk for 3 months; 65%–90% VO$_{2\,max}$	+33% +5%	+9% −1%	—	—	—
Frick et al., 1970 (56)	20 Men (18–19)	Running, marching daily for 2 months	+6%	+2% (NS)	+1% (NS)	—	—
DeMaria et al., 1978 (43)	15 Men, 11 women (20–34, X̄ = 26)	Walking, running 60 min/day, 4 days/wk for 11 wk; 70% max HR	+15%[a]	—	+11%[a]	+4%[a]	+21%[a]
Wolfe et al., 1979 (194)	20 Men (29–48, X̄ = 37)	Jogging, ergometer 30 min/day, 4 days/wk for 6 months; 80% max HR	+18%[a]	—	+1% (NS)	+1% (NS)	+3% (NS)
Peronnet et al., 1980 (130)	14 Men	Ergometer; 30 min/day 3 day/wk for 20 wk	+21%[a]	—	−4% (NS)	+1% (NS)	−4% (NS)
Stein et al., 1980 (170)	7 Men, 7 women (18–25, X̄ = 20)	Ergometer; 34 min/day 3 day/wk for 14 wk 70% max HR	+31%[a]	—	—	+6%[a]	—
Adams et al., 1981 (2)	22 Men (19–24, X̄ = 22)	Jogging, 50 min/day 5 day/wk for 11 wk 86% max HR	+16%[a]	—	−6% (NS)	+8%[a]	+3% (NS)

Note: Values represent the percentage difference from pretraining values.

[a] $p < 0.05$ compared with pretraining.

NS = not significant compared with pretraining.

is not the case in studies of athletes where both measurements normally increase in unison (96,110,141). The discordant results in studies of trained nonathletes may be due to the lesser magnitude of the hypertrophy.

An important consideration in interpreting findings of increased left ventricular internal diameter following training is the degree to which the training-induced bradycardia and prolongation of diastolic filling may contribute to the results. This possibility is more important to evaluate in serial studies of normal subjects, since the degree of hypertrophy, when observed, is generally within normal limits (43) and is not always associated with an increase in wall thickness. Adams et al. (2) plotted individual resting heart rate changes against end-diastolic dimensional changes and found no correlation. Although DeMaria et al. (44) have found a linear correlation between heart rate and end-diastolic dimension, their data would indicate that a change in resting heart rate approximating that of a training bradycardia (about 10 beats/min) would account for a 2.7% change in end-diastolic dimension (2). Therefore, an increased diastolic filling period secondary to a resting bradycardia may account for a portion of the observed increase in left ventricular internal diameter following training, but to what degree remains uncertain. However, it seems likely that at least part of the increase in left ventricular chamber volume represents an intrinsic cardiac adaptation.

It remains unclear whether or not training leads to changes in blood volume (157), and it is more uncertain whether an increase in left ventricular end-diastolic diameter due to training may be related to an increased blood volume. Few studies have made simultaneous measurements of changes in ventricular dimension and blood volume. One early study (55) reported increased heart volume by X-ray without an increase in central blood volume; however, the radiographic evidence could not determine whether an increase in end-diastolic volume had occurred. Future studies using more precise techniques should readdress the possible contribution of hypervolemia to training-related changes in cardiac dimensions.

One factor that may account for the inconsistent documentation of hypertrophy in longitudinal studies may relate to the level of fitness prior to the training program, the possibility being that subjects with lower base-line levels of conditioning would be more likely to demonstrate cardiac adaptations to training. The study of Saltin et al. (146) supports this possibility. They separated their population into two previously active subjects and three previously inactive subjects. As shown in Table 2, the three inactive subjects demonstrated a much greater increase in VO_2 max subsequent to exercise training and, in contrast to the active subjects, evidence for cardiac enlargement. Furthermore, Saltin et al. studied their subjects after a period of absolute bedrest, and when comparing values obtained after training to values obtained after bedrest, all subjects showed an increase in heart volume. These results suggest that the base-line sedentary state in studies of training may truly represent a partially conditioned state. Therefore, the training regimens used in longitudinal studies, which are generally of less intensity and duration compared with those of champion athletes, may not be sufficient to elicit adaptations in cardiac size and dimension. Indeed, the studies of Frick et al. (55,56) have shown that after 2 months of intense basic training of infantrymen, significant increases in heart volume resulted, but not after 2 months of less intense basic training of signal troops. Thus, as we suggested earlier, intensity of the workload may be important in determining the degree of stimulus for hypertrophy.

This survey of longitudinal training studies would suggest that future work should examine cardiac adaptions in normal subjects to a full spectrum of activity levels. Furthermore, measurements of hemodynamics and left ventricular diastolic and systolic function during exercise should be performed in order to define qualitative and quantitative aspects of the load placed on the heart. Studies conducted under more rigorously controlled conditions may provide more insight into cardiac adaptations to exercise in normal men and women.

Left Ventricular Function at Rest and During Exercise in Trained Subjects

Virtually all training studies in humans have shown that chronic exercise conditioning leads to an increase in VO_2 max. Increases in VO_2 max can be quite pronounced in highly trained athletes, the highest values having been reported in cross-country skiers (70,145). The relative contributions of cardiac adaptations and peripheral adaptations to this increase in aerobic capacity have been assessed. Most studies have shown that the arteriovenous oxygen difference in working skeletal muscle increases at maximal exercise conditions following training, for the most part because of an increase in respiratory capability of the cells (9,80). Saltin et al. (146) and Rowell (142) have shown that this adaptation could account for approximately 50% of the increased oxygen supplied to the tissue of trained male subjects. The remainder of the increase in oxygen consumption is accounted for by an increase in oxygen delivery to the skeletal muscle, that is, an increase in cardiac output. Normally, oxygen consumption and cardiac output increase in parallel with an increase in workload, and at any given submaximal workload, values are similar in trained and untrained subjects (9). However, the hallmark of the trained state is that the conditioned subject maintains a normal submaximal cardiac output at a lower heart rate. Implicit in these findings then is that training leads to an augmentation of stroke volume.

The mechanisms underlying the adaptive increase in stroke volume following training have been the subject of intensive investigation. Basically, an increase in stroke volume can be accomplished by (a) left ventricular chamber enlargement leading to a larger end-diastolic volume (Frank-Starling effect) and a larger stroke volume for similar degrees of myocardial shortening (similar inotropic state); (b) an increase in myocardial shortening (increased inotropic state) at a similar end-diastolic volume; or (c) a combination of the two mechanisms.

As we have already discussed and shown in Table 1, the majority of cross-sectional studies have reported increases in end-diastolic diameter and volume at rest in athletic populations. These findings are invariably associated with an increased resting stroke volume in the athletes (21,84,121,201). Therefore, it would appear that enlargement is an important intrinsic cardiac adaptation underlying the augmented stroke volume in trained subjects. On the other hand, measurements of indexes of cardiac contractility at rest in trained individuals have reported variable results. Using velocity of circumferential fiber shortening as an index, various studies have reported no change in contractility (60,84,141,183,202), an increase in contractility (6,121), or a decrease in contractility (90,114). Differences in methods of calculations, training programs, or age of the subjects may explain the variable results (114,122).

As several animal studies have shown, effects of training on myocardial contractility are not apparent unless the heart is stressed. Several studies have demonstrated a correlation between VO$_2$ max and heart volume (10,64) or end-diastolic dimension (201) determined at rest. Although these studies suggest that cardiac enlargement may contribute to maximal performance, they cannot separate the relative importance of intrinsic cardiac adaptations to those of peripheral adaptations. Furthermore, Blimkie et al. (25) have shown that if the results are expressed relative to fat-free weight, the correlation is not significant. Recent studies have also measured systolic time intervals in well-trained individuals. At rest, the ratio of preejection period to left ventricular ejection time was normal in long distance runners (183,202) but was found to be slightly increased (193), unchanged (1), or reduced (59) in trained subjects during exercise. Thus, these indirect measurements of left ventricular performance during exercise have not produced consistent results.

As we have already discussed, evidence for cardiac enlargement at rest may be secondary to the relative bradycardia in trained subjects and whether cardiac enlargement is maintained to the same degree at higher heart rates with exercise is not known. Therefore, studies of cardiac size and function in trained subjects during exercise may uncover cardiac adaptations to training which have not been observed under resting conditions. Only recently have such investigations been reported, primarily because of the advent of radionuclide techniques to measure cardiac function and volume during exercise.

Table 3 shows results from five recent studies that have examined cardiac size and function at rest and during exercise. This table is comprised of studies using both echocardiographic and radionuclide techniques and both longitudinal and cross-sectional designs. For the most part, the evidence demonstrates that cardiac enlargement observed at rest was also maintained during exercise (122,138,170), even when the heart rate during exercise was similar between untrained and trained subjects (138). The study of Bar-Shlomo et al. (16) is of interest, since these authors found that untrained subjects increased end-diastolic volume during exercise whereas trained subjects did not. However, the athletes constituted a group of rowers and it cannot be certain whether their responses to exercise represent adaptations to dynamic or static training (see further on). Evidence for enhanced contractility in trained subjects during exercise is somewhat contradictory. For example, the studies by Stein et al. (170) and Anholm et al. (6) showed increased myocardial shortening in trained subjects during exercise which may or may not have been present under resting conditions. The study by Bar-Shlomo et al. (16) showed no differences in shortening at rest or during exercise, and the study by

TABLE 3. Noninvasive studies of cardiac dimension and function in trained and untrained subjects at rest and during exercise

Study and type of design (ref.)	Subjects	Methods		Rest			Exercise		
				ED Heart size	Shortening	Velocity	ED Heart size	Shortening	Velocity
Stein et al., 1980 (long) (170)	Normals	E	U	47[1]	0.32[4]	—	46	0.37	—
			T	50[a]	0.35[a]	—	50[a]	0.41[a]	—
Rerych et al., 1980 (long) (138)	Swimmers	R	U	133[2]	73[5]	—	166	87	—
			T	167[a]	67	—	204[a]	86	—
Paulsen et al., 1981 (cross) (122)	Marathon runners	E	U	52[1]	—	164[6]	53	—	2.71
			T	56[a]	—	140[a]	55	—	2.36[a]
Anholm et al., 1982 (cross) (6)	Speed-skaters bicyclists	R	U	—	68[5]	3.6[7]	—	68	5.2
			T	—	72	4.1	—	75[a]	7.5[a]
Bar-Shlomo et al., 1982 (cross) (16)	Rowers	R	U	100[3]	65[5]	—	124	77	—
			T	100	65	—	100[a]	80	—

Abbreviations: E = echocardiography; R = radionuclide; long = longitudinal; cross = cross-sectional; ED = end-diastole; U = untrained; T = trained.

Units: [1]ED internal diameter (mm); [2]ED volume (ml). [3]Values represent relative changes in volume at rest and during exercise in U and T; [4]fractional shortening; [5]ejection fraction; [6]peak velocity of circumferential fiber shortening (circ/s); [7]ejection rate (sec^{-1}).
[a]$p < 0.05$ for results obtained in trained compared to untrained.

Rerych et al. (138) showed a decreased shortening in trained subjects at rest but no difference during exercise. Interestingly, the studies by Paulsen et al. (122) and Anholm et al. (6) demonstrated a decrease and an increase, respectively, in measurements of velocity of shortening in trained subjects both at rest and during exercise. However, Paulsen et al. attributed their finding of decreased velocity to a lower pressure rate product in their athletes so that it does not reflect a decreased myocardial contractility (122).

To draw conclusions from these studies of cardiac function during exercise would be premature, since they are so few in number and a consistent picture has not emerged. Future studies should be careful to compare function at the same heart rate during exercise. Hopefully, as noninvasive investigational procedures are refined and more data become available, a better understanding of function in the athletic heart during exercise may be forthcoming.

Animal Studies

As we have discussed so far, a clear definition of the cardiac morphological and contractile adaptations to training in humans has not emerged. A cause may be the heterogeneity of study populations, insensitivity of experimental techniques, and the obvious investigational limitations imposed by medical ethics. As a consequence, studies of physical conditioning in animals have been of great importance in the understanding of how the heart adapts to chronic exercise. Studies in animals allow the investigator greater control over extraneous experimental variables and enable the study of physiological, biochemical, and histological adaptations. This section focuses specifically on the contractile and morphological adaptations in cardiac muscle elicited by exercise.

Perhaps some insight into the effects of chronic activity on cardiac mass may be drawn from studies comparing hearts from wild and domesticated species of animals. It has been observed that the heart of the wild hare is substantially enlarged, by nearly 400%, over that of the domestic rabbit when expressed per kilograms of body weight (185). In wild and domesticated rats of similar body weight, a 50% increase in heart mass was noted in the wild species (133). Similarly, greyhounds have substantially enlarged hearts, with an increase in myocardial cell diameter of 50% when compared with mongrel species (30). Although an enlarged heart has been associated with existence in the wild, one cannot be sure of the nature of the stimuli responsible for this. Thus, it is necessary to physically train domesticated species at well-controlled exercise loads.

Animal studies have not arrived at a single definition of cardiac hypertrophy; rather, results for cardiac mass are expressed either in terms of absolute heart weight or heart weight relative to body weight. Quite often investigators have concluded that cardiac hypertrophy has resulted from exercise training by virtue of an increase in heart/body weight ratio even though cardiac weight remained unchanged. This result can only occur because of an absolute decrease in body weight or a slowing of the normal growth rate. This effect of training on body weight in animals is commonly reported (7). Training has been shown to cause cardiac cellular hyperplasia in very young animals (27), but since most exercise studies are performed in adult animals after the capacity of the myocardial cells to undergo mitosis has been lost (200), hearts of equal weight presumably have the same number of cells (157). Since hypertrophy denotes an increase in cell size, it is not legitimate to conclude that hypertrophy has occurred when training does not promote an increase in absolute heart mass.

Many studies have examined cardiac growth and functional adaptations to exercise training in dogs. Dogs quickly learn to run on a treadmill and show many of the common training effects reported in humans. These include a decrease in heart rate at rest (195) and at submaximal workloads (28,35,181), an increase in maximal workload (195), and an increase in skeletal muscle oxidative capacity (15,35). Furthermore, dogs may be chronically instrumented with ventricular pressure catheters and aortic and coronary flow probes so that serial comparisons can be made (173).

The majority of studies have shown that exercise training leads to a small increase in cardiac mass in dogs. The largest reported increase in heart mass due to training is 28% by Reidhammer et al. (136), although other studies report values of less than 10% (15,195). Interestingly, studies employing beagles (28,35,140,152) have not demonstrated increases in heart mass subsequent to training. Whether this is due to the breed or to inadequate exercise intensity is not known. Wyatt and Mitchell (195) have shown no change in resting end-diastolic volume although end-diastolic wall thickness and left ventricular mass increased following training in dogs. Conversely, Ritzer et al. (140) demonstrated an increase in end-diastolic volume at rest without an increase in left ventricular mass. In the latter study, no differences in end-diastolic volume were observed with pacing-induced tachycardia. These few studies do not provide a clear picture of cardiac dimensional changes after training in dogs. However, when positive changes are reported they are usually of small degree and may be sensitive to changes in heart rate.

Several studies in exercise-trained dogs would suggest that training enhances the inotropic state of the left ventricle. Often, evidence for an increased contractility is not apparent until the heart is stressed. Thus, Barnard et al. (15) observed increases in the rate of left ventricular pressure development (dP/dt) in trained animals at submaximal and maximal exercise but not at rest. Similarly, in anesthetized trained dogs, dP/dt and calculated velocity of contractile element shortening were increased during pacing-induced tachycardia but not at spontaneous heart rate (140). These changes in dP/dt would appear to be specific for the trained state since Stone (172) has shown dP/dt to be increased in trained dogs but not in dogs only partially trained (no decrease in heart rate at submaximal workloads). In these studies, increases in dP/dt in trained dogs were observed when end-diastolic pressure and volume, aortic pressure, and heart rate were similar to controls. Thus, these increases probably present a true increase in contractility.

In response to acute volume overloads, trained dogs have demonstrated improved pumping ability at similar heart rates compared with controls and require greater volume infusions to achieve similar left atrial pressures (28). However, in the volume-overloading studies reported by Stone (172), trained dogs showed a reduced cardiac output, associated with a reduced heart rate, but a similar stroke volume. Since these results were obtained in the same animals before and after training, it was felt that the reduced heart rate response to volume loading reflected a reflex adaptation of the nervous system. Stone concluded that these results represented a greater cardiac reserve capacity subsequent to training. In response to acute pressure overload induced by methoxamine, Reidhammer et al. (136) showed that trained dogs demonstrate lesser increases in end-diastolic pressure and volume compared with controls, indicating a lesser encroachment on the Frank-Starling mechanism after training. By and large, then, physical training in dogs has been associated with a modest degree of hypertrophy, an increased contractility, and improved responses to acute pressure and volume overload.

For several reasons, the laboratory rat constitutes the most often studied animal model in cardiac conditioning studies. Their genetic constitution is well-defined, they are economical, and they can be trained in large numbers. Furthermore, by virtue of their small size, hearts are amenable to being studied by isolated techniques. Studies employing isolated intact hearts (156) and isolated papillary muscles (115) are important in uncovering mechanical adaptations in cardiac muscle, since loading conditions and heart rate can be precisely controlled. However, there are disadvantages in using rats as well. The rapid heart rate of the animal may obscure measurements that are frequency dependent. In addition, their small size precludes chronic instrumentation so that comparisons of trained groups must be made cross sectionally to sedentary groups.

Rats can be conditioned by either running or swimming programs. Normally, running programs are performed on a treadmill and electrical stimulation is occasionally used to encourage running. Tipton and co-workers (17) recently designed treadmills to measure oxygen consumption while running so that the intensity of exercise can be precisely quantitated. Rats may be made to swim in large tanks, but the temperature of the water must be well regulated (33–35°C). The best results are obtained when rats are made to swim in groups, since the interaction between animals promotes maximum effort.

Some controversy has centered on whether cardiac adaptations to chronic swimming in rats represent a response to a pure exercise stimulus or whether some of these adaptations result from psychological or thermal stresses or to intermittent hypoxia due to submersion for short periods of time. A recent report by Flaim et al. (53) compared acute cardiovascular responses in untrained rats that were exercised either by running on a treadmill or by swimming. During running, rats demonstrated many of the expected cardiovascular responses to exercise, including increased heart rate and cardiac output, and increased blood flow to the exercising skeletal muscles. In contrast, rats acutely subjected to swimming showed no increase in heart rate or cardiac output and lesser increases in flow to skeletal muscle. Although these data suggest different cardiovascular responses to the two modes of exercise, they must be interpreted with caution since the acute responses were measured in inexperienced animals. Swimming in rats involves a significant learning component (191) so that rats exposed to swimming for several weeks respond differently to an acute swim than rats not familiar with swimming. Indeed, rats chronically trained by swimming show training effects common to those described in rats trained by running. These include a resting bradycardia (148,191) and a reduced heart rate at submaximal workload when running on a treadmill (191). Swimming rats can achieve oxygen consumptions that are 75% of the VO_2 max reported in running rats (103,164). Therefore, although the possibility that nonexercise-related stresses may contribute to cardiac adaptations in swim-trained rats has not been dispelled, it would seem that exercise is a major component of the swimming effect on the heart.

Assessing cardiac hypertrophy in trained rats is often confounded by the rather large effects of training on growth rate. Decreases in growth rate during training invariably occur in male rats (7) but only in female rats undergoing very intense training (149). Lower body weights in trained male rats are associated with the caloric expenditure of exercise and a decrease in food intake; in contrast, female rats increase food intake during training (71). Some studies have employed groups of sedentary rats that have food intake restricted in order to keep body weight similar to that in trained rats (117,118,149). In these studies heart weight was greater in trained rats (149). However, use of food-restricted control groups is questionable since heart weight may be affected by undernutrition and body composition and lean body mass is not the same as in trained rats (117). An exhaustive review of the effects of different training programs on body weight and heart weight in the rat has recently appeared (71).

Most studies in male rats have shown that training by running leads to an increase in the heart/body weight ratio, yet no increase in heart weight (71). An increase in heart weight relative to lean body mass has also been reported in treadmill-trained male rats (46). A few studies have shown small increases in heart mass in male rats following training by swimming (71). For reasons delineated at the outset of this section, an increase in heart/body weight ratio without an increase in cardiac mass cannot be construed as evidence for cardiac enlargement. This conclusion is supported by the findings of Dowell et al. (48) and Nutter et al. (116) who have shown that despite an increased heart/body weight ratio in male rats trained by running, cardiac mass, RNA concentration, and myocardial fiber size were not different from controls. In female rats it appears that the mode of training is critical in determining the response of cardiac mass to training. Female rats trained by running generally do not show an increase in heart mass. However, training female rats by swimming almost always leads to an increased cardiac mass. Hickson et al. (79) have followed the time-course of the development of hypertrophy and associated biochemical changes in swimming female rats. Heart weight and total protein increased after 2 days and plateaued after 14 days. An increase in RNA concentration occurred within 1 day and preceded the increase in heart weight. DNA and hydroxyproline concentration were decreased once heart weight stabilized, although total content was slightly increased, suggesting a small degree of connective tissue hyperplasia. These increases in total cardiac DNA and hydroxyproline content in exercise hypertrophy are quite small compared with those seen in studies of pressure-overload hypertrophy (67,68). On cessation of training, complete regression of heart weight occurred after 14 to 21 days, although hydroxyproline content remained increased (71). Mechanisms underlying the morphological dichotomy in response to the mode of training in females have not been investigated. However, this difference in female rats provides experimental models to examine cardiac functional adaptations to training with and without hypertrophy.

Studies in isolated left ventricular papillary muscle and trabeculae provide information regarding the effects of training on intrinsic myocardial contractility and passive muscle stiffness. This method allows loading conditions to be precisely controlled and geometric assumptions need not be made. Studies in male and female rats that have been trained by running or swimming have been performed. In none of these has an alteration in passive muscle stiffness been reported subsequent to training. On the other hand, active mechanics in papillary muscles and trabeculae of trained rats have shown a full spectrum of results. Several studies reported increases in isometric tension development and/or isotonic shortening velocity in trained animals with (178,180) or without hypertrophy (108,168). Other studies have reported no change in isometric mechanics (5,65), and one study (116) has shown a decrease in peak tension and rate of tension development in young rats which was not observed in adult rats. The disparate nature of these findings is difficult to explain but may be due to differences in duration or intensity of training, to age, or to subtle differences in animal strains. Furthermore, it is uncertain whether changes in contractility evident in papillary muscles represent similar changes in the whole ventricle. However, the general finding of unaltered or improved mechanics in muscles from hypertrophied hearts of exercise-trained rats is quite different than the depressed mechanics in muscles from hypertrophied hearts of chronically pressure-overloaded rats (24,29).

Scheuer and co-workers (19,20,126,148,149,150,154) have studied isolated perfused working hearts in several rat exercise models. In contrast to isolated muscle techniques, their method studies intact hearts at physiological temperatures and heart rate. Preload, afterload, and heart rate can be controlled, although assumptions regarding ventricular shape must be made. In addition, an indirect calculation of end-diastolic volume can be made so that differences in pump performance may be attributed to alterations in compliance and/or contractility. Therefore, intrinsic adaptations in pump and muscle function may be examined in intact hearts. Studies in hearts from male swimmers have shown increased pumping ability which was evident at high left atrial pressures (19,26,148). The increase in pump performance was due to an increased myocardial contractility (19,148) and may also have been due to an increase in left ventricular compliance (19). The mechanical adaptations were no longer observed after 2 weeks of deconditioning (61). These studies also showed that in swim-trained rats, but not treadmill-trained rats, ventricular relaxation was enhanced (19,148). Teleologically, this adaptation to training would be important, since a faster relaxation could allow more complete ventricular diastolic filling at rapid heart rates, such as during exercise. Virtually all the intrinsic cardiac adaptations observed in hearts from male swimming rats which did not have hypertrophy were also observed in hearts from female swimming rats with hypertrophy (150).

These same investigators have also examined the effect of the mode of training and sex on cardiac training effects. In studying the effects of running and swimming programs of approximately similar intensity and duration, qualitatively similar intrinsic mechanical adaptations were observed in hearts from male rats with the exception of the aforementioned differences in relaxation (148). When male and female rats of similar age were trained by the same running regimen, improved function was observed in hearts from male runners but not in hearts from female runners (149). From these studies using the same investigational methods, it would appear that exercise training, for the most part, promotes increased myocardial contractility in the rat. However, effects of training mode and sex may modulate the extent to which cardiac adaptations to training are observed in rats.

Studies of cardiac function in open-chested rats perhaps provide a more physiological setting in which to study cardiac mechanical adaptations to exercise conditioning. Evidence for a shift of the end-diastolic pressure-volume relationship to the right in trained animals has been reported (78). However, these findings were observed in hypertrophied hearts, so it is likely they represent the effect of cardiac enlargement and not a decrease in diastolic tone. Studies in open-chested rats also support the notion that the conditioning effects on the heart are most apparent when the heart is stressed. Thus Codini et al. (33) have shown that hearts from swimming rats develop greater pressures only during graded degrees of aortic constriction. Cutilletta et al. (41) showed that trained rats demonstrated an improved recovery of cardiac output after acute increases in afterload. This same group has shown that when subjected to substained (1–3 days) aortic constriction, exercised animals maintained or increased myocardial contractility whereas contractility was depressed in sedentary animals (47). With acute volume overloading, ventricular function curves tend to be enhanced after training in open-chested rats, despite their having lower heart rates (58,131).

This survey of studies of cardiac conditioning in rats demonstrates that although the data are not always consistent, the bulk of the evidence is consistent with the hypothesis that training leads to an adaptative increase in myocardial contractility in the rat. Although improved contractile performance is observed occasionally under base-line conditions, it is more often observed when the heart is stressed. Thus, it is better to consider this adaptation as an increase in inotropic reserve, which is called on only as demand requires.

Other animal exercise models, besides those of rats and dogs, have been used infrequently. Studies in cat right ventricular papillary muscles (189,197) have reported no change in active or passive mechanics resulting from training. Studies in guinea pigs have been few. Investigations in other animal species should be pursued, particularly in species that have lower base-line inotropic states than rats. Cardiac effects of physical training may be more prominent when imposed on a lower base-line functional state.

EFFECTS OF STATIC EXERCISE TRAINING ON CARDIAC ADAPTATIONS

So far we have discussed cardiac adaptations to dynamic physical training. However, many athletic disciplines involve exercise that is predominantly of a static nature, that is, they require contraction of skeletal muscle groups against fixed objects. Weight-lifting, wrestling, and field events such as the shot-put and hammer throw constitute sports of this type. Quite often the term "isometric" is used to describe this type of exercise, implying an increase in skeletal muscle tension with little change in length. It is also important to point out that few physical activities can be described as purely dynamic or static; indeed some athletic endeavors (e.g., rowing) probably represent significant contributions of both dynamic and static exercise (106). A symposium on the cardiovascular response to and the neural control mechanisms involved in static exercise has recently been published (107).

As we shall describe, the heart of athletes engaged in predominantly static exercise shows distinct differences in cardiac morphology when compared with findings in athletes involved in dynamic activities. However, to better understand these differences, an awareness of the differences in the hemodynamic response to static and dynamic exercise is a helpful prerequisite. In the experimental setting, hand-grip exercise is often used to produce isometric effects. The workload can be quantitated as force development or as a percentage of the maximal voluntary contraction (MVC). There is a marked increase in systolic, diastolic, and mean arterial pressure elicited by contraction of even a small mass of skeletal muscle (50), with further increases in pressure as the contraction is sustained. Aortic systolic pressure may reach 300 mm Hg during weight-lifting (87). The important factor in determining the blood pressure response to static effort is the percentage of maximal contraction by a given muscle group—the mass of muscle involved does not seem to matter (106). Thus, Lind and McNichol (94) and Donald et al. (50) have shown that similar mean blood pressures were achieved at 20% MVC of the thigh muscles or of the individual fingers. In comparison, when the same subjects perform static and dynamic exercise which evokes similar increases in oxygen consumption, an increase in mean arterial pressure occurs only during the static effort (8). During static exercise, heart rate and cardiac output increase, although much less than during dynamic exercise (40). Thus, although systemic resistance invariably decreases during dynamic exercise, it remains within normal limits during static exercise (72,124). The increased arterial diastolic pressure is thought to be due to the increase in cardiac output (106), but may also be due to reflex effects originating in the active muscles (125). Studies of left ventricular function in normal subjects during static exercise have been reported. Crawford et al. (40) have reported that the left ventricle performs as it would to an afterload stress. Thus, these workers observed decreases in the velocity and extent of shortening and stroke volume while end-diastolic volume did not change. These alterations seemed to be related to the intensity of the stress. Others have reported similar directional findings although of lesser degree (72,124,167). These responses to static exercise differ markedly to those observed in dynamic exercise where shortening, velocity of shortening, and stroke volume increase while end-diastolic volume remains the same or increases (see earlier section). The finding that shortening and velocity change little during static exercise despite a considerable increase in afterload also suggests that as in dynamic exercise, the inotropic state of the myocardium is increased (167). With these hemodynamic alterations in mind, it would appear that static exercise results in a pressure overload as compared with the volume overload associated with dynamic exercise.

A few studies have specifically compared cardiac size and dimension in athletes engaged in dynamic and static activities. Morganroth et al. (110) compared echocardiographic findings in college-age long distance runners, swimmers, wrestlers, and shot-putters. Each group of athletes demonstrated an increase in left ventricular mass; however, the swimmers and runners, but not the wrestlers or shot-putters, showed an increased left ventricular internal dimension. In contrast, only the wrestlers and shot-putters showed significant increases in posterior and septal wall thickness. Similar, but less striking differences were observed by Longhurst et al. (96) in comparing weight-lifters and long distance runners. Furthermore, these workers showed that the weight-lifters had greater lean body masses than controls or runners so that the relative increase in heart mass was probably less in weight lifters than in runners. Keul et al. (87) have reported on a set of identical twins, one a long distance runner and the other a power athlete. Radiographic heart volume was 560 ml in the power athlete and 710 ml in the runner. Thus, the two forms of training can change the phenotype in men who have the same genotype. In athletes involved in activities requiring both dynamic and static efforts the effects on cardiac dimension seem to be additive. Thus, in ballet dancers who perform movements of both a dynamic and static nature, increases in both internal dimension and wall thickness were observed (34).

Animal studies have also helped elucidate cardiac morphological adaptations to chronic training with static exercise. Rats have been trained to climb wire ladders for several weeks duration, and the completion of this regimen resulted in an increased heart mass (102). Muntz et al. (112) used operantly conditioned cats chronically performing isometric work to investigate the effects of this training on cardiac dimensions and fiber size. Their results showed increases in left and right ventricular mass, left ventricular wall thickness and left ventricular fiber diameter, but no alteration in left ventricular internal diameter. The increase in left ventricular wall thickness was correlated with the amount of isometric work performed.

Therefore, depending on the nature of the exercise, the manner in which the heart enlarges subsequent to training can be quite different. The heart of athletes engaged in endurance sports typifies that of a chronic volume overload (eccentric hypertrophy) whereas that of the athlete involved in sports requiring static exercise typifies that of a chronic pressure overload (concentric hypertrophy, i.e., similar chamber volume but increased wall thickness, ref. 66). However, left ventricular function in response to afterload stress is normal in the power athlete (97), but is depressed in patients with long-standing systemic hypertension (175). Therefore, although a chronic pressure overload is normally associated with eventual pathological sequelae, the intermittent nature of the overload in the power athlete results in a hypertrophy representing a physiological adaptation that is probably without pathological significance.

THE EFFECTS OF EXERCISE TRAINING ON CORONARY FLOW AND VASCULARITY

Since myocardial oxygen demand and coronary flow increase dramatically during exercise (37), it is reasonable to postulate that adaptations occur in the coronary vasculature when exercise is performed on a regular basis. Few studies have examined coronary perfusion in normal trained humans because of the invasive nature and relative insensitivity of the available investigational tools. The recent advent of radionuclide techniques is promising in this regard (159). Nevertheless, studies in animals have provided valuable insight into how the coronary vasculature adapts to exercise conditioning. Detailed reviews on this subject by Scheuer (159) and Cohen (37) have recently appeared.

By measuring the weights of coronary casts, several studies in rodents have demonstrated that physical training can increase the volume of the coronary vascular space relative to the myocardial mass (42,171,176). These effects were observed with as little as 2 days of exercise per week (42,73,176). In exercise models that produced hypertrophy, increases in cast weight relative to heart weight were or were not observed (171,176). However, a similar ratio in the hypertrophied heart would imply an absolute increase in the coronary vascular volume in pace with the increase in heart mass. Tepperman and Pearlman (176) also observed that after an 8-week deconditioning period in male swimmers, cast weight/heart weight ratios remained elevated even though heart weight had returned to normal. Whether the increased vascular volume in these studies depended on a vascular neoformation at the capillary level or to a widening of the coronary arteries, or to both, was not determined.

Wyatt and Mitchell (196) have examined longitudinally the effects of physical conditioning and deconditioning on the diameter of the circumflex artery of dogs. Using coronary angiograms obtained at similar heart rates, they observed a small but significant increase in diameter of the left circumflex artery after 12 weeks of training which decreased from trained values after 6 weeks of deconditioning. Similar effects of training and detraining on large vessel diameters have been observed in rats by Leon and Bloor (92). They found an increase in the combined cross-sectional area of the left and right coronary arteries in rats that had been swimming daily, but not in rats swimming only twice weekly.

Numerous studies using several animal species have reported on the effects of exercise training on capillary density and capillary/muscle fiber ratios. Studies in rats would suggest that the effect of training on capillary growth occurs in animals of various ages, but is most prominent in young animals. Bloor and Leon (27) found that although capillary/fiber ratios were increased after training by swimming in young, adult, and old male rats, the increased ratio was associated with an increased number of total capillaries in the exercised young rats, but with an actual loss of myocardial fibers in the exercised old rats. Tomanek (182) also studied animals of similar age groups trained by running and observed that capillary density increased significantly only in the exercised young rats, although trends for higher values were also observed in the adult and old rats. However, the capillary/fiber ratio was significantly increased to about the same extent in all age groups. In contrast, Bell and Rasmussen (18) showed that capillary/fiber ratio increased in rats that were 4 weeks of age at the initiation of training but not in rats 14 weeks of age (18). Slight but significant increases in myocardial capillary density of adult dogs have also been reported (196). In contrast to the rather positive relationship between capillary density and physical conditioning described so far, one report has shown a decreased capillary density in conditioned guinea pigs (69). In addition to histological evidence, autoradiographic evidence suggests that training leads to a neoformation of capillaries. Ljungqvist and Unge (95) and Mandache et al. (100) using light and electronmicroscopic techniques, respectively, showed a highly significant increase in the nuclear incorporation of (^{3}H)thymidine in both ventricles of swim-trained rats with hypertrophy. The increased incorporation was mainly confined to the nuclei of cells in the capillary walls, suggesting active DNA synthesis and new growth of capillaries. Interestingly, these observations were not observed in hypertrophied hearts from rats with renal hypertension or aortic stenosis. Therefore, except for minor discrepancies, review of the data suggests that training promotes myocardial vascular growth. This adaptation may serve to normalize diffusion distance for oxygen to the hypertrophied myocardial cell.

Studies that have shown increased coronary cast weights (176) and capillary/ fiber (92) ratios after periods of deconditioning raise the interesting possibility that improved vascularity may be a residual benefit of training. In contrast, Leon and Bloor (156) and Wyatt and Mitchell (196) showed that the increased capillary density resulting from training regressed after a period of deconditioning. However, Leon and Bloor (93) observed that the increased number of capillaries induced by physical conditioning could be maintained by as little as 1 hr of exercise per week, suggesting that only minimal physical activity is necessary to maintain this training effect. Clearly, more studies are needed on the influences of physical deconditioning.

Whether the histological evidence of an increased vascularity is witnessed physiologically as an increased coronary capacity in the intact heart has been investigated. Scheuer and co-workers have shown that hearts from trained rats had greater coronary flows when perfused with an aqueous buffer in an isolated working-heart apparatus (19,126,149). Under their experimental conditions, coronary vasodilatation was nearly maximal, so an increased coronary flow suggested an increased coronary capacity. Studies in isolated perfused hypertrophied hearts from female swimmers demonstrated normal coronary flow per gram tissue (150). However, the increased coronary capacity observed *in vitro* does not prove that it is available to the blood-perfused heart *in vivo*. In studies of male swim-trained rats, Yipintsoi et al. (198) used hypoxia to produce partial vasodilatation and measured coronary flow and its distribution with microspheres. They found no differences between trained and control rats in coronary flow during control or hypoxic conditions. Spear et al. (166) used treadmill-trained rats in an experiment of similar design and observed greater coronary flow and coronary conductance in the trained animals during hypoxia. However, these differences were only observed at low aortic pressures and not when aortic pressure was maintained at normal values with methoxamine.

Several studies have reported on the effects of training in dogs on coronary flow at rest and during exercise. Resting coronary flows have been reported to be lower (15,139), unchanged (36), or increased (89). Lower coronary flows at similar submaximal exercise loads have been reported (15,139) in trained animals, although similar coronary flows were observed at maximal workloads (15). Stone observed that coronary flow velocity was reduced in partially trained animals but not in completely trained animals (174). Trained animals were observed to have a greater myocardial oxygen extraction (139,174) during exercise, but the significance of these findings is not certain. Lower coronary flows at submaximal exercise have also been observed by Heiss et al. (76) in athletes when compared with normal subjects. The lower coronary flows observed during submaximal exercise were associated with lower myocardial oxygen consumptions (76,139), so they probably reflect a lower myocardial oxygen demand subsequent to training. Furthermore, measurements of coronary flow during exercise do not represent the maximal coronary reserve, since it has been shown that coronary flows greater than those observed at maximal exercise could be achieved using vasodilator drugs (15).

Reactive hyperemia may be used to estimate the maximal coronary reserve. Using similar coronary occlusion times, Laughlin et al. (89) showed that peak reactive hyperemic flow was increased in trained dogs, but Stone (174) observed no difference in his trained dogs. The differences in results in these studies may have been due to the use of anesthetized (89) versus unanesthetized (174) animals. Coronary reserve capacity determined by injection of the vasodilator dipyridamole was found to be lower in a group of athletes (76), although the athletes seemed to be relatively resistant to the drug and dose-response curves were not performed.

Therefore, animal studies would indicate that increased myocardial vascularity, as determined histologically, is a real adaptation to training. Attempts to demonstrate by physiological or pharmacological maneuvers that this results in increased coronary capacity has produced equivocal results. This may be due to the inadequacy of current techniques.

MYOCARDIAL SUBCELLULAR AND BIOCHEMICAL ADAPTATIONS TO EXERCISE TRAINING

Over the past 10 years a number of studies have investigated biochemical alterations in the hearts of trained animals. These studies have provided valuable insights into mechanisms that may affect enhanced myocardial performance. Of course, it is essential to first document a training effect in contractile performance before undertaking examination of biochemical mechanisms. In this section we first discuss mechanisms involved in energy production, followed by a discussion of mechanisms involved in energy utilization.

Metabolic

Studies in isolated perfused hearts of physically trained rats have shown that increases in external work are met by proportional increases in myocardial oxygen consumption (126) when hearts are studied at similar heart rates, preloads, and afterloads. Under these conditions, the energy cost of performing external work was similar in hearts from trained and untrained animals. Studies in trained dogs and athletes performing submaximal exercise have reported a lower index (tension-time index) for myocardial oxygen consumption (14,15) and have measured lower myocardial oxygen consumptions as well (15,76). This is certainly related, in part, to the decreased heart rate during exercise in trained subjects. However, it also underscores the importance of determining the factors responsible for the increased stroke volume in training. Augmentation of stroke volume by chamber enlargement would be less costly in terms of energy requirement whereas augmentation by an increase in contractility would be more costly. Studies that stimultaneously measure myocardial oxygen consumption and left ventricular pressure and dimension should be performed to determine whether training favorably affects the relationship between myocardial oxygen consumption and cardiac work.

Hearts of physically trained rats had increased resting glycogen stores (153) while glycogen synthetase activity increased in hearts from trained guinea pigs (88). In severely exercised animals there is a reduction in cardiac glycogen content which is followed by a resynthesis to above normal levels (161). It is possible that during training, these wide oscillations in cardiac glycogen stores eventually result in a higher resting glycogen content, and this would confer a greater substrate reserve for cardiac activity during exertion (157). Lower endogenous triglyceride stores and increased turnover of fatty acids through the triglyceride pool have been observed in hearts from trained rats (57,153).

One of the few investigations of the glycolytic pathway in conditioned rat hearts showed no difference in carbohydrate utilization in arrested perfused hearts (155). Studies of the glycolytic enzymes revealed no change in phosphofructose kinase activity, but pyruvate kinase and lactate dehydrogenase activities were increased substantially (62,199). The functional significance of these alterations in glycolytic enzymes has not been demonstrated.

Mitochondria

In contrast to the rather profound effects of exercise training on skeletal muscle mitochondria, the effects of training on cardiac muscle mitochondria are of a lesser degree and still somewhat controversial. The levels of activity (expressed per gram of muscle) of the mitochondrial enzymes cytochrome oxidase, succinate oxidase, citrate synthetase, or malate dehydrogenase showed no changes following programs of running or swimming in male rats (118,119). The effects of training on cardiac mitochondrial mass are not clear and may depend on the method of quantitation. Electron microscopic studies have reported increases in mitochondrial mass in hypertrophied hearts from female rats (3,7), but this was related to the duration of exercise in one study (7). Furthermore, these techniques are based on sampling methods and hence may represent qualitative changes. An increase in mitochondrial protein was reported by Penpargkul et al. (128) in male swimmers without hypertrophy. However, Oscai et al. (118) reported no differences in mitochondrial protein, and Hickson et al. (79) reported no increase in cytochrome *c*, a mitochondrial marker, in the hearts of trained rats with or without hypertrophy. Whether an increase in mitochondrial protein, when it occurs, is due to an increase in the number of mitochondria or to a greater mitochondrial density of cristae is not known. Some reports have suggested that exhaustive exercise leads to ultrastructural damage in heart mitochondria (3,7).

Measurements of respiratory function in cardiac mitochondria have shown no change in exercise-trained dogs (165) and rats (7) when several substrates were employed. Penpargkul et al. (128) reported normal mitochondrial ADP:0 ratio and respiratory control index in exercised rats but a 15% decrease in state 3 oxygen consumption when expressed per milligram of mitochondrial protein. However, in this study, since a greater mitochondrial protein content was observed, a normal oxidative capacity per gram of tissue was calculated. Thus, although the effects of training on mitochondrial morphology are uncertain, it seems that training has little effect on the oxidative capacity of cardiac mitochondria. Therefore, it appears that the heart muscle cell has sufficient preexisting oxidative capacity to meet the energy demands associated with exercise.

Although it remains uncertain how Ca^{2+} from mitochondrial sources may contribute to myocardial excitation-contraction, some studies would suggest that training may alter Ca^{2+} kinetics in cardiac mitochondria. Sordahl et al. (165) observed that the ability to retain Ca^{2+} was decreased in mitochondria from hearts of trained dogs. Penpargkul et al. (128) showed a reduced ability for mitochondria from trained rats to take up Ca^{2+} when expressed per milligram protein, but not when expressed per gram tissue. Firm conclusions regarding the effects of training on mitochondrial Ca^{2+} kinetics would be premature because the data are few and derived from studies using different species and modes of training. However, they deserve further investigation, since they may represent a mechanism important in the long-term regulation of intracellular calcium concentration.

Cardiac Contractile Proteins

Alterations in cardiac contractile proteins have been associated with the velocity of muscle contraction in various chronic hemodynamic overloads (158). Early training studies were performed by Bhan and Scheuer (22,23) in hearts of male rats trained by swimming. These workers demonstrated that training resulted in increases in actomyosin and myosin ATPase activity, which may have been due to a conformational change in the heavy meromyosin component (5,158). These alterations in myosin enzyme activity were correlated with the duration of swimming and returned to normal after a deconditioning period (98). Myosin light chains did not appear to be affected by exercise training as studied by electrophoretic techniques (158). There does seem to be a shift toward a faster isoenzyme of heavy chain in cardiac myosin from swimming rats (144,160). The adaptations in contractile proteins have been documented in exercise models without exercise-induced hypertrophy, but also in swim-trained female rats, where a marked hypertrophy was present (99). Therefore, in contrast to hypertrophy resulting from pathological hemodyamic overloads where a decrease in cardiac contractile protein ATPase activity is observed, hypertrophy due to exercise training results in an increase (105,158).

As opposed to studies employing swimming exercise, evidence for adaptations in cardiac contractile proteins has been inconsistent in studies employing running exercise in rats (11,129) and dogs (35,49). Minimal or absent changes have been reported, even though enhanced contractile performance was observed in most studies (49,178). The failure to demonstrate alterations in contractile proteins by running may be related to the intensity of the running regimen. Baldwin et al. (12) showed in several groups of rats trained by running programs of varying intensity that an increased myosin ATPase occured only in the group undergoing the most intense training. Even so, the consistency of observations for increased myosin ATPase activity in swim-trained rats would suggest a specificity for the training mode. However, this does not appear to be due simply to water immersion, since immersion of rats sitting on a platform over several weeks duration produced no change in myosin ATPase (129). Therefore, exercise would seem to be an obligatory component of the swimming effect.

Sarcoplasmic Reticulum

A possible role for the sarcoplasmic reticulum (SR) in regulating myocardial intracellular Ca^{2+} concentrations in conditioned hearts has been investigated in several rat conditioning models by Penpargkul et al. (99,127,129). These investigators have shown in male and female rats trained by swimming that training leads to an increased Ca^{2+} uptake and binding in SR preparations (99,127). Thus similar adaptations in SR activity were observed when exercise training did (females) or did not (males) produce hypertrophy. In contrast, hypertrophy due to systolic overload has been associated with depressed SR function (99). The exercise-induced enhancement in SR activity has also been associated with faster relaxation in isolated perfused hearts from swim-trained male and female rats (19,148,150). Treadmill-training in male rats produced only minor increases in SR activity, which was commensurate with only a trend for improved ventricular relaxation (129,148). Thus, the adaptations in SR function and ventricular relaxation are most apparent in rats trained by swimming. This specificity related to training mode is supported by the findings of Sordahl et al. (165), who showed no increase in Ca^{2+} uptake or binding in SR from dogs training by running. However, these same investigators observed differences in rate of release of Ca^{2+} from SR of trained dogs, which implicates a possible role for adaptations in SR function to the altered functional state of the exercised-trained dog heart.

Sarcolemma

The sarcolemma provides an external source of Ca^{2+} for excitation-contraction coupling. It has been proposed that this organelle may serve as an important site of adaptation by providing increased Ca^{2+} availability for myofibrillar cross-bridge formation in the conditioned heart (180). However, data to support this hypothesis have come only from indirect evidence; a pure sarcolemmal preparation has not been studied in training experiments. The first evidence suggesting a role for the sarcolemma in the cardiac adaptation to training was provided by Tibbets et al. (178), who demonstrated that when papillary preparations were perfused with lanthanum to displace membrane-bound Ca^{2+}, the time-course for tension decay was significantly prolonged in the trained muscles. These same workers have also reported that the concentration of phosphatidyl serine, a major binding moiety of sarcolemmal Ca^{2+}, is increased in sarcolemmal preparations from trained animals (179). Using Scatchard analysis and assuming that cardiac tension generation is a function of the amount of sarcolemmal Ca^{2+} receptors that are occupied by Ca^{2+}, this group has also calculated a 63% increase in sarcolemmal Ca^{2+}-binding sites in preparations from trained rats (180). These results are very promising, but conclusive evidence must await methods for studying sarcolemmal function directly.

Sensitivity to Catecholamines

In recent years several reports have indicated that physical training alters the cardiovascular responsiveness to exogenous catecholamines, but the data are contradictory regarding the direction of these alterations. Studies in humans have shown that infusion of norepinephrine may cause greater (91) or lesser (123) increases in blood pressure when comparing trained subjects to untrained subjects. However, these alterations can not be explained in terms of central or peripheral effects or to differences in resting autonomic tone in the trained individuals. To specifically address whether intrinsic myocardial contractile sensitivity to catecholamines may be altered by physical training, several recent studies were performed in isolated papillary muscles from trained animals. Molé (108) showed that addition of iso-proterenol in the same concentration to the bathing medium increased the rate of tension development to a greater degree in left ventricular papillary muscles of trained rats. A similar hypersensitivity to isoproterenol was observed by Wyatt et al. (197) in right ventricular papillary muscles of trained cats, but not in response to norepinephrine by Williams and Potter (189), although they administered the drug during paired stimulation, which may have masked a possible effect.

Since the control of the catecholamines over myocardial contractility is via their interaction with the β-adrenergic receptors and the adenylate cyclase system, several recent studies have addressed the effects of physical training on myocardial adrenergic receptors and adenylate cyclase activity. Studies by Williams et al. (190,191) in male and female rats trained by swimming and by Moore et al. (109) in male rats trained by running have not shown discernable effects of training on β-receptor number or affinity in heart membrane particulate fractions. These findings were associated with no difference in isoproterenol-stimulated myocardial adenylate cyclase activity (109). Dohm et al. (45) observed a decrease in epinephrine-stimulated adenylate cyclase in the hearts from rats trained by running. Conversely, Wyatt et al. (197) observed that enhancement of myocardial adenylate cyclase was greater in heart extracts from trained cats during stimulation by either isoproterenol or norepinephrine; however, they did not investigate β-receptor number. Recently, Williams et al. (191) showed a down-regulation in α-adrenergic and muscarinic cholenergic receptor number in hearts from trained rats. However, the physiological significance of these findings is not certain.

Although some of these studies are suggestive of a training effect on myocardial sensitivity to catecholamines, it would be premature to draw conclusions whether they represent basic mechanisms that may enhance myocardial contractility during stress. Clearly, further studies are required to address this possibility.

Summarizing the cardiac biochemical adaptations that occur in training, it would appear that a variety of alterations can occur, encompassing mechanisms involved in both energy production and energy utilization. The alterations in energy-utilizing processes seem to be more prominent and all of these can be considered as potentially contributing to an increased contractile state of the myocardium. These changes appear to occur more often and to a greater magnitude in hearts from swim-trained rats, although this exercise model has received more scrutiny. It does not rule out the possibility that certain cardiac biochemical alterations in training experiments may be of relatively greater or lesser importance, depending on the exercise model that is studied. Finally, many of the salutary biochemical adaptations we have discussed have been documented in exercise-induced hypertrophy, which distinguishes it from hypertrophy due to pathological causes where alterations also occur but generally in the opposite direction.

FACTORS THAT MAY MODULATE CARDIAC RESPONSES TO TRAINING

Sex

Whether cardiac adaptations to training differ in males and females has not been systematically investigated. Much of what we know in humans must come from comparisons of reports that have separately examined training responses in males and females. Generally, female athletes do not achieve the same absolute levels of VO_2 max or work performance as seen in males (70,145,157,201). In comparing different studies it would appear that females achieve a higher VO_2 max after training almost purely by an increase in cardiac output (143,201), whereas trained males increase both cardiac output and peripheral oxygen extraction to an equal extent (142,146). Thus, relative contributions of central and peripheral adaptations to the trained state may differ in males and females. However, no sex differences were reported by DeMaria et al. (43) in the degree of cardiac hypertrophy found in subjects after endurance training. In addition, female field hockey players had similar end-diastolic internal dimensions when normalized for body surface area as did a group of similar age male college swimmers or runners (110,201). These measurements, however, were obtained in different laboratories.

In animal studies, we have discussed in a previous section the finding of a greater propensity for hypertrophy in female rats subjected to a swimming program. Schaible et al. (149) did not observe a cardiac functional adaptation in female rats trained by the same running program that elicited one in similar aged male rats. This sex difference occurred even though the training regimen produced equal increases in skeletal muscle oxidative capacity in the two sexes. In response to isometric training, Muntz et al. (112) observed a lesser hypertrophic response in hearts from female cats, but this may have been due to a lesser workload performed by the females.

These results are only suggestive of sex differences in the response to physical conditioning. Systemic investigations need to be performed in humans. Whether the sex hormones can account for sex differences in animal-training studies is not known.

Age

As older segments of the population become more actively involved in sports, and older athletes continue their careers in master competitions, the effects of age on cardiac responses to training take on added interest. There is a progressive decline in the functional capacity of the cardiovascular system with aging which is reflected in a decrease in the VO_2 max (74,157). Recently, Heath et al. (74) compared functional capacity and cardiac dimensions in a group of masters athletes with that in a group of young athletes. Although VO_2 max was greater in the masters athletes compared with an age-matched group of untrained subjects, it was lower when compared with that in the group of young athletes. This appeared to be due to a lower maximal heart rate in the masters athletes, since the oxygen pulse (oxygen consumed per heart beat) was the same as in the young athletes. Echocardiographic dimensions were similar except for the finding that calculated left ventricular end-diastolic volume was slightly greater in the masters athletes. Resting ventricular function (mean V_{cf}) was the same in young and old athletes. In contrast, Nishimura et al. (114) showed that the cardiac functional and hypertrophic responses may be different in athletes that have trained for many years duration. Examining three age groups of professional bicyclers, they observed that resting ventricular function, as determined by mean V_{cf}, was lower in the oldest group of athletes (40 to 49 years) when compared with an age-matched control group. Moreover, they observed increases in posterior and septal wall thickness and evidence for left atrial enlargement only in the oldest group of athletes. ECG abnormalities were more prominent in the older athletes. However, others have found increases in left ventricular wall thickness in young athletes (Table 1), so the significance of these findings in older athletes, but not young athletes, in this study is uncertain. Clearly, further studies in older trained populations are needed.

Few animal studies have investigated the effects of aging on cardiac training responses. We have discussed in an earlier section the effects of aging on the responses of myocardial vascularity to training in rats.

EFFECTS OF TRAINING ON CARDIAC RESPONSES TO PATHOLOGICAL EVENTS

Oxygen Deprivation

One may postulate that since training improves myocardial vascularity, it may exert a protective effect on the myocardium against acute ischemic insults. McElroy et al. (104) showed that infarct size was smaller in hearts from physically trained rats after ligation of the left coronary artery. They associated these findings with the observation of an increased capillary/fiber ratio in another group of rats trained on the same regimen. Other studies in *in situ* hearts and in isolated hearts from trained rats have shown improved functional responses to global hypoxia (31,154) and ischemia (20). In these studies, however, better function was maintained even though metabolic indexes of ischemia (levels of high-energy phosphates and lactate) were similar. Therefore, it is unlikely that increased vascularity and improved oxygen delivery could account for the findings of improved performance. A more likely explanation would involve an intrinsic contractile adaptation in the heart muscle that was maintained during the ischemic period.

Much attention has been focused on the effects of exercise conditioning on coronary collateral blood vessels. These are initially unused vascular pathways that are recruited only after failure of the normal vessel no longer permits normal flows (37). Lowered myocardial oxygen tension is a potent stimulus for coronary collateral formation. Since exercise increases myocardial oxygen consumption and therefore demand, one may speculate that chronic repeated exercise may serve as a stimulus for collateral formation. The end result would be that reserve channels for flow would be available to an area of the myocardium if the vessel normally perfusing that area were to be critically stenosed or occluded. To test this hypothesis, Cohen et al. (35) trained dogs with normal coronary arteries. At the completion of the training program the left anterior descending coronary artery was occluded and blood flow to the ischemic area was measured by the microsphere technique. No differences were observed in collateral blood flow between trained and sedentary dogs. Similarly, Sanders et al. (147) found no increase in coronary collateral blood flow in pigs with normal coronary arteries when studied during acute coronary occlusion after 10 months of physical training.

An early study by Eckstein (51) suggested that exercise training subsequent to coronary artery narrowing increased collateral blood flow to the ischemic region.

This was determined by directly measuring retrograde flow to the ischemic region. For any degree of narrowing, retrograde flow to the ischemic area was greater in trained dogs, indicating that training had promoted collateral flow to the ischemic area. Subsequent studies using more precise techniques in conscious dogs have not confirmed these findings or shown only minor effects of training on collateral blood flow to the ischemic region (38,75,85,113). In isolated blood-perfused dog hearts, Scheel et al. (152) observed a larger increase in collateral flow to the ischemic area in dogs where training was started 3 months after the left circumflex coronary artery was stenosed. Schaper (151) also studied isolated dog hearts, but in animals that had both left circumflex and right coronary arteries occluded. Training in these dogs had no effect on collateral conductances and did not affect mortality. Thus, the effects of training on coronary collateral development are not clear. It would appear that in the normal heart, exercise is not a potent enough stimulus to increase collateral formation, but in studies with ischemia, the ischemic stimulus for collateral formation may mask a possible physical training effect. The effects of training on coronary collateral blood flow have recently been reviewed (37,159).

Systolic Overload

Although many investigations have evaluated the effects of physical training on blood pressure in hypertension (for review see ref. 157), few studies have examined the effects of training on cardiac responses to chronic pressure overload. In one study (41) that examined the acute response to aortic constriction, hypertrophy developed more rapidly in animals that had been physically trained than in sedentary animals. The mechanisms involved in this more rapid response to normalize myocardial stress was not clear. In female spontaneously hypertensive rats, training by swimming exaggerated the hypertrophy due to the hypertension alone, but had no effect on blood pressure (131). Although function of the heart *in situ* seemed to be improved, the effects of training on intrinsic cardiac function in hypertension were not clear. Two recent studies examined the effects of training on cardiac contractile proteins in hypertension. Rupp and Jacob (144) trained male spontaneously hypertensive rats by swimming. They observed that training normalized the myosin isoenzyme pattern, which was shifted toward a slower myosin isoenzyme in hypertensive animals. However, the training also lowered the blood pressure, so the effect of training could not be attributed to either a primary effect on the myocardium or to a secondary effect of blood pressure reduction. Furthermore, in studies using genetic hypertensive animals, one may not be sure of a possible strain specificity for these results. Scheuer et al. (160) also examined contractile proteins, but in hearts from female renal hypertensive rats trained by swimming. They found no effect of training on blood pressure but did observe a normalization for the myosin isoenzyme pattern in the trained hypertensive rats even though hypertrophy was exaggerated by the training. Therefore, the superimposition of a training-induced hypertrophy on that due to a pathologic overload does not appear to be harmful and may, in fact, reverse contractile abnormalities associated with the pathological overload.

CONCLUSIONS

Studies in athletes have demonstrated cardiac hypertrophy associated with chamber enlargement. The greater volume capacity of the heart is an important adaptive mechanism which enables a larger stroke volume to be ejected, but whether an increase in contractility contributes to the increase in pump performance in athletes is uncertain. Longitudinal studies of training in normal subjects have not consistently demonstrated hypertrophy subsequent to training. Therefore it remains questionable to what extent cardiac hypertrophy in the athlete is genetically determined or is due to training. Training by dynamic or static exercise results in a ventricular hypertrophy that corresponds to the respective volume versus pressure nature of the overload. Studies in trained animals strongly suggest that training leads to an enhanced contractile state of the myocardium. Biochemical studies have shown that alterations in the contractile proteins and/or in cellular calcium regulating systems may contribute to the increased contractility. Histological studies suggest that training improves myocardial vascularity but the physiological significance of this finding remains to be defined. Although some evidence suggests that exercise stimulates coronary collateral growth, whether exercise conditioning can protect the myocardium against an ischemic insult is not well established. The effect of age or sex on the cardiac response to training remains to be investigated.

The nature of the stimulus or stimuli that enables the heart to enlarge in training while maintaining normal or enhanced function has eluded definition. It may involve the intermittent versus continuous presence of the mechanical overload. It also may be due to neural or humoral influences that occur during exercise. Not until these mechanisms are established will we understand the rather salutary hypertrophy of the athlete's heart.

ACKNOWLEDGMENT

This work was supported in part by the National Heart, Lung, and Blood Institute Grant HL-15498 and the Young Investigator Award HL-25372 to Thomas F. Schaible.

We gratefully acknowledge the dedicated assistance of Mrs. Carol Atror in the preparation of this manuscript.

REFERENCES

1. Adamovich, D. R., Lubell, D., and Gutin, B. (1975): Systolic intervals from sitting to exercise of varying intensity (Abstract). *Med. Sci. Sports*, 7:72.
2. Adams, T. D., Yanowitz, F. G., Fisher, A. G., Ridges, J. D., Lovell, K., and Pryor, T. A. (1981): Noninvasive evaluation of exercise-training in college-age men. *Circulation*, 64:958–965.
3. Aldinger, E. E., and Sohal, R. S. (1970): Effects of digoxin on the ultrastructural myocardial changes in the rat subjected to chronic exercise. *Am. J. Cardiol.*, 26:369–374.

4. Allen, H. D., Goldberg, S. J., Sahn, D. J., Schy, N., and Wojcik, R. (1977): A quantitative echocardiographic study of champion childhood swimmers. *Circulation*, 55:142–145.
5. Amsterdam, A., Choquet, Y., Segal, L., Arbogast, R., Rendig, S., Zelis, R., and Mason, D. T. (1973): Response of the rat heart to exercise conditioning: physical metabolic and functional correlates (Abstract). *Clin. Res.*, 21:399.
6. Anholm, J. D., Foster, C., Carpenter, J., Pollock, M. L., Hellman, C. K., and Schmidt, D. H. (1982): Effect of habitual exercise on left ventricular response to exercise. *J. Appl. Physiol.*, 52:1648–1651.
7. Arcos, J. C., Sohal, R. S., Sun, S.-C., Argus, M. F., and Burch, G. E. (1968): Changes in ultrastructure and respiratory control in mitochondria of rat heart hypertrophied by exercise. *Exp. Mol. Pathol.*, 8:49–65.
8. Asmussen, E., (1981): Similarities and dissimilarities between static and dynamic exercise. *Circ. Res.*, 48(Suppl. I):I-3–I-10.
9. Åstrand, P. O., and Rodal, K. (1970): *Textbook of Work Physiology*. McGraw-Hill, New York.
10. Åstrand, P. O., Engstrom, L., Erickson, B., Karlberg, P., Nylander, I., Saltin, B., and Thoren, C. (1963): Girl swimmers. *Acta Paediat.* [Suppl.] 147:43–63.
11. Baldwin, K. M., Winder, W. W., and Holloszy, J. O. (1975): Adaptation of actomyosin ATPase in different types of muscle to endurance exercise. *Am. J. Physiol.*, 229:422–426.
12. Baldwin, K. M., Cooke, D. A., and Cheadle, W. G. (1977): Time course adaptation in cardiac and skeletal muscle in different running programs. *J. Appl. Physiol.*, 42:267–272.
13. Barach, J. H. (1910): Physiological and pathological effects of severe exertion (the marathon race) on circulatory and renal systems. *Arch. Intern. Med.*, 5:382–405.
14. Barnard, R. J., MacAlpin, R., Kattus, A. A., and Buckberg, G. D. (1977): Effect of training on myocardial oxygen supply/demand balance. *Circulation*, 56:289–291.
15. Barnard, R. J., Duncan, H. W., Baldwin, K. M., Grimditch, G., and Buckberg, G. D. (1980): Effects of intensive exercise training on myocardial performance and coronary blood flow. *J. Appl. Physiol.*, 49:444–449.
16. Bar-Shlomo, B-Z., Druck, M. N., Morch, J. E., Jablonsky, G., Hilton, J. D., Feiglin, D. H. I., and McLaughlin, P. R. (1982): Left ventricular function in trained and untrained healthy subjects. *Circulation*, 65:484–488.
17. Bedford, T. G., Tipton, C. M., Wilson, N. C., Oppliger, R. A., and Gisolfi, C. V. (1979): Maximum oxygen consumption of rats and its changes with various experimental procedures. *J. Appl. Physiol.*, 47:1278–1283.
18. Bell, R. D., and Rasmussen, R. L. (1972): Exercise and the myocardial fiber capillary ratio. In: *Training—Scientific Basis and Application*, edited by A. W. Taylor, pp. 123–130. Charles C Thomas, Springfield.
19. Bersohn, M. M., and Scheuer, J. (1977): Effects of physical training on end-diastolic volume and myocardial performance of isolated rat hearts. *Circ. Res.*, 40:510–516.
20. Bersohn, M. M., and Scheuer, J. (1978): Effect of ischemia on the performance of hearts from physically trained rats. *Am. J. Physiol.*, 234:H215–H218.
21. Bevegard, S., Holmgren, A., and Jonsson, B. (1963): Circulatory studies in well-trained athletes at rest and during heavy exercise with special reference to stroke volume and the influence of body position. *Acta Physiol. Scand.*, 57:26–50.
22. Bhan, A. K., and Scheuer, J. (1972): Effects of physical training on cardiac actomyosin adenosine triphosphate activity. *Am. J. Physiol.*, 223:1486–1490.
23. Bhan, A., Malhotra, A., and Scheuer, J. (1975): Biochemical adaptations in cardiac muscle: effects of physical training on sulfhydryl groups of myosin. *J. Mol. Cell. Cardiol.*, 7:435–442.
24. Bing, O. H. L., Matsushita, S., Fanburg, B. L., and Levine, H. J. (1971): Mechanical properties of rat cardiac muscle during experimental hypertrophy. *Circ. Res.*, 28:234–245.
25. Blimkie, C. J. R., Cunningham, D. A., and Nichol, P. M. (1980): Gas transport capacity and echocardiographically determined cardiac size in children. *J. Appl. Physiol.*, 49:994–999.
26. Blomqvist, C. G., Lewis, S. F., Taylor, W. F., and Graham, R. M. (1981): Similarity of the hemodynamic responses to static and dynamic exercise of small muscle groups. *Circ. Res.*, 48(Suppl. I.):I-87–I-92.
27. Bloor, C. M., and Leon, A. S. (1970): Interaction of age and exercise on the heart and its blood supply. *Lab. Invest.*, 22:160–165.
28. Bove, A. A., Hultgren, P. B., Ritzer, T. F., and Carey, R. A. (1979): Myocardial blood flow and hemodynamic responses to exercise training in dogs. *J. Appl. Physiol.*, 46:571–578.

29. Capasso, J. M., Strobeck, J. E., Malhotra, A., Scheuer, J., and Sonnenblick, E. H. (1982): Contractile behavior of rat myocardium after reversal of hypertensive hypertrophy. *Am. J. Physiol.*, 242:H882–H889.

30. Carew, T. E., and Covell, J. W. (1979): Fiber orientation in hypertrophied canine left ventricle. *Am. J. Physiol.*, 236:H487–H493.

31. Carey, R. A., Tipton, C. M., and Lund, D. R. (1976): Influence of training on myocardial responses of rats subjected to conditions of ischemia and hypoxia. *Cardiovas. Res.*, 10:359–367.

32. Clausen, J. P. (1977): Effect of physical training on cardiovascular adjustments to exercise in man. *Physiol. Rev.*, 57:779–815.

33. Codini, M. A., Yipintsoi, T., and Scheuer, J. (1977): Cardiac responses to moderate training in rats. *J. Appl. Physiol.*, 42:262–266.

34. Cohen, J. I., Gupta, P. K., Lichstein, E., and Chadda, K. D. (1980): The heart of a dancer: noninvasive cardiac evaluation of professional ballet dancers. *Am. J. Cardiol.*, 45:959–965.

35. Cohen, M. V., Yipintsoi, T., Malhotra, A., Penpargkul, S., and Scheuer, J. (1978): Effect of exercise on collateral development in dogs with normal coronary arteries. *J. Appl. Physiol.*, 45:797–805.

36. Cohen, M. V., and Yipintsoi, T. (1979): Myocardial performance and collateral flow after transient coronary occlusion in exercising dogs. *Am. J. Physiol.*, 237:H520–H527.

37. Cohen, M. V. (1983): Influence of exercise and training programs on coronary vascularity and collateral blood flow. *Exerc. Sport Sci. Rev.*, 11:55–98.

38. Cohen, M. V., Yipintsoi, T., and Scheuer, J. (1982): Coronary collateral stimulation by exercise in dogs with stenotic coronary arteries. *J. Appl. Physiol.*, 52:664–671.

39. Crawford, M. H., and O'Rourke, R. A. (1979): The athlete's heart. *Adv. Intern. Med.*, 24:311–329.

40. Crawford, M. H., White, D. H., and Amon, K. W. (1979): Echocardiographic evaluation of left ventricular size and performance during handgrip and upright bicycle exercise. *Circulation*, 59:1188–1196.

41. Cutilletta, A. F., Edmiston, K., and Dowell, R. T. (1979): Effect of a mild exercise program on myocardial function and the development of hypertrophy. *J. Appl. Physiol.*, 46:354–360.

42. Denenberg, D. L. (1972): The effects of exercise on the coronary collateral circulation. *J. Sports Med. Phys. Fitness*, 18:76–81.

43. DeMaria, A. N., Neumann, A., Lee, G., Fowler, W., and Mason, D. T. (1978): Alterations in ventricular mass and performance induced by exercise training in man evaluated by echocardiography. *Circulation*, 57:237–243.

44. DeMaria, A. N., Neuman, A., Schubart, P. J., Lee, G., and Mason, D. T. (1979): Systemic correlation of cardiac chamber size and ventricular performance determined with echocardiography and alterations in heart rate in normal persons. *Am. J. Cardiol.*, 43:1–8.

45. Dohm, G. L., Pennington, S. N., and Baraket, H. (1976): Effect of exercise training on adenyl cyclase and phosphodiesterase in skeletal muscle, heart and liver. *Biochem. Med.*, 16:138–142.

46. Dohm, G. L., Beecher, G. R., Stephenson, T. P., and Womack, M. (1977): Adaptations to endurance training at three intensities of exercise. *J. Appl. Physiol.*, 42:753–757.

47. Dowell, R. T., Cutilletta, A. F., Rudnik, M. A., and Sodt, P. C. (1976): Heart functional responses to pressure overload in exercised and sedentary rats. *J. Appl. Physiol.*, 230:199–204.

48. Dowell, R. T., Tipton, C. M., and Tomanek, R. J. (1976): Cardiac enlargement mechanisms with exercise training and pressure overload. *J. Mol. Cell. Cardiol.*, 8:407–418.

49. Dowell, T., Stone, H. L., Sordahl, L. A., and Asimakis, G. K. (1977): Contractile function and myofibrillar ATPase activity in the exercise-trained dog heart. *J. Appl. Physiol.*, 43:977–982.

50. Donald, K. W., Lind, A. R., McNicol, G. W., Humphreys, P. W., Taylor, S. H., and Staunton, H. P. (1967): Cardiovascular responses to sustained (static) contractions. *Circ. Res.*, 20:(Suppl. I):I-15–I-30.

51. Eckstein, R. W. (1957): Effect of exercise and coronary artery narrowing on coronary collateral circulation. *Circ. Res.*, 5:230–235.

52. Eshani, A. A., Hagberg, J. M., and Hickson, R. C. (1978): Rapid changes in left ventricular dimensions and mass in response to physical conditioning and deconditioning. *Am. J. Cardiol.*, 42:52–56.

53. Flaim, S. F., Minteer, W. J., Clark, D. P., and Zelis, R. (1979): Cardiovascular responses to acute aquatic and treadmill exercise in the untrained rat. *J. Appl. Physiol.*, 46:302–308.

54. Fox, S. M. III, Naughton, J. P., and Haskell, W. L. (1971): Physical activity and the prevention of coronary heart disease. *Ann. Clin. Res.*, 3:404–432.
55. Frick, M. H., Konttinen, A., and Sarajas, H. S. S. (1963): Effects of physical training on circulation at rest and during exercise. *Am. J. Cardiol.*, 12:142–147.
56. Frick, M. H., Sjogren, A.-L., Perasalo, J., and Pajunen, S. (1970): Cardiovascular dimensions and moderate physical training in young men. *J. Appl. Physiol.*, 29:452–455.
57. Fröberg, S. O. (1970): Effects of training and of acute exercise in trained rats. *Metabolism*, 20:1044–1051.
58. Fuller, E. O., and Nuttler, D. O. (1981): Endurance training in the rat. II. Performance of isolated and intact heart. *J. Appl. Physiol.*, 51:941–947.
59. Gandee, R. N., Anthony, J. R., Bartels, R. L., Lanese, R. R., and Fox, E. L. (1972): Effect of interval training on systolic time intervals (Abstract). *Physiologist*, 15:141.
60. Gilbert, C. A., Nutter, D. O., Felner, J. M., Perkins, J. V., Heymsfield, S. B., and Schlant, R. C. (1977): Echocardiographic study of cardiac dimensions and function in the endurance-trained athlete. *Am. J. Cardiol.*, 40:528–533.
61. Guisti, R., Bersohn, M. M., Malhotra, A., and Scheuer, J. (1978): Cardiac function and actomyosin ATPase activity in hearts of conditioned and deconditioned rats. *J. Appl. Physiol.*, 44:171–174.
62. Gollnick, P. D., Struck, P. J., Bogyo, T. P. (1967): Lactic dehydrogenase activities of rat heart and skeletal muscle after exercise and training. *J. Appl. Physiol.*, 22:623–627.
63. Grant, C., Bunnel, I. L., and Greene, D. G. (1965): Left ventricular enlargement and hypertrophy. *Am. J. Med.*, 39:895–904.
64. Grimby, G., and Saltin, B. (1966): Physiological analysis of physically well-trained, middle-aged and old athletes. *Acta Med. Scand.*, 197:513–526.
65. Grimm, A. R., Kubota, R., and Whitehorn, W. V. (1963): Properties of myocardium in cardiomegaly. *Circ. Res.*, 12:118–124.
66. Grossman, W., Jones, D., and McLaurin, L. P. (1975): Wall stress and patterns of hypertrophy in the human left ventricle. *J. Clin. Invest.*, 56:56–64.
67. Grove, D., Nair, K. G., and Zak, R. (1969): Biochemical correlates of cardiac hypertrophy. II. Changes in DNA content: relative contributions of polyploidy and mitotic activity. *Circ. Res.*, 25:463–471.
68. Grove, D., Zak, R., Nair, K. G., and Aschenbrenner, V. (1969): Biochemical correlates of cardiac hypertrophy. IV. Observation on the cellular organization of growth during myocardial hypertrophy in the rat. *Circ. Res.*, 25:473–485.
69. Hakkila, J. (1955): Studies on the myocardial cappillary concentration in cardiac hypertrophy due to training. *Ann. Med. Exp. Fenniae.*, 33:1–82.
70. Hanson, J. S. (1973): Maximal exercise performance in members of the US Nordic Ski Team. *J. Appl. Physiol.*, 35:592–595.
71. Harpur, R. P. (1980): The rat as a model for physical fitness studies. *Comp. Biochem. Physiol.*, 66A:553–574.
72. Haskel, W. L., Savin, W. M., Schroeder, J. S., Alderman, E. A., Ingles, N. B., Jr., Daughters, G. T., II, and Stinson, E. B. (1981): Cardiovascular responses to handgrip exercise in patients following cardiac transplantation. *Circ. Res.*, 48(Suppl. I):I-156–I-161.
73. Haslan, R. W., and Stull, G. A. (1974): Duration and frequency of training as determinants of coronary tree capacity in the rat. *Res. Q. Am. Assoc. Health Phys. Ed.*, 45:178–184.
74. Heath, G. W., Hagberg, J. M., Eshani, A. A., and Holloszy, J. O. (1981): A physiological comparison of young and older endurance athletes. *J. Appl. Physiol.*, 51:634–640.
75. Heaton, W. H., Marr, K. C., Capurro, N. L., Goldstein, R. E., and Epstein, S. E. (1978): Beneficial effect of physical training on blood flow to myocardium perfused by chronic collaterals in the exercising dog. *Circulation*, 57: 575–581.
76. Heiss, H. W., Barmeyer, J., Wink, K., Hell, G., Cerny, F. T., Keul, J., and Reindell, H. (1976): Studies on the regulation of myocardial flow in man. I. Training effects on blood flow and metabolism of the healthy heart at rest and during standardized heavy exercise. *Basic Res. Cardiol.*, 71:658–675.
77. Henry, W. L., Clark, C. E., and Epstein, S. E. (1973): Asymmetric septal hypertrophy: echocardiographic identification of the pathognomonic abnormality of IHSS. *Circulation*, 47:225–231.
78. Hepp, A., Hansis, M., Gulch, R., and Jacob, R. (1974): Left ventricular isovolumetric pressure-

volume relations, "diastolic tone", and contractility in the rat heart after physical training. *Basic Res. Cardiol.*, 69:516–531.

79. Hickson, R. C., Hammons, G. T., and Holloszy, J. O. (1979): Development and regression of exercised-induced cardiac hypertrophy in rats. *Am. J. Physiol.*, 236:H268–H272.

80. Holloszy, J. O., and Booth, F. W. (1976): Biochemical adaptations to endurance exercise in muscle. *Ann. Rev. Physiol.*, 38:273–291.

81. Holmgren, A., and Strandell, T. (1959): The relationship between heart volume, total hemoglobin and physical working capacity in former athletes. *Acta Med. Scand.*, 163:149–160.

82. Hood, W. P., Jr., Rackley, C. E., and Rolett, E. L. (1968): Wall stress in the normal and hypertrophied human left ventricle. *Am. J. Cardiol.*, 22:550–558.

83. Horwitz, L. D., Atkins, J. M., and Leshin, S. J. (1972): Role of the Frank-Starling mechanism in exercise. *Circ. Res.*, 31:868–875.

84. Ikaheimo, M. J., Palatsi, I. J., and Takkunen, J. T. (1979): Noninvasive evaluation of the athletic heart: sprinters versus endurance runners. *Am. J. Cardiol.*, 44:24–29.

85. Kaplinsky, E., Hood, W. H., Jr., McCarthy, B., McCombs, H. L., and Lown, B. (1968): Effects of physical training in dogs with coronary artery ligation. *Circulation*, 37:556–565.

86. Keul, J. (1971): Myocardial metabolism in athletes. In: *Muscle Metabolism During Exercise*, edited by B. Pernow and B. Saltin, pp. 447–455. Plenum Press, New York.

87. Keul, J., Dickhuth, H.-H., Simon, G., and Lehman, M. (1981): Effect of static and dynamic exercise on heart volume, contractility and left ventricular dimension. Circ. Res., 48(Suppl. I):I-162–I-170.

88. Lamb, D. R., Peter, J. B., Jeffress, R. N., and Wallace, H. A. (1969): Glycogen, hexokinase and glycogen synthetase adaptations to exercise. *Am. J. Physiol.*, 217:1628–1632.

89. Laughlin, M. H., Diana, J. N., and Tipton, C. M. (1978): Effects of exercise training on coronary reactive hyperemia and blood flow in the dog. *J. Appl. Physiol.*, 45:604–610.

90. Laurenceau, J. L., Turrat, J., and Dumesnil, J. (1977): Echocardiographic findings in olympic athletes (Abstract). *Circulation*, 56(Suppl. III):III-25.

91. LeBlanc, J., Boulay, M., Dulac, S., Jobin, M., Lebrie, A., and Rousseau-Migneron, S. (1977): Metabolic and cardiovascular responses to norepinephrine in trained and untrained human subjects. *J. Appl. Physiol.*, 42:166–173.

92. Leon, A. S., and Bloor, C. M. (1968): Effects of exercise and its cessation on the heart and blood supply. *J. Appl. Physiol.*, 24:485–490.

93. Leon, A. S., and Bloor, C. M. (1976): The effect of complete and partial deconditioning on exercise-induced cardiovascular changes in the rat. *Adv. Cardiol.*, 18:81–92.

94. Lind, A. R., and McNicol, G. W. (1967): Circulatory responses to sustained hand-grip contractions performed during other exercise, both rhythmic and static. *J. Physiol. (Lond.)*, 192:595–607.

95. Ljungqvist, A., and Unge, G. (1973): The proliferation activity of the myocardial tissue in various forms of experimental cardiac hypertrophy. *Acta, Pathol. Microbiol. Scand. [A]*, 81,3:233–240.

96. Longhurst, J. C., Kelly, A. R., Gonyea, W. J., and Mitchell, J. H. (1980): Echocardiographic left ventricular masses in distance runners and weight lifters. *J. Appl. Physiol.*, 48:154–162.

97. Longhurst, J. C., Kelly, A. R., Gonyea, W. J., and Mitchell, J. H. (1980): Cardiovascular responses to static exercise in distance runners and weight lifters. *J. Appl. Physiol.*, 49:676–683.

98. Malhotra, A., Bhan, A., and Scheuer, J. (1976): Cardiac actomyosin ATPase activity after prolonged physical conditioning and deconditioning. *Am. J. Physiol.*, 230:1622–1625.

99. Malhotra, A., Penpargkul, S., Schaible, T., and Scheuer, J. (1981): Contractile proteins and sarcoplasmic reticulum in physiologic cardiac hypertrophy. *Am. J. Physiol.*, 241:H263–H267.

100. Mandache, E., Unge, G., Appelgren, L.-E., and Ljungqvist, A. (1973): The proliferative activity of the heart tissues in various forms of experimental cardiac hypertrophy studied by electron microscopic autoradiography. *Virchow Arch. [Cell Pathol.]*, 12:112–122.

101. Maron, B. J., Roberts, W. C., McAllister, H. A., Rosing, D. R., and Epstein, S. E. (1980): Sudden death in young athletes. *Circulation*, 62:218–229.

102. Mazher Jaweed, M., Herbison, G. J., Ditunno, J. F., Jr., and Gordon, E. E. (1974): Heart weight of rat in different exercises. *Arch. Phys. Med. Rehabil.*, 55:539–544.

103. McArdle, W. D. (1967): Metabolic stress of endurance swimming in the laboratory rat. *J. Appl. Physiol.*, 24:98–101.

104. McElroy, C. L., Gissen, S. A., and Fiskein, M. C. (1978): Exercise-induced reduction in myocardial infarct size after coronary artery occlusion in the rat. *Circulation*, 57:958–962.

105. Mercadier, J.-J., Lompre, A.-M., Wisnewsky, C., Samuel, J.-L., Bercovici, J., Swynghedauw,

B., and Schwartz, K. (1981): Myosin isoenzymic changes in several models of rat cardiac hypertrophy. *Circ. Res.*, 49:525–532.

106. Mitchell, J. H., and Wildenthal, K. (1974): Static (isometric exercise) and the heart: physiological and clinical considerations. *Annu. Rev. Med.*, 25:369–381.

107. Mitchell, J. H., Blomqvist, C. G., Lind, A. R., Saltin, B., and Shepherd, J. T., editors (1981): Static (isometric) exercise: Cardiovascular responses and neural control mechanisms. *Circ. Res.*, 48:I-1–I-188.

108. Mole, P. A. (1978): Increased contractile potential of papillary muscles from exercised-trained rat hearts. *Am. J. Physiol.*, 234:H421–H425.

109. Moore, R. L., Riedy, M., and Gollnick, P. D. (1982): Effect of training on B-adrenergic receptor number in rat heart. *J. Appl. Physiol.*, 52:1133–1137.

110. Morganroth, J. B., Marion, B. J., Henry, W. L., and Epstein, S. E. (1975): Comparative left ventricular dimensions in trained athletes. *Ann. Intern. Med.*, 82:521–524.

111. Morris, J. N., Adam, C., Chave, S. P. W., Sirey, C., Epstein, L., and Sheehan, D. J. (1973): Vigorous exercise in leisure-time and the incidence of coronary artery disease. *Lancet*, 2:333–339.

112. Muntz, K. H., Gonyea, W. J., and Mitchell, J. H. (1981): Cardiac hypertrophy in response to an isometric training program in the cat. *Circ. Res.*, 49:1092–1101.

113. Neill, W. A., and Oxendine, J. M. (1979): Exercise can promote coronary collateral development without improving perfusion of ischemic myocardium. *Circulation*, 60:1513–1519.

114. Nishimura, T., Yamada, Y., and Kawai, C. (1980): Echocardiographic evaluation of long-term effects of exercise on left ventricular hypertrophy and function in professional bicyclists. *Circulation*, 61:832–840.

115. Nutter, D. O., and Fuller, E. O. (1977): The role of isolated cardiac muscle preparations in the study of training effects on the heart. *Med. Sci. Sports*, 9:239–245.

116. Nutter, D. O., Priest, R. E., and Fuller, E. O. (1981): Endurance training in the rat. I. Myocardial mechanics and biochemistry. *J. Appl. Physiol.*, 51:934–940.

117. Oscai, L. B., and Holloszy, J. O. (1969): Effects of weight changes produced by exercise, food restriction, or overeating on body composition. *J. Clin. Invest.*, 48:2124–2128.

118. Oscai, L. B., Mole, P. A., Brei, B., and Holloszy, J. O. (1971): Cardiac growth and respiratory enzyme levels in male rats subjected to a running program. *Am. J. Physiol.*, 220:1238–1241.

119. Oscai, L. B., Mole, P. A., and Holloszy, J. O. (1971): Effect of exercise on cardiac weight and mitochondria in male and female rats. *Am. J. Physiol.*, 220:1944–1948.

120. Paffenberger, R. S., Jr., and Hale, W. E. (1975): Work activity and coronary heart mortality. *N. Engl. J. Med.*, 292:545–550.

121. Parker, B. M., Londeree, B. R., Cupp, G. V., and Dubiel, J. P. (1978): The noninvasive cardiac evaluation of long-distance runners. *Chest*, 73:376–381.

122. Paulsen, W., Boughner, D. R., Ko, D., Cunningham, D. A., and Persaud, J. A. (1981): Left ventricular function in marathon runners. *J. Appl. Physiol.*, 51:881–886.

123. Paulik, G., and Frankl, R. (1975): Sensitivity to catecholamines and histamine in the trained and in the untrained human organism and sensitivity changes during digestion. *Eur. J. Appl. Physiol.*, 34:199–204.

124. Perez-Gonzales, J. F., Schiller, N. B., and Parmley, W. W. (1981): Direct and non-invasive evaluation of the cardiovascular response to isometric exercise. *Circ. Res.*, 48(Suppl. I):I-138–I-148.

125. Perez-Gonzales, J. F. (1981): Factors determining the blood pressure responses to isometric exercise. *Circ. Res.*, 48(Suppl. I):I-76–I-86.

126. Penpargkul, S., and Scheuer, J. (1970): The effect of physical training upon the mechanical and metabolic performance of the rat heart. *J. Clin. Invest.*, 49:1859–1868.

127. Penpargkul, S., Repke, D. I., and Katz, A. M., and Scheuer, J. (1977): Effect of physical training on calcium transport by rat cardiac sarcoplasmic reticulum. *Circ. Res.*, 40:134–138.

128. Penpargkul, S., Schwartz, A., and Scheuer, J. (1978): Effect of physical conditioning on cardiac mitochondrial function. *J. Appl. Physiol.*, 45:978–986.

129. Penpargkul, S., Malhotra, A., Schaible, T., and Scheuer, J. (1980): Cardiac contractile proteins and sarcoplasmic reticulum in hearts of rats trained by running. *J. Appl. Physiol.*, 48:409–413.

130. Peronnet, F., Perrault, H., Cleroux, J., Cousineau, D., Nadeau, R., Pham-Huy, H., Tremblay, G., and Lebeau, R. (1980): Electro- and echocardiographic study of the left ventricle in man after training. *Eur. J. Appl. Physiol.*, 45:125–130.

131. Pfeffer, M. A., Ferrel, B. A., Pfeffer, J. M., Weiss, A. K., Fishbein, M. C., and Frohlich, E. D.

(1978): Ventricular morphology and pumping ability of exercised spontaneously hypertensive rats. *Am. J. Physiol.*, 235:H193–H199.

132. Poliner, L. R., Dehmer, G. J., Lewis, S. E., Parkey, R. W., Blomqvist, C. G., and Willerson, J. T. (1980): Left ventricular performance in normal subjects; a comparison of the responses to exercise in the upright and supine position. *Circulation*, 62:528–534.

133. Poupa, O., and Rakusan, K. (1966): The terminal microcirculatory bed in the heart of athletic and non-athletic animals. In: *Physical Activity in Health and Disease*, edited by K. Evang, and K. L. Anderson, pp. 18–29. Universitetsforlaget, Oslo.

134. Pyorala, K., Karvonen, M. J., Taskinen, P., Takkunen, J., Kyronseppa, H., and Peltokaillo, P. (1967): Cardiovascular studies on former endurance athletes. *Am. J. Cardiol.*, 20:191–205.

135. Raskoff, W. J., Goldman, S., and Cohn, K. (1976): The "Athletic Heart". Prevalence and physiological significance of left ventricular enlargement in distance runners. *JAMA*, 236:158–162.

136. Reidhammer, H. H., Rafflenbeul, W., Weihe, W. H., and Krayenbuhl, H. P. (1976): Left ventricular contractile function in trained dogs. *Basic Res. Cardiol.*, 71:297–308.

137. Rerych, S. K., Scholz, P. M., Newman, G. E., Sabiston, D. C., Jr., and Jones, R. H. (1978): Cardiac function at rest and during exercise in normals and in patients with coronary artery disease: Evaluation by radionuclide and angiocardiography. *Ann. Surg.*, 187:449–464.

138. Rerych, S. K., Scholz, P. M., Sabiston, D. C., and Jones, R. H. (1980): Effects of exercise training on left ventricular function in normal subjects: A longitudinal study by radionuclide angiography. *Am. J. Cardiol.*, 45:244–252.

139. Restorf, W. von, Holtz, J., and Bassenge, E. (1977): Exercise induced augmentation of myocardial oxygen extraction in spite of normal coronary dilatory capacity in dogs. *Pflugers Arch.*, 372:181–185.

140. Ritzer, T. F., Bove, A. A., and Carey, R. A. (1980): Left ventricular performance characteristics in trained and sedentary dogs. *J. Appl. Physiol.*, 48:130–138.

141. Roeske, W. R., O'Rourke, R. A., Klein, A., Leopold, G., and Karliner, J. S. (1976): Noninvasive evaluation of ventricular hypertrophy in professional athletes. *Circulation*, 53:286–292.

142. Rowell, L. B. (1962): Factors affecting the prediction of the maximal oxygen intake from measurements made during submaximal work with observations related to factors which may limit maximal oxygen intake. Thesis. Minneapolis.

143. Rowell, L. B. (1974): Human cardiovascular adjustments to exercise and thermal stress. *Physiol. Rev.*, 54:75–159.

144. Rupp, H., and Jacob, R. (1982): Response of blood pressure and cardiac myosin polymorphism to swimming training in the spontaneously hypertensive rat. *Can. J. Physiol. Pharmacol.*, 60:1098–1103.

145. Saltin, B., and Astrand, P.-O. (1967): Maximal oxygen uptake in athletes. *J. Appl. Physiol.*, 23:353–358.

146. Saltin, B., Blomqvist, G., Mitchell, J. H., Johnson, R. L., Wildenthal, K., and Chapman, C. B. (1968): Response to exercise after bedrest and after training. *Circulation*, 38(Suppl. VII):VII-1–VII-78.

147. Sanders, M., White, F. C., Peterson, T. M., and Bloor, C. M. (1978): Effects of endurance exercise on coronary collateral blood flow in miniature swine. *Am. J. Physiol.*, 234:H614–H619.

148. Schaible, T. F., and Scheuer, J. (1979): Effects of physical training by running or swimming on ventricular performance of rat hearts. *J. Appl. Physiol.*, 46:854–860.

149. Schaible, T. F., Penpargkul, S., and Scheuer, J. (1981): Differences in male and female rats in cardiac conditioning. *J. Appl. Physiol.*, 50:112–117.

150. Schaible, T. F., and Scheuer, J. (1981): Cardiac function in hypertrophied hearts from chronically exercised female rats. *J. Appl. Physiol.*, 50:1140–1145.

151. Schaper, W. (1982): Influence of physical exercise on coronary collateral blood flow in chronic experimental two-vessel disease. *Circulation*, 65:905–912.

152. Scheel, K. W., Ingram, L. A., and Wilson, J. L. (1981): Effects of exercise on the coronary and collateral vesculature of beagles with and without coronary occlusion. *Circ. Res.*, 48:523–580.

153. Scheuer, J., Kapner, L., Stringfellow, C. A., Armstrong, C. L., and Penpargkul, S. (1970): Glycogen, lipid, and high energy phosphate stores in hearts from conditioned rats. *J. Lab. Clin. Med.*, 75:924–929.

154. Scheuer, J., and Stezoski, S. W. (1972): Effect of physical training on the mechanical and metabolic response of the rat heart to hypoxia. *Circ. Res.*, 30:418–429.

155. Scheuer, J., Penpargkul, S., and Bhan, A. K. (1973): Effect of physical conditioning upon

metabolism and performance of the rat heart. In: *Recent Advances in Studies on Cardiac Structure and Metabolism*, edited by N. S. Dhalla and G. Ronna, pp. 145–149. University Park, Baltimore.

156. Scheuer, J. (1977): The advantages and disadvantages of the isolated perfused working rat heart. *Med. Sci. Sports*, 9:231–238.

157. Scheuer, J., and Tipton, C. M. (1977): Cardiovascular adaptations to physical training. *Annu. Rev. Physiol.*, 39:221–251.

158. Scheuer, J., and Bhan, A. K. (1979): Cardiac contractile proteins. Adenosine triphosphatase activity and physiological function. *Circ. Res.*, 45:1–12.

159. Scheuer, J. (1982): Effects of physical training on myocardial vascularity and perfusion. *Circulation*, 66:491–495.

160. Scheuer, J., Malhotra, A., Hirsch, C., Capasso, J., and Schaible, T. F. (1982): Physiologic cardiac hypertrophy corrects contractile protein abnormalities associated with pathologic hypertrophy in rats. *J. Clin. Invest.*, 70:1300–1305.

161. Segal, L. D., Chung, A., Mason, D. T., and Amsterdam, E. A. (1975): Cardiac glycogen in Long-Evans rats: Diurnal patterns and response to exercise. *Am. J. Physiol.*, 229:398–401.

162. Sembrowich, W. L., Knudson, M. B., and Gollnick, P. D. (1977): Muscle metabolism and cardiac function of the myopathic hamster following training. *J. Appl. Physiol.*, 43:936–941.

163. Sharma, B., Goodwin, J. F., Raphael, M. J., Steiner, R. E., Rainbow, R. G., and Taylor, S. H. (1976): Left ventricular function in ischemic heart disease. *Br. Heart J.*, 38:59–70.

164. Shephard, R. E., and Gollnick, P. D. (1976): Oxygen uptake of rats at different workloads. *Pfluegers Arch.*, 362:219–222.

165. Sordahl, L. A., Asimakis, G. K., Dowell, R. T., and Stone, H. L. (1977): Function of selected biochemical systems from the exercised-trained dog heart. *J. Appl. Physiol.*, 42:426–431.

166. Spear, K. I., Koerner, J. E., and Terjung, R. L. (1978): Coronary flow in physically trained rats. *Cardiovas. Res.*, 12:135–143.

167. Stefadourous, M. A., Grossman, W., El Shahawy, M., Stefadourous, F., and Witham, A. C. (1974): Noninvasive study of effect of isometric exercise on left ventricular performance in normal man. *Br. Heart J.*, 36:988–995.

168. Steil, E., Hansis, M., Hepp, A., Kissling, G., and Jacob, R. (1975): Cardiac hypertrophy due to physical exercise—an example of hypertrophy without a decrease in contractility. In: *Recent Advances in Studies on Cardiac Structure and Metabolism*, edited by A. Fleckenstein, and N. S. Dhalla, pp. 491–496. University Park Press, Baltimore.

169. Stein, R. A., Michielli, D., Fox, E. L., and Krasnow, M. (1978): Continuous ventricular dimensions in man during supine exercise and recovery: an echocardiographic study. *Am. J. Cardiol.*, 41:655–660.

170. Stein, R. A., Michielli, D., Diamond, J., Horwitz, B., and Krasnow, N. (1980): The cardiac response to exercise training: echocardiographic analysis at rest and during exercise. *Am. J. Cardiol.*, 46:219–225.

171. Stevenson, J. A. F., Feleki, V., Rechnitzer, P., and Beaton, J. R. (1964): Effect of exercise on coronary tree size in the rat. *Circ. Res.*, 15:265–269.

172. Stone, H. L. (1977): Cardiac function and exercise training in conscious dogs. *J. Appl. Physiol.*, 42:824–832.

173. Stone, H. L. (1977): The unanesthetized instrumented animal preparation. *Med. Sci. Sports*, 9:253–261.

174. Stone, H. L. (1980): Coronary flow, myocardial oxygen consumption and exercise training in dogs. *J. Appl. Physiol.*, 49:759–758.

175. Takahashi, M., Sasayama, S., Kawai, C., and Kotoura, H. (1980): Contractile performance of the hypertrophied ventricle in patients with systemic hypertension. *Circulation*, 62:116–126.

176. Tepperman, J., and Pearlman, D. (1961): Effects of exercise and anemia on coronary arteries of small animals as revealed by the corrosion cast technique. *Circ. Res.*, 11:576–584.

177. Thadani, U., and Parker, J. O. (1978): Hemodynamics at rest and during supine and sitting bicycle exercise in normal subjects. *Am. J. Cardiol.*, 41:52–59.

178. Tibbets, G., Koziol, B. J., Roberts, N. K., Baldwin, K. M., and Barnard, R. J. (1978): Adaptation of the rat myocardium to endurance training. *J. Appl. Physiol.*, 44:85–89.

179. Tibbits, G. F., Negatomo, T., Sasaki, M., and Barnard, R. J. (1981): Cardiac sarcolemma: Compositional adaptation to exercise. *Science*, 213:1271–1273.

180. Tibbets, G. F., Barnard, R. J., Baldwin, K. M., Cugalj, N., and Roberts, N. K. (1981): Influence

of exercise on excitation-contraction coupling in rat myocardium. *Am. J. Physiol.*, 240:H472–H480.

181. Tipton, C. M., Carey, R. A., Eastin, W. C., and Erickson, H. H. (1974): A Submaximal test for dogs: evaluation of effects of training, detraining, and cage confinement. *J. Appl. Physiol.*, 37:271–275.

182. Tomanek, R. J. (1970): Effects of age and exercise on the extent of the myocardial capillary bed. *Anat. Rec.*, 167:55–62.

183. Underwood, R. H., and Schwade, J. L. (1977): Noninvasive analysis of cardiac function of elite distance runners—echocardiography, vectorcardiography and cardiac intervals. *Ann. NY Acad. Sci.*, 301:297–309.

184. Vatner, S. F., Franklin, D., Higgins, C. B., Patrick, T., and Braunwald, E. (1972): Left ventricular response to severe exertion in untethered dogs. *J. Clin. Invest.*, 51:3052–3057.

185. Wachtlova, M., Rakusan, K., and Poupa, O. (1965): The coronary terminal vascular bed in the heart of the hare (Lepus Europeus) and the rabbit (Oryctolagus Domesticus). *Physiol. Bohemoslov.*, 14:328–331.

186. Weiss, J. L., Weisfeldt, M. L., Mason, S. J., Garrison, J. B., Livengood, S. V., and Fortuin, N. J. (1979): Evidence of Frank-Starling effect in man during severe semisupine exercise. *Circulation*, 59:655–661.

187. Wexler, B. C., and Greenberg, B. P. (1974): Effect of exercise on myocardial infarction in young vs old male rats: electrocardiograph changes. *Am. Heart J.*, 88:343–350.

188. Wikman-Coffelt, J., Parmley, W. W., and Mason, D. T. (1979): The cardiac hypertrophy process. Analyses of factors determining pathological vs. physiological development. *Circ. Res.*, 45:697–707.

189. Williams, J. F., and Potter, R. D. (1976): Effect of exercise conditioning on the intrinsic contractile state of the cat myocardium. *Circ. Res.*, 39:425–428.

190. Williams, R. S. (1980): Physical conditioning and membrane receptors for cardioregulatory hormones. *Cardiovas. Res.*, 14:177–182.

191. Williams, R. S., Schaible, T. F., Bishop, T., and Morey, M. (1982): Effects of endurance training on cholinergic and adrenergic receptors of rat heart. *J. Mol. Cell. Cardiol. (in press)*.

192. Williams, R. S., Eden, R. S., Moll, M., Lester, R. M., and Wallace, A. G. (1981): Mechanisms of training bradycardia: Studies of beta receptors in man. *J. Appl. Physiol.*, 51:1232–1237.

193. Wolfe, L. A., Cunningham, D. A., Davis, G. M., and Rosenfeld, H. (1978): Relationship between maximal oxygen uptake and left ventricular function in exercise. *J. Appl. Physiol.*, 44:44–49.

194. Wolfe, L. A., Cunningham, D. A., Rechnitzer, P. A., and Nichol, P. M. (1979): Effects of endurance training on left ventricular dimensions in healthy men. *J. Appl. Physiol.*, 47:207–212.

195. Wyatt, H. L., and Mitchell, J. H. (1974): Influences of physical training on the heart of dogs. *Circ. Res.*, 35:883–889.

196. Wyatt, H. L., and Mitchell, J. H. (1978): Influence of physical conditioning and deconditioning on coronary vasculature of dogs. *J. Appl. Physiol.*, 45:619–625.

197. Wyatt, H. L., Chuck, L., Rabinowitz, B., Tyberg, J. V., and Parmley, W. W. (1978): Enhanced cardiac response to catecholamines in physically trained rats. *Am. J. Physiol.*, 234:H608–H613.

198. Yipintsosi, T., Rosenkrantz, J., Codini, M. A., and Scheuer, J. (1980): Myocardial blood flow responses to acute hypoxia and volume loading in physically trained rats. *Cardiovasc. Res.*, 14:50–57.

199. York, J. W., Penney, D. G., and Oscai, L. B. (1975): Effects of physical training on several glycolytic enzymes in rat heart. *Biochim. Biophys. Acta*, 381:22–27.

200. Zak, R. (1973): Cell proliferation during cardiac growth. *Am. J. Cardiol.*, 31:211–219.

201. Zeldis, S. M., Morganroth, J., and Rubler, S. (1978): Cardiac hypertrophy in response to dynamic conditioning in female athletes. *J. Appl. Physiol.*, 44:849–852.

202. Zoneraich, S., Rhee, J. J., Zoneraich, O., Jordan, D., and Appel, J. (1977): Assessment of cardiac function in marathon runners by graphic non-invasive techniques. *Ann. NY Acad. Sci.*, 301:900–913.

Growth of the Heart in Health and Disease,
edited by Radovan Zak. Raven Press,
New York © 1984.

Functional Changes in Pathologic Hypertrophy

James F. Spann

*Department of Medicine, Temple University, Health Center,
Philadelphia, Pennsylvania 19140*

When disease causes severe pressure or volume overload of the heart, pathologic cardiac hypertrophy is produced and major changes occur in cardiac pump function, in cardiac muscle contractile function, and in cardiac sympathetic nervous system function. Whether there is a causal relationship between the pathologic hypertrophy and the function abnormalities, or whether both are only simultaneous results of the overload in the heart is unknown. This chapter discusses the abnormalities of cardiac pump, contractile and sympathetic functions that accompany pathologic hypertrophy in the pressure- and volume-overloaded heart.

PRESSURE OVERLOAD

Overview

The contractile and pump functions of the pressure-overloaded heart have been subjects of recent controversy. It is clear that hypertrophy and other compensations maintain pump function in the initial stages of pressure overload. It is equally clear that if overload is excessive and prolonged, pump function eventually fails. But whether systolic contractile function is normal or reduced, in each hypertrophied muscle unit of the pressure-overloaded nonfailing and failing heart has been hotly debated. A number of recent studies make it clear that there is no universally applicable answer to this issue. Rather, the data indicate that within a group of pressure-overloaded hypertrophied hearts, there is a pathologic continuum of systolic contractile muscle function which varies from normal in some hearts to depressed in other hearts. The continuum extends from the one extreme of normally functioning units of hypertrophied muscle in a pressure-overloaded heart with excessive pump function, across the middle ground of moderately dysfunctioned units of hypertrophied muscle in a pressure-overloaded heart which maintains basic pump function, to the other extreme of severely dysfunctioned units of hypertrophied muscle in a pressure-overloaded heart with poor pump function and congestive failure. This portion of the chapter discusses data on the ventricular systolic muscle function and performance in experimental animals and patients with pressure overload of the heart. The relationships among continuing overload, muscle dysfunction, compensatory mechanisms, and the manifestations of heart failure are considered.

Animal Models with Pressure Overload

The presence and degree of myocardial contractile dysfunction in experimental pressure overload vary in direct relation to the extent of the overload stress and correlate with the degree of hypertrophy. These relationships can be best demonstrated by subjecting one species of experimental animal to various degrees of overload.

Various degrees of acute pulmonary artery constriction in the cat have been used in a number of studies in which the right ventricular papillary muscle was isolated and its contractile function analyzed quantitatively. Table 1 provides a summary of the severity of constriction, degree of hypertrophy, and extent of contractile dysfunction in three such studies.

When the pulmonary artery is mildly constricted, hypertrophy is mild and there is no defect of contractile function. Pannier (41) acutely constricted the pulmonary artery of the adult cat to a remaining lumen of approximately 50% of normal and produced 38% hypertrophy of the right ventricle. There was no heart failure. The contractile functions of papillary muscle maximum isotonic shortening and isometric tension development were normal.

When the pulmonary artery is moderately constricted, hypertrophy is moderate and there is no heart failure. Contractile function is only moderately impaired (54) and may return to normal with time (65). Further, such contractile impairment may be limited to a reduction in isotonic shortening whereas isometric tension development remains normal (54). Williams and Potter (65) acutely constricted the pulmonary artery of the adult cat to a remaining lumen of approximately 30% of normal and produced 70% hypertrophy of the right ventricle without heart failure. Papillary muscle contractile function was reduced to approximately 72% of normal at 6 weeks after constriction, but contractile function was normal 24 weeks after constriction. Spann et al. (54) (Fig. 1) acutely constricted the pulmonary artery of the adult cat more severely than Williams and Potter (65) to a remaining lumen of approximately 20% of normal and produced a greater degree of hypertrophy, 91%, without heart failure. In papillary muscles from these hearts, velocity of isometric shortening was reduced to 72% of normal at 3 to 12 weeks after constriction (Fig. 1). The isometric active tension achieved at the apex of the length-tension curve was lowered to 85% of normal, which was not a significant reduction (Fig. 2).

When the pulmonary artery is very severely constricted, hypertrophy is severe, heart failure occurs, and contractile function is severely impaired. Spann et al. (54) also acutely constricted the pulmonary artery of adult cats to a severe degree, leaving a lumen of only 10% of normal. This caused heart failure as well as 142%

TABLE 1. *Relationship of severity and duration of adult cat acute pulmonary artery constriction, extent of right ventricular hypertrophy, and degree of right ventricular papillary muscle contractile dysfunction*

	Degree of PA constriction			Duration of constriction (weeks)	Extent of hypertrophy % increase RV weight	Contractile function % of normal	
Study	PA band size (mm ID)	% Remaining PA lumen	CHF			Isotonic velocity	Isometric tension
Pannier (1)	5.0	50	−	4–24	38	100	100
Williams and Potter (2)	4.0	30	−	6	70	74	70
				24	69	100	100
Spann et al. (3)	3.5	20	−	3–12	91	72	85
Spann et al. (3)	2.8	10	+	3–13	142	38	38

PA = pulmonary artery; CHF = congestive heart failure; ID = internal diameter; RV = right ventricle.

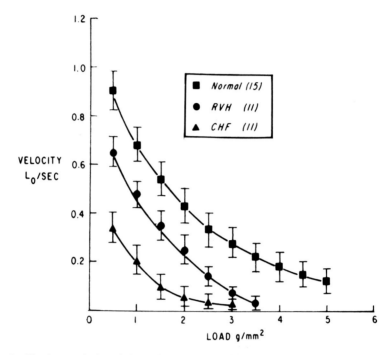

FIG. 1. The force-velocity relations of three groups of cat papillary muscles, normal, right ventricular hypertrophy (RVH), right ventricular hypertrophy and congestive heart failure (CHF). Average values with ± SEM are given for each point. Velocity has been corrected to muscle lengths per second (L_0/sec). Numbers in parentheses indicate number of animals. (Spann et al., ref. 54.)

hypertrophy of the right ventricle. When these animals were studied 3 to 13 weeks after constriction, severe reductions of velocity of isotonic shortening and isometric tension were found (Figs. 1 and 2). Both shortening velocity and active tension development were reduced to 38% of normal.

Two serious questions have been raised concerning the cat model used in the above-mentioned studies. Bishop and Melson (4) questioned the suitability of a model in which sudden and severe strain is placed on the myocardium in a fashion that is not similar to the usual course of events in man. They found areas of focal muscle cell degeneration 30 to 200 μm in diameter 3 to 5 days after banding the pulmonary artery. There was fibroblast activity 7 through 10 days after constriction, and collagen formation occurred by 14 days after constriction. The second question, raised by Williams and Potter (65), pertains to the possibility that the contractile changes are temporary and would resolve themselves over time. However, the results obtained by Williams and Potter (65) vary from the results obtained in four other studies in which acute overloading was used to produce hypertrophy. Bassett and Gelband (3) showed papillary muscle contractile deficits at 7, 21, and 110 days after banding and demonstrated further that the most marked deficit was present at 110 days. Spann et al. (54) showed that contractile deficits present at 3 weeks

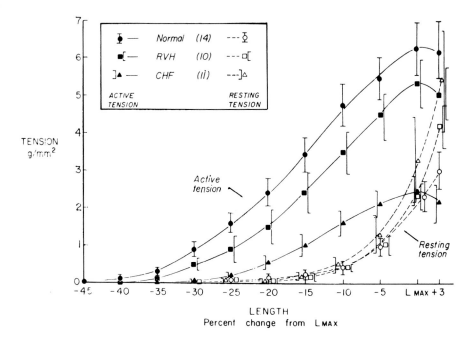

FIG. 2. Relation between muscle length and tension of papillary muscles from normal *(circles)*, hypertrophied (RVH, *squares*) and failing (CHF, *triangles*) right ventricles. *Open symbols* = resting tension; *solid symbols* = actively developed tension. Each value is the average of the group; *vertical lines with cross bars* = ± SEM. Tension is corrected for cross-sectional area (g/mm²). Numbers in parentheses indicate number of animals. (Spann et al., ref. 54.)

after constriction were also present at 13 weeks following acute constriction. Cooper et al. (18) showed contractile abnormalities present at 4 to 6 weeks and at 14 to 16 weeks after acute overload. Meerson and Kapelko (37) showed that contractile deficits were present 450 to 540 days after pressure overload.

Both the question of possible nonpathophysiologic acute damage imposed by sudden imposition of pressure overload and the question of return of function to normal with time were answered in the elegant study by Cooper et al. (20), using a chronic progressive pressure overload model. In this study, kittens were exposed to gradually increasing pressure overload as they grew into an initially nonconstricting band. Right ventricular systolic pressure gradually increased from 25 mm Hg to a stable value of 50 mm Hg at 16 weeks following placement of the pulmonary artery band. The animals were sacrificed 25 and 60 weeks after band placement. Hypertrophy became stable after the full extent of pressure overloading was reached. The right ventricle had 52% hypertrophy at 25 weeks and 44% hypertrophy at 60 weeks. The papillary muscle had contractile abnormalities of isotonic shortening and isometric active tension development at both 25 and 60 weeks after the placement of the pulmonary artery band (Fig. 3). At 25 weeks after banding, isotonic shortening velocity was reduced to 72% of normal, and maximum isometric active

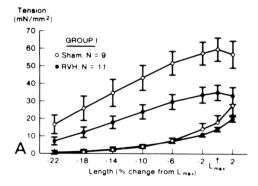

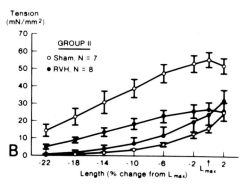

FIG. 3. Contractile function of papillary muscles from cats with gradual onset, chronic pressure overload (RVH). **A** and **B:** Average length-tension values ± SE for the sham-operated and RVH papillary muscles. In each instance, the upper pair of *lines* represents active tension, and the lower pair of *lines* represents resting tension. (Cooper et al., ref. 20.)

tension was reduced to 58% of normal. At 60 weeks after banding, isotonic velocity of shortening was reduced to 67% of normal and maximum isometric active tension was reduced to 46% of normal (Fig. 3). Since this model avoided acute injury produced by acute nonpathophysiologic pressure overload and demonstrated that defects of contractile state were clearly persistent 60 weeks after placement of the band and 44 weeks after development of full, stable pressure overload and hypertrophy, the concerns raised by Bishop and Melson (4) and by Williams and Potter (65) have been obviated.

A third possible question raised by these papillary muscle studies is whether the papillary muscle reflects abnormalities in the intact ventricular wall. Spann and co-workers (1972) determined contractile function of the intact right ventricle and of papillary muscles isolated from those same ventricles in cats. The cats studied were animals with pulmonary artery constriction causing severe ventricular hypertrophy and congestive heart failure. The intact ventricle was studied during isovolumic contractions. The relationship of contractile element velocity and wall tension was determined as one measure of muscle contractile state in the intact ventricle (Fig. 4A). Acute manipulation of end-diastolic volume was used to obtain Frank-Starling relationships of wall tension to mid-wall end-diastolic circumference as a second measure of muscle contractile state in the intact ventricles (Fig. 5). Papillary muscles were then removed from these hearts and isolated in a contraction chamber,

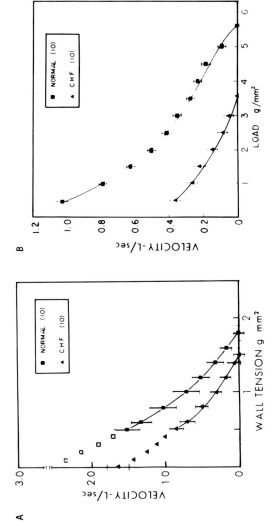

FIG. 4A: Muscle and pump function of the same failing ventricles. Tension-velocity relations of the normal and hypertrophied failing groups of cat right ventricles. Average values with ±SEM are given for each point. Velocity of contractile element is expressed in muscle lengths per second (L₀/sec). Wall tension is expressed in grams per square millimeter (g/mm²). *Points* through which a *line* has been drawn represent average of measured points, while *points* without a *line* represent average values of extrapolated points. Numbers in parentheses indicate number of animals. (Spann et al., ref. 55.) **B:** These are data from the same cats as in **A**. Average values with ±SEM are given for each point. Velocity has been corrected to muscle lengths per second (L₀/sec). Numbers in parentheses represent number of animals. (Spann et al., ref. 55.)

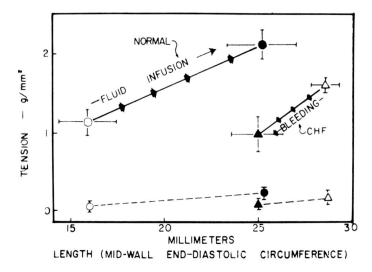

FIG. 5. Intact ventricle length-tension relationships. Acute manipulation of end-diastolic volume to obtain ventricular Frank-Starling curves. *Lines* represent segments of active and resting length-tension curves of five normal cats (normal, *circles*) and five failing cat ventricles (CHF, *triangles*). *Solid lines* represent active tension, while *dashed lines* refer to resting or diastolic tension. *Open symbols* refer to values obtained at spontaneously occurring end-diastolic volume, while *solid symbols* refer to values obtained after volume infusion in normal cats and bleeding of cats with heart failure. Average values $\pm$ SEM are shown. Active and resting tension are expressed as grams per square millimeter (g/mm²) on ordinate, and normalized end-diastolic circumference, or muscle length, is in millimeters on the abscissa. (Spann et al., ref. 55.)

and isotonic contractile velocity (Fig. 4B) and isometric contractile tension were determined. A marked depression of the contractile state of the heart muscle was observed in both the intact ventricles and the isolated papillary muscles removed from these ventricles, and the extent of reduction in the intact ventricle was similar to that found in the isolated muscle (Figs. 4A,B). Isotonic velocity of shortening was reduced by 64% in the papillary muscle whereas calculated velocity of contractile element shortening was reduced by 44% in the intact ventricle from which the papillary muscles had been removed. Isometric active tension was reduced by 54% in the isolated papillary muscle and by 50% in the intact ventricle. Thus, the papillary muscle contractile deficit is present to a similar degree in the intact ventricular wall.

The dog is a second species of experimental animal in which the ventricle has been subjected to various degrees of pressure overload with various degrees of hypertrophy. Again, the presence and degree of myocardial contractile dysfunction vary in direct relation to the extent of the overload stress and correlate with the degree of hypertrophy.

When there is a mild overload, hypertrophy is mild, pump function is increased or normal, and muscle contractile function is normal. Sasayama et al. (45) produced 36% left ventricular hypertrophy by 17 days of acute aortic constriction to a degree that initially increased the calculated peak wall stress by 55%. At first, the left ventricle was dilated by the mild increase in wall stress; it then responded to the pressure overload with increased wall thickness and a resultant fall in wall stress to near normal values. Based on isovolumic and ejection phase indexes, they concluded there was no depression of myocardial contractile function. In addition, in a later study, when Sasayama et al. (46) further examined this model using force-velocity relations, wall stress-diameter loops, and length-tension relations at end-systole, they found a normal level of inotropic state. Carabello et al. (7) produced gradual and mild aortic constriction by allowing puppies to grow into an initially nonconstricting subcoronary aortic band. After 37 weeks growth of the puppies, there was a 29-mm peak systolic gradient across the band, and the aortic lumen was 65% of normal size. This mild overload produced 27% hypertrophy. There was normal myocardial contractile performance as judged by ejection fraction, dP/dt, resting ventricular function (V_{cf}), and stroke work per gram of myocardium. Thus, in two dog models with a mild degree of pressure overload and mild hypertrophy (7,45,46) there was no defect of cardiac contractile function.

Newman and Webb (39) produced a more severe degree of acute aortic constriction and pressure overload in dogs. After 65 days, left ventricular weight was 45% greater than normal. Left ventricular contractile function was determined from quantitative isometric length-tension curves in a segment of the intact ventricle by a specially modified strain gauge. Ventricular muscle function was reduced. At all lengths along the Frank-Starling curve, the hypertrophied heart had a reduced length-active tension relationship.

Pfeffer et al. (42) studied spontaneously hypertensive rats at 6 and 18 months of age compared with normal rats of similar ages. After the rat had systemic hypertension for 6 months, there was a 25% increase in left ventricular weight. After 18 months of pressure overload due to systemic hypertension, there was a 60% increase in left ventricular weight. Left ventricular contractile function was estimated by the Frank-Starling relationship of peak stroke volume ejected from a variable end-diastolic volume and by ejection fraction indexes. In the 6-month-old animals with 25% hypertrophy, left ventricular contractile function was normal as was diastolic volume and end-diastolic pressure. At age 18 months with 60% hypertrophy, there was a depression of left ventricular contractile function with an increase in diastolic volume and end-diastolic pressure. In all cases, the hypertensive animals were compared with age-matched controls. Thus, the left ventricle of the hypertensive rat appears to have an initial compensated phase of normal cardiac performance with normal cardiac contractile function. With time, and in association with a more severe degree of hypertrophy, pump performance of the heart and cardiac contractile function become depressed.

Alpert et al. (2) and Hamrell and Alpert (27a) produced 30% to 60% right ventricular hypertrophy by acute pulmonary artery constriction of 37 to 80 days' duration in rabbits. Papillary muscles from these hearts show a consistent reduction in unloaded shortening velocity but no depression of active tension at the apex of the length-tension curve. Alpert et al. (2) has shown a correlation between this reduction of maximum contractile element velocity and reductions in myosin ATPase. Similar reductions of cardiac myosin ATPase in the hypertrophied heart have subsequently been observed in our laboratory, and the correlation between cardiac myosin ATPase activity and the velocity of isotonic shortening has been described (9–12).

Coulson et al. (21) in our laboratory have examined right ventricular papillary muscles in cats following relief of 2° of pressure overload (Fig. 6). Group I, consisting of cats with 30% remaining pulmonary artery lumens, had right ventricular hypertrophy without heart failure. Their muscle velocity of shortening and ability to develop tension were both depressed, but following relief of the pressure overload, these animals regained normal muscle shortening velocity and load-bearing ability. Group II, consisting of cats with a 13% remaining pulmonary artery lumen, had right ventricular hypertrophy complicated by congestive heart failure. There was severe reduction of both shortening velocity and load-bearing ability. However, when the pressure overload was relieved in the animals with the more severe degree of constriction, unloading shortening velocity returned to normal but the load-bearing ability remained depressed. We concluded that myocardium from animals with congestive heart failure as well as right ventricular hypertrophy was the subject of a double lesion, which reduced both contractile activation and the effective numbers of participating contractile units. When the recovery period was over, the activation defect had been corrected but the depleted numbers of effective contractile units had not been restored.

The notion that systolic muscle function of pressure-overloaded hearts forms a continuum from normal, in some hearts, to depressed, in other hearts, is partially consistent with the earlier work of Meerson (36). He defined three stages of cardiac hypertrophy in response to pressure overload. The first stage of isometric hyperfunction, described as the damage stage, lasts 510 days and is characterized by hyperfunction of the still nonhypertrophied heart with an increase in the breakdown of myocaridal proteins. The second stage is described as a state of relatively stable hyperfunction lasting 410 months in rabbits and rats and 12 years in dogs. Meerson characterized this stage as having normal intensity of function of the cardiac structures with hyperfunction of the organ as a whole and a stable hypertrophied mass. The third stage is that of gradual exhaustion and progressive cardiosclerosis, or a complex of wear. In this stage there is decreased functional capacity of the myocardium. For a time, this decrease in functional capacity is compensated for by the increase in myocardial mass, but later it is progressive and leads to a decreased contractile capacity of the entire heart.

Patients with Pressure Overload

Recent controversy over whether cardiac muscle contractile function is depressed or normal in patients with pressure-overloaded and hypertrophied hearts appears resolved, as many studies now show that it is normal in some patients, mildly depressed in other patients, and severely depressed in others. More severe degrees

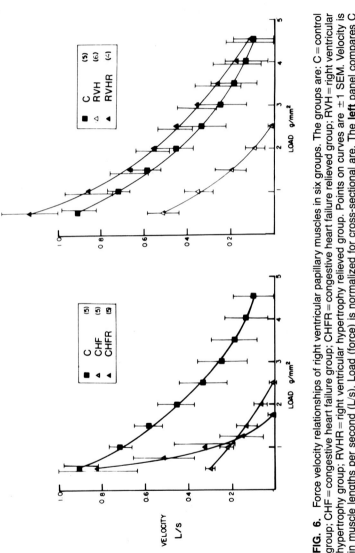

FIG. 6. Force velocity relationships of right ventricular papillary muscles in six groups. The groups are: C = control group; CHF = congestive heart failure group; CHFR = congestive heart failure relieved group; RVH = right ventricular hypertrophy group; RVHR = right ventricular hypertrophy relieved group. Points on curves are ±1 SEM. Velocity is in muscle lengths per second (L/s). Load (force) is normalized for cross-sectional are. The **left** panel compares C group with the CHF and CHFR groups. The **right** panel compares the same C group with the RVH and RVHR groups. Note the CHFR curve which has depressed isometric load but normal unloaded velocity of shortening (see text for detail). Numbers in parentheses represent number of animals. (Coulson et al., ref. 21.)

of pressure overload are associated with the more severe degrees of ventricular hypertrophy, the presence of muscle dysfunction, and the presence of congestive heart failure. While animal studies are limited by the necessity of using models, studies in patients are limited by the difficulties of measuring cardiac muscle contractile function and excluding the effects of afterload and preload alterations. Nevertheless, there are at least 10 well-conducted recent studies that use many different angiographic and echocardiographic methods of measuring cardiac muscle contractile function in patients with aortic stenosis or systemic hypertension (6,13,30,31,33–35,56,57,60). Each of these studies shows at least two groups of patients with ventricular pressure overload. One group has normal cardiac muscle contractile performance. The other group has depressed cardiac muscle performance and often has heart failure. The pathologic continuum from normal to depressed contractile function, which was demonstrated in animal models, is present in patients with naturally occurring pressure overload.

Four recent studies have utilized angiographic techniques in patients with aortic stenosis. Spann et al. (56), in our laboratories, examined ventricular performance and the relationship of compensatory mechanisms to symptoms in 11 patients with severe aortic stenosis and congestive heart failure symptoms, in 10 patients with significant aortic stenosis but no heart failure symptoms, and in 12 normal subjects. The techniques used included computer-assisted analysis of quantitative left ventriculograms and ventricular pressures obtained by either catheter tip micromanometers or fluid filled catheters. Four methods of estimating left ventricular performance were used to account for or avoid problems caused by altered afterload, preload, and wall thickness. Group performance diastolic volume curves (Frank-Starling) and end-systolic pressure-volume relationships (Sagawa) were determined. The slope of the linear regression lines that estimated both the group Frank-Starling relationship and the group end-systolic stress-volume index show statistically significant depression of left ventricular contractile function in the patients with severe aortic stenosis and congestive heart failure ($p > 0.01$). These indexes of ventricular contractile function were relatively normal in patients with significant but compensated aortic stenosis where there were no heart failure symptoms. The relationship of left ventricular end-systolic stress to end-systolic volume index in each patient group is shown in Fig. 7. Although this contractile index is thought to be independent of both preload and afterload, and end-systolic stress was calculated to correct for differences in wall thickness, these techniques have limitations. Naturally occurring variations in end-systolic volume within each group of patients were used to calculate linear regressions to estimate the E_{max} line for each group, and comparisons were made between groups by statistical techniques. Although the demonstrated relationship would have been better defined if each heart had been manipulated through a range of volumes and individual curves obtained, such manipulation would have required mulitple ventriculograms which was not considered safe in patients with aortic stenosis. The left ventricle was hypertrophied to 33% greater than normal ventricular mass in the patients with significant aortic stenosis but no heart failure symptoms and to 127% greater than normal mass in the patients with severe aortic stenosis and congestive heart failure. End-diastolic

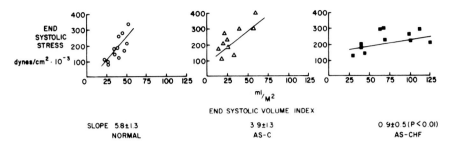

FIG. 7. The relationship of left ventricular end-systolic stress to end-systolic volume index in each patient group. The individual points are shown for each patient. The sloping *solid lines* through the points are the linear regressions. The slope of these linear regressions and their standard errors are shown below panel. The *p* value denotes the significant difference of the AS-CHF slope from both the AS-C and normal slopes. AS-C = patients with aortic stenosis and no symptoms of heart failure; AS-CHF = patients with severe aortic stenosis and heart failure. (Spann et al., ref. 56.)

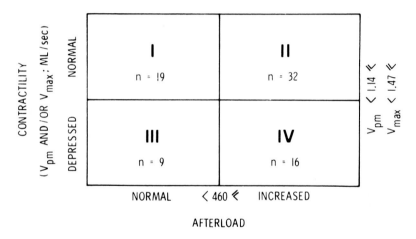

FIG. 8. Grouping of the 76 patients with aortic stenosis into four groups (I–IV) based on peak measured velocity of contractile elements (V) and/or total pressure V (measures of myocardial contractility) and on peak systolic wall stress; dynes·10^3/cm^2 (measure of left ventricular afterload). (Huber et al., ref. 30.)

volume index and pressure were significantly increased ($p > 0.01$) only in the patients with aortic stenosis and congestive failure. Peak systolic wall stress, ejection fraction, resting cardiac index, and the ratio of ventricular mass to volume were not different from normal in either group of aortic stenosis patients.

Huber and colleagues (30) studied 76 patients with valvular aortic stenosis by left ventricular micromanometry and quantitative cineangiography. Ventricular contractile performance was assessed in terms of mean normalized systolic ejection rate, total pressure V_{max}, and peak measured velocity of shortening. Peak systolic circumferential wall stress was also determined. These workers defined four groups of patients with aortic stenosis (Fig. 8). In Group 1 contractility and wall stress were both normal; in Group 2 contractility was normal and wall stress was increased; in Group 3 contractility was depressed and wall stress was normal; and in Group 4, contractility was depressed and wall stress was increased. At normal or increased wall stress, the mean normalized systolic ejection rate was significantly smaller ($p<0.01$) in patients with reduced contractility. Thus, in many patients with aortic stenosis, both depressed contractility and increased afterload or depressed contractility alone are operative in depressing left ventricular ejection performance. As also shown previously by Gunther and Grossman (27), some patients can have normal muscle contractile function with depressed ventricular ejection performance owing to an excessive afterload. The two groups of patients with depressed contractility had ventricular hypertrophy of 149% and 140% of normal mass, significantly greater than in the two groups of patients with normal contractility (88% and 97% ventricular hypertrophy). Left ventricular end-diastolic volume and left ventricular end-diastolic pressure were significantly greater in patients having reduced contractility indexes, even after excluding the effects of variable wall stress.

Carabello et al. (6) also showed that either excessive afterload or depressed contractility may result in depressed ejection performance in patients with aortic stenosis. These workers related ejection fraction to the mean circumferential left ventricular wall stress in 13 patients who had severe aortic stenosis and congestive heart failure. Three of the four patients who had severely depressed contractile function did not survive cardiac surgery owing to inability to be weaned from the heart-lung machine or to postoperative ventricular failure. The other one remained severely symptomatic with New York Heart Association (NYHA) functional class IV symptoms of congestive heart failure. The symptoms of all nine other patients improved after aortic valve replacement.

Levine et al. (34) used three measurements of contractile element velocity to assess the contractile state of the left ventricle in 12 patients with aortic stenosis. Eight patients had normal indexes of contractility, and none of these patients had congestive heart failure. Four patients had depressed values for all three indexes of contractility, and three of these four had clinical and hemodynamic evidence of congestive heart failure.

In addition to these angiographic assessments of contractile function, McDonald (35) used echocardiography to study left ventricular contraction in 45 patients with aortic stenosis. Left ventricular measurements included end-diastolic internal dimension, mural thickness, and fractional shortening, which is an index of circumferential myocardial contraction. In the absence of left ventricular failure in aortic stenosis, there was a normal fractional shortening and a normal end-diastolic internal dimension. When left ventricular failure was present in aortic stenosis, fractional shortening was usually reduced and left ventricular end-diastolic dimension was increased.

A very recent study by Donner et al. (24) at our institution assessed ventricular wall stress, muscle function and pump function in children with severe aortic stenosis but no heart failure. Left ventricular muscle contractile function was estimated by the ratio of end-systolic wall stress to end-systolic volume index, calculation of the ventricular wall stress volume loops, and calculation of the slope of the linear regression lines for group relationships of end-systolic stress to end-systolic volume. Left ventricular muscle contractile function was found to be relatively normal or moderately depressed. Ventricular pump performance, however, was supernormal. Ejection fraction and velocity of fiber shortening were increased, and end-systolic volume index was less than one-half of normal. Over-compensation for the increased left ventricular pressure by extensive ventricular hypertrophy caused a reduction in peak wall stress to less than one-half of normal in the children with aortic stenosis. The extensive reduction in wall stress throughout the stress volume loop resulted in supernormal pump performance despite the normal or moderately reduced muscle contractile function.

Other studies by Wroblewski et al. (67) in our laboratory have examined the dynamic geometry and pump function of the right ventricle subjected to moderate pressure overload due to mitral stenosis. Right ventricular stroke volume was plotted against end-diastolic volume to obtain a ventricular performance index. Calculations revealed that the right ventricle performs normally in patients with moderate pulmonary hypertension resulting from mitral stenosis.

Five recent studies have assessed the contractile performance of the hypertrophied ventricle in patients with left ventricular pressure overload due to systolic hypertension. These studies show results similar to those found in patients with pressure overload and ventricular hypertrophy caused by aortic stenosis. Left ventricular contractile performance was found to be normal in certain patients with systemic hypertension and reduced in others. Coronary artery disease was excluded in the patients in these studies.

Strauer (57) examined left ventricular function at rest and during exercise by angiographic techniques during cardiac catheterization in 88 patients with systemic hypertension. In patients who had compensated essential hypertension without coronary disease, he found left ventricular performance to be either normal or supernormal at rest and during exercise. However, when end-diastolic left ventricular volume increased, there was considerable global contraction disturbance of the left ventricle even at rest.

Takahashi et al. (60), using echocardiography to measure ventricular diameter and posterior wall thickness while simultaneously recording brachial artery pressure, assessed the contractile state of the hypertrophied ventricle in 22 patients with chronic systemic hypertension. The end-systolic wall stress diameter relationship was obtained during several levels of acute pressure reduction by nitroprusside infusion. Lines relating end-systolic wall stress to end-systolic diameter at several different diameters and stresses were then constructed for each patient. The slope of the line relating end-systolic wall stress to end-systolic dimension is a contractile index that is thought to be independent of both preload and afterload. The results showed that there were two groups of patients; one with normal contractile state and one with reduced contractile state. The patients with reduced contractile state had more extensive hypertrophy. In 15 patients with end-diastolic wall thickness up to 1.1 cm, the linear wall stress diameter relationship did not differ from the control group, indicating a normal inotropic state. In the seven patients with end-diastolic wall thickness of 1.3 cm or more, the end-systolic wall stress diameter relationship had a less steep slope, indicating depressed myocardial contractile function.

Chakko et al. (13) in our laboratory recently extended the investigations of Takahashi and colleagues to the study of ventricular contractile function, pump function, and compensatory mechanisms in two groups of patients with systemic hypertension. In one group, the hypertension had caused congestive heart failure; in the other group there was no heart failure. No patient in this study had evidence of coronary artery disease. Arterial pressure and echocardiographic left ventricular volume were measured first in the resting state, then with the legs raised, then during systemic arterial pressure increase by hand-grip, and then during pressure and volume decrease by amyl nitrite inhalation. End-systolic ventricular wall stress was plotted against end-systolic volume index for each of the four states in each patient. This allowed determination of the slope of the relationship between left ventricular stress and volume at end systole in each patient. This determination provided a cardiac contractile index that is felt to be independent of alterations in preload and afterload. This contractile index was significantly depressed in patients with systemic hypertension complicated by congestive heart failure, but it was normal in those patients with hypertension but no congestive heart failure. Peak systolic wall stress and ejection fraction were normal in both groups of hypertensive patients. End-diastolic volume was more than doubled when heart failure complicated hypertension. We interpreted these data as indicating that in systemic hypertension, left ventricular muscle function is initially normal, hypertrophy initially corrects wall stress, and pump function is initially maintained without increased preload or heart failure symptoms. However, left ventricular muscle function eventually becomes depressed, and then, despite the apparently adequate hypertrophy, pump function is maintained by increased end-diastolic volume and heart failure symptoms result.

Similar results were found by Karliner et al. (31) who used echocardiography to study 18 patients with systemic arterial hypertension. Ejection phase indexes of left ventricular performance (mean V_{cf}, fractional shortening, normalized posterior wall velocity, and ejection fraction) were normal at rest in the 16 patients without heart failure. The other two patients, who had recently recovered from an episode of congestive heart failure associated with accelerated hypertension, had reduced values of ejection fraction, mean V_{cf}, and fractional percent shortening.

The above 10 studies use many different methods of assessing ventricular contractile function by angiographic and echocardiographic techniques in patients with ventricular pressure overload of three different types. The data from these studies are consistent with one another and with the previously described animal experiments.

The following conclusions can be derived: At one extreme, when ventricular pressure overload is chronic and severe, hypertrophy becomes extensive, pump function is abnormal, heart failure occurs, and cardiac muscle contractile function is clearly depressed. At the other extreme, when pressure overload is less severe, hypertrophy is less extensive, pump function is normal or even supernormal, there is no heart failure, and muscle contractile function is usually normal. Between these two extremes is a pathologic continuum in which myocardial contractile function and pump function may be normal or abnormal. There may be moderately depressed muscle contractile function in an adequately hypertrophied pressure-overloaded heart which has normal pump function. At times there may be normal muscle contractile function in an excessively overloaded heart where hypertrophy does not normalize ventricular wall stress and systolic ejection pump function is thereby reduced. In children with severe aortic stenosis but no heart failure, pump function may be supernormal, muscle contractile function is normal or moderately reduced, and hypertrophy is extensive, resulting in a striking reduction of ventricular wall stress throughout the systolic contraction together with and an increase in ventricular ejection performance.

Relationship of Muscle Dysfunction, Compensatory Mechanisms, Pump Function, and Manifestations of Heart Failure in Pressure Overload

The pathophysiology that underlies congestive symptoms of heart failure in patients with ventricular pressure overload has been clarified by recent investigations. Five studies in patients (6,13,30,35,56) and three in experimental animals (42,54,55) support the concept that an increase in the end-diastolic volume activates the Frank-Starling mechanism to maintain pump function when muscle function is decreased in the pressure-overloaded heart. Further, the data support the clinical concept that when compensation of pump function and cardiac output is maintained by increased end-diastolic volume, the related rise of end-diastolic pressure precipitates congestive symptoms. If the data are to support these concepts, they should show decreased muscle function, increased diastolic volume, increased diastolic pressure, and relative preservation of resting cardiac output in patients with congestive symptoms of heart failure complicating pressure overload. They do.

As described in detail earlier, cardiac muscle function is usually depressed in patients with pressure-overloaded hearts and congestive heart failure. Muscle function usually is normal, despite pressure overload, when heart failure is absent.

Consistently, end-diastolic volume and pressure are increased in patients and experimental animals with pressure-overloaded hearts and congestive heart failure but are not increased in patients and experimental animals with pressure overload but no heart failure. Spann et al. (56) found a significantly ($p<0.01$) elevated end-diastolic volume index of 147 ml/M^2 (normal 94) in patients with aortic stenosis, congestive heart failure, and depressed myocardial contractile function. Patients with compensated aortic stenosis, no heart failure, and relatively normal myocardial contractile function had a normal end-diastolic volume index of 98. The end-diastolic pressure was significantly elevated in patients with aortic stenosis and congestive heart failure but was not different from normal in patients with aortic stenosis but no heart failure.

Huber et al. (30) found end-diastolic volume indexes of 123 and 137 ml/M^2 in two groups of patients with aortic stenosis and depressed cardiac muscle contractile performance. These values were significantly ($p<0.05$) higher than the end-diastolic volume index of 81 in a group of normal individuals and values of 91 and 107 in two groups of patients with aortic stenosis and normal cardiac muscle contractile function. There were significant increases in end-diastolic pressure and circumferential wall stress in the patients with increased end-diastolic volumes.

McDonald (35) demonstrated echocardiographically that the end-diastolic ventricular dimension was significantly increased ($p<0.01$) to a value of 5.7 cm in a group of patients with severe aortic stenosis and congestive heart failure compared with a value of 4.6 cm in a group of patients with equally severe aortic stenosis but no heart failure.

Carabello et al. (6) found end-diastolic volume indexes of 119 and 174 ml/M^2, values that were higher than the normal value of 64, which was previously reported from that laboratory (27) in two groups of patients with severe aortic stenosis and left ventricular failure. One group had severe left ventricular dysfunction, a poor response to surgical replacement of the aortic valve, and a significantly higher ($p>0.005$) end-diastolic volume (174 ml/M^2) than this volume (119 ml/M^2) in the group of patients with less ventricular dysfunction and a good response to surgery.

In a very recent echocardiographic study from our laboratory by Chakko et al. (13), hypertensive patients with heart failure had end-diastolic volumes that were twice the end-diastolic volumes of normal individuals or of patients with hypertension but no congestive heart failure.

Three experimental animal studies showed similar results. Spann et al. (55) determined right ventricular end-diastolic volume in cats with congestive heart failure and depressed ventricular muscle contractile function due to severe pressure overload; end-diastolic volume was increased ($p<0.01$) from the normal value of 2.0 ml to a value of 3.7 ml in these cats. High end-diastolic volume was associated with a significant ($p<0.01$) elevation of right ventricular end-diastolic pressure (7.0 mm Hg) above the normal value (1.7 mm Hg). Pfeffer et al. (42) found an increased left ventricular end-diastolic pressure in spontaneously hypertensive rats that had depressed ventricular function. End-diastolic volume was also increased in these animals, since the passive pressure volume relations of the failing hearts showed an increased volume compared with normal to equivalent pressures. Spann et al. (54) found an end-diastolic right ventricular pressure of 13 mm Hg in a group of cats with acute severe pulmonary artery constriction and congestive heart failure. This pressure was significantly greater than the values seen in animals with less severe pulmonary artery constriction, right ventricular hypertrophy and no congestive heart failure (5 mm Hg), and in normal animals (2 mm Hg).

Although it is quite variable, cardiac output is often normal at rest in patients and experimental animals with pressure overload, depressed ventricular muscle function, increased diastolic volume, and heart failure. Cardiac output was normal in 14 of 21 cats with congestive heart failure and severe cardiac muscle dysfunction due to pulmonary artery constriction (54,55). Cardiac indexes were normal at rest in 8 of 11 patients with severe aortic stenosis, symptoms of congestive heart failure, depressed cardiac muscle function, and increased end-diastolic volume and pressure (Spann et al., 1976). McDonald (35) found that the cardiac output of patients with aortic stenosis, heart failure, and increased diastolic dimensions was similar to the cardiac output of patients with aortic stenosis, no heart failure and normal diastolic ventricular dimensions. It is important to point out that these concepts refer only to cardiac output at rest. Reduced response of cardiac output to exercise has been demonstrated in such patients (1).

VOLUME OVERLOAD

Overview

The contractile and pump functions of the volume-overloaded heart, like those of the pressure-overloaded heart, have been controversial. A number of facts have now become clear. Total and forward cardiac output is sustained in the initial stages of volume overload, but forward output may deteriorate in later stages. Cardiac muscle contractile function is normal in certain forms and degrees of volume overload but is severely depressed in patients with chronic and severe aortic insufficiency or mitral regurgitation. Thus, like the pressure-overloaded heart, within a group of volume-overloaded hearts, muscle contractile function varies from normal in some hearts to depressed in others. In certain types of volume overload, even though myocardial contractile function is normal, there is a circulatory congestion that mimics heart failure.

Animal Models with Volume Overload

In experimental animals with volume overload, there appears to be a pathologic continuum of systolic contractile muscle function that varies from normal in some hearts to depressed in other hearts.

Four different animal models of volume overload have been used. A large defect in the atrial septum has been utilized as an animal model of severe right ventricular volume overload without heart failure or circulatory congestion (12,19). Cooper and colleagues (19) increased the load on the right ventricle of cats to three times the normal for 29 to 113 days by creating an atrial septal defect. Sixty-four percent hypertrophy of the right ventricle occurred. The velocity of isotonic shortening and the development of isometric tension were normal in papillary muscles from these right ventricles. In our laboratory, Carey and co-workers (12) produced large atrial septal defects by a tranvenous biopsy catheter. The right ventricles pumped three times the normal flow for an average of 50 days and ventricular hypertrophy was extensive. Function of papillary muscle from these hearts was normal.

Two studies utilized complete atrioventricular block to slow the ventricle and increase stroke volume. Congestive heart failure was not present in either study. Terina and colleagues (62) produced moderate myocardial hypertrophy by complete atrioventricular block of 50 to 96 days' duration in dogs. Force-velocity curves showed normal contractile function in these animals. When contractility was increased by paired pulse stimulation, the animals with heart block had normal potentiation of contractility. Newman (37a) evaluated the effects of 4 to 36 months of atrioventricular blockade in dogs. Ventricular weight was approximately 25% greater than normal. Contractile function, determined by a specially modified Walton-Brodie strain gauge arch, was normal.

A large aorta-caval fistula in dogs was used as a third model of volume overload. Ascites, pleural effusion, and edema are indicators of circulatory congestion in these animals. The severity and duration of the volume overload appear to determine the effects on myocardial contractile function. In less severe and less chronic volume overload, contractile function is normal; in more severe and more chronic volume overload, it is depressed.

Taylor and colleagues (58) produced moderate (20%) left ventricular hypertrophy in dogs by aorta-caval fistula of 29 to 49 days' duration. Seven of the nine animals had ascites, edema, and increases in body weight despite skeletal muscle wasting. Cardiac output increased by 192%. End-diastolic volume and pressure were increased. Ventricular contractile function was estimated from the tension-velocity relationship during isovolumic left ventricular contractions. Extrapolated velocity at zero tension, V_{max}, was unchanged, averaging 3.0 circ/sec in normal animals and 2.9 in the seven dogs with aorto-caval fistula and fluid retention.

Newman (38) subjected dogs to aorto-caval fistula for longer periods of time than Taylor (6 weeks to 7 months—average 3.5 months). At the time of study, all animals had elevated pulmonary artery wedge pressure, ascites, and limb edema. Mild left ventricular hypertrophy (13%) was observed. Ventricular myocardial contractile function was determined by measuring length-tension curves in a segment of left ventricle. A modified Walton-Brodie strain gauge arch attached to the free wall of the left ventricle in open-chest animals was used to make these measurements. The forces were corrected for the cross-sectional area of the muscle within the gauge. In the animals with chronic volume overload, mild hypertrophy, and circulatory congestion, there was a significant ($p<0.05$) reduction of contractile force at all muscle lengths.

Aortic insufficiency in dogs was used as a fourth animal model of volume overload. Taylor and Hopkins (59) found two groups of dogs with aortic insufficiency; one with normal contractile function and one with depressed contractile function. None of these animals had edema, ascites, or other evidence of congestive heart failure. Myocardial contractile function was estimated from the relationship of velocity of contractile element shortening to wall tension during isovolumic contractions. In seven animals, with moderate aortic insufficiency of less than 100 days' duration, contractile function was normal. In a second group of six dogs with more severe lesions or with lesions of longer duration, contractile function was less than normal ($p<0.025$). The duration of aortic insufficiency was greater than 450 days in three of these latter six animals.

Patients with Volume Overload

Hemodynamic effects of volume overload caused by mitral regurgitation are very different from hemodynamic effects of volume overload caused by aortic insufficiency. Both lesions increase preload. However, only mitral regurgitation reduces ventricular afterload as blood flows into the low pressure left atrium during systole. Controversy of whether cardiac muscle contractile function is normal or depressed in patients with volume-overloaded and hypertrophied hearts has been resolved. A number of recent studies now show that it is normal in some patients, mildly depressed in other patients, and severely depressed in others. Thus, the pathologic continuum from normal to depressed contractile function, which is seen in patients with pressure overload, appears to be present in patients with volume overload. Severe and prolonged volume overload is associated with cardiac muscle dysfunction and heart failure. Less severe and less prolonged volume overload is associated with normal cardiac muscle function and no heart failure.

Mitral Regurgitation

Pump function

Urschel and co-workers (63) examined the acute hemodynamic effects of mitral regurgitation in animals. There is increased preload and decreased afterload in mitral regurgitation. Myocardial wall tension is determined by the product of intraventricular pressure and ventricular radius. Since ventricular pressure and radius diminish more rapidly than normal during systole in mitral regurgitation as blood flows into the atrium, left ventricular wall tension falls more rapidly than normal during systole (Fig. 9). At any preload, mitral regurgitation reduces integrated left ventricular systolic wall tension. Since oxygen consumption is related to the integrated wall tension during systole, the ventricle would be expected to maintain the increased stroke volume without increased oxygen consumption.

Eckberg et al. (25) determined that regurgitant volume was 41% of the total stroke volume in patients with mitral regurgitation. These workers also found that 46% of the regurgitant volume was ejected into the left atrium prior to aortic valve opening and, thus, prior to antegrade stroke volume.

Wong and Spotnitz (66) studied patients with chronic mitral regurgitation in an open-chest state during operation for valve replacement. They measured left ventricular dimensions and pressure immediately before and after replacement of the mitral valve. The dimensional measurements were obtained by M-mode and two-dimensional echocardiography. Simultaneous pressure measurements were obtained by high-fidelity micro catheter-tip transducer. Elimination of the low-impedance left atrial pathway by mitral valve replacement caused a significant ($p<0.02$) increase in systolic wall stress (Fig. 10). The average integrated systolic wall stress increased from 25.9 ± 6.2 g/cm^2 to 36.0 ± 6.8 ($p<0.02$).

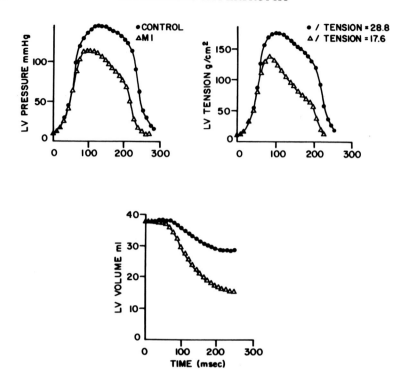

FIG. 9. Comparison of a control beat and MI at the same end-diastolic volume. (Modified from Urschel et al., ref. 63.)

The ejection fraction is an unreliable indicator of myocardial contractile function in mitral regurgitation. End-diastolic volume is elevated to greater than twice normal in mitral regurgitation (3a,64a). This increased end-diastolic volume (preload) and the lowered systolic wall stress (afterload) causes an artificial increase in ejection fraction. Immediately following replacement of the mitral valve for mitral regurgitation, when no change in myocardial contractile function is believed to have occurred, ejection fraction declines from the valve measured immediately before valve replacement (66). Phillips et al. (43) found that the ejection fraction determined by cardiac multigated nuclear imaging fell significantly ($p<0.001$) from a preoperative value of 0.62 ± 0.09 to an average postoperative value of 0.50 ± 0.15 in 34 patients having mitral valve replacement for isolated mitral regurgitation.

Although the total stroke volume is increased in both compensated and decompensated mitral regurgitation, forward stroke volume and cardiac output are often reduced in compensated and decompensated mitral regurgitation (64a).

Ventricular muscle contractile function

Recent controversy over whether cardiac muscle contractile function is normal or depressed in patients with mitral regurgitation appears resolved. It may be normal, mildly depressed, or severely depressed (5,7,25,47,66).

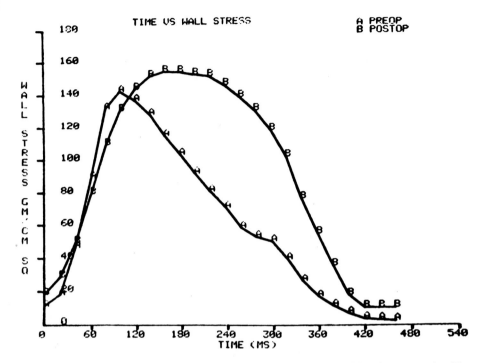

FIG. 10. Time-course of left ventricular (LV) wall stress preoperative (A) and postoperative (B) valve replacement for chronic mitral regurgitation. (Modified from Wong and Spotnitz, ref. 66.)

The previously described alterations in loading conditions in mitral regurgitation make it difficult to assess cardiac muscle contractile function in this disease and, in part, led to previous controversy. The preload increase and afterload decrease cause a rise in the values for ejection phase indexes of contractile performance such as ejection fraction. Such an artificial elevation of ejection fraction can mask a true decrease in myocardial contractile function. The recently described relationship between end-systolic ventricular volume and pressure is an index of myocardial contractile function that is independent of preload and is a linear function of afterload. End-systolic volume can be corrected for varying body size with the use of end-systolic volume index, and variations in ventricular wall thickness can be corrected for by using myocardial wall stress instead of ventricular pressure. Several recent studies have utilized these end-systolic relationships to more accurately assess myocardial contractile function in mitral regurgitation.

Carabello and colleagues (8) determined the ratio of end-systolic wall stress to end-systolic volume index (ESWS/ESVI) in normal patients and in patients with chronic mitral regurgitation who subsequently underwent mitral valve replacement. Before operation all patients had symptoms of congestive heart failure, and 15 of these 21 patients were NYHA class III or IV. Group A consisted of 16 patients who subsequently became NYHA functional class I or II following mitral valve replacement. Group B consisted of one patient who remained in NYHA functional class III postoperatively and four patients who died of left ventricular dysfunction perioperatively. The preoperative ESWS/ESVI ratio was significantly lower in both groups of patients with mitral regurgitation (group A, 3.3 ± 0.4; group B, 2.2 ± 0.2) than it was in normal individuals (5.6 ± 0.9) ($p < 0.025$). The values for ESWS/ESVI were significantly lower in group B than in group A mitral regurgitation patients ($p < 0.025$) (Fig. 11). There was considerable overlap of values for preoperative ejection fraction between groups A and B (Fig. 12).

Borow and colleagues (5) used end-systolic volume as a predictor of postoperative left ventricular performance in patients with mitral regurgitation who subsequently underwent mitral valve replacement. The echocardiographically determined percent ventricular dimension change from diastole to systole was used as the postoperative indicator of left ventricular function. Preoperatively, 13 of 16 patients with mitral regurgitation had an end-systolic volume index greater than the normal value of 30 cc/M². Patients with normal preoperative end-systolic volume index had normal postoperative percent ventricular dimension change. All patients with preoperative end-systolic volume index of greater than 30 cc/M² had postoperative percent dimension change below the normal value. Preoperative irreversible myocardial dysfunction secondary to chronic volume overload was proposed as the most likely explanation for the failure of these patients to show improvement postoperatively.

Wong and Spotnitz (66) assessed contractile function immediately after relieving mitral regurgitation by mitral valve replacement. Since the alterations of preload and afterload, which are present in mitral regurgitation, were no longer present following valve replacement, they could accurately assess ventricular muscle con-

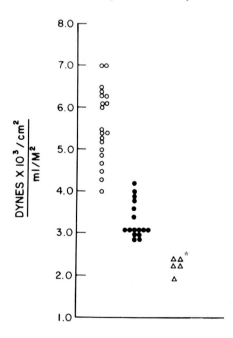

FIG. 11. End-systolic wall stress/end-systolic volume index ratio (ESWS/ESVI) for normal subjects *(open circles)*, group A *(closed circles)* and group B *(triangles)*. ESWS/ESVI was significantly lower in group A than in normal persons and lower in group B than in group A, suggesting left ventricular dysfunction in group A and more severe left ventricular dysfunction in group B. The asterisk denotes patient 21 who had an ejection fraction of 0.8 but in whom severe left ventricular dysfunction is suggested by the ESWS/ESVI. (Carabello et al., ref. 7.)

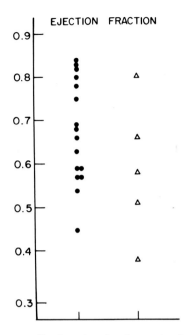

FIG. 12. Preoperative ejection fractions (EF) for members of group A *(circles)* and B *(triangles)*. Although EF tended to be higher in group A, there is considerable overlap between groups. EF alone was not a good predictor of surgical outcome. (Carabello et al., ref. 7.)

tractile function by determination of a postoperative ejection phase index. They compared the values of left ventricular shortening fraction observed in patients immediately following correction of mitral regurgitation by valve replacement with those observed in patients without mitral regurgitation who were undergoing coronary bypass surgery. The left ventricular shortening fraction was reduced in patients who had just had mitral valvular replacement for mitral regurgitation whereas shortening fraction was normal in patients who had not had mitral regurgitation (Fig. 13). The results were interpreted as consistent with preoperative depression of left ventricular function in chronic mitral regurgitation.

Eckberg and co-workers (25) estimated left ventricular contractile function by measuring the velocity of circumferential fiber shortening (V_{cf}) at maximum wall stress normalized for instantaneous left ventricular circumference. Such a measurement should account for variations in both preload and afterload. Maximum wall stress (afterload) was similar in the normal and mitral regurgitant ventricles. Despite an increase in resting fiber length (preload) in chronic mitral regurgitation, a change that would have been expected to increase maximum V_{cf}, the average value for V_{cf} at maximum wall tension in these patients was 1.01 ± 0.08 circ/sec compared with the average normal value of 1.74 ± 0.1 circ/sec ($p < 0.001$). These authors concluded that left ventricular contractile function was reduced in patients with mitral regurgitation.

Schuler and colleagues (47) found two groups of patients with mitral regurgitation. One group of patients had moderate left ventricular dilitation and a normal ejection fraction preoperatively. This group subsequently had regression of myocardial hypertrophy and almost normal left ventricular shortening following mitral

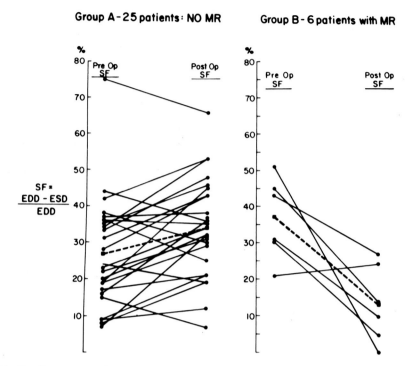

FIG. 13. Preoperative (Pre Op) and postoperative (Post Op) shortening fractions (SF) compared in 25 patients with no mitral regurgitation (MR) (group A) and 6 patients with chronic mitral regurgitation (group B). The *dashed lines* represent the average change in SF. Shortening fraction increases significantly in group A and decreases significantly in group B ($p<0.01$, unpaired t-test compared with the rise in group A). (Wong and Spotnitz, ref. 66.)

valve replacement. A second group had severe left ventricular dilitation and low normal or depressed ejection fraction preoperatively. This group had persistent myocardial hypertrophy, severe reduction in left ventricular ejection fraction, and severe chamber dilitation following mitral valve replacement. One can conclude that the second group had preoperative depression of left ventricular contractile function.

Based on the above six recent studies, the following conclusions can be made. There is a pathologic continuum of systolic contractile muscle function which varies from normal or mildly dysfunctioned in early mitral regurgitation, across the middle ground of moderately dysfunctioned muscle in chronic mitral regurgitation, to the extreme of severely dysfunctioned muscle in advanced severe mitral regurgitation with heart failure.

Assessment of ventricular contractile performance in mitral regurgitation by techniques that are independent of altered afterload and preload helps identify patients at high risk for residual postoperative ventricular dysfunction or perioperative death. The degree of cardiac muscle dysfunction before mitral valve replacement appears to be the major determinant of perioperative risk and postoperative cardiac function. For example, Borow and colleagues (5) found that patients with mitral regurgitation and an end-systolic volume index of greater than 90 cc/M^2 had an 80% mortality during the perioperative period, and all such deaths occurred in patients with end-systolic volume index of greater than 60 cc/M^2. Carabello et al. (8) found that patients with the lowest preoperative ratio of ESWS/ESVI had the highest perioperative mortality at the time of mitral valve replacement. All five patients with the worst ventricular contractile dysfunction (group B of Fig. 11, *open triangles*) did poorly after valve replacement, and four died in the perioperative period. Similar conclusions can be made from additional studies (25,43,47,64,66). In the future, serial measurement of ventricular contractile performance and detection of early deterioration may allow medical or surgical therapy to be applied in time to prevent irreversible and life-threatening heart muscle damage.

Aortic Regurgitation

Pump function

Urschel and co-workers also examined the acute effects of aortic regurgitation in animals (63). With onset of aortic regurgitation there was an immediate increase in end-diastolic volume, stroke volume, and ejection fraction. Left ventricular integrated systolic wall tension rose owing to a modest increase in intraventricular pressure and a substantial increase in ventricular radius. Since oxygen consumption per beat is largely related to the integrated wall tension during systole, oxygen consumption by the ventricle would be expected to increase with aortic regurgitation. When equal degrees of aortic and mitral regurgitation were compared, the aortic lesion imposed a greater burden on the myocardium.

In patients, Osbakken et al. (40) in our laboratory (Table 2) found that peak systolic wall stress was increased in aortic regurgitation by 19% in patients without heart failure and by 42% in patients with heart failure. End-diastolic stress was twice normal in patients with heart failure. Total cardiac output (forward plus regurgitant) was considerably increased in patients with aortic regurgitation whether or not heart failure was present. Total stroke work was increased but, owing to hypertrophy, stroke work per gram of heart muscle was normal.

Ventricular muscle contractile function

Controversy over whether ventricular muscle contractile function is depressed or normal in patients with aortic regurgitation appears resolved. Again, it may be normal in some patients, mildly depressed in other patients, and severely depressed in many patients with chronic and severe aortic regurgitation. Alterations in ventricular loading conditions make it difficult to assess cardiac muscle function in aortic regurgitation.

The relationship between end-systolic wall stress and volume index has been used to assess myocardial contractile function in aortic regurgitation. As described

TABLE 2. *Data in normal patients, asymptomatic patients with aortic regurgitation, and patients with aortic regurgitation and heart failure*

	Normal (n = 12)	Aortic regurgitation	
		Asymptomatic (n = 10)	Heart failure (n = 11)
Mean AoP (mm Hg)	87 ± 3	95 ± 4	99 ± 4[a]
LVSP (mm Hg)	121 ± 5	146 ± 8[a]	163 ± 5[a]
EDP (mm Hg)	10 ± 1	9 ± 2	23 ± 2[a]
ESP (mm Hg)	97 ± 6	111 ± 6	125 ± 5[a]
EDVI (ml/m²)	93 ± 6	159 ± 19[a]	247 ± 18[a]
ESVI (ml/m²)	37 ± 3	62 ± 14[a]	132 ± 14[a]
SVI (ml/m²)	58 ± 5	97 ± 8[a]	114 ± 8[a]
EF (%)	62 ± 3	65 ± 4	48 ± 3[a]
CI (liters/m²)			
Dye dilution	3.3 ± 0.3	3.3 ± 0.4	3.0 ± 0.4
Angiographic	3.7 ± 0.4	7.6 ± 0.7[a]	9.1 ± 0.8[a]
CI Fick	2.1 ± 0.1	2.3 ± 0.2	2.1 ± 0.18
LVMI (g/m²)	83 ± 6	180 ± 14[a]	212 ± 24[a]
LVM/EDV (g/ml)	0.92 ± 0.10	1.28 ± 0.20	0.83 ± 0.10
h/R	0.31 ± 0.02	0.43 ± 0.05[a]	0.33 ± 0.02
SWI (joule/m²)	0.76 ± 0.07	1.44 ± 0.2[a]	1.76 ± 0.19[a]
SW/g heart muscle	0.010 ± 0.001	0.008 ± 0.001	0.009 ± 0.004
PS (dynes/cm² × 10⁻³)	360 ± 33	428 ± 50	511 ± 55[a]
ESS (dynes/cm² × 10⁻³)	169 ± 23	191 ± 21	247 ± 20[a]
EDS (dynes/cm² × 10⁻³)	39 ± 3	33 ± 6	76 ± 10[a]

All values are mean ± SEM.

Abbreviations: AoP = aortic pressure; CI = cardiac index; EDP = left ventricular end-diastolic pressure; EDVI = end-diastolic volume index; EF = ejection fraction; ESP = end-systolic pressure; ESS = end-systolic stress; ESVI = end-systolic volume index; LVSP = left ventricular systolic pressure; SVI = stroke volume index; EDVI = end-diastolic volume index; h = wall thickness; LVMI = left ventricular mass index; R = radius of minor axis; SW = stroke work; SWI = stroke work index; EDS = end-diastolic stress; ESS = end-systolic stress; PS = peak stress.

[a] $p < 0.05$ compared with values in normal group.

From Osbakken et al. (40).

above, this index is independent of preload and is a linear function of afterload. The use of wall stress and volume index correct for variations in wall thickness and body size.

Osbakken and co-workers (40) determined the ESWS/ESVI ratio in normal individuals, patients with significant aortic regurgitation but minimal symptoms, and patients with aortic regurgitation and symptoms of heart failure (Fig. 14). Asymptomatic patients with significant aortic regurgitation had normal ESWS/ESVI, but this contractile index was significantly reduced in patients with aortic insufficiency and heart failure.

Borow and colleagues (5) utilized the end-systolic volume to estimate left ventricular contractile performance in patients before valve replacement for aortic regurgitation. This index does not correct for possible changes in wall stress but does have the advantage of being independent of preload. In these same patients

AORTIC INSUFFIENCY

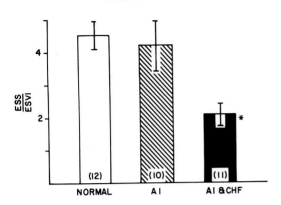

FIG. 14. Mean values ± SE of the mean for end-systolic wall stress/end-systolic volume index ratio (ESWS/ESVI) in normal subjects, patients with severe aortic insufficiency but no symptoms (AI) and patients with severe aortic insufficiency and congestive heart failure (AI & CHF). Numbers in parentheses equal number of patients. $* = p < 0.05$, AI & CHF group is significantly different from the normals and AI groups. (Osbakken et al., ref. 40.)

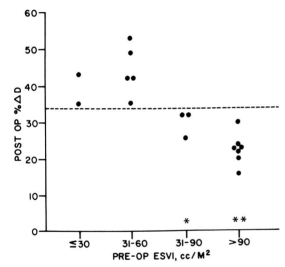

FIG. 15. The relationship between postoperative left ventricular function (percent dimension change = % ΔD) and preoperative end-systolic volume index (ESVI). Patients with aortic regurgitation. Patients are grouped according to the degree of enlargement in end-systolic volume index (on the horizontal axis). Patients who died perioperatively from heart failure are demarcated by an asterisk at the bottom of the graph in the appropriate preoperative end-systolic volume index group. Normal left ventricular function is marked by the area above the horizontal dashed line at % ΔD = 34. (Borow et al., ref. 5.)

the postoperative left ventricular performance was evaluated with ejection phase indexes, since the preload and afterload alterations that interfere with preoperative determination of ejection phase indexes were no longer present. A large preoperative end-systolic volume correlated well with poor postoperative left ventricular performance (R = 0.77) (Fig. 15) and with the persistence of heart failure symptoms after operation. It appeared that two groups of patients were present. Seven of 17 patients with aortic regurgitation had normal contractile function both before and after operation whereas 10 patients had depressed contractile function at both times. The presence or absence of cardiac muscle contractile dysfunction before aortic valve replacement appeared to be the major determinant of perioperative risk. The three patients who died in the perioperative period were patients having large preoperative end-systolic volumes of 31 to greater than 90 cc/M².

Henry and colleagues (28,29) used echocardiography to determine end-systolic left ventricular dimension in patients with aortic regurgitation. The end-systolic dimension should reflect left ventricular contractile function independently of pre-load and should be fairly reliable when there are no large differences in systolic wall stress. When this dimension was greater than 55 mm in preoperative patients with symptoms due to aortic regurgitation, these patients were found to be at high risk. Nine of 13 such patients died of congestive heart failure following aortic valve replacement. In contrast, of 32 similar patients with symptoms due to aortic regurgitation but with left ventricular end-systolic dimension of less than 55 mm, only two died following valve replacement. In a group of five asymptomatic patients with significant aortic regurgitation, and an end-systolic dimension greater than 55 mm, four subsequently developed heart failure and required operation during a 39-month follow-up. In 20 asymptomatic patients with significant aortic regurgitation and an end-systolic dimension 50 mm or less, only four subsequently developed symptoms and required aortic valve replacement during the follow-up period ($p<0.002$). Again, the presence or absence of cardiac muscle dysfunction before aortic valve replacement appeared to be the major determinant of perioperative risk and may even be a predictor of subsequent deterioration in medically treated patients.

ABNORMALITIES OF THE CARDIAC SYMPATHETIC NERVOUS SYSTEM IN THE HYPERTROPHIED AND FAILING HEART

Background

The sympathetic nervous system represents a major control mechanism in the moment-to-moment regulation of the normal circulatory responses to the changing metabolic requirements of the tissues. This system provides a sensitive mechanism for rapid alteration of myocardial contractility, heart rate, and peripheral venous and arterial tone. It occupies a crucial role in the response of man to physical exercise; the increase in heart rate, stroke volume, cardiac output, left ventricular work, and velocity of muscle fiber shortening that occur with exercising are due, in part, to augmented sympathetic activity. Nerve terminals from the network of sympathetic nerves that supply the cardiovascular system are found in arteries, veins, and all chambers of the heart. Stored in the nerve terminals are large concentrations of the neurotransmitter, norepinephrine. Stimulation of the sympathetic nerves to the heart results in discharge of this norepinephrine which acts upon the cardiac cellular β-receptor mechanism to exert effects dependent on the site of stimulation. Increases in heart rate occur with stimulation of the sinoatrial node, increased velocity of conduction occurs through the atrioventricular junctional tissues, and augmentation of myocardial contractility occurs when the β-receptors of the myocardium are stimulated. The synthesis of norepinephrine, as well as uptake and binding of the circulating norepinephrine, is also accomplished within these cardiac sympathetic neurons. Synthesis of norepinephrine by these nerve endings accounts for 80% to 90% of the catecholamine in the heart. Tyrosine hydroxylase is the major enzyme normally regulating the rate of synthesis. Circulating norepinephrine is taken up by these nerve endings and accounts for the remaining 10% to 20% of cardiac norepinephrine. The catecholes from both synthesis and uptake are retained in a physiologically inactive form in the storage vesicles. These vesicles bind and store norepinephrine and retard its diffusion into the neuronal cytoplasm, protecting it from enzymatic destruction by monamine oxidase which is present within the neuron. The vesicles also prevent inappropriate release of the catecholamine into the extra-neuronal space where the enzyme catechol-O-methyltransferase is the major norepinephrine metabolizing enzyme. Stimulation arrives as an action potential along the sympathetic nerve terminals, and the vesicles release the stored catecholamine from the neuronal cells. This released catecholamine then is bound to the β-receptor of the cardiac muscle and causes effects that are mediated indirectly through the activation of the adenylate cyclase and AMP system.

Depletion of Cardiac Norepinephrine in Cardiac Hypertrophy and Failure

The sympathetic nervous system is quite abnormal in the hypertrophied and failing heart. Myocardial stores of norepinephrine are severely reduced in the hypertrophied heart whether or not congestive failure is present. The reduction was first noted in atrial tissue from patients with congestive heart failure by Chidsey et al. (15,17) (Fig. 16). It was also found in left ventricular papillary muscles removed

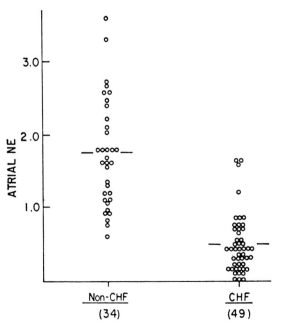

FIG. 16. Norepinephrine concentrations in biopsy specimens of atrial appendage obtained from 34 patients with no congestive heart failure (non-CHF) and from 49 patients with congestive heart failure (CHF). (Chidsey et al., ref. 15.)

from patients at the time of mitral valve replacement for mitral regurgitation with left ventricular failure (17).

There is abundant evidence of such reduction in experimentally induced ventricular hypertrophy in several animal models, with and without congestive heart failure (Fig. 17). In left ventricular hypertrophy and left heart failure produced by constriction of the ascending aorta of the guinea pig (51,52) in right heart failure induced by production of pulmonary stenosis and tricuspid insufficiency in the dog (16), and in right ventricular hypertrophy with or without heart failure produced by different degrees of pulmonary arterial constriction in the cat (54), a profound reduction in cardiac norepinephrine concentration and content occurs. Thus, both a volume overload and a pressure overload can cause this depletion in either man or animals. Norepinephrine depletion is present in both ventricles regardless of which ventricle is subjected to the primary hemodynamic burden. The reduced total cardiac content of norepinephrine proves that there is a true depletion of catecholamine, rather than dilution of the normal complement of norepinephrine by the hypertrophy of the heart.

The time required for depletion of cardiac norepinephrine after imposition of severe ventricular pressure overload was determined in the guinea pig by Spann et al. (52) (Fig. 18). In this study, average ventricular norepinephrine concentration fell to 22% of normal by the fifth day after aortic constriction and remained depressed for the 65-day observation period.

Mechanisms of Cardiac Norepinephrine Depletion

Cardiac sympathetic nerve terminals are complex structures involved in synthesis, uptake, binding, storage, and release of norepinephrine. In ventricular hypertrophy and heart failure, at least two defects of the cardiac sympathetic nerves cause norepinephrine depletion: a defect in neuronal uptake and binding of norepinephrine

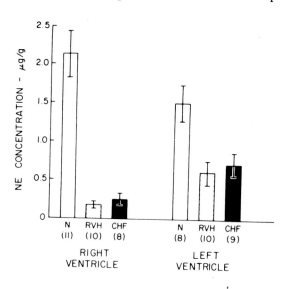

FIG. 17. The average norepinephrine concentration of the right and left ventricles of normal cats and cats with right ventriclar hypertrophy (RVH) and congestive heart failure (CHF). *Vertical lines with cross bars* = ±1 SEM. Numbers in parentheses represent number of animals in each group. (Spann et al., ref. 54.)

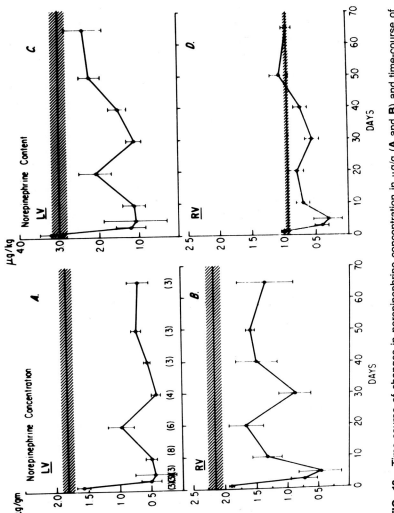

FIG. 18. Time-course of changes in norepinephrine concentration in μg/g (**A** and **B**) and time-course of changes in total norepinephrine content in each ventricle expressed as μg/kg body weight (**C** and **D**). *Solid circles* and *vertical bars* represent the mean values ±1 SEM obtained from animals with congestive heart failure. *Horizontal lines* and *hatched areas* represent the mean ±1 SEM obtained from 15 normal animals. Numbers in parentheses refer to the number of animals sacrificed at each point in time which provided the data shown in all four panels. LV, left ventricle; RV, right ventricle. (Spann et al., ref. 52.)

and a defect in norepinephrine synthesis. The defect in neuronal uptake and binding of norepinephrine was defined by Spann et al. (52) by measurement of the nor-epinephrine retained in the hearts and kidneys after infusion of nonradioactive *l*-norepinephrine in guinea pigs with left ventricular hypertrophy and congestive heart failure compared with the level of norepinephrine in a control group of normal guinea pigs. The results of such comparisons in 14 control animals and 13 guinea pigs with left ventricular hypertrophy and failure are shown in Fig. 19. In the normal animals, the renal and left and right ventricular concentrations of norepinephrine rose to peak values at the completion of the infusion, and the concentrations declined over the ensuing 3 hr to values that approached the control levels. The increase in ventricular concentrations in the animals with left ventricular hypertrophy and heart failure was minimal whereas the renal norepinephrine in this group increased in a manner similar to normal. When tracer quantities of tritium-labeled DL-norepinephrine were injected into animals with ventricular hypertrophy and failure, a depressed uptake of the tritium-label by the hypertrophied and failing heart were observed. These results were confirmed by Fischer et al. (26) who observed a decrease in the uptake of tritiated norepinephrine in the hearts of rats with severe hypertrophy but no congestive heart failure.

To rule out the possibility that the decrease in uptake and binding had been caused by a rapid turnover of infused norepinephrine, the net turnover rate of intraneuronal norepinephrine was investigated by administering a small amount of radioactive norepinephrine to normal guinea pigs and to those with left ventricular hypertrophy and heart failure. The turnover rate was determined by monitoring the specific activity in the left ventricle of both groups for 72 hr (52). In both groups, the decline of specific activity was complex and exhibited two exponential components. These findings, similar to the observations of Kopin et al. (32), are compatible with the presence of a multicompartmental distribution of norepineph-rine. The absolute level of specific activity and the rate of disappearance were essentially identical in both groups, which indicated that the relative turnover rate was the same as normal in the animals with ventricular hypertrophy and failure. Thus, the smaller increment of norepinephrine in the heart after infusion in the animals with hypertrophy and failure cannot be explained by a more rapid net turnover of norepinephrine, but must be interpreted as an abnormality of uptake or binding or both. This defect in uptake or binding is, in part, responsible for the observed depletion of norepinephrine stores in the hypertrophied and failing heart. The presence of a normal net turnover rate in hearts depleted of norepinephrine also indicates that the rate of synthesis in the ventricle must actually be reduced in the group with hypertrophy and heart failure.

A defect in the synthetic pathway for norepinephrine in the failing heart was first reported by Pool and co-workers (44), who demonstrated a severe defect in tyrosine hydroxylase, the rate-limiting enzyme for the synthesis of norepinephrine. In the right ventricles of dogs with right ventricular hypertrophy, congestive heart failure, and severe norepinephrine depletion, tyrosine hydroxylase activity was significantly reduced from the normal value of 3.3 ± 0.7 to 0.4 ± 0.1 μmoles/g/hr.

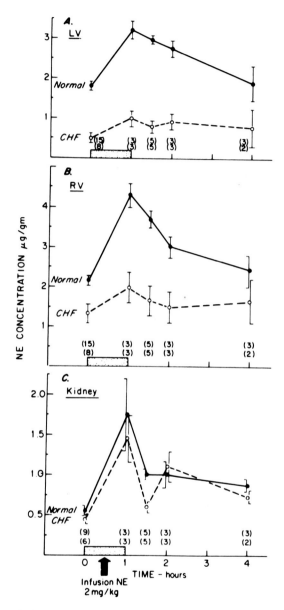

FIG. 19. Effects of infusion of norepinephrine (NE) on the concentrations of norepinephrine in the left ventricles (LV) **(A)**, right ventricles (RV) **(B)**, and kidneys **(C)** of normal guinea pigs (*solid lines* and *circles*) and guinea pigs with congestive heart failure (CHF, *open circles* and *broken lines*). *Verticle bars* represent ±1 SEM. *Stippled area* represents duration of infusion, and the numbers in parentheses refer to the number of animals in each group sacrificed at the various times. (Spann et al., ref. 52.)

Similar reductions in man have been observed by DiCuatro and co-workers (23) in biopsies of myocardium obtained from patients with hypertrophy and congestive heart failure. DiCuatro et al. (23) also showed a relationship in man between the extent of cardiac norepinephrine depletion and the extent of reduction of tyrosine hydroxylase activity in the hypertrophied and failing heart. Both norepinephrine and tyrosine hydroxylase were more severely reduced in patients with class III and IV heart failure than in patients with class I or II heart failure.

The cardiomyopathic Syrian hamster differs in certain ways from the guinea pig and dog models of hypertrophy and failure as well as from myocardium obtained from patients with hypertrophy and failure. This animal shows an increase in the rate constant for cardiac norepinephrine turnover, approaching the rate seen with maximum sympathetic stimulation due to immobilization stress (48). Also, during heart failure, an increase in the tyrosine hydroxylase activity was noted in this animal (50). The high concentration of dopamine found in the myopathic Syrian hamster implies that in this animal, the rate-limiting enzyme for norepinephrine synthesis in the hypertrophied and failing heart may have been dopamine betahydroxylase (49).

Possible Relationship Between Depleted Cardiac Norepinephrine and Depressed Intrinsic Contractile Function of the Hypertrophied and Failing Heart

As described in detail in the first two sections of this chapter, within a group of pressure- or volume-overloaded hypertrophied hearts, there is a pathologic continuum of systolic contractile muscle function which varies from normal in some hearts to depressed in other hearts. The continuum extends from the one extreme of normally functioning units of hypertrophied muscle in a pressure- or volume-overloaded heart with excessive pump function, across the middle ground of moderately dysfunctioned units of hypertrophied muscle in a pressure- or volume-overloaded heart which maintains basic pump function, to the other extreme of severely dysfunctioned units of hypertrophied muscle in a pressure- or volume-overloaded heart with poor pump function and congestive failure. Since cardiac sympathetic nerve activity has positive inotropic effects, it is reasonable to wonder if the depletion of cardiac catecholamines causes the depression of the intrinsic contractile function of the hypertrophied and failing heart. To assess the possibility that the cardiac norepinephrine depletion seen in ventricular hypertrophy and congestive heart failure was also responsible for the intrinsic depression of contractile performance in the failing heart muscle, the contractile state was determined by Spann et al. (52) in cardiac muscle removed from experimental animals whose hearts were depleted of norepinephrine by a mechanism other than heart failure. In 12 cats, cardiac norepinephrine depletion was produced by chronic cardiac denervation and contractile function of papillary muscles isolated from these hearts was determined. Cardiac norepinephrine concentration in the cardiac denervated animals was reduced to levels of 0.006 ± 0.003 μg/g, values even lower than those in the hypertrophy and heart failure groups, but the contractile function of cardiac muscle from the norepinephrine-depleted denervated heart was not depressed (Fig. 20). Thus, cardiac norepinephrine stores are not necessary to maintain the basic contractile state of the myocardium, and cardiac norepinephrine depletion that occurs in ventricular hypertrophy and congestive heart failure is not responsible

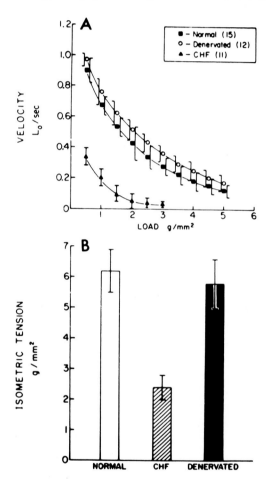

FIG. 20. Ventricular contractile state. **A:** Average force-velocity relation in right ventricular papillary muscles isolated from normal cats (N), from cats with total chronic cardiac denervation (denervated), and from cats with congestive heart failure (CHF). Velocity is expressed on the ordinate as muscle lengths (L_0/sec), and total load is expressed on the abscissa as g/mm. All *vertical bars* equal + SEM, and each number in parentheses represents the number of animals in that group. **B:** Average maximal active tension developed at the apex of the length-tension curve in isolated cat right ventricular papillary muscles from the three groups of cats, expressed as g/mm. (From Rutenberg and Spann.)

for the intrinsic depression of cardiac contractility in failing heart muscle. These conclusions have been confirmed in a series of experiments in rats by Dhalla et al. (1971).

Cardiac Norepinephrine Depletion and Transmission of Cardiac Sympathetic Nerve Impulses

Whether cardiac norepinephrine depletion interferes with the transmission of sympathetic impulses to the failing heart was examined by Covell et al. (22) in dogs with severe cardiac norepinephrine depletion, right ventricular hypertrophy, and right heart failure due to tricuspid insufficiency and pulmonary stenosis (Fig. 21). The chronotropic and inotropic responses to graded stimulation of the sympathetic nerves in six dogs with right ventricular hypertrophy and chronic right ventricular failure were compared with the responses of 13 normal animals. In dogs with heart failure, the heart rate and right ventricular contractile force response to stimulation of the right cardioaccelerator nerve were sharply reduced. However, the myocardium of dogs with heart failure responded normally to the direct effects of exogenously administered norepinephrine. These observations demonstrate that the quantity of neurotransmitter released per nerve impulse is dramatically reduced by the cardiac norepinephrine depletion that accompanies experimental ventricular hypertrophy and heart failure.

Similar results in man have been reported by Goldstein et al. (26a). In 38 patients with heart failure, the reflex chronotropic response to upright tilt and to hypotension induced by nitroglycerin was impaired. Since this abnormality persisted after atropine administration, the sympathetic reflex system of such patients was demonstrated to be defective.

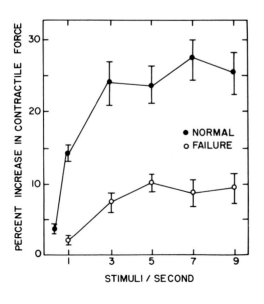

FIG. 21. Mean percentage increases in right ventricular contractile force at five frequencies of right cardio-accelerator nerve stimulation in control dogs and dogs with heart failure. (Covell et al., ref. 22.)

Thus, sympathetic nervous control of the heart is seriously impaired in the hypertrophied and failing heart both in experimental animals and in man. The heart has lost full use of an important mechanism which, if it had remained intact, could have improved myocardial force development and velocity of contraction in the failing heart and thus provided compensation for the depression of intrinsic cardiac muscle function.

Support of the Heart and Circulation by Circulating Norepinephrine in Patients with Heart Failure

Since a portion of norepinephrine released at the nerve terminals enters the circulating blood, augmented sympathetic activity can be estimated by the extent of increases in arterial plasma norepinephrine concentration which occur with exercise. In normal subjects, moderate muscular exercise causes an elevation of arterial norepinephrine from an average control level of 0.28 μg/liter to an exercise level of 0.46 μg/liter. In patients with congestive heart failure, the resting values of arterial plasma norepinephrine concentration are increased, and moderate exercise elevates the arterial norepinephrine from a control level of 0.36 μg/liter to an exercise level of 1.73 μg/liter (Fig. 22) (14). Levels in patients with heart disease but without evidence of heart failure do not differ from normal. These observations of resting plasma norepinephrine concentration elevations in patients with congestive heart failure have recently been confirmed by Thomas and Marks (61). Further, the level of plasma norepinephrine concentration is directly related to the degree of left ventricular dysfunction as indicated by systolic time-interval techniques. The

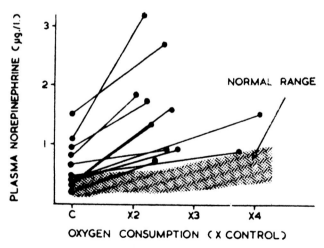

FIG. 22. Changes (from each left-hand *circle* to each right-hand *circle*) in plasma norepinephrine during exercise in congestive heart failure. Oxygen consumption during the exercise period is expressed in multiples of the resting oxygen consumption. C = control or resting values. The normal range is represented by *stippled area*. (Adapted from Braunwald et al.)

excessive augmentation of plasma norepinephrine concentration during exercise in patients with heart failure reflects an increased response of the sympathetic nervous system to exercise. This increased response may have an important supportive effect on hemodynamic function and distribution of blood flow in such patients.

The daily urinary excretion of norepinephrine provides an estimate of the total body level of sympathetic activity. Excretion of norepinephrine averaged 22 μg/day in normal persons and in patients with heart disease without congestive failure, but was significantly increased in patients with heart failure (17). Patients with NYHA functional class III status excreted 46 μg/day, whereas patients with class IV status excreted 58 μg/day (Fig. 23).

Papillary muscles removed from the heart with right ventricular hypertrophy, congestive heart failure, and norepinephrine depletion due to pressure overload are supersensitive to the positive inotropic effects of norepinephrine (Fig. 24) (54). Positive chronotropic and inotropic responsiveness of the hypertrophied, failing, and norepinephrine-depleted heart to exogenous norepinephrine was observed in the dog right ventricular model by Covell and co-workers (22). The number of cardiac α_1 and β-adrenoceptors is increased in guinea pigs with ventricular hypertrophy and heart failure due to pressure overload (31).

Since the circulating arterial norepinephrine concentration is increased in heart failure, and since the failing heart muscle is not only responsive to exogenous norepinephrine but may even be supersensitive to its positive inotropic and chronotropic effects, the circulating catecholamines play an important role in supporting

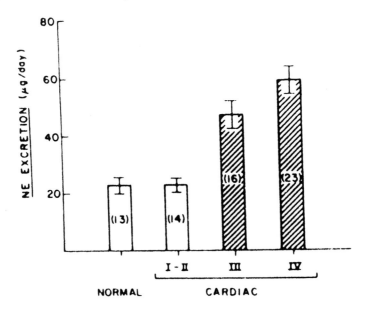

FIG. 23. Urinary norepinephrine (NE) excretion in normal control subjects, in cardiac patients without heart failure (NYHA classes I and II), and in patients with failure (classes III and IV). Average values ±SEM are shown. (Adapted from Braunwald et al.)

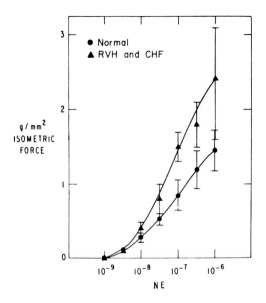

FIG. 24. Effects of exogenous norepinephrine on isometric tension of right ventricular papillary muscles from normal cats and from cats with right ventricular hypertrophy, heart failure, and cardiac norepinephrine depletion. *l*-Norepinephrine was added to the muscle bath at 5-min intervals in increasing concentrations starting at 10 M, while isometric force achieved at each concentration was recorded. The increment in isometric force is shown on the ordinate and the concentration of added norepinephrine (NE) on the abscissa. *Solid circles* = muscles from normal hearts; *solid triangles* = muscle from the norepinephrine-depleted hearts of animals with ventricular hypertrophy and failure. *Vertical lines* with *cross bars* = ±1 SEM. (Spann et al., ref. 54.)

the contractile function of the failing heart. Agents that block the cardiac β-sympathetic receptor sites may intensify congestive heart failure. Clinical experience with propranolol, a β-adrenergic receptor blocking agent, has shown that in certain patients with advanced cardiac disease, congestive heart failure can appear or increase if propranolol is administered (57a).

Prevention of Cardiac Norepinephrine Depletion in Ventricular Hypertrophy and Failure

Sole and co-workers (48) found that ganglionic blockade of cardiomyopathic Syrian hamsters completely restored the levels of cardiac norepinephrine to control values. They postulated that the ganglionic blockade prevented the progressive increase in cardiac sympathetic tone, which they believed was causing a decrease in cardiac norepinephrine. However, an increased turnover of cardiac norepinephrine is necessary to prove their hypothesis, and such an increased turnover has been demonstrated only in the cardiomyopathic Syrian hamster and not in other animal models of ventricular hypertrophy and congestive heart failure.

When digoxin was administered to cats by Carey et al. (10) in our laboratory prior to banding of the pulmonary artery and was continued after the imposition of this pressure overload, the reduced contractile function and reduced myosin ATPase activity usually seen in such hearts did not occur. However, the use of digoxin does not prevent the cardiac catecholamine depletion caused by this pressure-overload lesion (Fig. 25).

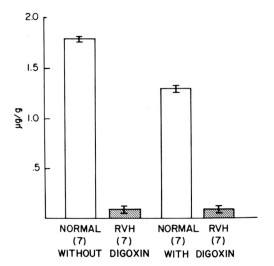

FIG. 25. Right ventricular nor-epinephrine in four groups of cats. One group of normal cats did not receive digoxin. One group of nor-mal cats received digoxin. One group of cats did not receive di-goxin before and after being sub-jected to pulmonary artery banding which caused right ventricular hy-pertrophy (RVH) without heart fail-ure. One group of cats received digoxin before and after being sub-jected to pulmonary artery band-ing which caused RVH without heart failure. (Carey et al., ref. 10.)

Reversal of Cardiac Norepinephrine Depletion Following Relief of Cardiac Hypertrophy and Failure

There has been limited study of whether relief of the overload on the heart with resultant relief of the hypertrophy and the heart failure also relieves the cardiac norepinephrine depletion. Coulson and co-workers (21) examined the recuperative potential of cat hearts subjected to experimental right ventricular pressure overload for a 10 to 14 day period which provoked hypertrophy with and without congestive heart failure. Five groups of cats were studied: a normal control; one group with a 70% pulmonary artery constriction which produced right ventricular hypertrophy; one group with an 87% constriction which produced right ventricular hypertrophy with congestive heart failure; and two groups that had been similarly subjected to pressure overload but that had been allowed a recovery period of 30 days after relief of the pressure overload. Both the 70% and the 87% pulmonary constrictions were associated with extensive right ventricular hypertrophy, depression of myo-cardial contractile function, and severe reduction of cardiac norepinephrine stores.

In cats in which the right ventricular hypertrophy had been relieved, right ventricular weight and contractile function returned to normal, but the depletion of cardiac catecholamine persisted. Cats with relieved congestive heart failure showed persistent depression of contractile function and myocardial norepinephrine depletion, and their right ventricular weight did not return to normal. Cardiac muscle of all pressure-overloaded, nonrelieved hearts showed depressed velocity of shortening and depressed ability to sustain load. Cats with right ventricular hyper-trophy alone regained normal muscle shortening velocity and load-bearing ability after relief, but cardiac muscle from the congestive heart failure relieved group recovered only unloaded shortening velocity while the ability to sustain load re-mained depressed. Cardiac catecholamine depletion persisted in both the right and left ventricles of cats relieved of right ventricular hypertrophy and relieved of congestive heart failure. Thus, hypertrophy due to pressure overload in the cat, with or without congestive heart failure, leads to a catecholamine depletion that is not reversed by relief of the overload.

The only other reported study that attempted to determine if there was recuperation of catecholamine deficit in the hypertrophied and failing heart is a report by Vogel et al. (64) on two calves that had right ventricular hypertrophy and heart failure produced by ligation of one pulmonary artery while existing at a high altitude. In such animals where there is right heart failure and depletion of cardiac catecholamines, the hypertrophy and heart failure regress if they are subsequently removed to sea level. Heart failure had disappeared and cardiac catecholamines were found to be normal 30 days after these animals were returned to sea level. It is not known whether cardiac catecholamine depletion returns to normal after relief of overload and heart failure in patients with ventricular hypertrophy and congestive heart failure.

ACKNOWLEDGMENT

The author wishes to express his appreciation to James A. Weiss, Esq. for editorial assistance and to Maxine Blob and Carol Barnette for typing the manuscript.

REFERENCES

1. Aderson, A., Hellestad, L., Rasmussen, K., and Myhre, E. (1971): The cardiac response to exercise in aortic valve disease before and after ball valve replacement. *Acta Med. Scand.*, 190:251–259.
2. Alpert, N. R., Hamrell, B. B., and Halpern, W. (1974): Mechanical and biochemical correlates of cardiac hypertrophy. *Circ. Res.*, 34,35 [Suppl. II]:II–71–II–82.
3. Bassett, A. L., and Gelband, H. (1973): Chronic partial occlusion of the pulmonary artery in cats. *Circ. Res.*, 32:15–26.
3a. Baxley, W. A., Kennedy, J. W., Feild, B., and Dodge, H. T. (1973): Hemodynamics in ruptured chordae tendineae and chronic rheumatic mitral regurgitation. *Circulation*, 48:1288–1294.
4. Bishop, S. P., and Melsen, L. R. (1976): Myocardial necrosis, fibrosis, and DNA synthesis in experimental cardiac hypertrophy induced by sudden pressure overload. *Circ. Res.*, 39:238–244.
5. Borow, K. M., Green, L. H., Mann, T., Sloss, L. J., Braunwald, E., Collins, J. J., Jr., Cohn, L. H., and Grossman, W. (1980): End-systolic volume as a predictor of postoperative left ventricular function in volume overload from valvular regurgitation. *Am. J. Med.*, 68:665.
6. Carabello, A. B., Green, L. H., Grossman, W., Cohn, L. H., Koster, J. K., and Collins, J. Jr. (1980): Hemodynamic determinants of prognosis of aortic valve replacement in critical aortic stenosis and advanced congestive heart failure. *Circulation*, 62:42–48.
7. Carabello, B. A., Mee, R., Collins, J. J. Jr., Kloner, R. A., Levine, D., and Grossman, W. (1981): Contractile function in chronic gradually developing subcoronary aortic stenosis. *Am. J. Physiol.*, 240:H80–H86.
8. Carabello, B. A., Nolan, S. P., and McGuire, L. B. (1981): Assessment of preoperative left ventricular function in patients with mitral regurgitation: Valve of the end-systolic wall stress-end-systolic volume ratio. *Circulation*, 64:1212–1217.
9. Carey, R. A., Bove, A. A., Coulson, R. L., and Spann, J. F. (1978): Recovery of myosin ATPase after relief of pressure-overload hypertrophy and failure. *Am. J. Physiol.*, 3(6):H711–H717.
10. Carey, R. A., Bove, A. A., Couslon, R. L., and Spann, J. F. (1978): Normal cardiac myosin ATPase and mechanics in pressure overload with digitalis treatment. *Am. J. Physiol.*, 234(3):H253–H259.

11. Carey, R. A., Bove, A. A., Coulson, R. L., and Spann, J. F. (1979): Correlation between cardiac muscle myosin ATPase activity and velocity of muscle shortening. *Biochem. Med.*, 1062:1–11.

12. Carey, R. A., Natarajan, G., Bove, A. A., Coulson, R. L., and Spann, J. F. (1979): Myosin adenosine triphosphatase activity in the volume-overloaded hypertrophied feline right ventricle. *Circ. Res.*, 45:81–87.

13. Chakko, S., Troy, A., Gash, A., Bove, A. A., and Spann, J. F. (1982): Decreased ventricular contractile function, normal pump function and compensatory mechanisms in patients with systemic hypertension. (Abstract). *Am. J. Cardiol. (in press).*

14. Chidsey, C. A., Harrison, D. C., and Braunwald, E. (1962): Augmentation of the plasma norepinephrine response to exercise in patients with congestive heart failure. *N. Engl. J. Med.*, 267:650–654.

15. Chidsey, C. A., Braunwald, E., Morrow, A. G., and Mason, D. T. (1963): Myocardial norepinephrine concentration in man: Effects of reserpine and of congestive heart failure. *N. Engl. J. Med.*, 269:653–658.

16. Chidsey, C. A., Kaiser, G. A., Sonnenblick, E. H., Spann, J. F., and Braunwald, E. (1964): Cardiac norepinephrine stores in experimental heart failure in the dog. *J. Clin. Invest.*, 43:2386–2393.

17. Chidsey, C. A., Braunwald, E., and Morrow, A. G. (1965): Catecholamine excretion and cardiac stores of norepinephrine in congestive heart failure. *Am. J. Med.*, 39:442–451.

18. Cooper, G., Satava, R. M., Harrison, C. E., Coleman, H. N. (1973): Mechanism for the abnormal energetics of pressure-induced hypertrophy of cat myocardium. *Circ. Res.*, 33:213–223.

19. Cooper, G., IV, Puga, F. J., Zujko, K. J., Harrison, C. E., and Coleman, H. N., III. (1973): Normal myocardial function and energetics in volume-overload hypertrophy in the cat. *Circ. Res.*, 32:140–148.

20. Cooper, G., IV, Tomanek, R. J., Ehrhardt, G. C., and Marcus, M. L. (1981): Chronic progressive pressure overload of the cat right ventricle. *Circ. Res.*, 48:488–497.

21. Coulson, R. L., Yazdanfar, S., Rubio, E., Bove, A. A., Lemole, G. M., and Spann, J. F. (1977): Recuperative potential of cardiac muscle following relief of pressure overload hypertrophy and right ventriclar failure in the cat. *Circ. Res.*, 40:41–49.

22. Covell, J. W., Chidsey, C. A., and Braunwald, E. (1966): Reduction of the cardiac response to postganglionic sympathetic nerve stimulation in experimental heart failure. *Circ. Res.*, 19:51–56.

23. Dequattro, V., Nagatsu, T., Mendez, A., and Verska, J. (1973): Determinants of cardiac noradrenaline depletion in human congestive failure. *Cardiovasc. Res.*, 7:344–350.

24. Donner, R. M., Carabello, B. A., Black, I., and Spann, J. F. (1982): Diminished wall stress, normal muscle function and supranormal pump function in children with severe aortic stenosis. *N. Engl. J. Med. (Submitted).*

25. Eckberg, D. L., Gault, J. H., Bouchard, R. L., Karliner, J. S., and Ross, J., Jr. (1973): Mechanics of left ventricular contraction in chronic severe mitral regurgitation. *Circulation*, 47:1252–1259.

26. Fischer, J. E., Horst, W. D., and Kopin, I. J. (1965): Norepinephrine metabolism in hypertrophied rat hearts. *Nature*, 207:951–953.

26a. Goldstein, R. E., Beiser, G. D., Stampfer, M., and Epstein, S. E. (1975): Impairment of autonomically mediated heart rate control in patients with cardiac dysfunction. *Circ. Res.*, 36:571–578.

27. Gunther, S., and Grossman, W. (1979): Determinants of ventricular function in pressure-overload hypertrophy in man. *Circulation*, 59:679–688.

27a. Hamrell, B. B., and Alpert, N. R. (1977): The mechanical characteristics of hypertrophied rabbit cardiac muscle in the absence of congestive heart failure. The contractile and series elastic elements. *Circ. Res.*, 40:20–24.

28. Henry, W. L., Bonow, R. O., Borer, J. S., Ware, J. H., Kent, K. M., Redwood, D. R., McIntosh, C. L., Morrow, A. G., and Epstein, S. E. (1980a): Observations on the optimum time for operative intervention for aortic regurgitation. I. Evaluation of the results of aortic valve replacement in symptomatic patients. *Circulation*, 61:471–482.

29. Henry, W. L., Bonow, R. O., Rosing, D. R., and Epstein, S. E. (1980b): Observations on the optimum time for operative intervention for aortic regurgitation. II. Serial echocardiographic evaluation of asymptomatic patients. *Circulation*, 61:484–492.

30. Huber, D., Grimm, J., Koch, R., and Krayenbuehl, H. P. (1981): Determinants of ejection performance in aortic stenosis. *Circulation*, 64:126–134.

30a. Karliner, J. W., Barnes, P., Brown, M., and Dollery, C. (1980): Chronic heart failure in the guinea pig increases cardiac adrenoceptors. *Euro. J. Pharmacol.*, 67:115–118.
31. Karliner, J. W., Williams, D., Corwit, J., Crawford, M. H., and O'Rourke, R. A. (1976): Left ventricular performance in patients with left ventricular hypertrophy caused by systemic arterial hypertension. *Br. Heart J.*, 89:1239–1245.
32. Kopin, I. J., Hertting, G., and Gordon, E. K. (1962): Fate of norepinephrine-H^3 in the isolated perfused rat heart. *J. Pharmacol. Exp. Ther.*, 134:34.
33. Krayenbuehl, H. P., Brunner, H. H., Riedhammer, H. H., Mehmel, H. C., and Senning, A. (1976): The influence of hypertrophy on myocardial function. *Eur. J. Cardiol.*, 4:123–130.
34. Levine, H. J., McIntyre, K. M., Lipana, J. C., and Bing, O. H. L. (1970): Force-velocity relations in failing and nonfailing hearts of subjects with aortic stenosis. *Am. J. Med. Sci.*, 259:79–89.
35. McDonald, I. G. (1975): Echocardiographic assessment of left ventricular function in aortic disease. *Circulation*, 53:860–864.
36. Meerson, F. Z. (1965): A mechanism of hypertrophy and wear of the myocardium. *Am. J. Cardiol.*, 15:755–760.
37. Meerson, F. Z., and Kapelko, V. I. (1972): The contractile function of the myocardium in two types of cardiac adaptation to a chronic load. *Am. J. Cardiol.*, 57:183–199.
37a. Newman, W. H. (1978a): Contractile state of hypertrophied left ventricle in long-standing volume overload. *Am. J. Physiol.*, 234(1):H88–H93.
38. Newman, W. H. (1978b): Volume overload heart failure: length-tension curves, and response to beta-agonists, Ca^{2+}, and glucagon. *Am. J. Physiol.*, 235(6):H690–H700.
39. Newman, W. H., and Webb, J. C. (1980): Adaptation of the left ventricle to chronic pressure overload: response to intropic drugs. *Am. J. Physiol.*, 238:H134–H143.
40. Osbakken, M., Bove, A. A., Spann, J. F. (1981): Left ventricular function in chronic aortic regurgitation with reference to end-systolic pressure, volume and stress relations. *Am. J. Cardiol.*, 47:193–198.
41. Pannier, J. L. (1971): Contractile state of papillary muscles obtained from cats with moderate right ventricular hypertrophy. *Arch. Intern. Physiol. Biochim.*, 79:743–752.
42. Pfeffer, J., Pfeffer, M., Fletcher, P., and Braunwald, E. (1979): Alterations of cardiac performance in rats with established spontaneous hypertension. *Am. J. Cardiol.*, 44:994–998.
43. Phillips, H. R., Levine, F. H., Carter, J. E., Boucher, C. A., Osbakken, M. D., Okada, R. D., Akins, C. W., Daggett, W. M., Buckley, M. J., and Pohost, G. M. (1981): Mitral valve replacement for isolated mitral regurgitation: Analysis of clinical course and late postoperative left ventricular ejection fraction. *Am. J. Cardiol.*, 48:647–654.
44. Pool, P. E., Covell, J. W., Levitt, M., Gibb, J., and Braunwald, E. (1967): Reduction of cardiac tyrosin hydroxylase activity in experimental congestive heart failure. Its role in the depletion of cardiac norepinephrine stores. *Circ. Res.*, 20:349–353.
45. Sasayama, S., Ross, J., Franklin, D., Bloor, C. M., Bishop, S., and Dilley, R. B. (1975): Adaptations of the left ventricle to chronic pressure overload. *Circ. Res.*, 38:172–178.
46. Sasayama, S., Franklin, D., and Ross, J., Jr. (1977): Hyperfunction with normal inotropic state of the hypertrophied left ventricle. *Am. J. Physiol.*, 232(4):H418–H425.
47. Schuler, G., Peterson, K. L., Johnson, A., Francis, G., Dennish, G., Utley, J., Daily, P. O., Ashburn, W., and Ross, J., Jr. (1979): Temporal response of left ventricular performance of mitral valve surgery. *Circulation*, 59:1218–1231.
48. Sole, M. J., Lo, C-M., Laird, C. W., Sonnenblick, E. H., Wurtmann, R. J. (1975): Norepinephrine turnover in the heart and spleen of the cardiomyopathic Syrian hamster. *Circ. Res.*, 37:855–862.
49. Sole, M. J., Kamble, A. B., and Hussain, M. N. (1977a): A possible change in the rate-limiting step for cardiac norepinephrine synthesis in the cardiomyopathic Syrian hamster. *Circ. Res.*, 41:814–817.
50. Sole, M. J., Wurtman, R. J., Lo, C-M., Kamble, A. B., and Sonnenblick, E. H. (1977b): Tyrosine hydroxylase activity in the heart of the cardiomyopathic Syrian hamster. *J. Mol. Cell. Cardiol.*, 9:225–233.
51. Spann, J. F., Chidsey, C. A., and Braunwald, E. (1964): Reduction of cardiac stores of norepinephrine in experimental heart failure. *Science*, 145:1439–1441.
52. Spann, J. F., Chidsey, C. A., Pool, P. E., and Braunwald, E. (1965): Mechanism of norepinephrine depletion in experimental heart failure produced by aortic constriction in the guinea pig. *Circ. Res.*, 17:312–320.
53. Spann, J. F., Jr., Sonnenblick, E. H., Cooper, T., Chidsey, C. A., Willman, V. L., and Braunwald,

E. (1966): Cardiac norepinephrine stores and the contractile state of heart muscle. *Circ. Res.*, 19:317–325.

54. Spann, J. F., Jr., Buccino, R. A., Sonnenblick, E. H., and Braunwald, E. (1967): Contractile state of cardiac muscle obtained from cats with experimentally produced ventricular hypertrophy and heart failure. *Circ. Res.*, 21:341–354.

55. Spann, J. F., Covell, J. W., Eckberg, D. L., Sonnenblick, E. H., Ross, J. Jr., and Braunwald, E. (1972): Contractile performance of the hypertrophied and chronically failing cat ventricle. *Am. J. Physiol.*, 223:1150–1157.

56. Spann, J. F., Bove, A. A., Natarajan, G., and Kreulen, T. (1980): Ventricular performance, pump function and compensatory mechanisms in patients with aortic stenosis. *Circulation*, 62:576–582.

57. Strauer, B. E. (1978): The heart in hypertension. I. Left ventricular function at rest and during exercise. *Zeit. Kardiol.*, pp. 375–383.

57a. Stephen, A. (1966): Unwanted effects of propranolol. *Am. J. Cardiol.*, 18:463–468.

58. Taylor, R. R., Covell, J. W., and Ross, J., Jr. (1968): Left ventricular function in experimental aorto-caval fistula with circulatory congestion and fluid retention. *J. Clin. Invest.*, 47:1333–1342.

59. Taylor, R. R., and Hopkins, B. E. (1972): Left ventricular response to experimentally induced chronic aortic regurgitation. *Cardiovasc. Res.*, 6:404–414.

60. Takahashi, M., Sasayama, S., Kawai, C., and Kotoura, H. (1980): Contractile performance of the hypertrophied ventricle in patients with systemic hypertension. *Circulation*, 62:116–126.

61. Thomas, J. A., and Marks, B. H. (1978): Plasma norepinephrine in congestive heart failure. *Am. J. Cardiol.*, 41:233–243.

62. Turina, M., Bussmann, W. D., and Krayenbuhl, H. P. (1969): Contractility of the hypertrophied canine heart in chronic volume overload. *Cardiovasc. Res.*, 3:486–495.

63. Urschel, C. W., Covell, J. W., Sonnenblick, E. H., Ross, J., Jr., and Braunwald, E. (1968): Myocardial mechanics in aortic and mitral valvular regurgitation: the concept of instantaneous impedance as a determinant of the performance of the intact heart. *J. Clin. Invest.*, 47:867–883.

64. Vogel, J. H. K., Jacobowitz, D., and Chidsey, C. A. (1969): Distribution of norepinephrine in the failing bovine heart. Correlation of chemical analysis and fluorescence microscopy. *Circ. Res.*, 24:71–84.

64a. Vokonas, P. S., Gorlin, R., Cohn, P. F., Herman, M. V., and Sonnenblick, E. H. (1973): Dynamic geometry of the left ventricle in mitral regurgitation. *Circulation*, 48:786–796.

65. Williams, J. F. Jr., and Potter, R. D. (1974): Normal contractile state of hypertrophied myocardium after pulmonary artery constriction in the cat. *J. Clin. Invest.*, 54:1266–1272.

66. Wong, C. Y. H., and Spotnitz, H. M. (1981): Systolic and diastolic properties of the human left ventricle during valve replacement for chronic mitral regurgitation. *Am. J. Cardiol.*, 47:40–50.

67. Wroblewski, E., James, F., Spann, J. F., and Bove, A. A. (1981): Right ventricular performance in mitral stenosis. *Am. J. Cardiol.*, 47:51–55.

Subject Index

Subject Index